Teratology of the Central Nervous System

Teratology of the Central Nervous System

Induced and Spontaneous Malformations of Laboratory, Agricultural, and Domestic Mammals

Harold Kalter

The University of Chicago Press

Chicago and London

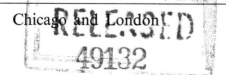
RELEASED
49132

636.089
K 81t

Library of Congress Catalog Card Number: 68-14628

The University of Chicago Press, Chicago 60637
The University of Chicago Press, Ltd., London W.C.1

© 1968 by The University of Chicago. All rights reserved
Published 1968
Printed in the United States of America

To my Wife
Bella Briansky Kalter

Preface

Teratology is the study of monstrosities. The prefix of the word derives from the Greek *teras*, meaning wonder, in the dual sense of prodigy and portent. Beginning with the earliest records of his consciousness, man traced his awe of the phenomena of malformed creatures and his bewilderment at their signification.

Of course we no longer regard such beings as visitations and omens, but our bewilderment has not greatly lessened.

We are perplexed at many points all at once. For instance, so seemingly elementary a task as defining the term *congenital malformation* has not yet been satisfactorily accomplished.

Let us first deal with the word congenital. The *Shorter Oxford English Dictionary on Historical Principles* (Onions 1956, p. 369) states that the word, which made its first appearance in English in 1796, means "existing from birth or born with." Though one part of this definition would seem to exclude existence before birth, the other does not; and the latter sense is made explicit by *Funk and Wagnalls Standard College Dictionary* (1963, p. 285), where the word is said to mean "existing prior to or at birth ...." Accepting this extension disposes of the possible objection of ornitho- and herpetoteratologists that their subjects are not "born."

Having thus made life a bit easier, Funk and Wagnalls lessens this achievement by adding to its definition " ... but not inherited ... " and " ... distinguished from *hereditary* ... ," thereby resurrecting a usage that had almost expired. For among modern biologists congenital simply indicates presence at birth and connotes nothing of origin.

The second word of the term—malformation—presents two difficulties. First, while all agree that malformations are departures from normality, it is not generally agreed what limit to set to the normal. This is less a difficulty for some than for others. To physicians the limit is that beyond which life is impossible or imperiled or physical, and perhaps social, function impaired. But when no such exigencies intrude the decision is necessarily somewhat arbitrary.

The second difficulty is more complex because it involves the essential nature of the phenomena themselves. In a sense there is agreement here already, too, since all maintain that congenital malformations are abnormalities of structure. The dispute turns on the word structure, or, more precisely, on the structure's size.

For many investigators, malformations are simply abnormalities perceptible to the unaided senses or recognizable by conventional clinical instruments. Some would also admit histological abnormalities detectable with the light microscope. And others would go further and, like Tatum (1961), include "molecular abnormalities detected in any organism from virus to man."

While it is true that the difficulty of knowing where to draw the dividing line seems to make all these views legitimate, other considerations help in setting limits for the present. It appears that the last—the molecular—opinion is based (Tatum 1961) on the premise that all characters—including morphological ones—are ultimately determined by the genetic complement and that "defective development . . . represents failure of particular genes to express themselves. . . ." This standpoint is weakened by there being little doubt that in man—and probably most other vertebrates as well—congenital malformations that are strictly genetic in etiology form but a relatively small proportion of all that occur. As Neel (1961), a medical geneticist, has stated, ". . . I acknowledge my deep respect for the role of nongenetic factors in eliciting congenital defect . . . ."

Indeed, it is such acknowledgement that distinguishes the predominant beliefs of the origin of congenital malformations today from those prevailing earlier in this century among many geneticists and others. Today it is generally recognized that congenital malformations are a thoroughly mixed bag etiologically, developmentally, and clinically.

Although at some future time a synthetic stage will undoubtedly be reached in the pursuit of understanding of congenital malformations, the most profitable approach now is an analytic one: differentiating entities and establishing patterns and interrelations; categorizing and classifying. Taking the broad view may help define future possibilities of research and understanding, but its present effect would be to jumble together disparate phenomena and obscure their diverse and manifold causation.

Hence for the time being it is preferable to regard as congenital malformations only gross structural departures from the norm having their origin before birth. And this has been the definition applied in this book.

There is also practical importance to the decision what shall be considered a malformation and what not. With the resurgent interest in human congenital malformations in recent years and the realization that investigators do not all understand alike what they mean by the term, it has become plain that the incidence of such conditions in man is poorly known. There is no doubt that to some extent this situation is due to absence of agreed standards of examination, interpretation, and nomenclature. Were such standards to be adopted and used, a great advance would have been made toward allowing studies to be compared with each other for the purposes of evaluating causative factors and preventive measures.

As far as animals are concerned, there is the additional necessity—most conspicuous in teratology testing—of having baselines against which to judge the effects of teratogenic agents and procedures. This means that, in addition to being well acquainted with the spontaneous defects our test animals show proclivities toward, we must be agreed upon what are to be considered malformations—and not merely retardation, microsomia, edema, extravasation, or even death—so that we will all be talking the same language.

Spontaneous congenital malformations of the central nervous system are especially common and severe in practically all mammalian species, and central nervous system defects are among the most frequent types of malformations induced by experimental teratogens. Why this is so is difficult to say. Perhaps it is a reflection of the vital place of the central nervous system in the body's economy; perhaps of its large size and distribution; perhaps of delicate balances of numerous events in time and space during its development that may easily be disturbed. Whatever the reasons, pathological genes, environmental teratogens, chromosomal aberrations, and multifactorial etiological situations all appear to exert an outsized influence on the central nervous system. A book devoted to the subject of congenital malformations of the central nervous system is thus amply called for.

The book is divided in two parts. The first, consisting of seven chapters, deals with malformations induced by external teratogens, usually experimentally applied. The second part, comprising fourteen chapters, most devoted to only one species, is concerned with spontaneous malformations, i.e., those not resulting from intervention of known extrinsic agents or conditions. Chapter 9, on the mouse, is entirely taken up by the many gene-induced central nervous system malformations in this species; whereas the others deal largely or completely with sporadic defects, i.e., those with no clearly identified cause.

H. KALTER

Cincinnati, May 1967

Acknowledgments

It is with gratitude that I record my debt to the National Association for Retarded Children, New York, for their support during the writing of this book.

The cooperation of many librarians throughout the United States and in several other countries is acknowledged. Part of this work could not have been put together at all without the good-humored and unstinting help of the chief librarian, Miss Alma Slagle, and the assistant librarian, Mrs. Jean Stern, of the medical library of the Children's Hospital Research Foundation, Cincinnati. The assistance of Mrs. Eva Takacs and Mrs. Mildred Floyd with the illustrations is appreciated.

The writing of this book was undertaken at the suggestion of Dr. Josef Warkany, but it is probably not quite what he had in mind.

Contents

Part One

Experimentally Induced Malformations

1

Principles and Techniques of Experimental Mammalian Teratology

The science of experimental mammalian teratology is young. Its birth dates from the studies of the radiation workers of the 1930's (Job, Leibold, and Fitzmaurice 1935; Kaven 1938*a*) and the nutritional experiments of the same decade (Hale 1933; Warkany and Nelson 1940). From the results of these investigations came a concept whose arena until then had largely been restricted to the spheres of human activity and frailty labeled speculative philosophy and superstition: that mammalian embryos are subject to laws of nature, and that they, too—as fishes, birds, and amphibia—could be deformed in systematic fashion by environmental circumstances, indeed by abnormal conditions of physiological consequence.

But the world in which these first discoveries were made took little note of them—the political fabric, as it seems in each age, no doubt, was being rent; and medical and biological science was absorbed in the predominant problems and achievements of the time.

Thirty years have passed since then. Unthought-of scientific progress has occurred and already seems commonplace. The field of experimental mammalian teratology has won a modest place; and this recognition is due to the work of a small group of people who erected a set of guiding principles and thereby created a new biological discipline. It is with these principles and related matters that this chapter deals.

Teratologic Susceptibility and Gestation Periods

The type and degree of responsiveness of conceptuses to the induction of congenital malformations by teratogens depends on, and varies with, their gestational age. So far as teratologic susceptibility is concerned, the time from conception to birth is roughly divisible into 3 periods, which are, of course, not absolutely demarcated: (1) the period before germ layer formation, (2) the period of embryo, and (3) the period of the fetus.

The Pregerm-Layer Stage

The first of these periods is sometimes known as the preimplantation period, but should be called the pre-early-germ-layer formation stage. Wilson (1965) has termed it the predifferentiation period.

The duration of the interval between fertilization and implantation, about the time of which germ-layer formation occurs, is remarkably similar in widely divergent mammalian species despite their total gestation periods being quite different. For example, this interval is approximately $4\frac{1}{2}$ days in hamsters and mice, 6 days in rats, $6\frac{1}{2}$ days in men, 7 days in rabbits, 9 days in rhesus monkeys, and 10 days in sheep, while the entire gestation period of these species ranges from 16 days in hamsters to 267 days in human beings (Monie 1965).

During the predifferentiation period conceptuses are generally resistant to the production of congenital malformations, as has been shown in the great majority of teratological studies in which exposure of animals was made early in pregnancy. In a very small number of experiments, however, some defective offspring were found after such treatment; these results have been magnified in importance because they are conspicuous exceptions to the general rule. It is interesting to note that most of these exceptional results occurred in radiation studies. They are discussed in detail in the chapter on congenital malformations produced by irradiation (see pp. 111–15).

One X-ray experiment that allegedly had such results was that of Woollam, Pratt, and Fozzard (1957), who stated, and were cited by at least 3 authors (who will remain anonymous) as so doing, that they produced malformations in rats by irradiating on day 2 of pregnancy. Certain inconsistencies in the article made it seem that an inadvertent error had been made, which was confirmed by Woollam in a personal communication to me. The explanation was that an 11 had been misinterpreted and printed as a Roman numeral 2.

Very few nonactinic teratogens have caused defects by preimplantation treatment, although in all fairness it must be said that not all such teratogens have been used acutely in early pregnancy. Female rats kept at reduced atmospheric pressures for 48 hours during the first 8 days of pregnancy bore several offspring with eye abnormalities (Werthemann and Reiniger 1950). With but 2 exceptions the anomalies occurred in stillborn specimens, and it is possible that at least some of the defects were actually postmortem artifacts.

Randombred white mice subjected to hypoxia on the 4th day of pregnancy had 2 offspring with vertebral defects (Ingalls, Curley, and Prindle 1952). A female golden hamster frozen for 45 minutes on the 3rd day of pregnancy and subsequently resuscitated had a litter of 11 all of which were alive but malformed and undersized (Smith 1957). Triparanol injected as early as the 4th day of pregnancy in rats produced severe malformations (Roux 1964). Actinomycin D given before implantation was teratogenic (Wilson 1966).

Teratogenic antiserum produced malformations in rats when injected as early as 3 days after insemination (Brent 1966a). Thus, but for these and perhaps several other scattered exceptions, the predifferentiation period has been found to be one of teratologic unresponsiveness.

It may of course be discovered, as a result of more intense investigation, that many other agents are also capable of having malformative effects when they are administered before implantation; but it may also come to be realized that, like trypan blue (see p. 87), some act by waiting in maternal structures for embryos to become susceptible.

Embryonic Period

The next period, that of the early embryo, is the time when conceptuses are most easily, often, and drastically deformed by teratogens. The onset of susceptibility occurs suddenly at about the time of germ-layer formation and is sometimes greatest at just this stage or shortly afterward. This sensitivity is due to the fact that numerous complex, crucial, and closely integrated events are simultaneously taking place in embryos, especially young ones, and that the least disturbance in this developmental network can have far-reaching and irreversible consequences.

In general, the teratologic malleability of embryos decreases as they age; but during the time of early differentiation (and later as well) particular organs and parts are chemically and morphologically developing at their own paces and according to their own timetables, and each therefore has its characteristic temporal shifts in proneness to damage, or, as it has been called, its "critical period." However, the critical period does not necessarily coincide with the time an organ or part first physically appears or undergoes some embryological step but may merely be the shortest interval during which minimal exposure to a teratogen will deflect it from its normal developmental pathway. Critical periods for the production of various malformations by a large number of teratogens in mice were listed by Dagg (1966) in a recent, excellent review of teratogenesis in that species.

Attempts at understanding some of the fundamental processes involved in teratogenesis have led to concentration on the possible relations between susceptibility and such phenomena as cell division and cellular differentiation (see, e.g., Hicks and D'Amato 1966). These topics have been most intensively looked into by radiation workers, whose ideas are discussed elsewhere (see pp. 134–37).

Fetal Period

As differentiation and organogenesis proceed, prenatal creatures become progressively less susceptible to teratogens, since ever fewer structures remain open to environmental interference. As embryos are transformed into fetuses, only those parts disturbance of whose growth, movement, or maturation can result in deformity are subject to maldevelopment, such as palate, cerebellum, some cardiovascular and urogenital structures, and so on.

The Agent

Dose

In order to produce congenital malformations with teratogens, it is necessary to discover empirically the more or less narrow dose zone that lies between amounts (positive or negative) harmless to conceptuses and amounts that destroy them. The teratogenic dose range thus malforms some, but does not kill all, offspring; and by adjusting the dose, it becomes possible to maximize the deformity rate while minimizing the mortality rate. E.g., in studies with pantothenic acid-deficient diets (Lefebvres-Boisselot 1955), all embryos were resorbed when pregnant rats consumed less than 10 μg/day of the vitamin, and all were normal when the diet contained 50 μg/day or more, while the highest incidence of defects occurred with 20 to 25 μg/day. The dose needed to produce a defect of a structure during its critical period of development, as defined above, is smaller than needed to induce the "same" defect at conterminous times. This fact was best demonstrated in studies with X rays (Russell 1950, 1956).

Another aspect of the topic of dosage is the effect of long-term multiple or continuous treatment versus short-term or single treatment. A common result of the former is the production of multiply deformed offspring, caused by interfering with development at many critical periods. An example of this situation is the study (Wilson, Roth, and Warkany 1953) in which the syndrome of defects produced by unrelieved vitamin A deficiency was modified by administering the missing vitamin at various times during pregnancy. Illustrative also are observations (Kalter, unpublished) that malformations produced by single doses of excess vitamin A given at particular times in pregnancy occurred together when multiple treatments were made.

An important finding, with regard to the comparative efficacy of acute and chronic treatment, is that short-term administration of a drug may be highly teratogenic, while long-term administration may be virtually without effect (King, Weaver, and Narrod 1965), and that the basis for this situation is the induction by some drugs of enzymes for their own metabolism. The lessened effects of chronic treatment with some drugs, however, are probably due to other mechanisms; with actinomycin D, e.g. (Wilson 1966), chronic small doses accentuated rather than lightened the teratogenic effects of a large final dose. The comparative effects of single versus fractionated and acute versus chronic X irradiation are discussed elsewhere (see pp. 130−33).

Administration

The mode of administering teratogens or the means of exposing pregnant animals to them varies, of course, with the type of agent and its properties.

Nutrient-deficient dietary regimes are fed; and in order to deplete animals of the substance the effects of whose absence are being tested, it is usually necessary to maintain animals on the diet for extended periods prior to conception as well as during pregnancy.

The addition of specific antagonists to deficient diets and, where needed, antibiotics to suppress endogenous synthesis makes possible the rapid production of a deficient state, and hence permits short-term treatment during pregnancy only, in some cases for as short as 36 hours (Nelson *et al.* 1956*b*). Where antagonists are injected, a far shorter period of exposure may be teratogenic (Pinsky and Fraser 1960). When antagonists, or any agent incorporated into diets, are fed, the dose received will of course depend on the amount of diet consumed; thus, spill-proof containers must be used and the diet must be weighed to determine how much is eaten per unit time.

It is sometimes necessary to give a life-supporting or protective substance to render a procedure teratogenic or to increase its effectiveness. E.g., to prevent total fetal resorption, Hale (1933) added small amounts of codliver oil, and Cheng and Thomas (1953) small amounts of tocopherol acetate, to a vitamin A- and vitamin E-deficient diet, respectively; Grainger, O'Dell, and Hogan (1954) increased the teratogenicity of vitamin B_{12} deficiency by adding riboflavin to a deficient diet; and Thiersch (1954*a*) and Murphy (1965) permitted fetuses to survive and show defects by injecting protective substances.

Numerous types of agents are administered parentally—by the percutaneous, subcutaneous, intramuscular, intraperitoneal, and intravenous routes. The relative effectiveness of giving the same substance by different avenues has not been systematically probed, although it is to be expected that it varies with the speed of exit of the test material from the site of injection. The different teratogenic capacities of some azo dyes may in part be due to such factors (Lloyd, Beck, and Griffiths 1965). Oily solutions of large doses of vitamin A are teratogenic only if given orally, but if they are saponified or if aqueous preparations of the vitamin are given, parenteral administration is teratogenic (see p. 47). Some of the interlitter variability commonly encountered in teratologic studies may be due to differences among pregnant females in agents' getting evenly into the maternal circulation (while some intralitter variability may be due to differences in reaching embryos).

Specificity

Mammalian teratogenesis has clearly revealed that all means of creating embryonic deviations are not equivalent. I.e., in a large measure, each agent or class of agents probably causes a specific defect or combination of defects. This statement contradicts what was learned in early teratologic studies with lower forms of life, especially amphibia and fish (Stockard 1921); from which the dictum was derived that not the agent but only the time it is used during embryogenesis determines the part malformed and the type of defect produced.

It is undeniable that this rule does not hold for mammals—or birds, for that matter (Ancel 1950; Landauer 1954)—since a vast body of experimental results has established that the agent shares with the gestation stage the responsibility for the effect that results. Certainly, as was just declared, time cannot be ignored: it sets the stage—presents the array of vulnerability; but the agent chooses from among the parts at risk those it has special affinities for damaging.

In many cases, that agents have specific teratologic consequences is easily supported: e.g., when they are used under comparable conditions and have very different effects. But sometimes various agents produce malformations that are similar or overlap. The question that then arises is—how can the defects be shown to be unlike? The decision cannot be based solely on their appearance at or near birth; since primary but transient features marking their individuality may by then have long disappeared or been obscured by secondary alterations undergone during the relatively long fetal period. Offspring must therefore be studied not only at term but throughout ontogenesis. Such an investigation revealed, e.g., that although cleft palate induced in mice by cortisone and in rats by folic acid deficiency resembled each other in perinatal animals, the embryological basis for each was quite distinct (Walker and Fraser 1957; Asling *et al.* 1960).

The Influence of Genotype

Experimental studies have shown that embryos are not all equally responsive to teratogens and that part of the difference in susceptibility is due to hereditary factors. However, it is a universal finding that variability occurs within and between litters in the incidence and severity of malformed offspring; therefore, when genetically heterogeneous animals are used in teratologic studies it is difficult to estimate how much of the variability is due to hereditary and how much to nonhereditary influences.

The use of genetically uniform animals, such as long-inbred strains, makes it possible to hold environment accountable for intrastrain variability and genotype largely accountable for interstrain differences. Thus gene-based differences are easily recognized by the use of such strains—if not easily analyzed. Despite the existence of numerous inbred strains of mice (Staats 1964), and the many strain differences in teratologic sensitivity that have been found among them (see below), very few genetic studies of these phenomena have been made.

Based on various types of crosses among 2 strains of mice and their F_1 hybrids, susceptibility to cortisone-induced cleft palate was shown (Kalter 1954a) to be a quantitative hereditary trait, i.e., one with a multigenic basis. The number of gene loci involved was not estimated. A point of great importance that emerged from this study was that both the maternal and fetal genotypes played roles in the prenatal response to the agent, which was also true for galactoflavin teratogenesis (Kalter 1965a).

A recent analysis (Dagg, Schlager, and Doerr 1966) of the genetic basis of teratologic susceptibility to 5-fluorouracil revealed it also to be polygenic. Approximately 80 per cent of the response was genetically determined. The minimum number of loci controlling incidence of malformed hindfeet was 4, while for cleft palate it was 3, and, further, it appeared that the set of genetic factors influencing the first defect was not completely identical with that influencing the second.

Evidence for other types of genetic influence on teratogenesis has been collected. First, teratogens may increase the incidence of spontaneous malformations of multifactorial origin that occur in some stocks of animals (Andersen 1949; Miller 1958; Beck 1964a). It is not easy to generalize about this phenomenon, however, because in other cases rates of spontaneous anomalies were not influenced by teratogenic agents (Ingalls *et al.* 1953; Kalter 1954a; Warkany and Kalter 1962), or, although increased, the induced incidence was smaller in a strain manifesting the spontaneous defect than in one free of it (Dagg 1964). Caution, of course, must be exercised in diagnosing whether "induced" and "spontaneous" defects are in fact the same. Thus, while acetylsalicylic acid produced a higher incidence of cleft lip in A/J mice than occurred in controls (Trasler 1965), some of the defects in the experimental group may have been morphologically different from the spontaneous type.

Second, teratogens may interact with genes in heterozygous state to increase the penetrance of dominant ones or result in defects produced by recessive ones when homozygous (Barber 1957; Beck 1963, 1964b; Dagg 1965; Winfield 1966). It is to be expected that such possible relations of genes and teratogens are specific, and hence that interaction would not occur in all cases (Kobozieff *et al.* 1959; Kalter 1965b).

Experimentally-induced, nonhereditary morphological variants that greatly resembled genetic traits were called phenocopies by Goldschmidt (1935). The implication was that the hereditary trait and its induced copy are phenotypically identical or closely similar because they develop, at least partly, over a shared pathway. Landauer (1959, 1960) discussed this subject in its varied aspects and presented evidence for the appearance of phenocopies in insects and fowl. He felt that such work would clarify the mechanisms by which mutant genes produce their phenotypic effects.

So far as the mammalian work discussed above is concerned, that the induced defects represent phenocopies is in most of the cases only poorly supported, either by proof that the genetic and induced phenotypes were closely alike or that they shared a common pathway of development, even in part. Such twofold evidence, of phenotypic resemblance and pathogenetic congruence, was found in the hydrocephalus and associated defects in mice produced by maternal treatment during pregnancy with the riboflavin antagonist, galactoflavin, and the now, unfortunately, extinct gene, hydrocephalus-1 (see pp. 24 and 194).

Genetic involvement in teratogenesis is also made evident by studies of inter- and intraspecific differences in susceptibility. These differences can be of several types. First, an agent teratogenic in some species or groups of animals may be completely or almost completely without teratogenic effect in others. Second, a teratogen may produce similar defects in various species, stocks, or strains of animals, but with the anomalies occurring in very different frequencies, a situation that makes it possible to designate the different groups as having various grades of susceptibility. Third, a teratogen may induce one or more abnormalities in some species or groups but have entirely or somewhat different effects in others. This type of variability may be of kind or degree—or, as the geneticist puts it, of penetrance or expressivity— and thus groups may differ in the particular array and severity of defects they manifest. Of course, these are not mutually exclusive categories, and certain situations may contain features of more than one of them.

First I will discuss a few of the studies that permit comparison to be made among different species. Probably one of the most clear-cut species differences is represented by the responses to glucocorticosteroids. Cortisone acetate, hydrocortisone acetate, prednisolone acetate, triamcinolone acetonide, and so on have been given to mice of various strains and types in a large number of laboratories and have been found to produce the congenital malformation cleft palate, without cleft lip (Fraser and Fainstat 1951; Kalter 1954a, 1961; Ingalls and Curley 1957a; Kohno 1960; Pinsky and DiGeorge 1965; Walker 1965; and so on).

Rabbits and guinea pigs have also been treated with cortisone, hydrocortisone, and other corticosteroids in a limited number of studies. In these species, also, cleft palate and a few other malformations were produced (Fainstat 1954; Buck, Clavert, and Rumpler 1962; Hoar 1962; Walker 1966).

Studies with, and observations on, other species, however, have been less rewarding, fortunately in some cases. Probably a large number of pregnant women have been given therapeutic doses of corticosteroids at some time during the gestation period. But only 5 cases of cleft palate have been reported in the children of women to whom large doses of these substances were administered early in pregnancy (Fraser 1962). The total number of women so treated is unknown, and hence it is impossible to determine whether this number of abnormal children represents an incidence larger than the spontaneous frequency of the defect, which is about one in 2500 births. Even if this small number of abnormal children is greater than would be expected, it is obvious that treatment with steroids during pregnancy has a fairly low probability of harming human embryos, except possibly in cases of susceptible genotypes exposed to large doses very early in pregnancy.

A much more fully and reliably documented example of species resistance to the teratogenic effect of corticosteroids is that of the case of rats. A very large number of investigators working in laboratories scattered throughout the world have failed in all (e.g., Gunberg 1957; Mercier-Parot 1957; Lohmeyer 1961) but 2 studies (Jost 1956; Zunin, Borrone, and Cuneo 1960) to produce cleft palate in rats with corticosteroids. The results of these 2 studies are doubtful. In the first (Jost 1956), the fetuses were themselves injected, intra-abdominally. Since even slight puncturing of the mouse amniotic sac induced cleft palate (Trasler, Walker, and Fraser 1956; Walker 1959), probably by permitting leakage of fluid, it is likely that the same mechanism was responsible for the production of the abnormality in the rats. It was, in fact, recently demonstrated (Poswillo 1966) that amniotic-sac puncture in rats prior to palate closure results in nearly 100 per cent cleft palate.

In the second case (Zunin, Borrone, and Cuneo 1960), it was reported that prednisone caused cleft palate in rats. The related steroid, prednisolone, was ineffective in producing this defect (Kalter 1962), although certain other minor abnormalities were found. It appears, therefore, that rats are remarkably resistant to the teratogenic effects of corticosteroids, agents that readily produce cleft palate in several other species.

The thalidomide incident spurred comparative studies in teratogenesis. Let us discuss a bit of what was learned about species differences in response to this substance. As can be seen from Table 1, human embryos were deformed by as little of the drug as 0.5 to 1.0 mg/kg taken daily for several days (Mellin and Katzenstein 1962; Lenz 1964; Loosli and Theiss 1964; Kajii 1965). Lesser primates also seem to be susceptible to relatively small quantities. In

TABLE 1
COMPARATIVE THALIDOMIDE TERATOGENICITY
(mg/kg/day)

Species	Smallest Dose Producing Defects	Largest Dose Producing No Defects
Man	0.5–1.0	?
Baboon	5	—
Monkey, Cynomolgus .	10	—
Rabbit	30	50
Mouse	31	4000
Rat	50	4000
Armadillo	100	—
Dog	100	200
Hamster	350	8000
Cat	—	500

baboons, 5 mg/kg daily for 12 to 22 days was teratogenic (Hendrickx, Axelrod, and Clayborn 1966); cynomolgus monkeys were deformed by 10 mg/kg daily for 6 to 10 days (Delahunt and Lassen 1964); and 50 mg/kg daily for several days immediately after mating apparently prevented implantation in rhesus monkeys (Lucey and Behrman 1963).

Continuing down the table, it would seem that rats (King and Kendrick 1962; Moore, Dwornik, and Dalton 1964), rabbits (Somers 1962), and mice (Giroud, Tuchmann-Duplessis, and Mercier-Parot 1962a; DiPaolo 1963) are about equally susceptible, since malformations were induced in all 3 by as little as 25 to 50 mg/kg/day. But that is deceptive. First, it must be remembered that there are numerous strains, stocks, and breeds of these animals and that wide intraspecies differences in response to the drug have been demonstrated. For example, in the studies with rats just cited, abnormalities were produced in offspring of Sprague–Dawley females given 50 mg/kg daily. But in all except one or two other experiments with rats, no congenital malformations were produced at all, even with doses as great as 4000 mg/kg/day (Brent 1964a).

In general, mice are more susceptible than rats, and in several stocks and strains malformations were produced with relatively small doses (Giroud, Tuchmann-Duplessis, and Mercier-Parot 1962a; DiPaolo 1963). But in quite a few other experiments with mice, abnormalities were not produced, even when as much as 4000 mg/kg were given daily (Mauss and Stumpe 1963; Somers 1963). Rabbits are quite susceptible, and with only few exceptions malformations were produced in all of the many studies made with them. As can be seen from Table 1, as little as 30 mg/kg/day was teratogenic in rabbits, and the largest dose reported to be ineffective is only 50 mg/kg (Seller 1962).

Armadillos (Marin-Padilla and Benirschke 1963) and dogs (Weidman, Young, and Zollman 1963; Delatour, Dams, and Favre-Tissot 1965) are susceptible to moderate doses. Malformations were produced in hamsters (Homburger et al. 1965) with 350 mg/kg; but in another laboratory (Somers 1963) the stupendous dose of 8000 mg/kg daily given throughout pregnancy failed not only to cause abnormalities but even to cause a significant increase in the resorption rate or a decrease in the litter size. And, finally, cats proved quite resistant to doses as large as 500 mg/kg daily for 12 days early in pregnancy (Somers 1963). Thus, wide differences exist from species to species in susceptibility to thalidomide; and not only in the amount of the drug that will elicit developmental defects, but also in the types of abnormalities that can be produced.

Various species differences in all-or-none response to other teratogens were also noted, but not as thoroughly documented as those already discussed. One of these is the different effects of anoxia or hypoxia, which is teratogenic for mice and rabbits but is not clearly teratogenic for rats (see p. 178).

A second general type of species difference, the qualitative one, is represented by numerous examples, only several of which will be mentioned here. Riboflavin deficiency induced in rats either by dietary procedures (Warkany and Nelson 1940) or by an antagonist, galactoflavin (Nelson *et al.* 1956*a*), produced certain skeletal derangements, but in addition the antimetabolite caused numerous malformations of soft tissues that did not appear in the offspring of mothers subjected to the dietary regime alone.

When mice were treated (Kalter and Warkany 1957) with galactoflavin, certain defects occurred that were not found in rats, though other anomalies were shared. For example, the rats had cardiovascular and urogenital malformations (Nelson *et al.* 1956*b*), neither of which occurred in mice. On the other hand, the mice had esophageal atresia, types of brain abnormalities, and certain skeletal defects, which were not seen in the rats. Here then is an example of a substance teratogenic in 2 different species, producing similar malformations in both, but also having particular effects in one that it does not have in the second.

Other examples of the same sort of thing are provided by vitamin A deficiency. This teratogenic technique has been studied in pigs, rabbits, and rats, and while at least one type of malformation occurred in all 3 species, many defects were produced in some that did not appear in the others. For instance, eye defects were found in all 3 (pig: Hale 1933; Palludan 1961; rat: Warkany and Schraffenberger 1944; Jackson and Kinsey 1946; Roux *et al.* 1962; rabbit: Lamming *et al.* 1954). Cleft palate and limb and ear abnormalities occurred in pigs (Hale 1935; Palludan 1961), but not in rats (Warkany and Roth 1948; Roux *et al.* 1962) or rabbits (Millen, Woollam, and Lamming 1953). Hydrocephalus appeared in pigs (Palludan 1961) and rabbits (Millen, Woollam, and Lamming 1953), but not in most studies with rats (Warkany and Roth 1948; Roux *et al.* 1962). Diaphragmatic hernia and cardiovascular and urogenital defects were seen in pigs (Hale 1935; Palludan 1961) and rats (Warkany and Roth 1948; Roux *et al.* 1962), but not in rabbits (Millen, Woollam, and Lamming 1953). In some studies with rats only single defects were found: diaphragmatic hernia (Andersen 1941, 1949), eye defects (Jackson and Kinsey 1946), hydrocephalus (Rokkones 1955). Thus in pigs and rats vitamin A deficiency usually caused a large multitude of different defects, but in rabbits only eye defects and hydrocephalus were reported in some studies, and only hydrocephalus in others.

Other interesting differences involve the teratogenic effects of starvation. While rats (Brent 1963, p. 54), and possibly hamsters (Harvey 1963, p. 54), are apparently refractory to this situation, mice are susceptible. Runner (1954) and Runner and Miller (1956) fasted strain 129 mice for 24 hours at different times during pregnancy and produced vertebral and costal deformities and exencephaly. In other studies, starvation (Kalter 1954*b*) or feeding limited amounts of food (Kalter 1960*a*) produced only cleft palate. Thus fetal mice of different genotypes reacted to maternal starvation by the development of quite different congenital malformations.

Another example of this type of phenomenon is the following. Four different inbred strains of mice were subjected to acute riboflavin deficiency induced by the antimetabolite, galactoflavin (Kalter and Warkany 1957). While many skeletal defects occurred (albeit in very different frequencies) in all the strains, certain ones were found in 2 of the strains that did not appear in the others.

Far more common than such qualitative differences are quantitative ones. The azo dye trypan blue was discovered to be teratogenic by Gillman and coworkers in 1948, and a large number of studies of this property of the dye have been made since that time. Many different stocks of rats have been used and much variability found. This subject is discussed at length beginning on page 72. Many quantitative differences have also been found in mice, among the numerous inbred strains that exist. I will not discuss these but merely list (Tables 2 and 3) a number of strain differences in the incidence of various defects produced by a number of teratogens.

Environmental Bases of Variability

As was intimated, every experimental teratologist knows that the effects of teratogens vary to some extent, so that all or most offspring may be affected, perhaps severely, in one litter, while in the very next one few or no young may be affected or the abnormalities may be minimal. And since these things happen even when inbred strains are used, hereditary factors cannot be responsible for all the variability that occurs. Several attempts have been made to identify some of the environmental influences that underlie these common observations.

TABLE 2

PER CENT MALFORMATIONS PRODUCED IN FOUR INBRED STRAINS
OF MICE BY GALACTOFLAVIN

Strain	Cleft Palate	Skeletal Defects	Brain Defects	Atresia of Esophagus
A/J	3	38	55	78
DBA/1	41	92	44	83
129	8	84	9	30
C57BL/6	13	0	5	2

SOURCE: Kalter and Warkany 1957.

TABLE 3

SOME DIFFERENCES BETWEEN INBRED STRAINS OF MICE

Teratogen	Strain	Per Cent Defect	References
Cleft Palate			
5-Fu[a], 20 mg/kg 10th d[b]	129 BALB/c	92 4	Dagg 1960
VA[c], 10,000 IU/d 11th–12th d	A/J C57BL/6	96–100 37–57	Walker and Crain 1960
G[d], 12 mg/g diet 11th–15th d	DBA C57BL	42 0	Walker and Crain 1961
X ray, 300 r 12th d	A/J C57BL/6	99.5 73	Callas and Walker 1963
X ray, 150 r 11th d	BALB/c C57BL/Ks	35 1	Dagg 1964
6-AN[e], 19 mg/kg 14th d	A/J C57BL/6	76 11	Goldstein, Pinsky, and Fraser 1963
CA[f], 2.5 mg/d 12th–15th d	DBA/1 C3H C57BL/6 CBA	92 68 19 12	Kalter 1965a
Other Skeletal Defects			
H[g], 260 mm Hg 5 hr, 9th d	A/J DBA/1	75 17	Ingalls *et al.* 1953
24 hr. fast 9th d	129 C57BL/6	37 9	Miller 1963a
Skeletal Defects and Exencephaly			
PZI[h], 4–5 unit/d 10th d	129 BALB/c	62 3	Smithberg and Runner 1963
T[i], 1 mg/g 10th d	129 BALB/c	56 44	Smithberg and Runner 1963

[a]5-fluorouracil, [b]d = day(s) treated, [c]Vitamin A, [d]Galactoflavin, [e]6-aminonicotinamide, [f]Cortisone acetate, [g]Hypoxia, [h]Protamine zinc insulin, [i]Tolbutamide.

Maternal Factors

The incidence of cleft palate induced by standard doses of cortisone declined as maternal weight, but not age, increased, in mice of several genotypes (Kalter 1956, 1957a; Trasler, Naylor, and Miller 1964); but not in C57BL animals (Trasler, Naylor, and Miller 1964). An inverse relation of maternal weight and cleft palate frequency was also found in studies using 6-amino-nicotinamide (Pinsky and Fraser 1959) and 5-fluorouracil (Dagg, Schlager, and Doerr 1966). On the other hand, a positive correlation occurred in the latter experiment between maternal weight and digital defects. The inverse relation with cleft palate may partly be explained by observations that pre-natal development was precocious in offspring of "heavy" mice compared with that in fetuses from "light" mothers (Trasler and Fraser 1958). In a study (Jaworska 1965) in which C57BL mice were given cortisone and excess vitamin A, a larger incidence of cleft palate was found in offspring of 7- to 9-month-old mice than in those of 3- to 5-month-old ones. Maternal weight was not mentioned.

Fetal and Uterine Factors

Fetal weight is often greatly reduced by teratogens (e.g., Kalter 1957a; Kalter and Warkany 1957; Beaudoin and Kahkonen 1963; Endo 1966). Furthermore, it was noted that malformed fetuses weighed less (Kalter 1957a, 1965a; Trasler and Fraser 1958; Endo 1966) and were more developmentally retarded (Trasler and Fraser 1958) than nonmalformed littermates. Thus it may be that embryos that lag developmentally are more sensitive to some teratogens than those keeping closer to the embryological timetable.

Litter size was apparently not associated with incidence of cortisone-induced cleft palate (Kalter 1956); but the number of fetuses occupying a uterine horn was positively correlated with the malformation rate in that horn (Woollam and Millen 1961; Kalter 1965a). The latter finding may be related to the fact that the average weight of fetal mice declines with increasing number in a horn (McLaren 1965). However, a positive relation also existed between the malformation rate in the 2 horns of the same female (Kalter 1965a) which may reflect the substantial negative influence of fetal number in one horn on fetal growth in the other horn (McLaren 1965).

Uterine site may be associated with differential fetal susceptibility to teratogenesis. Mouse fetuses situated at the ovarian end of uterine horns appeared to be less subject to the effects of hypervitaminosis A (Woollam and Millen 1961) and hypoxia (Woollam and Millen 1962) than those at the cervical end. It was postulated (Woollam and Millen 1962) that these results were due to developmental differences among fetuses owing to their being asynchronously implanted along the length of the uterus.

Contradictory results occurred in another study (Kalter 1963a), in which the malformation rate apparently increased in one series and decreased in a second with distance from the ovary. In a trypan blue study (Beaudoin and Kahkonen 1963), little difference in malformation rate was found between fetuses occupying the ovarian versus those in the cervical half of the uterus.

In relating uterine site with a spontaneous malformation, cleft lip with or without cleft palate (CL), in A/J mice, Trasler (1960) noted that defective fetuses were located more often nearest the ovary than at other positions in the uterus. However, in a private communication, Trasler reported the following: "Data on 485 embryos collected from 1953–59 and published (Trasler, *Science* 132 : 420, 1960) showed that within the A/Jax strain, embryos in the uterine site nearest the ovary develop cleft lip significantly more often than embryos in other positions in the uterus. Data on 561 embryos collected in the two subsequent years showed that along with a rise in the overall frequency of CL, the excess of CL embryos at the ovarian site disappeared, that is the frequency at the non-ovarian sites rose to equal that at the ovarian site."

If the reported uterine site–malformation rate associations are real, they may be based on fetal weight differences that may also exist in relation to uterine site. Three types of fetal weight–uterine site associations have been reported. First, Hashima (1956) and Healy, McLaren, and Michie (1960) found that fetal mice occupying the ovarian position were lighter than those elsewhere; but the latter authors noted this situation only in crowded horns. Second, Rosahn and Greene (1936), working with rabbits, and McLaren (1965), with mice, found that fetal weight decreased progressively from the ovary to the cervix; in the mice, however, the fetal weight gradient reflected the marked relation between uterine position and placental weight, with which fetal weight was also closely correlated. Last, in guinea pigs (Ibsen 1928), swine (Waldorf *et al.* 1957), and mice (McLaren and Michie 1959), the weight of fetuses at the ovarian and cervical ends was greater than of those between. The last pattern was felt (McLaren 1965) to support the hemo-dynamic theory of fetal growth, which states that the quantity of nutrients available for growth depends in part on the pressure at which maternal blood reaches fetuses, and that this pressure tends to be greater at the ends of the uterine horn than in the middle.

Uterine factors in teratogenesis may have been involved in several other observations (Kalter 1965a). First, the incidence of predisolone-induced cleft palate in mice was greater in fetuses lying next to those with the defect than in those next to fetuses without it; and, second, the weight of normal-palated fetuses lying next to normals was greater than of those next to fetuses with cleft palate, and their weight increased with distance from those with the defect.

Amount and Type of Diet

Teratogenic action may be influenced by dietary factors. Since the food intake of teratogen-treated pregnant animals may be reduced (e.g., Takaori,

Tanabe, and Shimamoto 1966) or increased (Kalter 1955), such aspects must be considered when probing into the origin of variability of results.

A short-term fast, which is itself teratogenic in mice (Kalter 1954b; Runner 1954), was combined with several other procedures and substances (Runner 1954, 1959; Runner and Dagg 1960). In a number of instances dual treatment had an additive or potentiative effect, but in others was no more teratogenic than either agent alone. The incidence of cortisone-induced cleft palate in mice was increased by fasting pregnant mice prior to (Miller 1958, 1962b) or concurrent with (Kalter and Warkany 1959a) cortisone administration. Insulin plus fasting also resulted in increased cleft palate production (Kalter and Warkany 1959a). Fasting plus trypan blue had additive effects in rats (Setokoesoema and Gunberg 1966), although food deprivation itself was reported to be nonteratogenic in this species (Brent 1963, p. 54; Takaori, Tanabe, and Shimamoto 1966).

Limiting the food consumption of pregnant mice for several days or administering small doses of cortisone produced a small percentage of cleft palate; and both together had a highly synergistic effect (Kalter 1960a).

Trypan blue teratogenesis was modified by altering the proportions of dietary constituents (Gilbert and Gillman 1954; Gunberg 1955). In a study in which 2 commercially obtained diets were used (Warburton et al. 1962), the offspring of A/J mice were more susceptible to low doses of cortisone when the pregnant females were fed one of the diets, and C57BL mice more susceptible when fed the other diet. Adding large amounts of casein, folic acid, or riboflavin to the diet did not alter the incidence of cortisone-induced deformity (Kalter 1959a).

Season

Seasonal variability in experimental teratogenesis has been reported infrequently, but may not be rare. In summarizing studies made over a $5\frac{1}{2}$-year period, in which mice of a uniform genotype were given a standard schedule of cortisone injections, a cyclic rise and fall in percentage of young with cleft palate was noted, with the mean incidence being much greater during the winter-centered 6 months than in the summer-centered ones (Kalter 1959b). In a study of the effects of cortisone plus excess vitamin A on mice, the incidence of cleft palate obtained during the winter was higher than during the other seasons of the year (Jaworska 1965). In unpublished observations, I noted that the severe teratogenic effects produced in mice by excess vitamin A during November to January, 1959–60, became much milder in the following few months. In several experiments the fetal mortality rate in the winter was greater than in the summer (Ingalls et al. 1953; Kalter 1959b; Jacobsen 1965).

Multiple Agents

A favorite type of teratologic experiment is that in which 2 or more agents or an agent and some other procedure are used concurrently. In general, such experiments have been made for 2 reasons: (1) to simulate multifactorial etiological situations (Wilson 1964), believed to be responsible for the bulk of congenital malformations in man (Fraser 1961); and (2) to clarify the mechanisms of teratogens by modifying their actions (Runner and Dagg 1960). The purpose of the first is to determine whether and under what conditions combined administration of 2 or more agents in subteratogenic or only slightly teratogenic doses can intensify each other's actions and produce significant teratogenic effects. In the second the purpose is to increase or decrease an agent's effectiveness by interfering with its metabolic or other consequences.

Many such experiments are discussed in following chapters and need not be mentioned here. I merely wish to make the following remarks. It must be recognized that the entire basis for deciding whether multiple treatments have different effects from single ones has been the incidence of malformations produced. And since variability of results is expected in teratologic studies, differences that may occur between groups of experimental animals will be satisfactorily demonstrated to be due to the differences in their treatment only if precautions are taken to eliminate or hold constant factors making for variability. Furthermore, since experimenters these days are rarely willing to repeat exactly (even when this is possible) the studies of others, it is incumbent on the worker himself to see whether his results are reproducible.

Pregnancy Timing and Its Designation

Studies relating teratogenesis and embryonic age require that pregnancy be timed, i.e., its time of onset be known. With mice and rats—the most common subjects of such experiments—a usual practice is to place males and females together overnight. If copulation occurs (as indicated the next morning by the presence of a vaginal plug or by sperm in the vaginal smear), gestation is often considered to have begun at midnight. The question then is, what shall the time of this positive diagnosis of pregnancy be named? It has been called day 0, day 1, and 1st day. Obviously the different designations are frequently confusing, especially when, as sometimes happens, an author uses them interchangeably. In our laboratory the day (morning) the vaginal plug or sperm-positive smear is seen is called the 1st day of pregnancy, and the time 240 hours later, e.g., is called the 11th day. In the following pages I have taken the liberty of transforming other practices to this one, hoping that confusion will thus be minimized and comparison facilitated.

It is well recognized that embryos of a group of females impregnated during the same hours of mating, although considered to be of the same chronological age, will vary in developmental age. This variability may be due in part to the spread in time over which mating is allowed to occur and hence may to some extent be reduced when this time is shortened. But to believe (Rugh *et al.* 1964) that allowing mating for only a relatively short interval will thereby provide knowledge of exact gestational age is erroneous, since this practice does not control numerous other variables influencing gestational age, some of which may not be completely controllable insofar as an individual is concerned. Some of these factors are interval between coitus and ovulation, interval between ovulation and fertilization, time taken for complete ovulation in any one female, as well as various other factors regulated by light cycles, natural or artificial, and the genetic control of response to them (Braden and Austin 1954; Braden 1957).

2

Nutrient Deficiency

In this chapter are included discussions of the teratogenic effects of deficiencies of nutrients induced by feeding deficient diets or by administering counteracting substances, such as analogues, antimetabolites, and antagonists.

Riboflavin Deficiency

Riboflavin deficiency was one of the earliest teratologic techniques used in mammals (Warkany and Nelson 1940). The original method of obtaining a maternal riboflavin deficiency—long-term feeding of a diet containing little or none of the vitamin—had widespread deformative effects, but with rare exceptions produced only skeletal abnormalities (Warkany and Nelson 1941). However, short-term feeding of a riboflavin-deficient diet to which the riboflavin-antagonist galactoflavin was added regularly produced various nonskeletal malformations as well as the usual skeletal ones. Among the soft tissue defects was hydrocephalus.

The modified technique was introduced by Baird *et al.* (1955) and Nelson *et al.* (1956a). Stock female Long–Evans rats were placed for their entire gestation period or for several days during gestation on a basal riboflavin-deficient diet containing various levels of galactoflavin. A small but unstated percentage of offspring showed congenital hydrocephalus, which was not described. No other congenital malformation of the central nervous system was apparently seen in these studies with rats.

A similar technique was used by Kalter and Warkany (1957) with several inbred strains of mice. The animals were fed riboflavin-deficient, galactoflavin-containing diets for 4 days beginning the 10th or 11th day of pregnancy and killed near the end of the gestation period. Among the malformations produced was a syndrome of abnormalities of the brain, which included a form of hydrocephalus. The incidence of brain defects differed from strain to strain, being about 5 and 9 per cent, respectively, in C57BL/6J and 129/J mice, 55 per cent in A/J mice, and over 80 per cent in DBA/IJ animals (Kalter and Warkany 1957; Kalter 1963*b*, 1965*a*). The conditions varied in severity, but generally the more susceptible strains were also more extremely affected.

The heads of abnormal late-fetal and near-term offspring, with few exceptions, appeared externally normal, i.e., they were not visibly enlarged. Occasionally they were transilluminable. In histological sections, however, the entire ventricular system was found to be greatly expanded (figs. 1–4). This was especially true of the 4th ventricle, often to the extent that the condition resembled hydranencephaly. The increase in volume of this ventricle was due partly to thinning of the mid- and hindbrain and atrophy of the tela chorioidea, but mainly to its extreme dilatation. The tissue changes in the region of the 4th ventricle included completely absent or greatly reduced cerebellum, thin tectum mesencephali, and reduced medulla oblongata, pons, and tegmentum mesencephali.

Evidence of excessive pressure within the 4th ventricle was twofold: (1) upward bulging of the thin tectum mesencephali, which pulled the superior medullary velum upwards, stretching and closely flattening it against the region of the squama occipitalis; and (2) rostral inclination of the tegmentum mesencephali. The latter feature, combined with the thinning of the structures forming the floor of the 4th ventricle, increased the usually acute angle of the rhomboid fossa (as seen in median sagittal section) to an obtuse one. In the most pronounced instances, the dilated 4th ventricle pouched into the spinal cord and enlarged the cranial end of the central canal.

The lateral ventricles, in addition to being variably enlarged, were often bizarrely shaped and sometimes approached each other owing to distortion and reduction in width of the septum pellucidum. The foramina of Monro and the 3rd ventricle were also frequently expanded and the massa intermedia often absent or reduced in size. In most cases the aqueduct of Sylvius was greatly dilated, but in several cases it was only barely patent. In one case hydrocephalus was present on both sides of a minute aqueduct.

Many other anomalies were often found. The corpus callosum was usually absent. The body of the fornix was commonly small and cleft, or otherwise distorted, and the choroid plexus of the 3rd ventricle entered deeply into the cleft. The cavum septi pellucidi was often large. Cerebral areas dorsal to the lateral ventricles were thin, and these regions as well as the thin septa pellucida contained numerous cavities, which appeared as rosette-like formations. In other sections it could be seen that these cavities communicated with the ventricles.

Many of the brain defects, especially those of the 4th ventricle, greatly resembled a rare condition seen in children, known as the Dandy–Walker syndrome (Dandy 1921; Taggart and Walker 1942). Summaries of known cases were recently presented by Vichi and Bufalini (1962) and D'Agostino,

Kernohan, and Brown (1963). In affected children a huge cystlike, much-dilated 4th ventricle is present, which is expanded posteriorly and laterally and also projects downward into the cervical spinal canal. The cyst is lined by a greatly thinned posterior medullary velum and associated tela chorioidea and upwardly displaced tentorium. The choroid plexus is small or absent. The cisterna magna is underdeveloped or obliterated. Midline structures of the cerebellum are deficient or entirely absent. The pons, medulla, and upper cervical cord are flat, broad, and displaced anteriorly. There may be symmetrical internal hydrocephalus involving the anterior ventricles and aqueduct.

The abnormalities in the mice were remarkably like those just described in children. The 4th ventricle was greatly dilated and often extended into the cervical spinal canal. It was bounded posteriorly by a very thin and upwardly displaced tectum and stretched, thin medullary vela and tela chorioidea. The choroid plexus was small, with diminished floridity. The cerebellum was absent or greatly reduced, especially in the midline. The pons and medulla were small and pushed forward. The rest of the ventricular system was also enlarged.

The pathogenesis of the Dandy–Walker syndrome is unknown. Essentially there are 2 ideas as to its embryological basis: (1) the foramina of Magendie and Luschka fail to appear, and hydrocephalic enlargement of the 4th ventricle results and interferes with cerebellar development; (2) abnormalities of the roof of the 4th ventricle and cerebellum arise long before the time of formation of the foramina and thus can have nothing to do with their failure to appear. Instead the anomalies are due to (a) cleft formation of the cerebellum and a meningocele-like sac replacing part of the ventricular roof (Benda 1954); (b) increased intraventricular pressure of unknown origin (Brodal and Hauglie-Hanssen 1959).

The prenatal development of the galactoflavin-induced condition was studied (Kalter 1963b) in 12th- to 17th-day-old mouse fetuses. No obvious brain defects were present in younger specimens, but a syndrome of brain abnormalities was found in fetuses on the 14th and later days of gestation. This syndrome comprised most of the encephalic abnormalities seen in near-term young, as described above, but the defects at the early fetal stages were less severe than those present at the end of pregnancy. Little change in degree of the hydrocephalus occurred between the 14th and 17th days of pregnancy, and it therefore appeared that the extreme defects noted near birth (Kalter and Warkany 1957) developed in the last 2 days of pregnancy and hence were late phenomena.

The most revealing feature discovered in the embryological study (Kalter 1963b) was persistence of the area membranacea superior. This is a pear-shaped, median, normally transitory structure, composed of a single layer of flattened cells, which lies between the posterior fold of the cerebellum (metencephalon) and the anterior fold of the choroid plexus of the 4th ventricle.

Usually it is incorporated into the forewall of the plexus before the 12th day of uterine life (Bonnevie 1943). In 14th-day and older abnormal animals, however, the membrane remained an identifiable structure, long, thin, and bulging outward. It was postulated on the basis of this feature that the cause of this early sign of hydrocephalus is abnormality of elaboration or secretion of primitive, i.e., prechoroidal, cerebrospinal fluid, excess of which cannot leave the ventricle because the anterior membrane is normally impermeable and remains so owing to its later maldevelopment.

The similarities between the galactoflavin-induced hydrocephalus and that caused by the hydrocephalus-1 gene in mice are discussed in the chapter dealing with the latter (see p. 194).

Folic Acid Deficiency

The role of folic acid in reproduction and prenatal development has been studied in a large number of laboratories in the past 15 years or so (Kalter and Warkany 1959a). The present discussion will be confined to experiments in which maternal deficiency of the vitamin had teratogenic effects on the central nervous system. The studies of Hogan and colleagues, in which hydrocephalus was produced by folic acid or vitamin B_{12} deficiency, will be discussed below.

Although folic acid deficiency has widespread and potent teratogenic effects—so much so that it has been called a universal teratogen (Nelson 1955)—its harmful effects on the prenatal development of the central nervous system were less dramatic than on other parts of the body. Probably for this reason, although several authors have noted central nervous system defects, in only few reports were detailed statistical, anatomical, or embryological data concerning these abnormalities presented. Most studies were done with rats, which were usually fed a synthetic diet deficient in folic acid to which was added either an antibiotic, usually succinylsulfathiazole (SST), to suppress intestinal synthesis of the vitamin, or the antibiotic plus an antimetabolite of folic acid. The duration and time of feeding the regime varied.

Hydrocephalus was found in rats after such treatment by Evans, Nelson, and Asling (1951); Giroud, Lefebvres, and Dupuis (1952); Sansone and Zunin (1953, 1954); Thiersch (1954a); Nelson et al. (1955, 1956b); Obbink (1955–57); Monie, Armstrong, and Nelson (1961); and Stempak (1965). Most of these authors described the condition only briefly.

A fairly detailed description of hydrocephalus produced in rats by maternal folic acid deficiency was given in a preliminary communication by Monie, Armstrong, and Nelson (1961). Long–Evans rats were fed a folic acid-deficient diet to which was added 9-methylfolic acid (25 mg/kg diet) from the 9th to 11th days of pregnancy. This regime produced no visible congenital abnormalities; but histological study of 21st-day fetuses in some cases showed thinness of the cerebral cortex and concomitant enlargement of the lateral ventricles. The cerebral aqueduct was patent and the 4th ventricle and its roof were normal.

The postnatal development of the condition was also studied. Thirty-one offspring were autopsied between the ages of 15 and 65 days, 21 because of recognizable abnormality of the head region. Fourteen had hydrocephalus of various degrees of severity. In some the cortex of the cerebral hemispheres was so thin that perforation had occurred, usually in the occipital region. In a few the distended lateral ventricles were continuous across the midline. Absence or retarded growth of the corpus callosum and deformities of olfactory processes were occasionally seen. In older hydrocephalic animals, in addition to cortical thinness, the aqueduct was closed, and this was associated with reduced width of the midbrain. The latter finding suggested that closure of the aqueduct, in older abnormal cases, was a secondary feature, possibly related to compression of the brain by the distended cerebral hemispheres, and indicated that the hydrocephalus apparently resulted from retarded development of the cerebral cortex and related structures.

Quite different results were obtained by Stempak (1965). Female Wistar rats were fed a folic acid-deficient diet containing x-methylfolic acid (28 mg/kg diet) or 9-methylfolic acid (30 mg/kg) for 48 hours beginning the 8th or 9th day of pregnancy. The deficiency was terminated by an intraperitoneal injection of 0.5 mg folic acid. A relatively low incidence (13/193 = 6.7%) of hydrocephalus was found in offspring examined on the 20th and later days of pregnancy. Frank hydrocephalus was not exhibited by fetuses removed from the uterus on the 18th and 19th days (0/124), although incipient signs were observed. The condition was not clearly described; illustrations showed dilatation of the lateral ventricles, but the state of the other ventricles was not mentioned.

In all 13 hydrocephalic offspring the aqueduct was occluded or extremely stenotic, contrary to the findings of Monie, Armstrong, and Nelson (1961). Stempak (1965) suggested that the occlusion was caused by reduction in growth of the neural plate prior to its closure and that this reduction was due to altered mitotic rates. This supposition was entirely unsupported, since measurements of mitotic rates or of the size of neural structures in embryos and young fetuses were not made. Nor was evidence presented for the suggestion that the patent aqueducts found by Monie, Armstrong, and Nelson (1961) in their hydrocephalic offspring were the result of secondary reopening, a suggestion which could have been checked by examining hydrocephalic offspring at postnatal ages.

By feeding AEC Commentry rats a mixture consisting of a folic acid-deficient diet and 5 per cent antibiotic for 21 to 64 days before breeding and throughout pregnancy, it was possible to produce some congenital malformations without an antagonist; but so far as those of the central nervous system are concerned, only a few young with exencephaly and hydrocephalus resulted

(Giroud and Lefebvres 1951; Giroud, Lefebvres, and Dupuis 1952). A small amount of folic acid added to the mixture abolished the teratogenic effects. The addition of the crude antagonist, methylfolic acid (10–40 mg/kg), to a folic acid-deficient diet, in addition to greatly increasing the incidence of hydrocephalus produced by long-term feeding of the diet alone, resulted in occasional cases of exencephaly (O'Dell, Whitley, and Hogan 1951).

When a folic acid-deficient diet containing 1 per cent SST and 0.5 per cent x-methylfolic acid was fed to pregnant Long–Evans rats, beginning not later than the 10th day of gestation, all litters were resorbed; when instituted on the 11th to 14th days of pregnancy congenital malformations were produced, but those of the central nervous system were not noted (Nelson, Asling, and Evans 1952). Treatment before the 10th day resulted in the production of live young some of which had microscopic defects only if the level of the antagonist was reduced or the duration of the treatment shortened or both (Evans, Nelson, and Asling 1951; Nelson *et al.* 1955). When 0.15 to 0.2 per cent antagonist was given (Nelson *et al.* 1955) for 72 hours beginning the 8th day of pregnancy, young with hydrocephalus, exencephaly, and acephaly were produced (the incidence of all defects of the central nervous system being 49%, 38/77). Various cerebral defects, including hydrocephalus, exencephaly, and craniorachischisis, were also produced by as short as 36 hours of feeding the regime with 0.5 per cent antagonist beginning at this early time (Nelson *et al.* 1956*b*; Nelson 1957).

Pregnant Wistar rats (Tuchmann-Duplessis and Lefebvres-Boisselot 1957*a*) fed x-methylfolic acid had less severely deformed young than did the Long–Evans rats of Nelson *et al.* (1955). No abnormalities of the central nervous system were produced, but the antagonist was given relatively late in pregnancy (10th–11th or 11th–12th days).

Various congenital malformations were produced in the offspring of Long–Evans rats given different doses of 2,4-diaminopyrimidine antagonists of folic acid by intubation between the 5th and 11th days of gestation (Thiersch 1954*a*). The most common malformation induced by the methylpyrimidine derivative was exencephaly, described as failure of the cranium to close over the brain. In several instances the entire cranium was only rudimentarily developed, and in one case the brain was eroded and not covered by meninges or cranial bones. The largest frequency of malformed young and the greatest variety of defects of the central nervous system occurred in offspring of females given both the antagonist and leucovorin in an attempt, paradoxically, at counteracting the effect of the antagonist. The combined treatment produced hydrocephalus, microcephaly, and spina bifida, as well as exencephaly. It is likely that the variety of defects and their relatively great incidence were due to the leucovorin's salvaging deformed young that would otherwise have been entirely destroyed. Malformations were produced by much smaller doses of the methylpyrimidine derivative than of the ethylpyrimidine one.

The ethylpyrimidine derivative was also used by others. Dyban, Akimova, and Svetlova (1965) produced various congenital malformations in rats; those of the central nervous system, which included exencephaly and craniorachischisis, resulted from intraperitoneal and oral treatment on the 9th day of gestation with 3 to 10 mg/kg. Subcutaneous treatment somewhat later in pregnancy resulted in noncentral nervous system defects (Anderson and Morse 1966). Thiersch (1964) tested several other 2,4-diaminopyrimidines and found that some of them produced hydrocephalus and underdevelopment and abnormalities of the cranium.

Aminopterin (4-amino folic acid), a more powerful antagonist of folic acid than the x-methyl one, was used by several investigators. In an early study (Thiersch and Philips 1950), it destroyed all embryos. In other studies some congenital malformations were produced, but except for hydrocephalus (Sansone and Zunin 1953, 1954; Obbink 1955–57), no defects of the central nervous system were found (Murphy and Karnofsky 1956; Kotani *et al.* 1958; Kosterlitz 1960, pp. 155–56; Kinney and Morse 1964). Recently Baranov (1965, 1966) succeeded in producing exencephaly and microcephaly in rats; treatment was made at the relatively early time of the 6th day of gestation and the highest incidence of defects was obtained with a dose of 0.1 mg/kg.

Several studies were made of the teratogenic effects of folic acid deficiency in other species, namely mouse and cat. Inbred mice of the 129 strain were fed a semisynthetic folic acid-deficient diet for 24 hours on the 9th day of gestation. By itself the diet was not teratogenic, but when x-methylfolic acid was added or animals were given antibiotic and the antagonist, 9-methylfolic acid, exencephaly was produced (Runner 1954, 1959; Runner and Dagg 1960).

Albino mice of unspecified origin were given a mixture of a commercial stock diet and 0.5 per cent x-methylfolic acid from the 6th or 7th to the 9th days of pregnancy (Tuchmann-Duplessis and Mercier-Parot 1957). More severe and frequent congenital malformations were caused by the earlier-instituted treatment. The majority of defects were of the brain and consisted of exencephaly of the entire brain or occasionally only of a more limited region. Mice of several inbred strains and other genotypes were given single or multiple injections of various doses of another folic acid antagonist, 4-amino-pteroylaspartic acid, at different times in gestation. Although numerous types of congenital malformations resulted, no defects of the central nervous system were found (Kalter 1953; Trasler 1958).

In a study of the effects of folic acid deficiency on embryonic development of cats (Tuchmann-Duplessis and Lefebvres-Boisselot 1957b), only a few, noncentral nervous system defects were noted.

The effects of a short period of folic acid deficiency on the early embryology of rats was studied by Johnson, Nelson, and Monie (1963). Experimental 10th-day embryos were indistinguishable from controls; 11th-day and older embryos were reduced in size; 11th-day ones had partial or complete absence of closure of the neural folds; the most severe defects in 12th-day specimens were located in the cranial portion of the neural tube; 13th-day embryos had many abnormal diverticula in various parts of the brain. Fewer mitotic figures were found in the wall of the neural tube than in controls (Johnson 1964).

Vitamin B$_{12}$ and Folic Acid Deficiency

A series of papers by Hogan and colleagues that appeared between 1946 and 1962 dealt with studies of the teratogenic effects of deficiencies of folic acid and vitamin B$_{12}$. Because of the difficulty of separating the effects of deficiency of one vitamin from those of the other, these reports are perhaps best discussed chronologically.

During a study of the adequacy of a synthetic basal diet (diet A) for reproduction and lactation in rats, Richardson and Hogan (1946) observed that about 2 per cent of the offspring of females fed the diet were hydrocephalic. The animals used were albino rats of a closed, noninbred colony at the University of Missouri. Diet A contained casein as the protein source and was supplemented with all then-known water-soluble vitamins except folic acid. Vitamin B$_{12}$ was not a recognized vitamin at the time, but it was later learned (Grainger, O'Dell, and Hogan 1954) that the diet used by Richardson and Hogan (1946) contained (in the casein) a significant amount of this vitamin. Why this point is mentioned will soon become apparent. In the earliest studies the diet was apparently fed from weaning (Richardson and Hogan 1946; Richardson and DeMottier 1947), but placing the females on the experimental diet only a short time before mating produced the same incidence of hydrocephalus (O'Dell, Whitley, and Hogan 1948).

The hydrocephalus occurred in 30/1756 (1.7%) offspring weaned from females receiving the diet, but was not observed in young whose mothers were fed the diet supplemented with liver extracts (Richardson and Hogan 1946). The condition was not recognized in animals less than 10 days old; most cases were first observed between 14 and 20 days of age, some even later. In typical cases the head was domeshaped and greatly enlarged. In doubtful cases transillumination was used as a diagnostic aid. It was later found (Newberne and O'Dell 1958) that the incidence of hydrocephalus was approximately doubled, by detection of less severe cases, when animals were grossly sectioned. In this way, also, younger affected animals could be discovered. The only other abnormalities noted were some eye defects (Richardson and Hogan 1946).

In typical cases (Richardson and Hogan 1946), the amount of brain tissue was reduced and the ventricles were filled with straw-coloured or pink serum. Gross dissection showed that the hydrocephalus was internal, and measurement of the cerebrospinal-fluid pressure indicated it to be of the communicating type (O'Dell, Whitley, and Hogan 1948). The condition apparently did not interfere with reproduction, and crosses of hydrocephalic parents produced normal offspring if the females were fed a stock diet (Richardson 1951).

A low incidence of hydrocephalus, some cases of which were congenital, was also produced in rats of another closed colony (of the Texas Agricultural Experiment station), by feeding diet A (Richardson and DeMottier 1947). The conclusion was thus strengthened that the hydrocephalus was caused by a nutritional deficiency, and efforts were made to identify the deficient nutrient.

Suspecting folic acid of being the missing ingredient, O'Dell, Whitley, and Hogan (1948) placed females of the Texas colony on diet A, or diet A supplemented with this vitamin, shortly before mating. The offspring were examined at the end of the second, third, and fourth weeks of age, by trans-illumination, for symptoms of hydrocephalus. Females given diet A had 532 weaned offspring, 10 (1.9%) of which were hydrocephalic, while the incidence was 0.1 per cent in those weaned from females given the folic acid-supplemented regime, approximating that found in offspring of animals fed the stock ration (0.2%). The protective effect of folic acid was confirmed by Richardson (1951), and it thus seemed that maternal folic acid deficiency was responsible for the hydrocephalus.

In an attempt at increasing the frequency of hydrocephalus, a diet (2087) containing soybean oil meal, instead of casein, as the protein source was fed from weaning onwards (Hogan, O'Dell, and Whitley 1950). But the incidence of the condition remained low, possibly because of intestinal synthesis of folic acid, and in further studies the crude folic acid antagonist (probably x-) methylfolic acid (10 or 20 mg/kg) was added to diet 2087. Apparently once more confirming that folic acid deficiency was etiologically involved, this procedure generally succeeded in raising the incidence of the condition. In this study (Hogan, O'Dell, and Whitley 1950), all cases of hydrocephalus were congenital. Furthermore, it seems that the condition was more severe than that found earlier, since almost all defective young died by 3 to 4 days after birth.

Up to this point the results seemed fairly straightforward: diets deficient in folic acid caused low frequencies of hydrocephalus. It was decreased by adding folic acid and was increased by intensifying the deficiency through use of an antagonist of the vitamin.

A question that remained was the role of the casein-containing diet A in lowering the frequency of hydrocephalus (Hogan, O'Dell, and Whitley 1950). It was suspected that this effect was due to a protective factor in casein, and when it was found (O'Dell, Whitley, and Hogan 1951) that casein usually contains more vitamin B_{12} than does soybean meal oil, it seemed that a deficiency of this vitamin might also be implicated in the abnormality. In other words, it appeared as though deficiency not only of folic acid but of vitamin B_{12} as well was involved. Some support for this position was supplied by Richardson (1951), who found that addition to diet A of folic acid or of a vitamin B_{12} concentrate reduced the incidence of hydrocephalus, and further that the antagonist methylfolic acid (10 mg/kg) produced only a small incidence of the abnormality in the presence of added vitamin B_{12}.

Confirmation of these general findings came from the study of O'Dell, Whitley, and Hogan (1951), who found that when diet 2087 was fed from weaning (= pre-experimental depletion) and methylfolic acid (10, 20, or 40 mg/kg) added during the experimental period, the incidence of hydrocephalus was 23.4 per cent (222/949), whereas it was 15.1 per cent (237/1568) when no pre-experimental depletion was made. This difference was striking among first and second litters but was little present after third litters. When a vitamin B_{12} concentrate, supplying 22 μg/kg, was added to the diet, no hydrocephalus occurred (0/1261), despite the presence of methylfolic acid.

When the females were depleted of vitamin B_{12} by being fed diet 2087 from weaning, the addition of folic acid to the diet did not prevent hydrocephalus, and it made little difference whether methylfolic acid was included or not. It thus appeared that hydrocephalus was the outcome of deficiency of either vitamin or of both of them. However, since neither the dietary depletions nor the levels of antagonist used were intense enough to produce marked deficiencies, the effect of absence of either nutrient in the presence of adequate supplies of the other was not studied, and hence interpretation of the results is precarious.

The study of Grainger, O'Dell, and Hogan (1954) attempted to remedy some of these drawbacks. The animals used were rats of Wistar origin, but whether of the same University of Missouri colony as previously used was not mentioned. The females were usually placed on the experimental diets at weaning. They were allowed to deliver and were bred again. The incidence of congenital hydrocephalus in offspring from females fed by the Steenbock–Black rachitogenic diet supplemented only with viosterol (the same diet used by Warkany and Nelson 1940) was 23.7 per cent (24/101). When folic acid was added the incidence decreased to 14.8 per cent (67/452), and when both folic acid and vitamin B_{12} were added no hydrocephalus was found. Clear-cut confirmation of the teratogenicity of vitamin B_{12} deficiency was obtained by long-term feeding of a folic acid-supplemented, B_{12}-deficient diet (Newberne and O'Dell 1958; Woodard and Newberne 1966) to Wistar rats, 10.3 per cent (96/897) of whose offspring were hydrocephalic.

An extremely interesting finding of Grainger, O'Dell, and Hogan's (1954) was that addition of riboflavin to a vitamin B_{12}-deficient diet permitted a much more severe deficiency of the latter vitamin to occur than when both vitamins were absent; and consequently, although no hydrocephalus was produced in the absence of both vitamins, when riboflavin was added and an apparently uncomplicated and severe vitamin B_{12} deficiency resulted, 11.7 per cent (44/375) of the offspring were hydrocephalic.

Although, as mentioned above, Warkany and Nelson (1940) used the Steenbock–Black diet, hydrocephalus was not noted in their (Sprague–Dawley) rats. Grainger, O'Dell, and Hogan (1954) believed that this stock is less readily depleted of vitamin B_{12} than Wistar rats and less subject to congenital malformations when depleted.

Little was added to the facts summarized in the past few pages by the study of Erickson and O'Dell (1961), who investigated the effects of varying the concentration of different dietary components on the frequency of vitamin B_{12} deficiency-induced hydrocephalus. The study of Woodard and Newberne (1966), which investigated the relation of 1-carbon metabolism and vitamin B_{12} deficiency-induced hydrocephalus, was weakened by the fact that the newborn young were fixed in formalin, a procedure that may distort the ventricular spaces.

Several papers by different members of this group of investigators were devoted to descriptions of the morphological features of the hydrocephalus. The ventricular system was studied in sectioned material by Overholser *et al.* (1954), who found that the middle part of the cerebral aqueduct became occluded between the 16th and 18th days of gestation; and thus presumed that the condition was a result of this closure. Surprisingly, however, in 1-day-old hydrocephalics the aqueduct was usually open, although abnormally-shaped and smaller than normal. The authors speculated that this was due to a reopening, sometime between the 18th day of gestation and birth, caused by pressure of accumulated cerebrospinal fluid in the lateral and 3rd ventricles.

In 1-day-old animals the lateral ventricles, interventricular foramina, and 3rd ventricle were greatly enlarged, but the size of the posterior part of the aqueduct and the 4th ventricle was normal. The enlargements, according to the authors, apparently developed between the 16th and 18th days of gestation, since they were not found in 16th-day fetuses but were present in 18th-day ones (Overholser *et al.* 1954). However, these datings of fetal events cannot be taken too seriously since they were based on a very limited number of observations. Somewhat different results, in fact, were obtained by Newberne and O'Dell (1959), who found signs of hydrocephalus and marked alterations in the aqueduct in some 16th-day fetal brains from rats fed a vitamin B_{12}-deficient diet. In their opinion, the abnormal pattern developed between the 14th and 16th days of gestation, which matched the finding of O'Dell, Whitley, and Hogan (1951) that parenteral administration of vitamin B_{12} to pregnant vitamin B_{12}-deficient rats prevented congenital hydrocephalus if given before the 14th day of gestation.

Overholser *et al.* (1954) examined sections of 50 neonatal, normal-appearing littermates of hydrocephalic animals. Twelve had partially closed cerebral aqueducts and histological abnormalities, some with moderate enlargement of the 3rd and lateral ventricles; and 23 had slight constriction of the anterior portion of the aqueduct but no histological abnormalities. Thus, 70 per cent of young without observable hydrocephalus from vitamin B_{12}-deficient mothers also had brain defects.

In control brains there was present (Overholser *et al.* 1954) a specialized group of high columnar ependymal cells in the roof of the posterior part of the 3rd ventricle and anterior part of the aqueduct. These cells, later identified (Newberne 1962) as the subcommissural organ, were partly or completely absent in hydrocephalic brains (Overholser *et al.* 1954). The appearance of these cells suggested that they have a secretory function that is active before full development of the choroid plexus. Their absence would therefore result in closure of the ventricular system at its narrowest portion, i.e., the aqueduct, because of lack of hydrostatic pressure. When the choroid plexuses of the 3rd and lateral ventricles become functional, the authors contended, pressure would build up in these spaces and hydrocephalus would develop.

The tall columnar cells of the subcommissural organ were also absent in most of the vitamin B_{12} deficiency-induced hydrocephalics examined by Newberne and O'Dell (1958). However, these cells were present in some animals with completely occluded aqueducts. This was confirmed by Newberne (1962). It seems unlikely, therefore, that their absence was the primary defect in the hydrocephalus of these animals.

Whitley (1952, unpublished thesis cited by Overholser *et al.* 1954) considered that the possible cause of the aqueductal stenosis was an abnormal growth rate of glial tissue surrounding the aqueduct, but no evidence for this supposition was presented. Newberne and O'Dell (1959) noted a larger than normal number of mitotic figures in the aqueductal ependyma of 16th-day fetuses from vitamin B_{12}-deficient mothers, which they interpreted, in the light of the general developmental retardation of such fetuses, not as evidence of increased, but of reduced, cell division with consequent piling up of mitoses, analogous to those seen in colchicine-treated tissues.

Other histological findings of Newberne and O'Dell (1959) were areolization of the extremely thin cerebral cortical parenchyma, areas of absent ependyma, loss of normal architectural appearance of choroid plexuses, and mild glial changes around the 3rd and lateral ventricles and aqueduct. Unaffected littermates of hydrocephalics showed no distention of ventricles but had irregularly-shaped aqueducts and slight histological changes in choroid plexus and ependyma.

Aside from these studies of Hogan and his colleagues, only Montanari (1961) has studied the teratogenic effects of vitamin B_{12} deficiency. He found that chronic vitamin B_{12} deprivation of Sprague–Dawley rats produced mild dilatation of the 3rd and lateral ventricles and moderate atrophy of choroid plexus in newborn offspring.

Pantothenic Acid Deficiency

A mammalian teratogenic method that was introduced relatively early is deficiency of the B vitamin pantothenic acid (Boisselot 1948); its most frequent effects were eye anomalies and exencephaly (Boisselot 1949). A synthetic diet deficient in pantothenic acid was fed (Lefebvres-Boisselot 1951) to female rats of 3 origins—AEC Commentry, Oxford Wistar, and Parisian piebald. No differences were noted among the stocks in teratologic response to the deficiency. The diet was started 3 to 38 days before breeding and continued during pregnancy. When the diet was begun more than 10 days before breeding nearly all young were resorbed, and when begun 3 to 10 days before breeding resorption of entire litters occurred in half the females. Of 49 females that received the diet, 21 aborted or failed to implant, and 19 resorbed their litters. The remaining 9, killed between the 13th and 20th days of gestation, had 65 offspring, 61 (94%) of which were malformed, 13 (20%) with exencephaly.

The external appearance of the exencephaly was very characteristic. The top of the head was covered by an irregular convex protuberance, consisting of the herniated brain, which never extended to the nape. The anomalies of the exencephalic brain were generally severe and affected the telencephalon, diencephalon, and mesencephalon. Further, the disorganization of the brain was sometimes of such a degree that its state could only be described by the term pseudencephaly. Only one case of hydrocephalus, which was of the lateral ventricles, was found. It appeared to be correlated with obstruction of the cerebral aqueduct (Lefebvres-Boisselot 1951).

The morphology of the exencephaly in late fetal specimens was analyzed in great detail (Giroud *et al.* 1957). There was a general torsion of the brain and a strongly marked mesencephalic curvature accentuated by the projection of the brain at the vertex. The telencephalon was not subdivided into hemispheres, i.e., a single anterior ventricle was present; the 3rd and 4th cranial nerves were abnormal; and accessory nervous tissue occurred, mainly in the region of the midbrain.

By adding graded amounts of calcium pantothenate to a pantothenic acid-deficient diet, fed to "albino" rats, it was found (Lefebvres-Boisselot 1955) that the presence of less than 10 μg/day of the vitamin caused all embryos to resorb. Above that amount, the incidence of resorption decreased and the incidence of congenital malformations increased as more pantothenate was added to the diet, the highest level of abnormalities occurring with 20 to 25 μg/day. A minimum of 50 μg/day was necessary for completely normal development.

Despite the marked teratogenicity of pantothenic acid deficiency, only a slight reduction in the content of the vitamin was found in maternal liver (Giroud, Lefebvres-Boisselot, and Dupuis 1961). This finding seems to point to the precarious balance prenatal development is subject to and reveals how slight a disturbance of maternal physiology can affect the embryo. The same situation was true of riboflavin deficiency (Giroud *et al.* 1952).

Nelson *et al.* (1957) also found that the incidence of completely resorbed litters increased with length of time on a pantothenic acid-deficient diet before breeding. The largest frequency of malformed offspring (29%) resulted when the diet was started 4 days before breeding. This was far lower than resulted (94%) in Lefebvres-Boisselot's (1951) experiment, and the difference may have been due to any of several possibilities. Nelson *et al.* (1957) used Long–Evans rats, and killed them late in gestation; while Lefebvres-Boisselot (1951) used other stocks, which were killed at various times during the last half of pregnancy. Stock differences or the obtaining of severely deformed fetuses relatively early in pregnancy that may not have survived to later pregnancy may thus account for the difference in frequency of abnormal offspring. The latter possibility is supported by the fact that a far smaller rate of malformed offspring was also obtained by Giroud, Lefebvres-Boisselot, and Dupuis (1957) when the mothers were killed near the end of pregnancy.

Addition of the antimetabolite, omega-methylpantothenic acid (5–10 μg/kg deficient diet), for 2 or 3 days, between the 10th and 15th days of gestation (Nelson *et al.* 1957), intensified the teratogenic effect and hence made it unnecessary to give the deficient diet before breeding. Many more types of malformations were produced in this study than in that of Lefebvres-Boisselot (1951), which again may have been due to stock differences or, as is more likely, to the use of the antagonist. Nelson *et al.* (1957) did not indicate whether the malformations produced by the deficient diet alone were in any way different from those induced by the antagonist. Exencephaly and hydrocephalus were found in 13 per cent of 102 abnormal offspring by Nelson *et al.* (1957) after pantothenic acid deficiency, but the separate incidence of each of these abnormalities was not stated nor were the conditions described.

A different antagonist of pantothenic acid, pantoyltaurine, was used by Zunin and Borrone (1954). Brain abnormalities produced were called "dehiscence of cerebral material." In this condition brain tissue was found spread outside the cranial cavity between the calvaria and skin, and in some cases the ectopic brain tissue was connected by a stalk to the brain. This anomaly may have been similar to that found by Giroud *et al.* (1957), who described accessory nervous tissue lying alongside certain areas of the brain. Apparently, frank exencephaly was not produced (Zunin and Borrone 1954).

Several abnormal offspring were found in other studies in which the role of pantothenic acid in reproductive performance and prenatal development was being investigated. Pfaltz and Severinghaus (1956) and Barboriak *et al.* (1957), using rats, and Kimura and Ariyama (1961), using mice, found a small number of young with exencephaly. No abnormalities of the central nervous system apparently occurred in another study with rats (Cooper 1962), and no malformations at all in a different study with mice (Coggi 1965). In testing the combined action of dietary-induced pantothenic acid deficiency and thalidomide feeding (Fratta, Sigg, and Maiorana 1965), the exencephalies found (in Long–Evans rats, percentage unstated) were probably the result only of the vitamin deficiency.

In studies with pigs (Ullrey *et al.* 1955; Davey and Stevenson 1963), some offspring of females fed suboptimal levels of pantothenic acid exhibited locomotor incoordination and irregularities of gait. Some young could not stand at all and lay with their legs outstretched, while others moved with outspread rear legs or with a typical "goosestep." Occasional individuals exhibited a persistent tremor of the head and body, resembling paralysis agitans. These symptoms were sometimes present at birth or developed soon afterward. A characteristic syndrome of locomotor disturbances was also produced in Long–Evans rats by prenatal maternal pantothenic acid deficiency (Ershoff and Kruger 1962). Histological examination of brains from abnormal animals revealed no evidence of pathology beyond a reduction in the fissural pattern of the cerebellum.

Vitamin A Deficiency

Vitamin A deficiency was the first nonactinic method discovered of causing congenital malformations in well-controlled experiments with mammals (Hale 1933). In these early studies, which were made with pigs (Hale 1933, 1935, 1937), as in later ones made with pigs (Goodwin and Jennings 1958) and rats (Warkany and Schraffenberger 1944; Andersen 1949; Wilson, Roth, and Warkany 1953; Roux *et al.* 1962), no congenital malformations of the central nervous system were reported. It was not until the work with rabbits and the newer work with pigs described below was performed that such defects were found. In several other studies (summarized by Mason 1935), contemporaneous with and earlier than those of Hale, on the effects of vitamin A deficiency on reproduction in rats, fetal death and other phenomena resulted, but congenital malformations were not produced.

The first congenital malformations of the central nervous system induced by vitamin A deficiency were found in experiments with rabbits reported by Millen, Woollam, and Lamming (1953). Female rabbits fed a synthetic diet containing less than 1 μg carotene (provitamin A) per gram of diet had offspring with hydrocephalus. When the females were given this diet from 14 weeks before mating to delivery, the condition was apparently first manifested by the young 2 to 8 weeks after birth (Millen, Woollam, and Lamming 1953). Thirty-five offspring from vitamin A-deprived females were examined between the ages of 10 and 74 days, by which latter time all were dead, and of these, 26 (74.3%) had hydrocephalus (Lamming, Woollam, and Millen 1954). When the diet was given for longer periods, from 14 to 38 weeks before mating to the end of pregnancy, congenital hydrocephalus resulted. This condition occurred in 47/51 (92.2%) newborn young and late fetuses, 21 cases being considered severe, 17 moderate, and 9 slight (Millen, Woollam, and Lamming 1954). The frequency of hydrocephalic offspring was greater the longer the females were kept on the deficient diet before mating, being approximately 14 per cent in young from mothers fed the diet from 12 to 15 weeks before mating, 58 per cent 16 to 19 weeks, 67 per cent 20 to 23 weeks, and 82 per cent 24 to 28 weeks (Millen and Woollam 1956).

It should be noted that in this study, despite the long periods of time the diet was given to some females, the hydrocephalus was apparently not congenital, but appeared postnatally. The fact that in one experiment (Millen, Woollam, and Lamming 1954) prolonged ingestion of the deficient diet resulted in congenital hydrocephalus, while in another (Millen and Woollam 1956) it produced postnatally-appearing hydrocephalus, may be related to the fact that in these 2 studies animals of different origins were used: in the earlier experiment, inbred rabbits from a colony closed for many years; and in the later study, commercially obtained rabbits of mixed breeds, mostly of a small Dutch variety. That genetic differences between the 2 groups of animals may account for the discrepancy is supported by the fact that in the earlier study, in which inbred animals were used (Millen, Woollam, and Lamming 1954), a 14-week deprivation period before mating produced 74 per cent malformed young, whereas in the later study with animals of mixed breeds (Millen and Woollam 1956), a comparable deprivation period produced only 14 per cent abnormal young.

Millen and Woollam (1956) diagnosed young for hydrocephalus at postmortem examination but usually failed to say how old the offspring were when examined. It would be valuable to know not only that the incidence of the defect was related to the degree of maternal deprivation of vitamin A, but whether its onset and severity were also so related. On these points there was no information. In this paper a photograph of a section through the head of a 1-day-old control rabbit is compared with that of a 20-day-old hydrocephalic specimen. Surely a more convincing demonstration would have been made by comparing control and experimental animals of the same age.

Measurements were made of the cerebrospinal-fluid pressures of nonhydrocephalic (Millen and Woollam 1956) and hydrocephalic young (Millen and Dickson 1957), from vitamin A-deficient females. In the former, pressures ranged from 120 to 265 mm water and in the latter from about 120 to 470 mm water, whereas the average normal pressure in rabbits is less than 100 mm water. These findings suggested that increase in cerebrospinal-fluid pressure was one of the earliest signs of vitamin A deficiency, preceding the occurrence of ventricular dilatation (Millen and Woollam 1956).

Administration to 28 hydrocephalic young of 10,000 to 20,000 IU (international units) synthetic vitamin A acetate by mouth or subcutaneous injection at weekly intervals led to rapid fall in cerebrospinal-fluid pressure, which in general continued until normal limits were reached (Millen and Dickson 1957). Some hydrocephalic animals survived almost indefinitely provided vitamin A was given regularly (Millen and Woollam 1958a).

The first signs of postnatally-developing hydrocephalus, occurring 3 to 6 weeks after birth, were retraction of the head, paralysis of the hindquarters, convulsions, and emaciation, but these symptoms did not appear in all animals later found to be hydrocephalic (Lamming, Woollam, and Millen 1954). Externally, the vault of the skull was expanded, the calvaria was very thin, and the anterior fontanelle was wide open (Millen and Woollam 1956; Millen and Dickson 1957). In no hydrocephalic animal examined after death was any congenital abnormality discovered other than hydrocephalus (Millen and Woollam 1956). One offspring with exencephaly was found in a different study (Millen and Woollam 1959).

In sectioned material (Millen, Woollam, and Lamming 1953) from offspring with late-developing hydrocephalus, the lateral and 3rd ventricles were found to be greatly dilated, and in some specimens the cortex and white matter were reduced to an extremely thin layer lining the interior of the skull. The authors stated that it was surprising to find such a condition compatible not only with life but even with the comparatively few signs of hydrocephalus. In one case the brain had herniated through the skull and formed a slight swelling under the skin. The 4th ventricle was grossly and histologically normal, even in the presence of herniation of the cerebellum through the foramen magnum. No deformity of the foramen magnum itself or of the base of the skull was found, but the optic nerves were markedly constricted at the optic foramina.

Pronounced stenosis of the cerebral aqueduct was present at the level of the superior colliculus. Rostral to the constriction the lumen of the aqueduct was enlarged, but distal to it appeared normal. Colloidal carbon injected in vivo into the anterior ventricles apparently did not pass beyond the stenotic aqueduct, since no carbon particles were found in the 4th ventricle. It was therefore concluded that the signs of the nervous disorder could be attributed to hydrocephalus produced by stenosis of the aqueduct (Millen, Woollam, and Lamming 1953). But this opinion had to be modified when it was found in several animals that carbon did pass through the aqueduct (Millen and Woollam 1958a).

The congenital hydrocephalus closely resembled in many details the postnatally-developing condition, with one significant exception (Millen, Woollam, and Lamming 1954). Again, the 3rd ventricle and, especially, the lateral ventricles were greatly dilated; and the 4th ventricle was normal—despite, in severer cases, the posterior part of the cerebellum and medulla oblongata being displaced into the upper part of the cervical canal. Retardation of ossification of the skull was noted. But the difference was that in the congenital condition the lumen of the aqueduct in the region of the superior colliculus was not appreciably smaller in experimental animals than in controls (Millen, Woollam, and Lamming 1954). In the light of this finding, the stenosis of the aqueduct in the later-appearing hydrocephalus was probably a secondary occurrence and not of primary significance in its development. Other features were also probably secondary.

The sequence of pathogenetic events was considered to be as follows (Millen and Woollam 1958a). Overproduction of cerebrospinal fluid and the consequent dilatation of the lateral ventricles forced the hindbrain downwards and caused the cerebellum to herniate through the foramen magnum. This secondary displacement, in itself, and by producing a narrowing and distortion of the aqueduct, interfered with escape of the cerebrospinal fluid from the 4th ventricle and increased the severity of the hydrocephalus. In several animals, however, the aqueduct was not completely occluded, since carbon passed through it. The basic cause was thus felt to be increased cerebrospinal-fluid pressure due to overproduction of cerebrospinal fluid by the choroid plexuses of the anterior ventricles.

These studies with rabbits were in large measure recently confirmed by Carton, Pascal, and Tennyson (1961). The breed of rabbit used was not specified. A diet containing 9.67 mg carotene per 100 lb. was fed beginning either 4 days before (group I) or immediately after (group II) mating and presumably continued throughout pregnancy. Group I females had 69.0 per cent (107/155) and group II females 29.3 per cent (12/41) hydrocephalic offspring, and the abnormality was congenital in some cases and appeared postnatally in others. The offspring of females kept on the deficient diet for the longer period (group I) were apparently more severely damaged than those of the group II females, since in addition to being more frequently affected, the incidence of congenital hydrocephalus was greater in them than in the latter; whereas some group II offspring did not become obviously hydrocephalic until the age of 1 to 2 months. Others that were apparently normal were found to be hydrocephalic when autopsied at 6 to 8 months of age.

In sections of abnormal brains, secondary aqueductal compression presumably due to intracranial pressure was sometimes found, but in the majority, particularly in early-expressed hydrocephalus, there was no obstruction anywhere in the ventricular system, including the foramina of Luschka.

In electron-microscopic studies of choroid plexuses of these hydrocephalic rabbits, certain nonspecific morphological changes were found, which may have been due to factors other than vitamin A deficiency (Tennyson and Pappas 1961).

Although, as stated above, Hale (1933, 1935, 1937) did not find congenital malformations of the central nervous system in his studies with pigs, in more recent work with this species such defects were produced by vitamin A deficiency. In preliminary studies (Hjarde *et. al.* 1961; Palludan 1961) a high incidence of multiply malformed offspring occurred. A detailed description of the defects noted in an expanded investigation recently appeared (Palludan 1966). Thirty-three females, mostly of the Danish Landrace breed, were fed a diet supplying 5 to 10 per cent of the minimum vitamin A required from about 2 months of age to the end of pregnancy. Nineteen of the females received one or more supplements of vitamin A alcohol (for a total of 0.4–1.2 million IU) at various times during pregnancy; 5 received small daily doses of vitamin A acid, usually throughout pregnancy; and 9 received no vitamin A supplement during pregnancy. Offspring of vitamin A-acid-supplemented females presented the same array and incidence of malformations as did those of females that received no supplement; whereas young from vitamin A-alcohol-supplemented females were in general less often and less multiply malformed. E.g., the last group was almost entirely free of malformations of the central nervous system (3/171 = 1.8%), while the other groups were almost all affected (127/128 = 99.2%).

There occurred two types of congenital defects of the central nervous system, internal hydrocephalus and defects of the spinal cord, and these varied in severity. The head of hydrocephalic young was more rounded and domed than normal. The calvaria was usually very thin with large fontanelles. The bones of the cranial base, on the contrary, were often far thicker than normal. The cerebrum was almost circular, and the convolutions were greatly flattened. The lateral ventricles were markedly expanded and both the gray and white matter of their walls much thinned. The rest of the ventricular system was usually also dilated. Compression of the cerebellum was frequently seen. One offspring had microcephaly combined with a small exencephaly, absent cerebellum, and other defects; it would be difficult to attribute these conditions to lack of vitamin A. The spinal cord defects consisted of reduction in size and narrow vertebral canal, with the cord thus tightly enclosed by meninges and vertebrae. These anomalies were most commonly present and most clear cut in the lumbar region.

The types of malformations found in this study (Palludan 1966) depended on the stage of pregnancy at which vitamin A supplementation was made, and the earlier in embryogenesis the deficiency was arrested the fewer were the malformations observed in the offspring. Defects of the central nervous system were not seen if supplementation was made before about the 90th day of gestation.

Bendixen (1944) described eye defects in pigs that may have been the result of vitamin A deficiency, and later (Bendixen 1950) reported eye defects produced by a vitamin A-poor diet, as did Schoop (1955). In studies (Bailey and Nelson 1965) of the effects of continual feeding of a vitamin A-devoid ration on successive litters in pigs, several young from the third and fourth litters of a sow had eye defects and one offspring had edematous brain and absent cerebral convolutions. Congenital malformations of the limbs, ataxia, and other abnormalities were found in offspring of pigs fed a diet deficient in some factor or factors necessary for normal reproduction and lactation. The deficient substance was not identified, nor was the basis of the ataxia determined (Ross *et al.* 1944). This report is mentioned here merely to keep all the pigs together.

Although, in the studies with rats cited above (Warkany and Schraffenberger 1944; Andersen 1949; Wilson, Roth, and Warkany 1953*c*; Roux *et al.* 1962), defects of the central nervous system did not occur, in another experiment with rats hydrocephalus was found. In this case, the hydrocephalic condition seems to have been produced by a relative deficiency of vitamin A (Rokkones 1955). Female rats (of unstated stock) were placed at weaning on a basal diet and given weekly supplements of vitamins A (105 IU), D, K, and E. They were usually bred at 6 months of age. Visible manifestations of abnormality in their offspring usually appeared at the age of 5 days and onward, and consisted of spastically contracted limbs, bendings of the tail, bloody exudate from the eyes, bristly fur, and a more or less pronounced swelling in the frontal region, giving a certain bulldog-like appearance to the head. Autopsy of diseased animals revealed enlargement of cerebral ventricles in all cases.

Daily supplements to the mothers of several B vitamins and linseed oil did not prevent the condition. But when the vitamin A supplied was increased from 105 IU/week to 105 IU/day visible symptoms of hydrocephalus did not appear.

Abnormal offspring of females receiving the weekly vitamin A supplement increased in frequency and severity in succeeding litters, reaching 100 per cent in the third litters of a small number of females.

Although only 5/24 (4.0%) young in first litters from females receiving weekly supplements of vitamin A showed slight symptoms of hydrocephalus, the cerebrospinal-fluid pressure of such offspring was significantly greater than that of first-litter young from females receiving daily supplements of vitamin A (204 ± 19 mm water vs. 97 ± 8 mm water, P < 0.001). A rise in the cerebrospinal-fluid pressure was thus demonstrated in apparently healthy animals and was therefore considered the initial symptom of the condition. No description of the hydrocephalus was given beyond the autopsy finding of "dilatation of the ventricles," nor was any mention made of other abnormalities.

Rokkones (1955) failed to record in any useful way the age of onset of the various external symptoms of the condition or to present a correlation of the age of onset with litter seriation. More serious, he apparently did not examine brains of nonhydrocephalic animals with elevated cerebrospinal-fluid pressure in order to see whether microsymptoms were present. To conclude, without such an examination, that elevated pressure was the initial symptom of the condition is unjustified.

Vitamin E Deficiency

Vitamin E has been a recognized antisterility factor for 40 years (Evans, Burr, and Althausen 1927). But its necessity for normal embryonic development was not established until fairly recently. Only a few studies were made before 1952 of the effects of vitamin E deficiency on prenatal morphogenesis (Kalter and Warkany 1959a), and only Shute (1936) reported an effect on the developing central nervous system of maternal lack of this vitamin. He found 2 hydrocephalic offspring from vitamin E-deficient female rats. In 1952, Thomas and Cheng reported the production of syndromes of congenital malformations in rats by the following procedure.

Sprague–Dawley female rats (Cheng and Thomas 1953) and, in later studies, Holtzman rats (Cheng, Chang, and Bairnson 1957) were placed on a vitamin E-depleting basal ration from about 3 weeks of age to maturity. They were then bred and continued on the deficient diet throughout pregnancy, either with no supplementation or with single orally-administered supplements of d,l-alpha-tocopherol acetate (vitamin E). In the first studies (Thomas and Cheng 1952; Cheng and Thomas 1953), a supplement of 1.2 mg vitamin E was given once on the 5th to 13th days of gestation. Later (Cheng, Chang, and Bairnson 1957; Cheng *et al.* 1960), supplements of 2 or 4 mg were also given and treatment was made only on the 11th day of gestation; but neither this increase nor the incorporation of the vitamin E antagonist, tri-o-cresyl phosphate, in the depleting ration significantly modified the results (Cheng, Chang, and Bairnson 1957).

The unsupplemented females, i.e., those with an unrelieved and severe deficiency of vitamin E, all resorbed their entire litters. Some of those that received the supplement on the 9th day of gestation or earlier maintained their pregnancies and produced live young, none of which was malformed. When the supplement was given on the 10th to 13th days offspring with various malformations were produced, with one or another defect predominating depending on the day of supplementation (Cheng and Thomas 1953). The defects included those of the central nervous system, with hydrocephalus commonest when vitamin E was given on the 10th day, and exencephaly commonest after therapy on the 12th day. The highest total incidence of abnormality occurred after addition of the vitamin on the 11th day (Cheng and Thomas 1953).

Females supplemented on the 10th day or later had a total of 121 near-term offspring. Hydrocephalus occurred in 11 and exencephaly in 2 of 60 young from 10th-day therapy; in 2 and 5, respectively, of 25 young from 11th-day therapy; and in 4 and 10, respectively, of 33 young from 12th-day therapy. Only 3 live young occurred after 13th-day therapy; one had hydrocephalus and another exencephaly. There thus were 36 (29.8 %) young with these defects of the central nervous system among the 121 survivors. In offspring collected (Cheng *et al.* 1960) at various fetal ages, after supplementation with 2 mg vitamin E on the 11th day, the incidence of such malformations was 15.6 per cent (35/224).

In a preliminary histological study of hydrocephalic specimens (Cheng and Thomas 1955), which, to my knowledge, has not been further amplified, it was stated that the thickness of the cerebral cortex was reduced and the lateral ventricles distended even in normal-appearing littermates of abnormal young, making it possible that the reported incidences of hydrocephalus, stated above, based on macroscopic examination, were underestimates. It was recently mentioned (Verma and King 1966) that abnormal fetuses contained defective choroid plexuses and that dilatation of lateral ventricles was accompanied by occlusion of the aqueduct.

An embryological study (Cheng, Chang, and Bairnson 1957) showed that exencephaly was recognizable on the 14th day of pregnancy. Hydrocephalus occurred infrequently, but it was not stated how early in development the abnormality could be detected. A later paper (Cheng et al. 1960) contained the information that hydrocephalus was noted in 16th-day fetuses.

Supplementation with d-gamma-tocopherol was not as effective in protecting embryos against the lethal and teratogenic effects of vitamin E deficiency as the d,l-alpha form (King 1964). The administration of progesterone, estrone, or both, appeared to reduce the incidence of vitamin deficiency-induced congenital malformations (Cheng 1959); however, since the hormones also increased the resorption rate, it may well be that the decreased frequency of surviving defective offspring resulted from their prenatal destruction.

Gortner and Ekwurtzel (1965) reported that in attempting to repeat the studies of Cheng and coworkers, discussed above, they were able to produce congenital malformations in only 3.7 per cent (11/297) of surviving offspring, and they thus questioned the validity of some of the original findings. They also pointed to apparent inconsistencies in some of these results; e.g., that in one study (Cheng 1956) a higher incidence of congenital malformations was found after 4 mg supplements of vitamin E than after 2 mg ones, while in another study (Cheng et al. 1960) the reverse occurred, when certain variations were introduced into the basal ration fed the pregnant rats.

These remarks indicated to me that Gortner and Ekwurtzel did not sufficiently understand the situation involved in vitamin E-deficiency teratogenesis and, further, that they expected the sort of rigid cause-effect relation in biology one has been told occurs in relatively simple physical phenomena.

As in many experimental teratologic studies, in order to produce congenital malformations by deficiency of vitamin E, a balance must be struck between a state severe enough to destroy all embryos and one so minimal as to harm no survivor. Furthermore, within this so-called teratogenic zone, the frequency of malformation varies in general with the severity of the state— whether negative or positive, according to the specific procedure. But, in vitamin E deficiency, as in, e.g., vitamin A (Wilson, Roth, and Warkany 1953), or pantothenic acid deficiency (see p. 33), the incidence may, paradoxically, be increased rather than decreased by administering small doses of vitamin, since a greater number of abnormal fetuses may thereby be enabled to survive—but only up to a point, since larger doses may prevent maldevelopment.

This may explain the low incidence of malformation found by Gortner and Ekwurtzel (1965), who used the relatively large vitamin E supplement of 10 mg, and the higher malformation rate produced by Cheng after 4 than after 2 mg.

In order to engender respect for the variability that is encountered in prenatal studies, it is worthwhile pointing out that an apparent inconsistency occurred in Gortner and Ekwurtzel's own study; which may (or may not) make one more tolerant of such occurrences in the studies of others. Their data revealed that after administration of 10 mg vitamin E by stomach tube on day 9, 10, or 11 of gestation (incidentally, they did not indicate how they timed pregnancy) the resorption rate was 84.1 per cent (487/579), while vitamin incorporation in the diet of 5, 10, or 20 mg/kg (and thus of its daily intake of about 0.075 to 0.3 mg) during the same period in pregnancy resulted in only 14.2 per cent (34/239) resorbed offspring. Thus the larger supplement (and presumably more complete dietary regime) was associated with a larger fetal death rate than a less satisfactory diet.

Niacin Deficiency

The teratogenic and other effects on prenatal development of niacin deficiency have been investigated in numerous laboratories (Murphy, Dagg, and Karnoisky 1957; Pike, Kirksey, and Callahan 1959; Pinsky and Fraser 1959, 1960; Chamberlain and Nelson 1963*a*, *b*; Goldstein, Pinsky, and Fraser 1963; Chamberlain 1964). Only in the studies of Chamberlain and Nelson, however, were defects of the central nervous system detected.

Administration to pregnant Long–Evans rats for different 3-day periods of the antimetabolite, 6-aminonicotinamide, by incorporation into the diet, resulted in relatively low incidences of exencephaly and hydrocephalus (Chamberlain and Nelson 1963*a*). Single injections of the antimetabolite during the last week of pregnancy resulted in hydrocephalus and associated abnormalities of the brain, with the highest incidence (64%) occurring after injection on the 14th day of pregnancy (Chamberlain and Nelson 1963*b*). The malformations consisted of dilatation of all ventricles, especially the lateral ones; expansion of the interventricular foramina and the cerebral aqueduct; and thinning of the cerebral cortex. The massa intermedia and corpus callosum were occasionally absent and often reduced in size. Although not mentioned in the text, a photograph of an abnormal brain (p. 295) also showed the cerebellum to be apparently absent and the choroid plexus of the 4th ventricle to be hypoplastic. In these respects and in the appearance of the cystic 4th ventricle, the condition greatly resembled that produced by galacto-flavin in mice (Kalter and Warkany 1957; Kalter 1963*b*).

The prenatal development of the condition was followed (Chamberlain 1964) in fetuses from the 15th to 22nd days of pregnancy following single injections of 6-aminonicotinamide on the 14th day. The earliest effect was reduction in the number of mitotic figures and vacuolization of neural epi-thelium. Progressive dilatation of all intracerebral lumina and passages was noted. Diminution of choroid plexuses also occurred.

It was claimed (Ingalls, Ingenito, and Curley 1963) that 6-aminonicotin-amide caused chromosomal aberrations in fetal mice, and it was intimated that the aberrations were causally related to the teratogenic effect of the antagonist.

Thiamine Deficiency

Very few studies have been made of the teratogenic effects of thiamine defi-ciency. Deficiency induced in rats by dietary deprivation resulted in some young with exencephaly in one laboratory (Pfaltz and Severinghaus 1956) and in normal young in another (Nelson and Evans 1955). Deficiency induced by the antimetabolite, oxythiamine, produced gross abnormalities, which were not named (Gottlieb, Frohman, and Havlena 1958), but another anti-metabolite, neopyrithiamine, may have caused no malformations (Kosterlitz 1960, p. 275).

Pyridoxine Deficiency

Exencephaly occurred occasionally in offspring of female rats fed a pyridoxine-deficient diet (Pfaltz and Severinghaus 1956), but no defects were found in studies with rats using the antagonist, desoxypyridoxine (Nelson and Evans 1948, 1951). Neither was another pyridoxine antagonist, hydroxymethypyri-midine, teratogenic, in mice of the ddN strain (Takekoshi 1965*a*). But when the latter substance was given in conjunction with the tuberculostatic agent, ethionamide, which by itself was also probably nonteratogenic, a significant incidence of malformation occurred, including about 10 per cent exencephaly.

Fasting

Depriving pregnant mice of all food for short periods during the middle third of gestation was found by several investigators to produce congenital mal-formations (Kalter 1954*b*; Runner 1954, 1959; Runner and Miller 1956; Runner and Dagg 1960; Smithberg 1961; Miller 1962*a, b*; Nishikawa 1963, 1964; Smithberg and Runner 1963). Even merely restricting the food intake of pregnant mice caused a small incidence of defects (Kalter 1960*a*). Abnor-mality of the central nervous system occurred only in some of these studies.

Runner (1954, 1959); Runner and Miller (1956); Runner and Dagg (1960); Smithberg (1961); Miller (1962*a, b*); and Smithberg and Runner (1963) found exencephaly after maternal starvation for 24 hours during various days of pregnancy. Starvation on the 9th day was apparently most effective

(Runner and Miller 1956), producing anomalies (rib, vertebra, and brain) in 28 per cent of offspring. The same spectrum of abnormalities, in lower frequencies, was also produced by starvation on other days of gestation. The incidence of malformations was reduced to the control level or greatly lowered by concomitant administration of carbohydrate, individual amino acids, or fat (Runner 1959).

Smithberg and Runner (1963) fasted prepubertal (induced to ovulate) and adult strain 129 mice for 24 hours on the 10th day of pregnancy. As was previously found (Runner and Miller 1956), starvation of pregnant adult mice on the 10th day produced only sporadic congenital defects; but the offspring of young (30–35 days old) mice had a relatively high total incidence (35%) of malformation, including 10 per cent exencephaly.

Rats appeared refractory to the induction of congenital malformations by maternal starvation (Brent 1963, p. 54), and severe food restriction (Takaori, Tanabe, and Shimamoto 1966), nor were hamsters harmed by starvation (Harvey 1963, p. 54).

Deficiency of Minerals

Maternal manganese deficiency has long been known to be associated in laboratory animals with congenital ataxia in offspring (see Hurley, Everson, and Geiger 1958, for references). The condition was prevented in rats by supplementation of the deficient maternal diet with manganese for 24 hours on the 15th day of pregnancy (Hurley and Everson 1963). No structural or histological defect of the nervous system was found (Hurley, Everson, and Geiger 1958), but retarded and anomalous ossification of the otic capsule (Hurley *et al.* 1960) and abnormalities of the otic labyrinth (Asling, Hurley, and Wooten 1960) may have been responsible for the ataxia. Low manganese levels were associated with slight leg deformities in calves. No neurological symptoms were mentioned (Dyer, Cassatt, and Rao 1964; Dyer and Rojas 1965).

Milk diets deficient in iron, manganese, or copper were tested in rats (O'Dell, Hardwick, and Reynolds 1961). A mild anemia was produced in pregnant females and offspring by an iron deficiency, but, as the authors commented, despite the presumed anemic anoxia thus produced, only a small number of young with possible malformations of the eye occurred. The manganese deficiency, which was not severe, caused some eye and bone defects. A few of the manganese-deficient young that were raised to weaning showed incoordination. The copper deficiency caused a high incidence of skeletal defects and many abdominal hernias.

A condition of sheep known as swayback or enzootic ataxia, which is widespread throughout the world, has been associated with copper deficiency. The clinical and pathological features of the disease and its etiology and pathogenesis, as well as its history and lore, were summarized by Innes and Saunders

(1962, pp. 577–90), whose admirable book should be consulted for references to the original observations. The condition consists of congenital demyelination with prenatal onset, probably in the last month of gestation, and a relatively rapid course. The pathological lesions are confined to the central nervous system. Grossly, the cerebral convolutions are flattened and poorly defined and the sulci are shallow. In coronal section the white matter is degenerated and largely replaced by a gelatinous network and extensive porencephalic-like cavitations. The cerebral gray matter is fairly well preserved but only as a thin shell around the degenerated white matter and cavities. The lateral ventricles are usually dilated and hydrocephalic, especially in more severe cases; the 3rd ventricle and aqueduct, only rarely so; and the 4th ventricle, never. All degrees of gradations of these features occur.

The role of copper deficiency in the etiology of the disease was reviewed by Barlow (1958). In Australia swayback occurred on pastures low in copper content and thus presented a straightforward relation to lack of the element, especially since it was prevented by administering copper supplements to pregnant ewes. But in some other parts of the world a more complex situation apparently exists. In England swayback occurred on pastures containing a fairly high level of copper and, in Iceland, in lambs whose mothers fed on seaweed with appreciable amounts of copper. Yet the copper content of liver and blood of affected lambs was far lower than in tissues of unaffected animals. It therefore appears that other factors are involved that may influence the availability or elimination of copper. Still, even in these areas, copper supplementation during pregnancy reduced the incidence of the disease (Pálsson and Grímsson 1953; Barlow 1958).

No effects on fetal development were noted in offspring of rats subjected to copper deficiency during pregnancy (Frick and Lampl 1953). A copper deficiency in guinea pigs resulted in brain abnormalities, including various degrees of agenesis of the cerebellar folia (Everson and Wang 1967). Various malformations were produced in rats by zinc deficiency. In a preliminary report (Hurley and Swenerton 1965) the defects were said to include spina bifida; but in a fuller account of the study (Hurley and Swenerton 1966), the only central nervous system defects mentioned were hydrocephalus and hydranencephaly, whose combined incidence was 65 per cent. The zinc content of term fetuses from deficient mother was lower than in control animals, suggesting that the fetal anomalies were direct effects of zinc deficiency on prenatal development.

Deficiency of Other Nutrients

Deficiency of numerous other nutrients has been inflicted on pregnant animals, including that of vitamins C, D, and K, fatty acids, choline, biotin, various amino acids, etc. (Kalter and Warkany 1959a). None of these efforts succeeded in producing congenital malformations of the central nervous system.

3

Hypervitaminosis A

The study of experimentally induced congenital malformations in mammals was greatly advanced by Cohlan's discovery (1953a, b) of the teratogenic action of large doses of vitamin A alcohol. The technique is simple and convenient, has been used by many investigators, and produces extensive embryonic damage.

Introduction

Several different procedures have been used. Cohlan (1953b) gave Wistar rats daily oral doses of 35,000 IU (international units) of an aqueous preparation of vitamin A from the 2nd, 3rd, or 4th to the 16th days of gestation. In most cases the pregnant animals were killed on the 20th or 21st day of gestation and the young were removed and examined. More or less the same procedure was also used, at first, by Giroud and Martinet (1954), who, however, administered the vitamin in oil. These authors later modified this schedule (Giroud and Martinet 1955a) and gave a larger daily dose (60,000 IU) for several different 3-consecutive-day periods during gestation. Various other teratogenic doses of the vitamin and times of administration were used with other species, such as rabbit, guinea pig, and mouse. These will be discussed below.

In attempting to duplicate Cohlan's results, Gebauer (1954) administered vitamin A intraperitoneally, not orally as Cohlan had done. He was unsuccessful in producing malformations and concluded that Cohlan's work could not be confirmed. Gebauer (1954) used 2 commercial brands of vitamin A but failed to state whether they were oily or aqueous preparations. In the light of subsequent investigations, it is most likely they were the former.

Woollam and Millen (1957), e.g., by contrasting the effects of subcutaneous and oral administration of excess vitamin A, conclusively demonstrated the nonteratogenicity of an oily preparation of vitamin A given parentally. Similar results were obtained by Mauer (1964a), who found intramuscular administration of an oily preparation of vitamin A to be ineffective, while aqueous vitamin A given by this route was teratogenic. More recently Millen and Woollam (1960) showed that when an oily preparation of vitamin A is saponified by suspension in Tween 80 it is teratogenic even when administered subcutaneously. Recently malformations were produced in rats and mice with fairly small doses of vitamin A (retinoic) acid (Monie and Khemmani 1967; Kalter, unpublished).

Malformations Produced in Rats

By his technique, Cohlan (1954) produced grossly observable abnormalities of the brain in 49 per cent (77/158) of offspring. Since all young were not cleared for inspection of the skeleton and none was sectioned for internal examination, it seems likely that this figure is an underestimate of the total incidence of malformed offspring. The most conspicuous and frequent malformation, which all 77 outwardly abnormal animals possessed, was a gross defect of the skull and brain, i.e., exencephaly. This condition consisted of protrusion of some or all of the forebrain through a defect in the parietal and frontal areas of the cranium. The bony defects were plainly seen in cleared specimens. The exposed brain mass lay like a cap or icebag on the top of the head and extended laterally, sometimes far enough to interfere with gross examination of the eyes.

This congenital malformation has been known by a large number of names, such as exencephaly, anencephaly, pseudencephaly, acrania, hemicephaly, cranium bifidum, extrakranielle Dysencephalie, cranioschisis, etc., which have all been used more or less synonymously by animal teratologists. However, one of these terms—anencephaly—though a misnomer, is often used in human pathology to designate the deteriorated condition of the exencephalic brain of late fetal or term children; and thus it may also be applied to the same state in animals.

Among the less deformed, viable offspring of a small number of treated mothers that were allowed to deliver their litters (Cohlan 1954), several had small hematoma-like discolorations in the region of the anterior fontanelle. These young were raised and examined again at 30 days of age, when they were found to have defects of various sizes in the continuity of the bony cranium. Therefore, in addition to the frank cranial and brain abnormality exencephaly, the treatment also produced defects of a lesser degree represented by the cranial lacunar opening.

By varying the dose of vitamin A and the duration of the treatment period, Cohlan (1954) was able to alter the incidence of grossly abnormal young and also to show that daily doses of 15,000 and 25,000 IU were nonteratogenic under his experimental conditions.

Intensive morphological and embryological analyses of the teratogenic effects of hypervitaminosis A were made by Giroud and his colleagues. Having confirmed Cohlan's discovery that large amounts of vitamin A given over an extended portion of the gestation period produced numerous and diverse congenital malformations (Giroud and Martinet 1954), they next demonstrated that treatment for shorter periods with a larger daily dose produced different defects or combinations of defects, depending on the period of treatment (Giroud and Martinet 1955a, 1956). Administration to pregnant Wistar rats of daily oral doses of 60,000 IU of vitamin A in oil for different 3-day periods produced the following: treatment on the 5th to 7th days, 9 per cent exencephaly, 4 per cent eye defects, such as microphthalmia and anophthalmia, and 4 per cent cleft palate; on the 8th to 10th days, 53 per cent exencephaly, 73 per cent eye defects, 3 per cent spina bifida, and 22 per cent cleft palate; on the 10th to 12th days, 5 per cent exencephaly, 30 per cent eye defects, 3 per cent spina bifida, and 71 per cent cleft palate; later treatment produced cleft palate, paw and digit defects, and cataract. Exencephaly was also produced in rats by Araki (1958), Inaba (1958), Cahen et al. (1964), Dumas (1964), Vichi et al. (1965b), and Langman and Welch (1966).

The exencephaly was described as follows (Giroud and Martinet 1956). The skin and vault of the cranium were missing. The rhombencephalon was generally intact, but the mesencephalon and diencephalon were very abnormal, their ventricles being open to the exterior and their walls continuous with the epidermis. Several areas of the brain were recognizable, but a large part of it was necrotic. At certain points there was an abundance of choroid plexus. Because the condition was not produced by treatment beginning later than the 10th day of gestation, it appeared that the exencephaly was not the outcome of some secondary effect, but resulted from arrest in closure of the anterior portion of the neural tube.

Cohlan (1954) first observed, and Giroud and Martinet (1955b) confirmed, that the exencephalic offspring were consistently associated with a large excess of amniotic fluid, which was frequently bloody. In young with lesser degrees of cranial or brain abnormalities (meningocele and encephalocele) the volume was not increased (Giroud and Martinet 1955b).

Minor brain and skull malformations, such as Cohlan (1954) noted, were also found by Giroud, Martinet, and Solère (1958). These defects, encephalocele and meningocele, occurred in the area of the midvertex of the head. Externally, encephalocele appeared as an oval projection of greater or lesser size in the region of union of the occipital and parietal bones. Histological sections showed a skin defect corresponding in extent to the size of the subjacent brain abnormality and that the latter consisted of herniation through the incompletely closed cranium. Meningocele was externally identical to the picture presented by encephalocele except in being smaller. Histologically, there was also great resemblance between the 2 types of malformation, but in meningocele nervous tissue was not herniated.

The minor defects had certain features in common with exencephaly, such as incomplete differentiation of epidermis and incomplete closure of the cranial vault. These similarities, combined with the fact that all 3 types of malformations occurred in the same litters, i.e., were produced simultaneously by treatment with hypervitaminosis A, indicated that the same embryonic processes were disturbed in all 3 and that they therefore represented different degrees of the same response to the teratogen (Giroud, Martinet, and Solère 1958). Such hypervitaminosis A-induced minor defects in rats were also described by McLaurin (1964).

Spina bifida aperta was produced in small to moderate incidences in rats (Cohlan 1954; Giroud and Martinet 1956; Inaba 1958; Baba and Tsuruhara 1959; Dumas 1964; Gonțea *et al.* 1964; Vichi *et al.* 1965*b*; Langman and Welch 1966). Its external features were described briefly by Giroud and Martinet (1956). The defect was always located in the lumbosacral area. The spinal canal was open and the 2 edges were continuous with the bordering epidermis. Apart from these aspects the structures usually seemed normal, except for some degeneration of nervous tissue.

Embryological Studies

The morphogenesis of hypervitaminosis A-induced exencephaly in rats was studied in detail by Giroud and Martinet (1957) and Giroud, Delmas, and Martinet (1959). Female Wistar rats were given 50,000 IU of the vitamin per day on the 8th, 9th, and 10th gestation days and killed on the 11th to 21st days of pregnancy. About 250 exencephalic offspring were collected at different stages of development and were sectioned and studied histologically. From observations on these specimens the following points were established.

In 12th-day embryos, i.e., at an age when the anterior part of the neural tube is normally already closed, the region of most of the telencephalon and all of the diencephalon and mesencephalon was still open, and the neural tissue persisted in continuity with the epidermis. The rhombencephalon closed more or less successfully, but its subsequent development was somewhat altered, apparently owing to disturbed cerebrospinal-fluid pressure (Rebollo 1958). Despite its failure to close, the brain (on the 13th–16th days) underwent fairly normal histogenesis and organogenesis. The hemispheres and their constituents—subcortical nuclei and olfactory bulbs—formed; the various layers—ependymal, mantle, and marginal—differentiated; the choroid plexuses developed; and the cortex appeared. The lateral hemispheres, however, were covered by the everted walls of the diencephalon and mesencephalon.

The fate of well-defined brain areas was indicated by the external location of choroid plexuses. Those normally of the lateral ventricles lay on the sides of the head near the orifice of each of the open hemispheres; that normally of the 3rd ventricle lay, continuous with skin, at the borders of each of the everted diencephalic sheets. Subsequently (on the 16th day), necrotic processes appeared, first in superficial parts of the brain and then in deeper parts, which soon led to the destruction of most of the fore- and midbrain, only some remnants and several nerves surviving. The resulting condition was called anencephaly, but it must be remembered that some of the forebrain and much of the hindbrain were still present even near term.

Many of the above-described pathogenetic phenomena were studied by means of reconstructions and described in great detail (Giroud, Delmas, and Martinet 1959). In addition the relations between nonclosure of the neural tube and abnormalities of epidermal differentiation and those of the osseous cranial vault were investigated (Giroud, Martinet, and Lefebvres-Boisselot 1960). The embryology of hypervitaminosis A-induced exencephaly in rats was also studied by other investigators (Baba and Araki 1959; Langman and Welch 1966), and, in general, the same pathogenetic events and sequences found.

Effects in Mice and Other Animals

These experiments were extended to mice (Giroud and Martinet 1959*a, b*; Kalter 1959*c*; Kalter and Warkany 1959*b*), in which hypervitaminosis A was also found (Giroud and Martinet 1959*c*; Kalter and Warkany 1959*b*; Mauer 1964*a*; Knudsen 1965; Murakami and Kameyama 1965) to produce exencephaly (fig. 5) as well as other congenital malformations, the frequency and type of which depended on the stage of gestation when the teratogen was administered (Giroud and Martinet 1960*a*; Kalter 1960*b, c*; Kalter and Warkany 1961). One of the many anomalies found in mice that were apparently not noted in rats is craniopharyngeal duct. This anomaly consisted of a narrow passage from the rear part of the nasopharyngeal canal through the center of the presphenoid, which ended at the base or in the parenchyma of the anterior lobe of the pituitary (Kalter and Warkany 1961). Another defect noticed was decreased size or obliteration of the periencephalic cisternas. In these cases the brain itself was morphologically normal except for a narrow or closed Sylvian aqueduct (Kalter 1963*c*).

The morphogenesis of the induced exencephaly in mice was analyzed (Giroud and Martinet 1960*b*), and also compared with the defect as it occurs in human beings. Swiss-Webster female mice, given daily oral administrations of 3000 IU vitamin A on the 8th to 10th days of gestation (Giroud and Martinet 1959*c*), had young 59 per cent of which were exencephalic. Contrary to the finding in rats (Giroud and Martinet 1956), the eyes in the mice were always well formed (Giroud and Martinet 1959*c*; Kalter and Warkany 1961). In general, the development of exencephaly in mice paralleled that in rats, with the anterior end of the neural tube remaining open, morphogenesis and differentiation of the brain nevertheless continuing, and necrotic processes destroying many structures secondarily (Giroud and Martinet 1960*b*). Despite the relatively short fetal period in mice, the exencephalic brain of near-term animals (fig. 5) had obviously degenerated, as was also true of rats, in comparison to its size and configuration in fetuses only a few days younger (fig. 6) (Kalter, unpublished observations).

The schedule used by Kalter and Warkany (1961), with inbred mice of 3 different strains, consisted of single oral administrations of 10,000 IU vitamin A during the middle third of pregnancy. Despite the extreme teratogenicity of this schedule (congenital malformations were produced in 98.5 per cent of the 196 offspring of females treated on the 9th or 10th day of pregnancy), exencephaly occurred in only 5/99 young from females treated on the 9th day, and in none from females treated 24 hours later. Although spina bifida aperta did not occur very often either (10 cases, 2 of which were also exencephalic, see fig. 7), 3 instances of spina bifida occulta were found in serial sections of 5 offspring with no outwardly overt defect of the spine. It is possible, therefore, that spina bifida occulta occurred fairly often. The structure of the spina bifida aperta was not unusual (figs. 8, 9), but the spina bifida occulta presented some novel features (figs. 10, 11). Murakami and Kameyama (1965) also produced very few instances of exencephaly and spina bifida aperta in mice. In Knudsen's (1965) study, in which treatment was made on the 7th, 8th, and 9th days of pregnancy, exencephaly was the most frequent malformation produced, but its incidence was not stated.

A syndrome of congenital malformations of the brain consisting of abnormalities of the prosencephalon, found in offspring of vitamin A-treated mice (Giroud, Delmas, and Martinet 1963; Giroud, Martinet, and Deluchat 1965), was termed cyclocephaly, thus indicating that it was considered to be a form of cyclopia. The telencephalon was not divided into hemispheres, the interhemispheric fissure being absent, and it contained one large ventricle, which communicated with the 3rd ventricle by a median foramen of Monro. The rhinencephalon was absent, and, though olfactory nerves were present, they did not reach the brain. The pituitary was absent and there was medial fusion of the eyes.

These abnormalities were produced by treatment with 500 IU vitamin A daily from the 8th to 10th days of pregnancy. Similar malformations were produced in inbred mice in my laboratory (unpublished observations) after single oral administrations of 5000 IU early on the 8th day of pregnancy. Univentricular telencephalon and associated malformations were also induced in mice by X irradiation (Murakami *et al.* 1961; Murakami, Kameyama, and Nogami 1963; Giroud *et al.* 1966; Degenhardt, cited by Lund 1966), in rats by pantothenic acid deficiency (Giroud *et al.* 1957) and vinblastine (DeMyer 1965a), and in sheep by the plant *Veratrum californicum* (Binns *et al.* 1959).

In another study, Giroud and Martinet (1962) produced malformations with smaller doses than had previously been used. Mice (of unstated type) were given 100, 250, or 500 IU vitamin A daily from the 8th to 10th days of pregnancy. The smallest dose was not teratogenic even when given for 5 instead of 3 days. But the larger doses produced various defects, among which was exencephaly (19% after 250 IU and 10% after 500 IU).

Rabbits, guinea pigs, and dogs have been used only in limited hypervitaminosis A studies. Exencephaly was produced in rabbits (Giroud and Martinet 1958), but no congenital malformations of the central nervous system occurred in guinea pigs (Giroud and Martinet 1959a) or dogs (Wiersig and Swenson 1967).

A wide spectrum of malformations was induced in golden hamsters (Marin-Padilla and Ferm 1965). Females were given single oral doses of 20,000 USP units of vitamin A on the 5th to 11th days of pregnancy. No defects were produced by treatment on the 5th or 11th day and very few by treatment on the 6th. Congenital malformations of the central nervous system occurred after treatment on the 7th or 8th day, predominantly the latter, after which exencephaly was found in 14/89 (15.7%) and spina bifida in 11/89 (12.3%). The latter defect was usually of the occult type, few fetuses showing an open neural plate.

The authors also killed a group of females at different intervals after treatment on the 8th day of pregnancy and examined the embryos microscopically. The first signs of damage were found in specimens obtained 12 hours after treatment, and reached their maximum 24 hours after treatment. The signs consisted of cellular necrosis in somites, restricted at first to those of the cephalic end of the embryos but later apparently more extensive and observed in all specimens. Embryonic tissues surrounding necrotic areas were unaffected. The necrosis was believed to be a basic and primary effect of the teratogen, from which various other anomalies (exencephaly, spina bifida occulta, and rib defects) stemmed. However, if massive necrosis occurred in all embryos, it is difficult to understand why all offspring treated on the 8th day of gestation in the first part of the study were not affected with abnormalities resulting from damage to somites. The most frequent of these defects (of the ribs) was seen in only 37 per cent of offspring. Using the same techniques, Marin-Padilla (1966) later noted other alterations as soon as 6 hours after treatment, which reached their maximum 4 hours later. Present only in mesodermal tissue, at first in cephalic regions, later spreading to other sites, the changes consisted of shrinkage of cytoplasm, enlargement of intercellular spaces through fluid accumulation, and reduction of mitotic rate. These changes thus preceded cellular necrosis, noted in the earlier study, which was hence relegated to a secondary role.

The Mechanism of Action of Excess Vitamin A

Numerous studies have been made investigating the teratogenic action of hypervitaminosis A combined with other substances or procedures, for the purpose of clarifying the mechanism of the vitamin in producing embryonic damage. Female Wistar rats given (Millen and Woollam 1957) 60,000 I U vitamin A daily from the 8th to 13th days of gestation had offspring, examined near term, 7.8 per cent (6/77) of which were exencephalic. Concurrent subcutaneous daily administration of 20 mg cortisone acetate from the 9th to 12th days apparently increased the incidence of this malformation to 36.6 per cent (15/41). Thus, although cortisone alone was found to be nonteratogenic (Millen and Woollam 1957; Woollam and Millen 1957), a fact often noted in rats (Kalter and Warkany 1959*a*), when given concurrently it seemed to potentiate the effect of the vitamin. Potentiation also occurred when incidence of cleft palate was taken as the index of teratogenicity (Woollam and Millen 1957).

The intensifying effect of cortisone on the production of exencephaly by hypervitaminosis A was next shown (Millen and Woollam 1958*b*) to be negated by simultaneous subcutaneous injection of protamine zinc insulin (1.5 units daily from the 9th–12th days of pregnancy); insulin also abolished the teratogenic effect of the vitamin alone. The influence of the thyroid on hypervitaminosis A teratogenesis was indicated by the potentiating effect of the antithyroid agent 4-methyl-2-thiouracil (Woollam and Millen 1958*a*; Takekoshi 1964), and by the protective effect of thyroxin (Woollam and Millen 1960). Finally, vitamin B complex reduced the teratogenic effects of large doses of vitamin A (Millen and Woollam 1958*c*). From their results Woollam and Millen (1960) concluded that "vitamin A exerts its teratogenic powers by interfering in some way at some level in the carbohydrate metabolism of the mother, placenta, or foetus."

The significance and validity of much of Woollam and Millen's work was clouded by the negative findings of others. Cohlan and Stone (1961), in experiments employing large numbers of Wistar rats, were unable to confirm some of the above-discussed results. A daily dose of 25,000 I U aqueous vitamin A or 60,000 I U vitamin A in oil was given from the 8th to the 13th days of gestation. Both vitamin A preparations produced quite consistent frequencies of exencephaly in offspring from 6 different groups of females (334/919, for an average of 36.3 % with a range of 34–39 %).

Vitamin A treatment was combined with administration of cortisone, insulin, cortisone and insulin, or growth hormone, and with maternal adrenalectomy, thymectomy, or parathyroidectomy. Without exception, these combined treatments failed to result in incidences of exencephaly significantly different from those produced by excess vitamin A alone (Cohlan and Stone 1961). Giroud (1960) noted that vitamin C, pantothenic acid, or a vitamin B mixture had no countereffect on the teratogenic action of vitamin A; and Kochhar (1965) found that treatment of rats with cortisone did not modify the incidence of cleft palate induced by hypervitaminosis A.

Several other experiments of this sort have been made. Härtel and Härtel (1960) investigated the effect of combined vitamin A and "stress." Holtzman rats were given 15,000 IU vitamin A daily from the 8th to 12th days of pregnancy or were immobilized or subjected to audiovisual stimuli for several hours daily from the 9th to 12th days of pregnancy. Different pregnant rats received the vitamin plus one or the other of the "stresses." Those only stressed had no abnormal offspring. Females receiving vitamin alone had 7.3 per cent (13/178) deformed young; 11 of them (6.2%) had deformities of the brain and calvaria, i.e., presumably, exencephaly. Treatment with vitamin plus audiovisual stimuli produced approximately the same incidence of abnormal offspring as vitamin alone; but vitamin A plus immobilization appeared to result in a higher total incidence (18/49 = 36.7%) of defect; however, only one exencephaly occurred. The authors (Härtel and Härtel 1960) concluded that while audiovisual stimulation did not potentiate the effects of vitamin A, possibly because it was not a severe enough stress, immobilization did do so, and they postulated that this synergism may have been mediated through the maternal pituitary-adrenal axis, an effect to be expected as "a result of emotional stress."

While it is almost hopeless to vanquish this oft-used argument, several contradictory lines of evidence may briefly be cited. Large doses of cortisone and hydrocortisone (Kalter and Warkany 1959*a*), and even of a much more potent glucocorticosteroid (Kalter 1962), have been time and time again found to be without teratogenic effect in rats; and an "emotional stress" had no effect on the embryonic development of mice (Warkany and Kalter 1962).

Most recently, it was suggested (Ferm 1967) that the potentiation of the teratogenic effects of hypervitaminosis A by protracted exposure to cold in hamsters may be due to hypersecretion of adrenal hormones resulting from the cold stress.

A study was made by Ishii, Kamei, and Omae (1962) of the combined effect of vitamin A and chondroitin sulfate in mice, but these substances together did not have a statistically significantly greater effect than the vitamin alone. In a paper in Japanese with an inadequate English summary, Amano *et al.* (1963) reported the synergism of concurrent administration of vitamin A, cortisone, and trypan blue. Takekoshi (1964) found trypan blue to intensify the effects of vitamin A, but the results were not convincing. However, in a more extensive study, Wilson (1964) also found a potentiating effect of trypan blue on hypervitaminosis A. Finally, Takekoshi (1965*b*) reported that pregnant mice treated with urethan and vitamin A had higher incidences of deformed offspring than those given either agent alone.

An interesting finding is that the teratogenic effect of vitamin A was influenced by the uterine position of the fetus, those situated at the ovarian end of the horn having cleft palate less frequently than those at the vaginal end (Woollam and Millen 1961). A second discovery (Woollam and Millen 1961), that the incidence of cleft palate increased as the number of young in the uterine horn increased, was also found true of cortisone-induced cleft palate (Kalter 1965*a*).

So far as the mechanism of the teratogenic action of hypervitaminosis A is concerned, little of certainty has been established, despite these studies. The vitamin has been presumed to have a direct effect on the embryo because elevated quantities of it were found in fetal livers after large amounts were given to pregnant females (Giroud, Gounelle, and Martinet 1957). Woollam and Millen (1960) believed their results indicated that vitamin A acts by interfering with carbohydrate metabolism. Härtel and Härtel (1960) invoked oversecretion of maternal corticoids induced by emotional stress. Takekoshi (1964), based on his finding that methylthiouracil intensified the action of vitamin A, postulated that hypervitaminosis A teratogenesis depends, in part at least, on the vitamin causing a fall in the maternal blood concentration of thyroid hormone.

It is obvious that much remains to be learned.

4

Trypan Blue

Introduction

In 1948 Gillman, Gilbert, Gillman, and Spence reported that injection of pregnant rats with trypan blue produced a spectrum of congenital malformations in the offspring, including defects of the brain, spinal cord, eye, ear, tail, skeleton, and anus. Subsequently, abnormalities of the cardiovascular and urogenital systems were also found (Wilson 1954a; Fox and Goss 1956; Goldstein 1957; Richman, Thomas, and Konikov 1957; Christie 1961; Wegener 1961; Smith 1963a; Monie, Takacs, and Warkany 1966).

Gillman *et al.* (1948) gave a large number of stock colony female rats, housed together continuously with males, subcutaneous injections of 1 ml of 1 per cent aqueous Grübler's trypan blue once every 2 weeks before conception and during pregnancy. When injected, therefore, some females were not yet pregnant and others were already pregnant for various unknown amounts of time. The females were allowed to deliver their young and raise them to weaning, and were then rebred. The times at which the females were treated during pregnancy were calculated by counting back from 22 days, which was estimated to be the duration of pregnancy in them. In later series of studies, injections were made only before or after conception, but still at 2-week intervals (Gillman *et al.* 1948, 1951). The modification of these procedures devised by Wilson (1954a, b) will be described below.

Malformations Produced

Hydrocephalus

Gillman *et al.* (1948, 1951) obtained 267 litters containing 1347 offspring from females treated before conception as well as during pregnancy. Four hundred and thirty-seven (32.4%) young displayed gross abnormalities at birth, the commonest of which, found in 236 (17.5%), was hydrocephalus (Gillman *et al.* 1951).

In the majority, hydrocephalus could be detected at birth (Gillman *et al.* 1948) and was characterized externally by a domeshaped head, widened suture lines, and transparency of the skull. In some instances of suspected hydrocephalus transillumination was used to aid the diagnosis. In offspring not otherwise diagnosable at birth the defect sometimes became clearly recognizable during the first week of life and in others only several weeks after weaning. No data were given by the authors as to the percentage in which the condition was detectable only later than at birth and the ages at which detection became possible.

They did state that at autopsy of 55 apparently normal rats, 10 exhibited mild symptoms of hydrocephalus such as moderately dilated ventricles and widely separated skull sutures. In fact, it would appear that postmortem examination of outwardly normal animals sometimes revealed very dilated ventricles and a much thinned cerebral cortex. The total incidence of hydrocephalus was therefore probably quite a bit higher than that stated (fig. 12).

In older hydrocephalic animals the eyes were usually deeply sunken, the snout was short and upturned, and the cranium bulged. Nevertheless they were able to move and feed, but their growth lagged. In severe cases, toward the end of the course of which they became blind, the animals did not live beyond 30 days of age; milder cases survived to over 100 days. The fertility of survivors was apparently not impaired. Both hydrocephalic males and females were able to reproduce and their offspring showed no abnormalities at birth, but the mortality rate was high (Gillman *et al.* 1951).

Gross dissection of hydrocephalic rats showed enormous distention of the lateral ventricles, which reduced the cortex to a thin membrane not more than 1 mm in thickness lining the interior of the skull. Serial sections of brains revealed a completely communicating ventricular system, suggesting the involvement of a disturbance in the relation between secretion and absorption of cerebrospinal fluid.

Of the 236 hydrocephalic offspring, the condition occurred alone in 159 (67.4%), and was combined in 38 cases (16.1%) with eye defect, in 8 (3.4%) with ear defect, in 16 (6.8%) with eye and ear defect, and in the remainder with one or more other defects. In only 2 cases was hydrocephalus combined with spina bifida.

Females given trypan blue only before conception bore 376 young of which one had hydrocephalus; but since a low incidence of hydrocephalus also occurred in control animals (5/5886 = 0.08%), this one case was probably of no significance. A relatively small number of animals were injected during pregnancy only. Their offspring had hydrocephalus if treated before the 9th day of pregnancy, but the condition was produced by treatment on almost every day between conception and that time. Females given the dye both before conception and during pregnancy had hydrocephalic offspring after treatment on every day of pregnancy, but the incidence was highest when made on the 5th or 6th day of gestation.

The explanation for the teratogenicity of trypan blue administered before implantation is probably that dye sufficient to affect embryonic development remains in the maternal body for days after its injection. It was indeed noted by Gillman *et al.* (1948) that dye was macroscopically visible for weeks after injection. Support for this explanation comes from the fact (Gillman *et al.* 1951) that the frequency of hydrocephalus induced by administration of trypan blue before implantation was higher if females had in addition received trypan blue before conception than if not (49/323 = 15.2% vs. 12/145 = 8.3%). This topic is discussed further below (see p. 87).

Soon after the initial report by Gillman *et al.* (1948), Hogan, O'Dell, and Whitley (1950), Lyngdoh (1950), and Stefanelli and Grignolo (1950) confirmed that trypan blue is teratogenic; Hogan, O'Dell, and Whitley (1950) produced an unstated incidence of hydrocephalus in stock colony rats, and Lyngdoh (1950), hydrocephalus in 4/268 offspring from treated Long–Evans rats, a far smaller incidence than found by Gillman *et al.* (1948, 1951). Lyngdoh's (1950) report, furthermore, was the first of many that described sharp quantitative and qualitative variability in the pathological effects of trypan blue on embryonic development. These aspects are discussed elsewhere (see pp. 72–78).

Other trypan blue studies in which hydrocephalus was produced were those of Wilson (1954*a*, *b*, 1955), Gunberg (1955), Gepts, Carpent, and Toussaint (1957), Kreshover, Knighton, and Hancock (1957), Richman, Thomas, and Konikov (1957), Warkany, Wilson, and Geiger (1958), Wilson, Beaudoin, and Free (1959), Vaupel, Nelson, and Roux (1961), Vickers (1961*a*), Beaudoin and Kahkonen (1963), Stempak (1964), and Kelly *et al.* (1964), in rats; Ferm (1956) and Langman and Drunen (1959), in rabbits; Kreshover, Knighton, and Hancock (1957) and Beck (1964*b*), in mice; Ferm (1958), in hamsters; and Hoar and Salem (1961), in guinea pigs.

On the other hand, hydrocephalus was apparently not produced by Fox and Goss (1956), Carpent (1958), Tuchmann-Duplessis and Mercier-Parot (1959*a*), Wegener (1961), and Cahen *et al.* (1964), in rats; Harm (1954), in rabbits; Hamburgh (1952, 1954), Waddington and Carter (1952, 1953), Murakami (1953), Barber (1957), and Kobozieff *et al.* (1959), in mice; and Conn and Hardy (1959), in dogs.

Wilson (1954*a*, *b*) introduced a modified procedure for studying the teratogenic effects of trypan blue. He administered the dye (1 ml of a 1% aqueous solution, subcutaneously) on each of 3 successive days of pregnancy (8th, 9th, and 10th days) and killed the females (Wistar stock) on the 21st day of pregnancy. Therefore, all defects noted were "congenital." Forty-five animals treated in this way had 228 offspring, 26.3 per cent of which had hydrocephalus, the most frequent and specific malformation found (Wilson 1954*a*, *b*, 1955).

The hydrocephalus was not always readily recognizable on external examination but was clearly visible in all degrees upon sectioning by razor blade. Dilation was confined to ventricles anterior to the cerebral aqueduct (Wilson 1954*a*, *b*). In the few hydrocephalic animals examined histologically, the mesencephalic aqueduct was either obliterated or reduced in calibre. The cause of the reduction was not apparent; no evidence of undue proliferation in the vicinity of the aqueduct was found. The ependymal lining was retained, although it was sometimes little more than a cord of atrophic epithelial cells (Wilson 1955). Apparently no other part of the brain was affected in hydrocephalic offspring.

Vickers (1961*a*) also made a morphological study of trypan blue-induced hydrocephalus. Using Wilson's (1954*a*) procedure, Sprague–Dawley rats were given a total of 24 to 30 mg of dye in 3 equal doses. Hydrocephalus was found in 7/123 offspring, but in only one was the condition externally diagnosable. In 3, the anterior portion of the aqueduct was obliterated at its junction with the 3rd ventricle; and the occlusion was due to narrowing of the lumen and to its being completely filled with ependymal cells. This observation is in apparent contradiction to the finding of Wilson (1955), who, though also finding obliteration, reported no excessive ependymal proliferation. In another offspring (Vickers 1961*a*) the lumen was patent but was greatly narrowed. In addition, the ependyma of the constricted segment was partly ragged and the subependymal areas appeared edematous. The author suggested that in this animal fixation shrinkage may have occurred and hence that during life the aqueductal constriction was significantly greater than when seen in sections. In these 4 specimens, as in the 3 discussed below, the ventricular enlargement was anterior to the aqueduct and was thus the result, seemingly, of the obliteration or narrowing of the Sylvian aqueduct.

In the other 3 hydrocephalics the condition was designated as mild to moderate and principally affected the lateral ventricles. In addition, the size of the aqueduct was normal. In 2 the size of the 4th ventricle was considered normal, but there was slight but definite enlargement of a short segment of central canal in the upper spinal cord. In the third the 4th ventricle was reduced in size, with an appearance of compression of the cavity, but the central canal was normal. Since the hydrocephalus in these 3 could not have been due to aqueductal constriction, it was believed to have resulted from associated factors, such as appear in the Arnold–Chiari malformation in man, especially since 2 of the animals had spinal dysraphic lesions and the third a cranial meningocele (Vickers 1961*a*).

Occlusion or stenosis of the aqueduct was also found in rats by Stempak (1964), who reported that the former could be seen as early as the 18th day of gestation, and the latter as early as the 17th day, but that hydrocephalus was not present for certain until the 19th day. The ventricular enlargement in hydrocephalic offspring was apparently restricted to the lateral ventricles.

Among 376 newborn offspring of Wistar females treated with certain samples of trypan blue, using Wilson's (1954a) schedule, Stempak (1964) found 35 (9.3%) with hydrocephalus. Thirty-three were sectioned and 24 found to have completely occluded or extremely stenotic aqueduct. Seven of the other 9 had lesser degrees of stenosis, one a possible forked aqueduct, and only one a patent aqueduct. Of 58 fetuses recovered on the 20th day, 9 (15.5%) were hydrocephalic; in 5 the aqueduct was occluded and in 4 it was extremely stenotic. Four of 36 fetuses obtained on the 19th day were possibly hydrocephalic. Thirty were sectioned; 3 considered hydrocephalic upon gross examination had occluded aqueduct, another also believed hydrocephalic had a stenosed aqueduct, and 21 of the remaining 26 may have had slight stenosis.

Therefore, because of the fairly good relation between reduction or obliteration of the aqueduct and hydrocephalus, Stempak (1964) believed that the aqueductal defects were the primary ones, and he hypothesized that stenosis, if severe enough, is transformed into occlusion by normal growth processes, since the diameter of the aqueduct normally becomes reduced during late fetal life. He did not discuss what may have caused the stenosis, except for the vague suggestion that the distended cerebral hemispheres may have been a factor, working through mesencephalic compression. In photographs of abnormal aqueducts there was no sign of ependymal proliferation. In a publication dealing with hydrocephalus induced by folic acid deficiency, Stempak (1965) proposed that stenosis may have been caused by growth inhibition due to reduction of the mitotic rate, and that this explanation may also apply to the trypan blue-induced defect.

Spina Bifida

Spina bifida was the second most frequent defect produced in the trypan blue studies of Gillman *et al.* (1948, 1951). It occurred in 76 offspring, or 5.6 per cent of the total born to females treated both before conception and during pregnancy. In 34 cases (44.7%) it was unassociated with any other defect, and in 42 cases (55.3%) was combined with one or more other defects, most commonly with tail defect (39/76 = 51.3%). In only 4 animals was spina bifida accompanied by another defect of the central nervous system, twice with hydrocephalus and twice with meningocele (Gillman *et al.* 1951).

In most of the defective offspring the malformation occurred in the lumbar region or at the lumbosacral junction. Externally, the affected area, composed in some cases of spinal cord completely exposed through a dermal defect, was in a few instances covered by vascular tissue while in others only a red-brown scab (area medullovasculosa) remained where an opening had previously existed. In still others the skin over the affected area was thinned and depressed (fig. 13).

In sectioned material the transformation of the spinal cord from normality above and below the area of the lesion to abnormality of the cord and its supporting and accessory structures in the region of the bifida could be followed in great detail (Gillman *et al.* 1948). The following is a description of a severe case. The spinal cord adjacent to the normal regions was reduced in size, elongated dorsoventrally, and elevated from the vertebral canal, so that its dorsal half lay exposed while the ventral half remained flanked by vertebral laminae. The elevation of the cord increased toward the patent region until the spinal cord was completely dislodged from the vertebral canal. The skin, which for a space formed the immediate dorsal boundary of the cord, was disrupted and the cord then lay exposed on the surface contiguous with the skin. Toward the center of the lesion the spinal cord became still smaller, the central canal more disorganized, and the lumen extremely narrow. In addition, the lesion became increasingly vascularized, dilated vessels gradually replacing neural tissue until the cord completely disappeared. So far as structures surrounding the cord are concerned, the posterior root ganglia migrated ventrally from their normally paired ventrolateral location to form a single, midline, continuous chain between cord and laminae; vertebrae were malformed and in the area of the lesion the laminae and other elements were missing and the bodies fused.

Different degrees of severity of spina bifida were noted. In cases with complete destruction of the cord, the condition was associated with unilateral or bilateral paralysis and interference with efficiency of sphincters (Gillman *et al.* 1948, 1951).

Spina bifida was also produced with trypan blue in rats by Lyngdoh (1950), Wilson (1954*a, b*, 1955), Gunberg (1954, 1955, 1956), Fox and Goss— "a questionable spina bifida"—(1956), Gepts, Carpent, and Toussaint (1957), Kreshover, Knighton, and Hancock (1957), Warkany, Wilson, and Geiger (1958), Tuchmann-Duplessis and Mercier-Parot (1959*a*), Wilson, Beaudoin, and Free (1959), Vaupel, Nelson, and Roux (1961), Vickers (1961*b*), Baba and Goda (1961), Carpent (1962), Beaudoin and Kahkonen (1963), Beck and Lloyd (1963*a, b*), Cahen *et al.* (1964), Gordon (1964), Kelly *et al.* (1964), Jelen *et al.* (1964), Stempak (1964), and Lorke (1965); in mice by Murakami, Kameyama, and Kato (1954), Kreshover, Knighton, and Hancock (1957), and Barber and Geer (1964); in guinea pigs by Hoar and Salem (1961); and in hamsters by Ferm (1965*a*).

Spina bifida was apparently not seen by Hogan, O'Dell, and Whitley (1950), Richman, Thomas, and Konikov (1957), and Wegener (1961), in rats; Hamburgh (1952, 1954), Waddington and Carter (1952, 1953), Murakami (1953), Barber (1957), and Kobozieff *et al.* (1959), in mice; Harm (1954), Ferm (1956), and Langman and Drunen (1959), in rabbits; and Conn and Hardy (1959), in dogs.

A detailed morphological study of trypan blue-induced spina bifida in rats was made by Gunberg (1956). Using a technique resembling that of Gillman *et al.* (1948), i.e., injecting trypan blue before conception and during pregnancy, Gunberg found in sectioned and dissected material from Long–Evans rats, 44/268 (16.4%) young with spina bifida, which were classified as having spina bifida occulta or spina bifida aperta. In spina bifida occulta there was no external sign of the condition, and internally it was characterized by failure of vertebral laminar fusion extending for a distance of 1 to 3 vertebrae in the sacral region. In addition there were minor malformations of the cord, cauda equina, and meninges, but the dorsal root ganglia were normal.

The offspring classified as having spina bifida aperta were those with an external defect consisting of a lesion or a dimple on the dorsal surface of the lumbosacral region. This defect was subdivided into 5 morphological groups, primarily on the basis of extent of the vertebral malformation. In the first 2 groups, in addition to failure of midline laminar fusion, there was abrupt termination of the spinal cord at or near the level of the laminar defect, with no eruption of the cord to the dorsal surface (group 1) or with a short (about 3 to 5 vertebrae long) exteriorized segment of cord caudal to the laminar defect (group 2). In the remaining 3 groups the cord was present cephalic and caudal to the bifid region, which was more extensive (8–10 vertebrae long) than in group 2. Microscopic examination of the cord in the bifid region showed it to be dysraphic, myeloschitic, and pseudoduplicated, and its edges to be continuous with the adjacent epidermis. Abnormalities of dorsal root ganglia were often found. A discussion of the Arnold–Chiari type of malformation also produced in these rats (Gunberg 1956) is presented below (see p. 70).

With regard to Gunberg's (1956) subdivision of spina bifida, Warkany, Wilson, and Geiger (1958) questioned whether some of his categories are to be properly considered as consisting primarily of spina bifida, since they included a more serious defect, such as agenesis of many vertebrae. Warkany, Wilson, and Geiger (1958), in their article on the anatomy and morphogenesis of spina bifida in offspring of trypan blue-treated rats, regarded as true cases of myeloschisis only those instances of midline abnormality possessing a skin defect, an enlarged subarachnoid space, and an open spinal cord. The purpose of their investigation was to obtain information that might resolve the controversy as to the nature and development of the lesion known in children as myelomeningocele.

Perhaps this is an appropriate place to discuss the nomenclature and definition of spina bifida and its variations. Cameron (1956) in a study of human spina bifida recognized 4 main subdivisions of the defect, which he named and described somewhat as follows: (1) Spina bifida occulta. There is a localized gap in one or more vertebral arches, but the spinal cord and meninges remain entirely within the vertebral canal. The cord, however, may exhibit a malformation (myelodysplasia), such as duplication (diastematomyelia) or dilatation of the central canal (hydromyelia). The overlying skin may be normal or the underlying defect may be revealed by a dimple or a pigmented hairy spot. (2) Meningocele. The dura and arachnoid maters protrude through a defect in the vertebral arches, forming a cystic swelling, but as in the occult condition the cord and nerves remain in the vertebral canal. The cord may exhibit some form of myelodysplasia. (3) Myelomeningocele. There is a cystic swelling and the spinal cord and nerves are raised from the vertebral canal and are closely apposed to the wall of the swelling or sac at its apex. (4) Myelocele (better named myeloschisis). The spinal cord takes the form of an open neural plate exposed to the external surface. Cameron (1956) grouped the last 3 types as spina bifida cystica, since they are characterized by a cystic swelling. This scheme is very much like that outlined by Patten (1953).

Warkany, Wilson, and Geiger (1958) would use "spina bifida" as the comprehensive term for any midline defect of the osseous elements enclosing the spinal cord; which therefore includes spina bifida anterior, a defect in the anterior wall of the vertebral column, as well as spina bifida posterior, the far more common abnormality, in which bilateral components of the neural arches remain separated. Spina bifida posterior they divided, more or less conforming to Cameron's (1956) scheme, into spina bifida occulta, meningocele, myelocystocele (cystic enlargement of the central canal), myelo-meningocele, and myeloschisis.

The spina bifidous condition that is seen most frequently in children and whose anatomy and prenatal development have been most puzzling and most debated is the defect known as myelomeningocele or meningomyelocele. According to one school of thought (see references in Warkany, Wilson, and Geiger 1958), in myelomeningocele the spinal cord is closed and is usually found flattened in the posterior wall of the sac with its central canal demonstrable in the neural tissue incorporated into the sac. Opposed to this concept is the belief of other observers (see references in Warkany, Wilson, and Geiger 1958) that myelomeningocele is merely a modified myeloschisis, i.e., a malformation in which the embryonic neural plate remains partly open and remnants of which are incorporated in the sac; therefore no central canal exists in the protruding sac. The latter concept was upheld by Cameron (1956) in his study of spina bifida cystica in children, and more conclusively demonstrated to be true by Warkany, Wilson, and Geiger (1958) in their experiment.

These authors used Wilson's (1954a) schedule of trypan blue administration with a commercially obtained stock of rats. Embryos and fetuses of various ages were examined in serial section. Externally recognizable spinal defects were observed in 76/1850 (4.1%) offspring. Twenty-five abnormal specimens, varying in age from the 12th to 22nd days of gestation, were studied microscopically.

The youngest specimen in which a form of myeloschisis was recognized was a 12th-day embryo. An extensive myeloschisis was observed in a 14th-day fetus, which had the typical eversion of the open neural tube onto the surface and an apparently marked increase in total quantity of neural tissue. Several degrees of myeloschisis were found in 17th-day fetuses. In one of the milder forms the defect was limited to the lumbar region, but extensive overgrowth and eversion of the exposed nervous tissue caused it to overhang the adjacent normal skin in all directions. In serial sections the central canal of the spinal cord was seen to open onto the surface at the cephalic end of the everted mass of nervous tissue, and the ependyma of the central canal to be continuous with the layer covering the outer surface of the open neural tube. At the level of the open tube spinal ganglia were fused in the midline forming single, median, ganglionic masses, which were also noted by Gillman *et al.* (1948). In the sacral region the spinal cord was reestablished around the central canal and came once again to lie within the vertebral canal.

Other significant features at this stage were best seen in sagittal sections. Between the open neural plate and the vertebral column there occurred an enlarged subarachnoid space filled with a loose network of meningeal tissues and capillaries, the latter being hypertrophic, particularly at the caudal end of the defect. Hence the excessive vascularity of the pia-arachnoid, characteristic of myeloschisis, made its appearance in early fetal life. The dilatation of the subarachnoid space was more severe in a sympodial specimen, with the entire neural plate being pushed above the general body surface.

Even in fetuses as young as the 17th day, signs of degeneration and tissue damage were present at the surface of the exposed neural plate. But towards the end of pregnancy such changes became more noticeable. The effects of these alterations were analyzed in several 21st-day fetuses, in which various stages were found in the transformation of myeloschisis, characterized by an open but intact neural plate, into a structure that showed increasing resemblance to the sac of a myelomeningocele. The sac was formed by shedding of exposed neural tissue and epithelialization and vascularization of the supporting meninges. In younger fetuses a meningeal meshwork was interposed between the pia of the neural plate and the dura covering the vertebrae. By the 21st day this meshwork was replaced by a fluid-filled space, which, with the various surrounding structures, simulated many of the elements characteristic of human myelomeningocele.

Finally, in an advanced case of spina bifida, found in a 22nd-day animal, i.e., about one day before birth, there was observed the ultimate transformation of myeloschisis into a sac almost devoid of nervous tissue (Warkany, Wilson, and Geiger 1958). (For further description and discussion, see Warkany 1960.)

Other forms of the abnormality, induced by trypan blue, were noted by Gordon (1964). He examined 145 offspring, of which 30 had spina bifida aperta and 39, spina bifida occulta. In those with the open defect 2 groups were identified, the first with the cord directly continuous with the superficial lesion, and the second with the cord ending abruptly several segments proximal to the superficial defect without evidence of connecting elements. Intermediate grades also occurred. In animals with the occult defect a similar range of abnormalities was found, but in these cases the anomaly was related to associated tail defects.

Exencephaly

Exencephaly (fig. 14) was usually produced by trypan blue in low frequencies. In rats, e.g., Gillman *et al.* (1951) found this condition in but 5/1347 offspring, and Lyngdoh (1950), who was not explicit, found "skull defects" and hydrocephalus in only 4/268 viable young. Wilson (1954*a*, 1955) considered it one of the "less frequent" defects; he found (Wilson, Beaudoin, and Free 1959) the following incidences: treatment, 7th to 9th days, 3/70; 8th to 10th days, 7/226; 9th to 11th days, 2/56; with treatments earlier or later than at these times virtually ineffective.

Others who also found exencephaly uncommon are Gepts, Carpent, and Toussaint (1957), Cahen *et al.* (1964), and Stempak (1964), in rats; and Murakami (1953), Kobozieff *et al.* (1959), Runner and Dagg (1960), Barber and Geer (1964), and McCafferty, Wood, and Knisely (1965), in mice. Kreshover, Knighton, and Hancock (1957), using rats of unspecified origin and randombred (Swiss) mice, stated exencephaly to be the "most frequent" defect in both species; but its absolute incidence, although not mentioned, could not have been large, since the highest total occurrence of malformed rat and mouse fetuses was only 12.3 and 8.1 per cent, respectively. The only study in which a fairly high level of exencephaly was produced was that of Barber (1957); but only a small sample was gathered. An appreciable incidence (19%) was found in Wistar rats by Beaudoin and Kahkonen (1963). Exencephaly was also produced in rats by Gunberg (1955, 1958), Tuchmann-Duplessis and Mercier-Parot (1959*a*), Vaupel, Nelson, and Roux (1961), Carpent (1962), Beck and Lloyd (1963*a*), and Inoue *et al.* (1964); in mice, by Hamburgh (1952, 1954), Waddington and Carter (1952, 1953), and Warkany, Kalter, and Geiger (1957); and in hamsters, by Ferm (1958, 1965*a*). Some of these studies will be discussed further below.

On the other hand, exencephaly was not explicitly reported by Fox and Goss (1956), Gunberg (1956), Warkany, Wilson, and Geiger (1958), Vickers (1961*a*, *b*), and Wegener (1961), in rats; by Harm (1954) and Langman and Drunen (1959), in rabbits (but Ferm 1956 noted the occurrence of small encephalocele in this species); and by Conn and Hardy (1959), in dogs.

Midline dorsal defects of the head produced in rats by trypan blue and hypervitaminosis A were described by McLaurin (1964). The anomalies were divided into 2 groups. (1) In encephalocele neural tissue was present on the surface or at least beyond the confines of the cranial vault. There sometimes occurred closure of mesodermal structures beneath pinched-off neural tissue with absence, therefore, of central connection. (2) Meningocele was characterized by herniation of meninges beyond the cranium. Here, also, the connection was sometimes lost, leaving an arachnoidal cyst beneath the skin. The skin over these lesions was always intact, but usually defective, in most instances being thin and devoid of hair folicles. Meningocele and meningo-encephalocele were also noted by Wilson (1955), Beck and Lloyd (1963*b*), and others.

Arnold–Chiari Malformation

The Arnold–Chiari malformation of children consists of congenital defects of the hindbrain region, the essential abnormalities being herniation of tongue-like processes of cerebellar tissue through the foramen magnum into the upper cervical spinal canal and elongation of the medulla oblongata. Three experimental studies have been reported in which offspring of trypan blue-treated pregnant rats exhibited abnormalities of the hindbrain more or less resembling the Arnold–Chiari malformation (Gunberg 1956; Warkany, Wilson, and Geiger 1958; Vickers 1961*b*).

Gunberg (1956) saw defects consisting of elongated brain and skull, flattened colliculi, and herniation of the posterior lobe of the cerebellum, medulla, or both through the foramen magnum. Warkany, Wilson, and Geiger (1958) found structures of the rhombencephalon compressed or crowded toward the foramen magnum. The roof and floor of the 4th ventricle were close together, the cerebellum was situated low in the posterior fossa, and the inferior vermis protruded through the foramen magnum. The normally spacious periencephalic cisternas of the hindbrain region were sometimes obliterated. These changes were collectively termed "crowding" of the brain. Vickers (1961*b*) noted a disturbed relation between structures of the hindbrain and cerebellum and the cranial fossa. Various grades of caudal displacement brought the medulla oblongata and cerebellum into close approximation to the cranial wall. These phenomena led to reduction or obliteration of subarachnoid cisternas. In 5/10 animals examined the obex of the medulla lay opposite or caudal to the margin of the first cervical vertebra. At the same time a considerable portion of the cerebellum passed through the foramen magnum. In addition, the choroid plexus of the 4th ventricle was partly or entirely caudal to the cerebellum in the midline. Other signs of caudal displacement of the hindbrain were the abnormal position of the inferior olivary nuclei and the irregular relation between the interpeduncular fossa and the basisphenoid.

The Arnold–Chiari malformation in human beings almost invariably accompanies spina bifida cystica, which has led to the assumption that they are causally related. One theory (Lichtenstein 1942) states that as a result of anchorage of the spinal cord by a low spina bifida and of the brain by its fixation in the cranium, the differential growth of the spinal column and cord during the middle trimester of gestation, resulting in the relative ascent of the cord, causes abnormal traction that pulls the medulla and cerebellum caudad through the foramen magnum.

Russell (1949) pointed out several contradictions that threw doubt on this mechanical explanation: (1) The Arnold–Chiari malformation may be absent in spina bifida occulta and meningocele despite the cord's being fixed in an abnormal, low position by these abnormalities. (2) The Arnold–Chiari malformation has occurred in association with spina bifida or meningocele at thoracic and other high levels where traction would not be expected to occur. (3) Several instances of the Arnold–Chiari malformation have been found in the absence of spina bifida. To these, Cameron (1957) has added several other objections.

In a recent experimental study, Goldstein and Kepes (1966) simulated the tethering presumably involved in myelomeningocele by ligating the lumbar spinal cord in newborn rats and opossum fetuses. In adult survivors of the surgical procedure, although the lumbar cord was fixed within the scar of the operation, none developed an Arnold–Chiari malformation.

A second theory explaining the association of the Arnold–Chiari malformation and spina bifida was advanced by Cameron (1957). He hypothesized that the herniation of the medulla and cerebellum is caused by pressure disturbances resulting from leakage of cerebrospinal fluid from the spina bifida into the amniotic cavity. He contended that in cases of the Arnold–Chiari malformation with no obvious spina bifida (1) some form of spinal or cranial deformity had not been completely excluded and, (2) the hindbrain anomalies were not typical of the Arnold–Chiari malformation; and that therefore these cases did not preclude his hypothesis.

A third theory states that the Arnold–Chiari malformation and spina bifida are both the outcome of generalized overgrowth of the central nervous system, which, continuing during differentiation of the brain and cord, involves different areas to different degrees (Barry, Patten, and Stewart 1957). Overgrowth may occur to such a degree in, e.g., the lumbosacral region, that it prevents normal closure of the neural tube and leads to spina bifida; or overgrowth of caudal parts of intracranial areas of the nervous system may displace the hindbrain and lead to the Arnold–Chiari malformation and its many accompanying defects. The rare occurrence of the Arnold–Chiari malformation without spina bifida, or vice versa, can therefore be explained as the result of overgrowth limited to the brain or cord, respectively. Supporting this theory was the finding (Barry, Patten, and Stewart 1957) of an apparently excessive hindbrain volume in a human fetus with the Arnold–Chiari malformation, and (Patten 1952, 1953) of excessive volume of nervous tissue in the area of the open neural plate in human myeloschitic fetuses.

A fourth theory, most recently enunciated by Gardner (1959), is more appropriately dealt with below in the discussion of the relation between the Arnold–Chiari malformation and hydrocephalus.

The final theory of the pathogenesis of the Arnold–Chiari malformation states that the condition is not the result of mechanical forces, such as traction, disturbed fluid relations, or overgrowth, but that in and of itself it is a congenital malformation in the same sense that spina bifida, e.g., is a congenital malformation; and hence that it is the product of abnormal embryonic development, albeit of as yet unknown morphogenesis.

This theory has not been vigorously defended by any investigator in the past, probably because its vagueness is not attractive. Several persons, however, have rather timidly offered this alternative because none of the other explanations mentioned above seemed entirely satisfactory (List 1941; Russell 1949; Feigin 1956). The main point supporting this interpretation is that the numerous associated defects and malformations are not explicable on any mechanical basis. Daniel and Strich (1958) agreed that the defects are developmental, starting in early embryonic life, and offered the opinion that their basis may in part be failure of formation of the pontine flexure and abnormal cerebellar development and growth.

It should be pointed out that a cerebello-medullary dislocation, simulating the Arnold–Chiari malformation, occurs in a deformity of the base of the skull, platybasia. Russell (1949) believed, however, that no intrinsic malformation of the neuraxis is present in such cases, and she would therefore restrict the term Arnold–Chiari malformation to cases with spina bifida. In addition, Lichtenstein (1959) stated that the Arnold–Chiari complex—as he called this set of hindbrain defects, regardless of associated phenomena—when present in the adult without evidence of spinal dysraphism is due in the majority of cases to platybasia or cervical spinal defects.

Spina bifida, especially the extreme form known as myelomeningocele, is frequently accompanied not only by the Arnold–Chiari malformation but by hydrocephalus as well. The first attempt to explain this association was made by Chiari (1891), who thought the downward dislocation of the cerebellum, pons, and medulla was the result of the hydrocephalus. This idea has been championed most recently by Gardner (1959), who, going a step further back in embryogenesis, theorized that the hydrocephalus is due to abnormal permeability of the roof of the 4th ventricle early in fetal development. Russell and Donald (1935), on the other hand, held the hydrocephalus not to be the cause but the effect of the hindbrain abnormalities. A communicating hydrocephalus, they believed, may arise from displacement of the foramina of Magendie and Luschka of the 4th ventricle into the spinal canal, which by plugging the foramen magnum causes an obstruction to the return of cerebrospinal fluid to the cranial cavity. Lichtenstein's (1942, 1959) interpretation was that the hydrocephalus is a sequela of the traction on the spinal cord exercised by the spina bifida, which in turn produces elongation and narrowing of the aqueduct of Sylvius, or, less often, obstruction in the 4th ventricle.

Undoubtedly, as it does of many other problems in human pathology, the examination of embryonic and fetal stages of the Arnold–Chiari malformation sheds much light on its pathogenesis and serves to clarify the relation of the hindbrain defects to spina bifida and hydrocephalus. However, adequate numbers of well-preserved human fetal specimens showing the condition in different stages of its development do not exist, and it is unlikely that such a series could be obtained by a single investigator.

As we have seen above, a condition closely simulating the Arnold–Chiari malformation in certain of its essential features is experimentally producible. Let us, then, return to a discussion of these experimental studies to see whether they can resolve some of the problems of the development of the Arnold–Chiari malformation.

As stated above, Gunberg (1956) grouped the abnormal offspring in his study into 6 categories, consisting of spina bifida occulta and 5 grades of spina bifida aperta according to linear extent of the lesion. The percentages of animals with the Arnold–Chiari malformation were 0 in those with spina bifida occulta, 27 and 83 in the 2 least extensive, and 100 in each of the 3 most extensive forms of spina bifida aperta. In addition, 3 animals without spina bifida, but which were tailless and consequently had abnormal termination of the spinal cord, also had the Arnold–Chiari malformation. With exception of these 3, it therefore appeared that the incidence of the Arnold–Chiari malformation was directly correlated with linear extent of the spina bifida, which Gunberg (1956) took to be a measure of its severity.

Gunberg suggested, on the basis of this correlation and of other features such as elongation of the skull, flattening of the braincase, and apparent deviation of spinal nerve angulation, that traction imposed on the cord by the myeloschitic lesion was the cause of the Arnold–Chiari malformation. The question of hydrocephalus was not touched on, since it apparently did not occur in this experiment. Overgrowth of nervous tissue as a possible etiological factor could not be substantiated, because there were no clear-cut examples of this phenomenon. Duplication of spinal cord and canal, which did occur, Gunberg regarded as possibly representing hyperplasia of ependymal elements.

Warkany, Wilson, and Geiger (1958) observed a condition they regarded as "reminiscent" of the Arnold–Chiari malformation in all late – fetal offspring with myeloschisis. The downward dislocation of the hindbrain and cerebellum into the cervical spinal canal was not as extreme as it is in children with the Arnold–Chiari malformation, but this less severe manifestation was regarded as an early form of the malformation. An important finding was that this sign did not occur in 17th-day myeloschitic fetuses, which may mean that the Arnold–Chiari malformation is not present in early embryonic life, as it was postulated to be by Schwalbe and Gredig (1906), but that it is a late fetal expression of growth disturbances.

None of the animals with myeloschisis in this study had hydrocephalus, but the aqueduct was narrow in 3 of them and it may have developed later if the animals had survived. On the other hand, trypan blue-treated pregnant females had many hydrocephalic offspring with no cord defect at all.

Vickers (1961*b*) emphasized the difficulties of comparing abnormal embryonic development of rats and human beings, difficulties that are due not only to species differences, but also to differences in developmental stages of parts being compared. He nevertheless concluded that the trypan blue-induced abnormalities of the rat hindbrain were remarkably similar in morphology to the human Arnold–Chiari malformation; but did not try to explain the relations among the various facets of the human syndrome that may have been permitted by the similarities between it and its counterpart in the rat.

These are the sole experimental studies that have so far been made on this complicated and perplexing syndrome of congenital malformations. We can thus see that, although a promising start has been made, the great potential that terato-embryological investigations hold for unravelling these problems has as yet been scarcely tapped.

Embryology of Defects in Mice

Embryological studies of trypan blue-induced developmental abnormalities were made in mice by Hamburgh (1952, 1954) and Waddington and Carter (1952, 1953). Hamburgh (1952) injected (route unstated) BALB/c female mice twice with 0.25 to 0.5 ml of 0.5 per cent trypan blue, first at about 8 days before and then at 7 to 8 days after fertilization. Females allowed to deliver had 67 offspring, and of these, 16 showed different types and degrees of tail abnormalities. Other females killed 10 to 14 days after fertilization yielded 118 embryos of which 68 were abnormal. The majority of the abnormalities were of the posterior axial (i.e., kinky, short, or curled tails) or anterior axial region (i.e., exencephaly). Abnormalities of the latter type were so severe that embryos with them could not have survived to birth, thus accounting for the absence of exencephaly among the newborn and for the small litter sizes from the females permitted to deliver.

In another study (Hamburgh 1954) BALB/c females were injected with 0.5 ml of 1 per cent trypan blue on the 8th day of pregnancy and the embryos were recovered on the 9th to 15th days; 571 embryos were examined and 332 found to have malformations of varying degrees. Again 2 major types of defects were found, involving the anterior and posterior axes. In anterior abnormalities the neural folds remained wide open throughout the head and neck regions. This resulted in microcephaly, in which the brain vesicles were either reduced in size or asymmetrical owing to abnormal growth on one side; or in exencephaly with heavy thickening and eversions of the roof of the hindbrain and anterior cord. Posterior abnormalities, i.e., tail defects, did not appear before the 10th day of gestation. In sectioned material gross tail defects were always found associated with a doubled neural tube or with the formation of irregular neural outgrowths in the posterior trunk and tail region only. The notochord was affected in only 11 cases. Anteriorly there occurred hypertrophy and thickening of the neural folds of the midbrain and other nervous tissues, and diverticulae and folds pushing into the ventricles thus narrowing these spaces.

Waddington and Carter (1952, 1953) used the CBA strain of mice. Females were given single subcutaneous injections of 0.5 ml of 1 per cent trypan blue on the 8th day of pregnancy, and embryos were removed at 24-hour intervals one to 9 days later. Dead embryos and retardation of live ones were perhaps already noted one day after injection, i.e., among 9th-day specimens. On the 10th day subectodermal blebs were found near somites. In addition the pericardium was enlarged, which apparently interfered with the turning of the embryo that normally occurs at this stage, with the result that the posterior part of the body failed to slip around the allantois and so remained deflected along the right side of the anterior part. These defects were still present on the 11th day; in addition, the anterior neural tube, which at that stage normally is closed, was sometimes still open, i.e., exencephalic. On the 12th day the abnormalities were more severe, and by the 13th day death intervened. After that time, in embryos that successfully completed the turning process, other abnormalities were noted, namely, hematomata on the head and tail.

Other phenomena noted (Waddington and Carter 1953) were rapid localization and great concentration of trypan blue in the yolk sac, and abnormalities of embryonic body fluids and circulation, such as subepidermal blisters and edematous enlargement of cardiac structures. To the former, via disturbed nutrition, was attributed the inhibition of growth and differentiation, which were marked features of abnormal 10th- and 11th-day embryos; while the latter were held responsible for certain specific malformations, such as tail defects and failure of neural-tube closure, through mechanical interference with normal processes.

The pathogenesis of trypan blue-induced malformations of the eye was studied by Gilbert and Gillman (1954) and Toussaint (1958), and defects of the internal ear were examined in fetuses by Myers (1955) and in neonates by Altmann (1955).

Variability of Trypan Blue Teratogenicity

Several studies have been made of some of the sources of the quantitative and qualitative variability of the teratogenic effects of trypan blue. Most obvious, of course, of the factors involved in such variability are the dose, sample, and quality of the dye itself. So far as dose is concerned, as is generally true of teratogenic agents, the greater the quantity given the greater was the incidence of congenital malformations (Beck and Lloyd 1964), up to the point of total embryonic destruction.

Trypan Blue Samples

Remarkable differences in yield of malformed offspring were obtained with samples of trypan blue of different origin. Several investigations of this aspect have been made. Tuchmann-Duplessis and Mercier-Parot (1959a) tested the teratogenicity of 4 samples of trypan blue, obtained from (1) National Aniline (lot no. 477–11003), (2) Coleman and Bell (lot no. B430–410.213), (3) Prof. J. G. Wilson, and (4) R.A.L. and found the percentage of abnormal young produced to be 4, 38, 28 and 6, respectively. No differences in type of malformation were found.

Carpent (1962) also obtained such results with other samples (Grübler, and National Aniline lot nos. 7286 and 9652), which produced 33, 50, and 37 per cent abnormalities, respectively. Different frequencies of specific defects occurred; e.g., among the abnormal young the 3 samples caused congenital malformations of the central nervous system in 18, 37, and 36 per cent, respectively; of the tail in 40, 21, and 8 per cent respectively; and of the cardiovascular system in 18, 8, and 11 per cent, respectively. Similarly, Stempak (1964) produced hydrocephalus with trypan blue obtained from the Matheson, Coleman and Bell Company, but not with that from the Chroma Gesellschaft.

Beck, Spencer, and Baxter (1960) and Beck (1961) emphasized that uncertainty exists as to the actual dose of trypan blue administered in past experiments since commercial samples of trypan blue contain highly variable amounts of the dye, owing to contamination with sodium chloride. The quantity of azo dye in the samples they tested ranged from 20 to 86 per cent. Kelly *et al.* (1964) stated that typical commercial samples of trypan blue may be expected to contain 50 to 80 per cent nominal dye, 4 to 14 per cent reddish dyes, and various amounts of inorganic salts and organic colored or colorless compounds.

Beck (1961) examined this source of variability by using 3 commercial preparations of trypan blue that were standardized by titration to contain the same amount of azo dye. One sample was obtained from G. T. Gurr and 2 others from Flatters and Garnett. Despite this standardization, the 3 samples were different in their effects, since the Gurr sample was not teratogenic at all while the Flatters and Garnett samples caused 18 and 19 per cent abnormalities, respectively, in the surviving young. Since variability persisted, Beck (1961) concluded that commercial trypan blue is a mixture of substances and that only one or a combination of several of the components of the mixture is teratogenic, and thus that it is likely that the variable potencies of samples used depends on the amount of teratogen(s) each contains. Probably the true explanation was revealed later, when it was discovered (Lloyd and Beck 1963) that the Gurr sample was nonteratogenic because it in fact contained almost no trypan blue.

Trypan Blue Fractions

Beck and Lloyd (1963a) made a study of which of the fractions present in commercial trypan blue is responsible for its teratogenic action. They started with a sample of Williams Limited trypan blue (batch 85333), and by separating and purifying its components obtained 3 colored fractions—pure blue, purple, and red. Tested on Wistar rats, only the blue fraction proved teratogenic; further, the impurities (i.e., the purple and red fractions) did not modify this property of the blue fraction.

Kelly *et al.* (1964) also investigated this aspect of the problem. Starting with 8 different samples of trypan blue (Direct blue 14, C.I.23850), they tested the whole dyes and their blue and red fractions for teratogenicity, using Sprague–Dawley and hooded King rats. The whole dyes were found to be most teratogenic, the blue fractions intermediate, and the red fractions least teratogenic, although the potency of all was variable. The incidence of anomalous young produced by the whole dyes ranged from 3.0 to 54.8 per cent, with a mean of 23.1 per cent, and those produced by the blue and red fractions ranged, respectively, from 0 to 30.8 per cent and 0 to 8.7 per cent, with means of 7.0 and 3.4 per cent. In 2 cases the blue fraction was more teratogenic than the whole dyes from which they were derived, but in these cases the whole dyes were those with the lowest activity of any whole dyes in the series. There was no relation between types of anomalies produced and any particular dye sample or fraction, and no distinct correlation was found between teratogenic and embryocidal activity. The authors (Kelly *et al.* 1964) suggested that, since the whole dyes were in general stronger teratogens than their fractions, other contaminants of commercial samples must be responsible for some of their teratogenic properties.

Barber and Geer (1964) broke a sample of National Aniline whole trypan blue (C.I.477) into blue, red, and water-soluble and sodium hydroxide-soluble purple fractions, and tested the effects of the whole dye and its components in DBA/2 mice. The whole dye and the blue fraction caused 55.5 and 57.1 per cent defective offspring, respectively. The red and sodium hydroxide-soluble purple fractions were nonteratogenic, whereas the water-soluble purple fraction was mildly teratogenic. As in Kelly *et al.*'s (1964) study, Barber and Geer (1964) noted no differences in the types of abnormalities caused by the teratogenic fractions and the whole dye.

Genetic Factors

Genetic influences on the teratogenic effects of trypan blue have been recorded. The discussion of this point will be limited to the work done with rats since this teratogen has been used predominantly with them. Only a few brief reports of work with mice on this aspect have appeared (Murakami and Kameyama 1954; Beck 1964*a*, *b*).

Gunberg (1958) gave subcutaneous injections of 1 per cent aqueous trypan blue (5 ml/kg) on the day of breeding and on the 4th and 7th days of gestation to 3 groups of rats: (1) Long–Evans rats of an inbred colony, (2) Long–Evans of commercial origin, and (3) Sprague–Dawley. The incidence of external congenital malformations in the offspring was 34, 12, and 67 per cent, respectively; exencephaly or cranial meningocele appeared in 17, 50, and 97 per cent, respectively, of the abnormal offspring. Similar results occurred in a later study (Gunberg *et al.* 1962).

Tuchmann-Duplessis and Mercier-Parot (1959*a*) also found such differences in the stocks they used. Employing Wilson's (1954*a*) schedule of treatment (and using Coleman and Bell trypan blue, which they found most potent) with 6 groups of rats—(1) stock, (2) commerical Wistar, and 4 types obtained from the CNRS: (3) Black, (4) August, (5) PVG, and (6) Long–Evans—they produced 11, 37, 80, 10, 32, and 54 per cent congenital malformations, respectively. No differences in type of defect were found among the 6 groups. The majority of abnormalities, about 90 per cent, affected the central nervous system (exencephaly, craniorachischisis, spina bifida, but apparently no hydrocephalus). Similar situations were also noted by Beck, Spencer, and Baxter (1960), Wegener (1961), and Carpent (1962) in the stocks of rats at their disposal.

In numerous instances certain congenital malformations of the central nervous system were produced in some studies that were virtually absent in others. However, only in the studies from 2 laboratories have almost no central nervous system defects appeared at all. Fox and Goss (1956, 1957, 1958), using a long-isolated "substrain" of Long–Evans rats, reported that the only external abnormalities noted in appreciable numbers were those of the eye, while high incidences of cardiovascular malformations were found in sectioned material; and Wegener (1961), using Sprague–Dawley, Wistar, and a mixed stock of rats, found that cardiovascular, eye, and tail abnormalities predominated.

Diet

Gunberg (1955) explored the influence of diet on the teratogenic action of trypan blue. Pregnant Long–Evans rats fed diets containing 24, 15, or 10 per cent protein were given 3 injections of the teratogen, and had young with 23, 46, and 41 per cent external congenital malformations, respectively. Tail defects and spina bifida occurred in all groups of offspring, but hydrocephalus, exencephaly, and umbilical hernia appeared only in the groups fed the low-protein diets. Gillman and his associates also modified the effects of trypan blue by dietary and endocrine influences on the mother (Gilbert and Gillman

1954). Fasting and trypan blue had additive teratogenic effects in mice (Runner and Dagg 1960) and rats (Setokoesoema and Gunberg 1966).

Time of Treatment

Time of treatment is also certainly influential. Gillman *et al.* (1948, 1951), and all who have followed them in this work, observed that treatment during pregnancy was most effective in producing congenital malformations when given after the time of implantation, which occurs in the rat on the 6th day of gestation. Gillman *et al.* (1951) found that trypan blue caused abnormalities when administered at any time during the first 9 days of pregnancy, but that none was produced by treatment later than this time, if injections were given during pregnancy only.

A study of the comparative teratogenicity of trypan blue injected at different times during the first half of pregnancy in the rat was made by Wilson, Beaudoin, and Free (1959). Treating on 3 consecutive days (each subcutaneous injection consisting of 1 ml 1 % trypan blue) beginning the 1st day of gestation, they found that teratogenic effectiveness increased steadily as the initial injection was given progressively later in pregnancy. The peak (49 % abnormal offspring) was reached when the first of the 3 injections was given on the 8th day; treatment beginning later than this time was far less effective, and no defects were produced by treatment beginning after the 11th day. In order to determine the time of maximal effect, single intravenous injections (1 ml, 2 % trypan blue; therefore, 2/3 of the total amount given subcutaneously) were given on the 7th to 13th days of pregnancy. The results closely paralleled those obtained with subcutaneous injection, with the peak of activity (32 % abnormal offspring) occurring after injection on the 9th day of pregnancy.

Although the total incidence of abnormal young varied considerably with the time of treatment, the relative frequency of the individual defects remained fairly constant. Thus, hydrocephalus was the most common defect and gastroschisis one of the rarest, regardless of when treatment was given. This consistency of the overall pattern of malformations suggested that trypan blue acts only within a limited span of time (Wilson, Beaudoin, and Free 1959). This subject will be discussed further below. Similar results were obtained in rats by Fox, Goss, and Bordeaux (1958); single injections were given on the 8th to 11th days of pregnancy, but defective fetal development was not produced by treatment after the 9th day.

Prenatal Mortality

Variability of the effects of trypan blue may also sometimes be due to prenatal death and resorption of severely damaged embryos and fetuses. In the studies of Hamburgh (1952, 1954), Waddington and Carter (1952, 1953), and Murakami (1953) with mice, pregnant females that were allowed to deliver or were killed in late pregnancy had small litter sizes and offspring with defects mostly of the tail or no defects at all. When the females were killed during pregnancy, however, many conceptuses were found with exencephaly and other brain defects. In these animals, therefore, such abnormalities or those associated with them were incompatible with intrauterine life, and hence young with them were not found at birth.

A similar situation was discovered by Beck and Lloyd (1963b). These workers gave pregnant Wistar rats single subcutaneous injections of trypan blue (50 mg/kg) on the 9th day of pregnancy, and killed them 3, 6, and 12 days later. At these times they found 48, 29, and 20 per cent of the young malformed, respectively. The same decline was true of the incidence of some particular malformations. For example, at these 3 times in gestation 44, 41, and 15 per cent of the malformed young had spina bifida, and 31, 16, and 5 per cent exencephaly, respectively. At the same time the shift in frequency was less consistent for other defects or, in fact, rose; e.g., the incidence of eye defects at these 3 times was 38, 25, and 75 per cent, respectively. With the general decline in the malformation rate there was a rise in the fetal resorption rate. Presumably, as some severely or multiply malformed fetuses were eliminated and less damaged ones preferentially survived, a distorted picture came to exist in late pregnancy of the incidence and spectrum of congenital malformations produced by trypan blue (Beck and Lloyd 1963b).

On the other hand, Smith (1963b) contended that his findings did not support the belief that fetal death is related to, or is a secondary effect of, malformations produced by trypan blue. He found 21.8 per cent of trypan blue-treated embryos and early fetuses undergoing resorption. Those showing even the slightest degree of resorption were always smaller than their living littermates, but in the absence of resorption the smallest embryos did not display the greatest degree of malformation and usually showed no evidence of abnormal development apart from growth retardation. Thus the lethal effect did not seem to be dependent on, or even related to, the teratologic effect. In using different samples and fractions of trypan blue, Kelly et al. (1964) also found no distinct correlation between teratogenic and lethal effects.

In a study of the synergistic action of trypan blue and excess vitamin A, Wilson (1964) obtained results that suggested that "mortality and teratogenicity are separable and therefore not merely different degrees of expression of the same reaction to injury on the part of the embryo." The same conclusion was reached (Kalter 1965a) in a study of the teratogenic effects of galactoflavin in several inbred strains of mice and a large number of types of their hybrids.

Nevertheless, evidence brought forth (Beck and Lloyd 1963b, 1966) is, I feel, convincing that some fraction of trypan blue-induced fetal death and resorption is associated with or consequent upon maldevelopment. But in all likelihood every death cannot be so explained. The problem, thus, is to identify other lethal situations and to assess the relative roles played by all of them in fetal wastage.

Until experiments such as those discussed above are made with 2 or more stocks or strains of animals simultaneously no definitive information will be had of the influence of heredity in producing variable pictures of the effects of teratogens such as trypan blue by means of differential, selective prenatal death. There can be little doubt that genetic factors are responsible for at least some of the discrepancies reported in the literature; such as the fact that Niagara blue 2B caused no malformations in some studies (Wilson, Beaudoin, and Free 1959; Beaudoin and Pickering 1960; Beaudoin and Ferm 1961), but was teratogenic in others (Lloyd and Beck 1964a, 1966); or that exencephaly was not found beyond late embryonic stages in some trypan blue-treated mice (Hamburgh 1952, 1954; Waddington and Carter 1952, 1953; Ferrario 1957), while in studies with mice of other genetic constitutions this anomaly appeared in near-term young (Kreshover, Knighton, and Hancock 1957; Warkany, Kalter, and Geiger 1957; Kobozieff *et al.* 1959).

The Mechanism of the Teratogenic Action of Trypan Blue

For no teratogen has the question of the mechanism by which it induces congenital malformations been so intensively pursued as for trypan blue. Three principal hypotheses have been proposed to explain its teratogenic action. The first assumes that the effects on the embryo are the indirect outcome of disturbances of maternal physiology by the dye; the second that dye molecules enter the placenta and interfere with transport of substances necessary for embryonic nutrition; and the third that the dye actually reaches the embryo itself and thus has a direct effect on development.

As in so many other aspects of the subject of trypan blue teratogenesis, so in this one Gillman and his coworkers in the first report of this subject (1948) made the initial observations and started the ball rolling. The effects of trypan blue on the embryo, they believed, cannot be dissociated from those on the maternal organism. They therefore paid considerable attention to the structural and biochemical changes in their trypan blue-treated pregnant rats. Some consistent findings were great loss of weight, severe anemia, increased red cell sedimentation, hyalinization of kidney glomeruli, fatty degeneration of liver cells and other hepatic changes, gross enlargement of the adrenals, spleen, and lymphatic glands, and partial blockage of the reticuloendothelial system owing to uptake of the dye by phagocytes. This latter point was substantiated by Wilson's (1955) observation of dye-laden macrophages in lung, liver, spleen, lymph nodes, and general connective tissue. Some of these changes were also observed by Langman and Drunen (1959).

Coupled with these effects, Gillman *et al.* (1948) noted that trypan blue did not enter the embryo—that although it became localized in the yolk-sac epithelium, other parts such as the amnion, amniotic fluid, and embryonic tissues proper remained unstained. Since trypan blue apparently does not exist in a leuco form, it cannot be present in the rat embryo in an invisible state, and presumably, therefore, it was reasoned, its teratogenic effects may be exerted indirectly through its influence on the physiology amd metabolism of the mother.

Maternal Disturbance

The first possibility is that congenital malformations are caused by one or more of the effects of the dye on the mother. Liver damage can probably be ruled out since malformed young were not found among the offspring of rats (Wilson 1954c) given carbon tetrachloride, a treatment that destroyed a large fraction of maternal liver tissue. This was recently confirmed in rabbits (Heine *et al.* 1964).

Hypoxia. In view of the maternal anemia produced by trypan blue, and because of the fact that hypoxia is teratogenic, it seemed reasonable to Barber (1957) to suspect that trypan blue-induced embryonic defects may be mediated via a maternal anemic anoxia. To some extent this belief was based on a misreading of Gillman *et al.*'s (1948) ideas. In a later publication Gilbert and Gillman (1954) explicitly rejected this hypothesis because, while they felt it may explain the maldevelopment of some parts of the body—e.g., of the eye, through disturbance of blood supply owing to vascular abnormalities— they believed it could not account for the widespread defects on the central nervous system and skeleton produced by trypan blue.

Evidence of the unlikelihood of the anemia-mediated hypoxia hypothesis was provided by Wilson (1953) and Moscarella, Stark, and de Forest (1962), who failed to affect embryonic development by massive maternal bleeding. It is also appropriate to recall that while anoxic anoxia is teratogenic in mice and rabbits, its effects on prenatal development of rats are equivocal (see p. 178).

Thyroid factors. The possible role of thyroid factors in trypan blue teratogenesis has been considered by several investigators. It was found (see Christie 1964 and Beaudoin and Roberts 1966, for references) that repeated injections of adult rats with trypan blue led to appearance of abnormal serum proteins, decrease in serum protein-bound iodine, suppression of thyroidal uptake of radioiodine, and lowered thyroid weight. Thyroid hormone secretion in these cases was restored by exogenous thyrotropin (TSH). These phenomena have been understood to mean that trypan blue competes with thyroxin for serum-protein binding sites, thus resulting in increased free thyroxin, which in turn inhibits TSH secretion and produces hypofunction of the thyroid gland.

Insofar as they relate to the teratogenic action of trypan blue, these effects of the dye on thyroid function have been variously interpreted. Hamburgh and Sobel (1960) treated female rats late in pregnancy with trypan blue or thyroxin and found that both reduced fetal thyroid weight and disorganized its follicular structure. They reasoned that the dye may have acted by displacing maternal thyroxin from its protein carrier, allowing it to cross the placenta and inhibit fetal TSH release, i.e., in effect, by producing maternal hyperthyroidism. They did not feel, however, that the presence of excess thyroxin in the fetus could explain the teratogenic role of trypan blue.

More audaciously, perhaps, Christie (1964) suggested that the teratogenic action of trypan blue is due to inhibition of secretion of thyroxin from the maternal thyroid gland, i.e,. hypothyroidism; which directly or indirectly leads to fetal maldevelopment through general decrease in oxidative metabolism and thus to reduction in the supply to the embryo of oxygen or essential nutrients. Subsequently, Christie (1966) reported that administration of trypan blue to pregnant thyroidectomized rats increased the fetal resorption rate and may have produced a higher incidence of malformations than it did in nonoperated females, and that these increases were abolished by thyroxin. He thus took these results to support his (Christie 1964) hypothesis. However, since no data were given as to the numbers of offspring obtained, the results cannot be objectively evaluated. Beck and Lloyd (1966) found that thyroxin had no effect on the incidence of malformation produced by trypan blue.

Beaudoin and Roberts (1966), studying the effects of TSH on trypan blue teratogenesis, found that the incidence of malformations produced by the former was significantly increased when it was combined with a nonteratogenic dose of trypan blue. However, they cautiously refrained from speculating about the nature of the interaction between these agents but merely commented that since the current literature suggests the placenta is impermeable to TSH, its site of action must be the placenta itself or the maternal organism.

Adrenal stimulation. Another theory concerns the effects of trypan blue on the maternal pituitary-adrenal axis. Hommes (1959) postulated that the effects of trypan blue on protein composition and prenatal development are secondary to its initial action, which is stimulation of adrenal overactivity. He based this hypothesis on several lines of evidence: (1) similar shifts in maternal serum composition produced by trypan blue and ACTH injections, (2) the maternal adrenal hypertrophy noted after trypan blue treatment by Gillman *et al.* (1948), and (3) the teratogenic effects of glucocorticosteroids (Kalter and Warkany 1959a). This hypothesis is contradicted by certain facts. First, although adrenal corticosteroids are teratogenic in mice and rabbits (Fraser and Fainstat 1951; Kalter and Fraser 1952; Kalter 1954a, 1961; Fainstat 1954; Ingalls and Curley 1957a; Clavert, Buck, and Rumpler 1961; Pinsky and DiGeorge 1965; Walker 1965, 1966), they have not produced congenital malformations in rats (Davis and Plotz 1954; Gunberg 1957; Mercier-Parot 1957; Haumont 1958; Lohmeyer 1961). Second, apparently nonteratogenic azo dyes also induced adrenal hypertrophy (Ferm 1959).

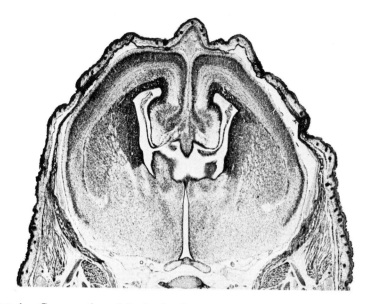

FIG. 1a. Cross section of the brain of a near-term control mouse at the level of the foramina of Monro. The narrow vertical median slit is the 3rd ventricle and at its base is the optic chiasm. The 3rd ventricle in this section is not yet quite in communication with the lateral ventricles via the broad transverse channel the foramina of Monro here comprise. The choroid plexuses of the lateral ventricles in this region each appear as a graceful filament that follows the general contour of the ventricle upward from its origin near the hippocampal fimbria. Hematoxylin and eosin stain. Thickness of section 20 μ. Magnification about 21 ×.

FIG. 1b. Cross section of the brain of a near-term mouse from a female treated with galactoflavin, a riboflavin-antagonist, during pregnancy. The region of the brain is approximately the same as that of the control animal in fig. 1a. As is abundantly evident, the lateral and 3rd ventricles are greatly expanded; further, the fornix is very narrow, possibly through compression, and the choroid plexuses are aplastic. Hematoxylin and eosin stain. Thickness of section 20 μ. Magnification about 18 ×.

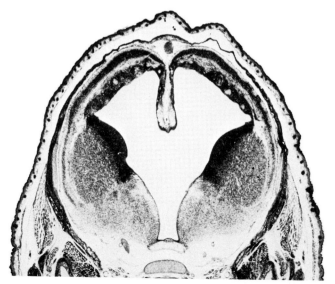

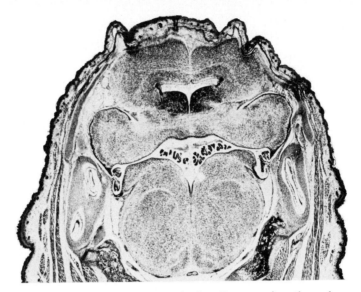

FIG. 2a. Near-term control mouse brain. Cross section through an anterior region of cerebellum. The 4th ventricle is seen above and below the superior medullary velum, lateral to which are rostral parts of the cerebellar hemispheres. In the lower section of the ventricle is the choroid plexus, and beyond the narrowed portions of the ventricle are its lateral recesses, just medial to the labyrinth of the inner ear. Hematoxylin and eosin stain. Thickness of section 20 μ. Magnification about 19 ×.

FIG. 2b. Cross section of the brain of a near-term mouse from a galactoflavin-treated female, matching the region in the control in fig. 2a. Here, again, the tremendous dilation of ventricle (4th ventricle, in this case) can hardly be overlooked. Accompanying this expansion is absence, except for possible vestiges, of the entire cerebellum. The choroid plexus, too, is missing with the exception of the fronds at the "lateral recesses" of the ventricle. Hematoxylin and eosin stain. Thickness of section 20 μ. Magnification about 18 ×.

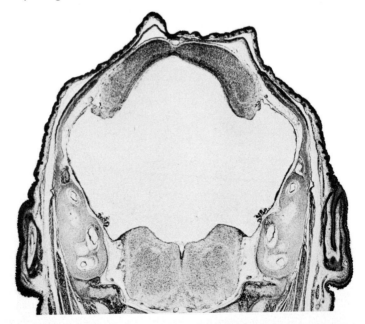

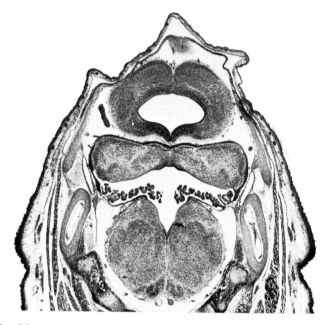

FIG. 3a. Near-term control mouse brain. Cross section through the cerebellum slightly posterior to the area shown in fig. 2a; thus the superior medullary velum is not present, and the cerebellum forms a wide transverse bar, completely separated from the mesencephalic parts superior to it. Hematoxylin and eosin stain. Thickness of section 20 μ. Magnification about 20 ×.

FIG. 3b. Cross section of the brain of a near-term mouse from a galactoflavin-treated female, matching the region shown in the control in fig. 3a. The abnormalities of this brain are less severe than of those shown in figs. 1b and 2b. The 4th ventricle is enlarged but far less so than in the extreme case illustrated in fig. 2b; though the cerebellum is present, it is much reduced in size, especially in the midline. Hematoxylin and eosin stain. Thickness of section 20 μ. Magnification about 21 ×.

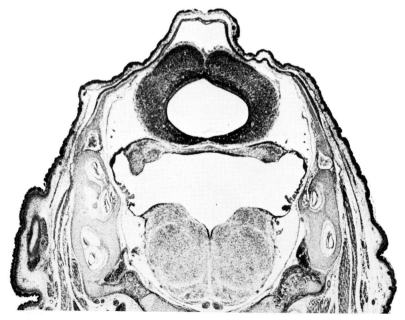

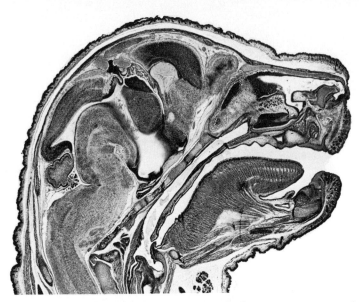

FIG. 4a. Median sagittal section of the head of a near-term control mouse. Contrast with fig. 4b. Hematoxylin and eosin stain. Thickness of section 20 μ. Magnification about 11×.

FIG. 4b. Median sagittal section of the head of a near-term mouse from a galactoflavin-treated female. The 3rd and 4th ventricles, especially the latter, are extremely dilated. Also enlarged are the aqueduct of Sylvius, seen here, and the foramina of Monro and the lateral ventricles, not seen here. Yet despite the marked ventricular enlargement the size and shape of the head are not appreciably different from those of the control head in fig. 4a, a situation reminiscent of hydranencephaly. The cerebellum, a conspicuous structure in the control, is missing, except perhaps for some cells of cerebellar origin in the thin membrane superior to the remnant of the choroid plexus that persists. See the text (p. 22) for a description of other abnormalities present. Hematoxylin and eosin stain. Thickness of section 20 μ. Magnification about 11×.

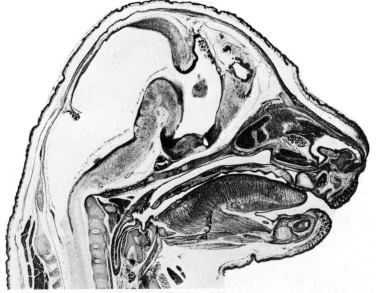

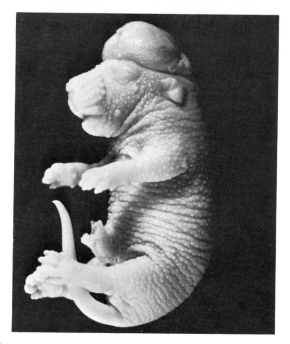

FIG. 5. Near-term exencephalic mouse from a female given a single oral dose of 10,000 IU vitamin A on the 9th day of pregnancy. Although the brain was exposed in utero for only the relatively short fetal period it shows unmistakable signs of degeneration, especially when contrasted with the well-preserved conformation of the brain of the exencephalic fetus shown in figs. 6a and 6b. Also contrast the rear view of the near-term exencephalic brain in fig. 7 with the rear view of the fetus in fig. 6b.

FIGS. 6a and 6b. Two views of an exencephalic 15th-day mouse fetus from a female given a large dose of vitamin A.

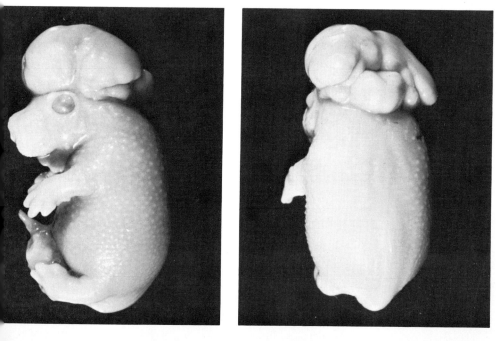

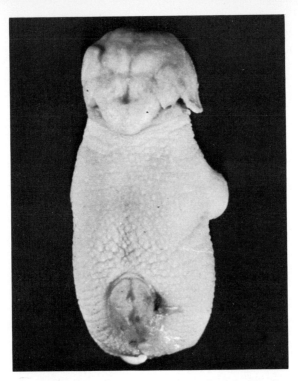

Fig. 7. Near-term mouse with hypervitaminosis A-induced exencephaly and lumbosacral spina bifida aperta.

Fig. 8. Near-term mouse with hypervitaminosis A-induced lumbosacral spina bifida aperta.

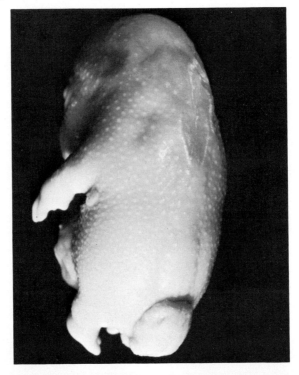

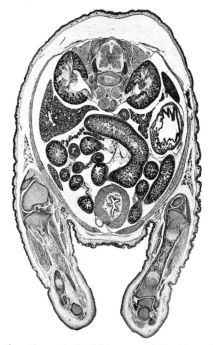

Fig. 9a. Cross section through the kidneys and bladder of a near-term control mouse. Compare the spinal cord with that in fig. 9b. Hematoxylin and eosin stain. Thickness of section 20 μ. Magnification about 9×.

Fig. 9b. Cross section of near-term mouse from a female given a single oral dose of 10,000 IU vitamin A on the 9th day of pregnancy; the area illustrated matches that of the control in fig. 9a. Dorsal to the midline fused kidney with its single dilated ureter are seen the open neural plate of the spina bifida aperta and its associated vertebral defects. Hematoxylin and eosin stain. Thickness of section 20 μ. Magnification about 13×.

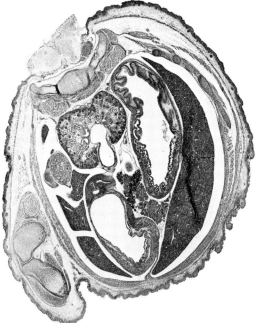

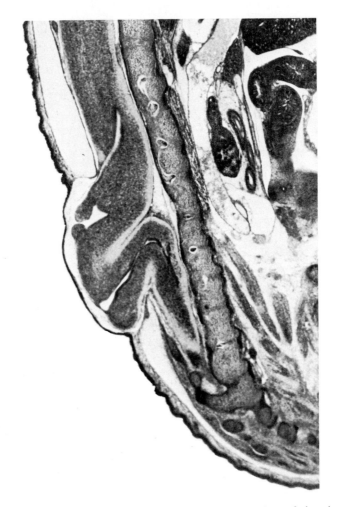

FIG. 10. Near-term mouse from a female given a large dose of vitamin A during pregnancy. Sagittal section of an unusual spina bifida occulta. The spinal cord is extensively folded and open, i.e., cleft, but covered by abnormal skin, which is only slightly elevated above the height of the animal's back; and thus was not discovered until the specimen was sectioned. Hematoxylin and eosin stain. Thickness of section 20 μ. Magnification about 27 ×.

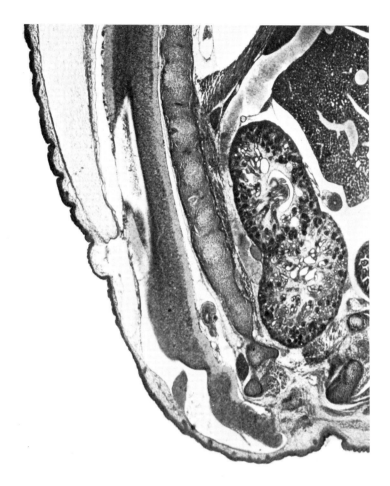

Fig. 11. Sagittal section of near-term mouse from a female given a large dose of vitamin A. Another example of an extensive and unusual but occult spina bifida, not discovered until sectioned. Hematoxylin and eosin stain. Thickness of section 20 μ. Magnification about 25 ×.

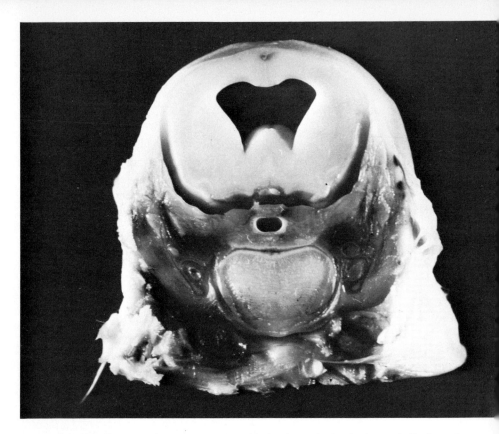

Fig. 12. Cross section cut by razor blade through the hydrocephalic lateral ventricles of a 32-day-old rat from a mother given trypan blue during pregnancy.

Fig. 13. Lumbosacral spina bifida in a late fetal rat from a trypan blue-treated female.

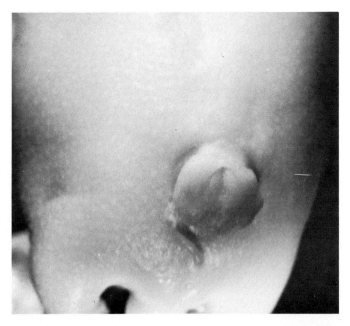

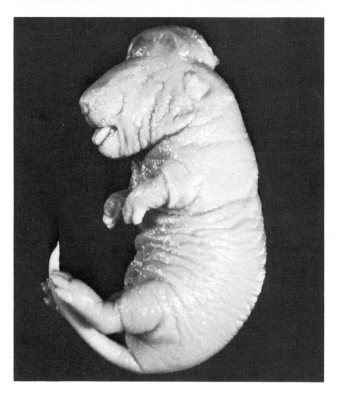

Fig. 14. Near-term rat with trypan blue-induced exencephaly.

Fig. 15. Craniorachischisis in near-term rats produced by maternal treatment with methyl salicylate.

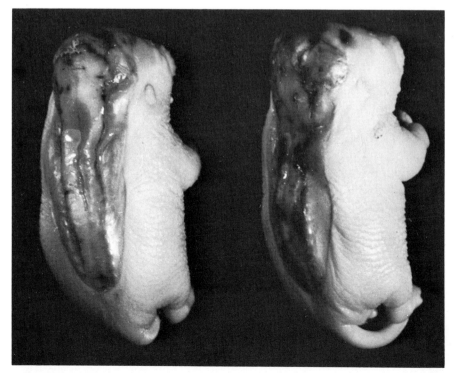

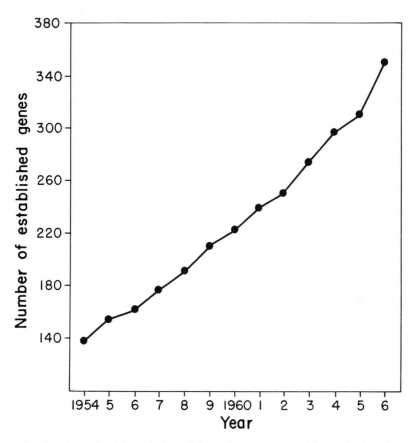

FIG. 16. Growth of knowledge of the mouse genome. This graph demonstrates the brisk increase in the number of established mutant genes in mice over the past several years. The chart is based on the lists of mutants appearing in the July numbers of the *Mouse News Letter* from 1954 to 1966.

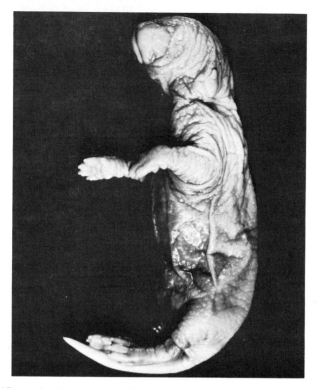

FIGS. 17a and 17b. Otocephalic newborn mice of the C57BL/6JKt inbred strain. They have relatively low grades of the condition, in which the predominant malformations consist of ectopic ears and defects of the lower jaw, mouth, pharynx, and nasal structures.

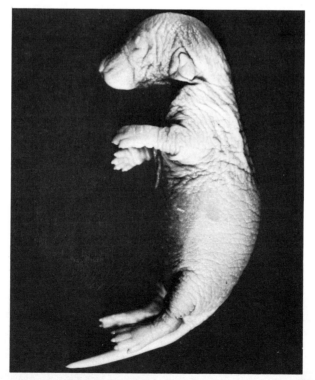

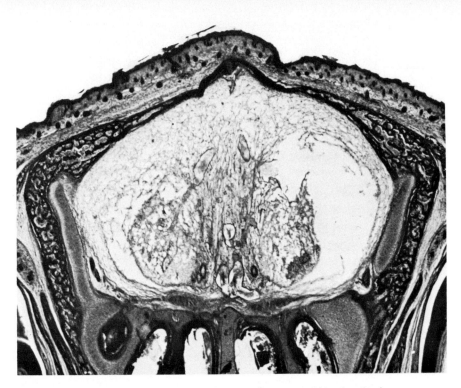

Fig. 18. Cross section through the anterior part of the head of a near-term polydactylous rat of the *po/po* genotype. The network-filled space is normally occupied by the olfactory bulbs. Hematoxylin and eosin stain. Thickness of section 20 μ. Magnification about 25 ×.

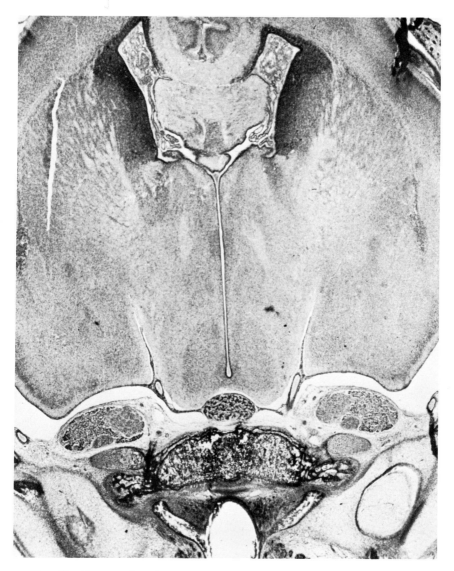

FIG. 19. Cross section through the brain of a *po/po* near-term rat at the level of the foramina of Monro. The eggshaped body below the 3rd ventricle is the aberrant pars anterior of the pituitary. The pars nervosa is absent.

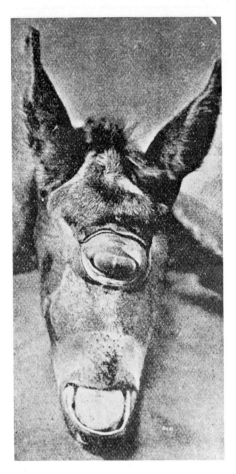

FIG. 20. Orr's (1888) cyclopic horse.

Finally, the administration of formalin to pregnant rats failed to produce congenital malformations (Ranström 1956; Schnurer 1963), although this substance is a well-known stressor that causes the classical stress-response signs such as adrenal hypertrophy, thymic involution, and so on.

The results of other studies also apparently implicated maternal adrenal function in trypan blue teratogenesis. It was found that pregnant mice (Ishii and Yokobori 1960) and rats (Shidara 1963) exposed to prolonged loud noise and injected with trypan blue had a higher incidence of malformed offspring than those treated with either noise or dye alone; and further (Shidara 1963) that bilaterally adrenalectomized pregnant rats treated with both noise and trypan blue had fewer malformed young than females not adrenalectomized.

An interesting finding, which may be considered as the reverse of some of the results discussed above, is that cortisone appeared to reduce the incidence of trypan blue-induced malformations of the cardiovascular system in rats to the control value (Agarwal *et al.* 1960). These workers also claimed that cortisone alone produced heart defects in their rats. This paper is difficult to appraise since numerous details were omitted.

RES blockade. The possibility that blockade of the reticuloendothelial system is somehow involved can also be eliminated because not only are teratogenic azo dyes taken up by this system but so are apparently nonteratogenic ones. Gillman *et al.* (1951) found that while trypan red was stored for a time in the maternal reticuloendothelial system, it did not produce reticulosis or congenital malformations; and that although methylene blue, Sudan IV, Bismarck brown, Niagara blue, and sky blue, like trypan blue, excited a maternal reticulosis and tumor formation in the liver, they were not teratogenic. Likewise, it was noted (Wilson, Beaudoin, and Free 1959) that India ink, a particulate suspension, and Niagara blue 2B, a dye with a chemical structure and colloidal properties similar to trypan blue, were both taken up in great quantities by the maternal reticuloendothelial system and other cells, but that neither caused congenital malformations.

Parenthetically, it may be mentioned that Lloyd and Beck (1964*b*) suggested that the relative lack of teratogenic effectiveness of a related dye, Niagara blue 4B, may be due in part to its quick removal from the maternal circulation, whereas a more teratogenic dye, Afridol blue, persisted in the maternal serum for a longer time. This aspect was pursued further (Lloyd, Beck, and Griffiths 1965; Lloyd and Beck 1966) by measuring maternal plasma levels of several azo dyes after subcutaneous administration on the 9th day of pregnancy to Wistar rats. Trypan blue reached and maintained levels (15–18 mg%) 3 to 4 times those attained by other dyes (Niagara blue 2B and 4B, Afridol blue, Evans blue), among which certain variations in this property were noted (such as the time taken to reach maximum concentration). These findings suggested that differences in teratogenic potency of these and other azo dyes are due to their different rates of release from the subcutaneous injection site and rates of removal from the circulation.

Several azo dyes and 2 synthetic compounds resembling trypan blue in molecular structure were also found to be similar to trypan blue in distribution in rat maternal tissues (Beaudoin and Pickering 1960), yet were not teratogenic or were only slightly so. According to results of this study, a certain molecular configuration was necessary for teratogenicity. Yet a compound satisfying these requirements was not teratogenic (Christie 1965).

Although a purple fraction was found (Dijkstra and Gillman 1961) to be the most effective component of commercial trypan blue in stimulating the maternal reticuloendothelial system, Beck and Lloyd's (1963a) purple fraction was incapable of producing congenital malformations, while Barber and Geer's (1964) purple fraction was only mildly teratogenic.

On the other hand, dyes such as Evans blue and Niagara blue 4B were found to be mildly teratogenic but were not accumulated by the maternal reticuloendothelial system (Wilson 1955).

Protein metabolism. Trypan blue may produce congenital malformations by inducing the formation in the mother of abnormal serum proteins or altered relative proportions of normal serum proteins, which may lead to interference with maternal metabolic processes or may cross the placenta and interfere with embryonic development. Gillman *et al.* (1948) again took the lead when they implied that, since trypan blue is bound to albumin fractions of serum proteins, disturbance of maternal protein metabolism may be involved in the dye's teratogenic effects.

Serum electrophoretic patterns of adult rats injected on several successive days with trypan blue revealed the presence of an aberrant protein (Yamada 1959; Paoletti, Riou, and Truhaut 1962). It appeared within an hour after treatment, appeared more rapidly the higher the dose, increased with repeated injections, and persisted for about 10 days. However, it did not appear in mice treated similarly (Paoletti, Riou, and Truhaut 1962); nor were any protein fractions found in trypan blue-treated pregnant rats or in their offspring (Beaudoin and Kahkonen 1963), or in adult male rats (Christie 1964) that did not occur in control animals.

Altered concentrations of normal serum protein components were induced in trypan blue-treated animals, which have been extensively analyzed for the purpose of establishing their possible relation to teratogenesis. Studies with rabbits (Hommes 1959; Langman and Drunen 1959; Beaudoin and Ferm 1961) showed that trypan blue induced marked elevations in maternal serum α and β globulin quantities and reduction in albumin; and that to some extent parallel changes occurred in yolk-sac fluid (Hommes 1959; Beaudoin and Ferm 1961). Incidentally, marked increase of β globulins occurred in yolk-sac fluid regardless of the degree to which the fluid was stained by the dye (Beaudoin and Ferm 1961).

The effects of trypan blue on protein composition of maternal serum and yolk-sac fluid in rabbits were compared (Beaudoin and Ferm 1961) with those of 2 other azo dyes, Evans blue, which in rats was about one-third as teratogenic as trypan blue (Wilson 1955), and Niagara blue 2B, which was nonteratogenic (Wilson, Beaudoin, and Free 1959; Beaudoin and Pickering 1960) or only moderately so (Lloyd and Beck 1964*a*, *b*). It was found that while the mild teratogen Evans blue resulted in alterations in the protein fractions of the same sort and in the same direction as did trypan blue, the latter produced larger shifts from normal, especially in β globulin values. The nonteratogenic dye Niagara blue 2B, however, caused only slight changes from the control values (Beaudoin and Ferm 1961). A correlation was thus demonstrated between the degree of teratogenicity of these dyes and the degree of their effect on protein composition.

Studies were also made of alterations in blood proteins of trypan blue-treated rats, but these did not yield as clear-cut results as those from rabbits appeared to be. While a transient rise occurred in maternal β globulins during the days following treatment (Beaudoin 1963), at first no differences were noted (Kahkonen and Beaudoin 1963) in concentration of α, β, and γ globulins and albumin between trypan blue-treated and control late fetuses. A more definitive analysis (Beaudoin and Kakhonen 1963) revealed that the concentration of serum β and α-1 globulins and albumin in treated late fetuses was decreased, which was later confirmed (Beaudoin 1966). To Beaudoin and Kahkonen (1963) this suggested interference with the transport of maternal proteins to fetuses or abnormality of protein activity.

Some of the results discussed above may thus be suggestive of a causal relation between altered serum protein composition and teratogenesis. But other studies have thrown great doubt on the existence of such a relation. Treatment of pregnant rats with serum α and β globulins derived from trypan blue-treated pregnant rats did not cause malformations in the offspring (Beaudoin and Roberts 1965). The authors felt that current information suggested altered serum proteins to be secondary manifestations of effects of trypan blue on rats, perhaps resulting from interference with normal hepatic function.

In addition, several apparent contradictions recently uncovered by Beaudoin (1964) cast even graver doubts on the hypothesis that the teratogenic action of trypan blue can be explained by its effects on maternal protein composition. Wilson (1955) found that Congo red was not teratogenic; he gave 30 mg of the dye per injected animal, which is about 140 mg/kg body weight. This dose was also found to be ineffective by Beaudoin (1964), but a larger one (200 mg/kg) was teratogenic. Malformations were produced in a total of 15.4 per cent of offspring (38/247), of which 13 (5.3%) had hydronephrosis, 13 (5.3%) eye defects, and 12 (4.8%) hydrocephalus. Only 4 were multiply affected, all others having single malformations. No heart or skeletal defects were seen.

While Congo red thus resembled trypan blue in teratogenicity, it differed from it in several important respects. In molecular structure it is less like trypan blue than any of the other related teratogenic disazo dyes. Congo red, unlike trypan blue, could not be found in maternal macrophages or in epithelial cells of the yolk-sac placenta. And finally, maternal serum protein changes produced by trypan blue were not found after treatment with the teratogenic dose of Congo red (Beaudoin 1964).

Combined treatment. Studies on the combined effects of trypan blue and other substances or procedures may prove valuable in the search for understanding of mechanisms. In addition to those already discussed (e.g., thyroid factor), several other agents have been tried. Alizarin red S, reported to be nonteratogenic, may have enhanced the effect of trypan blue (Laurenson and Kropp 1959). The prior administration of the nonteratogenic or only mildly teratogenic dye Niagara blue 2B reduced the teratogenicity of trypan blue (Beaudoin 1962). Additive effects occurred when trypan blue was administered to fasted animals (Runner and Dagg 1960, Setokoesoemo and Gunberg 1966), and potentiation when it was given with vitamin A or 5-fluorouracil (Wilson 1964) or TSH (Beaudoin and Roberts 1966), even when subteratogenic doses of the dye were used. Others reported the same to be true after simultaneous treatment with cortisone, vitamin A, and trypan blue (Amano *et al.* 1964), and with vitamin A and trypan blue (Takekoshi 1964). Chin, Nelson, and Monie (1963) found that the effects of trypan blue combined with folic acid deficiency or chlorambucil injection were additive and only sometimes synergistic.

Placental Clogging

The second hypothesis of the action of trypan blue to be considered is that dye accumulates in the placenta interfering with the passage of necessary metabolites and nutrients to the embryo (Waddington and Carter 1953; Hamburgh 1954). Almost all investigators have agreed that although trypan blue does not appear to enter mouse or rat embryos themselves, it quickly becomes concentrated in the yolk sac, which in association with other structures probably forms the main channel of nutrition of the early embryo, before the appearance of the chorioallantoic placenta.

Wilson (1955) studied the distribution and effects of 14 azo dyes in near-term specimens. Four of them were found to be strongly or mildly teratogenic, trypan blue producing congenital malformations in 49 per cent of surviving offspring, Evans blue in 14 per cent, Niagara blue 4B in 4 per cent, and Niagara sky blue in 3 per cent. Fetuses contained none of these dyes, nor did the chorioallantoic part of the placenta accumulate any of them in appreciable amounts. On the other hand, large numbers of trypan blue granules were collected in the yolk-sac epithelium, and smaller amounts of the less teratogenic dyes were found at this location in quantities roughly proportional to their teratogenic activity.

A more precise approach, using C^{14}-labeled trypan blue (Wilson, Shepard, and Gennaro 1963), also demonstrated that dye did not enter embryonic tissues, but was apparently trapped in placental structures. By scintillation spectrometry high levels of radioactivity were found in the yolk-sac placenta and several maternal tissues one to 12 days after administration of the dye, but in contrast embryos contained very little activity. For purposes of more precise localization, a relatively pure fraction of highly radioactive trypan blue was prepared. By radioautography it was found, 2 days after treatment, that embryonic tissue and the amniotic and exocoelomic cavities contained scarcely more than background levels of radioactivity, whereas considerable activity was noted in trophoblast, decidua, and other uterine tissues. But the greatest activity always occurred in the visceral epithelium of the extra-embryonic yolk-sac placenta. The only conclusion permitted by these results was that it appeared unlikely that the teratogenic effects of trypan blue resulted from direct influence on the embryo, but on the contrary that it acted by inter-fering with some essential transport, nutritive, or protective mechanism, pro-duced by accumulation of dye in certain parts of the yolk sac.

The same conclusion can be drawn from the results of 2 more recent studies. Johnson and Chepenik (1966) noted that after exposure to tritiated uridine, trypan blue-treated proximal yolk sac of rats contained fewer grain counts than control tissues, i.e., incorporation of uridine was reduced by trypan blue. However, the cranial neural tube and other parts of trypan blue-treated embryos also contained fewer grains. Nebel and Hamburgh (1966) found evidence of decreased acid phosphatase and monoamine oxidase, but not of alkaline phosphatase, in the yolk-sac epithelium of embryos from trypan blue-injected pregnant mice.

A contradictory bit of evidence was discovered by Tuchmann-Duplessis and Mercier-Parot (1955), who noted that although azo blue was just as intensively collected in the embryonic adnexa as trypan blue, it was not teratogenic. A claim (Wilson 1954*a*) that azo blue was teratogenic was with-drawn (Wilson 1954*b*) when it was discovered that through an error of the manufacturer trypan blue had actually been supplied. These contradictions make it dangerous to decide either for or against the hypothesis of placental clogging at our present imperfect and fragmentary stage of knowledge.

Direct Action

It may be that direct action of the teratogen on the embryo is the answer to this problem. The evidence for this thesis will now be examined. It has been found, with one exception (Barber and Geer 1964), that although trypan blue collects in the yolk-sac epithelium of rat and mouse embryonic membranes, it does not enter the amnion, amniotic fluid, or embryonic tissues themselves (Everett 1935; Gillman *et al.* 1948; Murakami 1953; Waddington and Carter 1953; Hamburgh 1954; Wilson 1955; Barber 1957; Wilson, Beaudoin, and

Free 1959; Beaudoin and Pickering 1960; Kelly *et al.* 1964; Nebel and Hamburgh 1966). It would thus appear at first sight that direct action cannot explain the effects of trypan blue in these species.

In continuing, let us first turn to the question of the time of action of trypan blue during gestation, which may shed some light on the problem of the mechanism of the dye. As mentioned previously, if administered only during pregnancy, trypan blue did not induce congenital malformations when given later than about the 9th day of pregnancy in rats, rabbits, and mice; and the highest incidence of defects in rats was caused by treatment begun on about the 7th day.

Wilson, Beaudoin, and Free (1959) found that, regardless of when the dye was given to rats during the first 9 or 10 days of gestation, the pattern of malformations produced and the relative frequency of the components of the syndrome were the same, only the absolute incidence varying with the time of treatment. This constancy in the overall pattern of malformations suggested that the dye acts (or is permitted to act) only within a limited period of embryogenesis, since if this were not so the pattern of defects would change as different parts of the embryo reached susceptible phases of development. Such changes of pattern have been commonly observed following the application of numerous teratogens at different times during pregnancy (Kalter and Warkany 1959*a*).

Additional evidence (Wilson, Beaudoin, and Free 1959) for the idea that the dye acts only during a limited span of time came (1) from analysis of the parts malformed by trypan blue, which indicated that the dye is effective late on the 8th and perhaps early on the 9th day of gestation, at the time of early embryogenesis, since it is at this time that the affected parts are susceptible to damage; and (2) from the negative results produced by direct exposure of embryos to trypan blue by intrauterine injections prior to or at the time of implantation, which meant that embryos younger than 8 days were refractory to the teratogenic action of the dye.

Three questions are raised by these results. (1) Why, if the dye has no action before the 8th day, do treatments before this time produce defects? (2) Why does the incidence of defects decline the later treatment is made between the 7th and 9th days? (3) Why does the dye produce no defects after the 9th day?

The first question was definitely answered by Wilson, Beaudoin, and Free's (1959) study. They found that very high maternal-serum levels of trypan blue were reached soon after injection and that the level then fell rapidly but still remained moderately high for several days following treatment. After 2 to 3 days the rate of fall slowed and measurable quantities of dye were present even 4 to 5 months later. Similar results were obtained by Barber and Geer (1964) and Lloyd and Beck (1966).

Knowing these facts it is not surprising that malformations were produced by treatment even early in pregnancy, since circulating trypan blue continues to be present in the mother. It can also be understood why teratologic effectiveness steadily rises with later treatment between conception and the 7th day, since the later a course of short-term treatment is begun during this period the greater the concentration of dye when the embryos become susceptible.

The explanation for the declining incidence of malformations produced by treatment begun after the 7th day must take into consideration the fact that there is a cutoff in teratogenic action on the 9th day. Therefore no great maternal concentration of trypan blue can be built up in the relatively short interval before the cutoff occurs, and hence a decrease in teratologic effects results.

Another possible reason for this decline (Wilson, Beaudoin, and Free 1959) is that between the 7th and 9th days of gestation there is progressive growth of the visceral layer of the yolk-sac endoderm, whose possible capacity of absorbing and accumulating the dye and preventing it from reaching the embryo thus also continually increases.

Before we discuss the third question let us review the course of certain events in rabbits and contrast it with possible events in rats, mice, and perhaps hamsters.

The first evidence in support of the direct action theory was Ferm's (1956) finding that trypan blue (and Congo red) entered the yolk-sac fluid of rabbit blastocysts soon after injection of the mother. The permeability of rabbit blastocysts to trypan blue has been confirmed in several laboratories (Hommes 1959; Langman and Drunen 1959; Beaudoin and Ferm 1961). But it was noted that not all specimens of yolk-sac fluid were equally intensively stained; occasionally no apparent color was found, and in other cases the color varied from pale to deep blue (Beaudoin and Ferm 1961).

But trypan blue was found (Ferm 1956) in rabbit yolk-sac fluid only when injections were made up to the 9th day of pregnancy. The period of permeability thus corresponded, unpropitiously, with the time of differentiation and early embryogenesis, just when the conceptuses are most responsive to abnormal environmental influences.

When injected during the period of permeability dye entered the yolk-sac fluid within 2 hours of its administration (Ferm 1956) and apparently remained there for many days, since the contents of the yolk sac were still stained when females were sacrificed on the 28th day of pregnancy (Langman and Drunen 1959). I have not found an explicit statement as to whether trypan blue was deposited in the rabbit yolk-sac wall early in embryogenesis; but Evans blue, which like trypan blue entered the yolk-sac fluid, was not found in the wall at this time (Brambell and Hemmings 1949).

On the other hand, trypan blue injected into rabbits after the 9th day of pregnancy did not stain the blastocyst fluid nor was it taken up by the yolk-sac epithelium until injected on the 16th day (Ferm 1956); but, again, once stained this membrane retained the dye for many days (Langman and Drunen 1959).

It is fairly well agreed that, as with rabbits, the chorion, amnion, amniotic fluid, and embryos of rats and mice are not stained with trypan blue. But aside from this similarity the situation is somewhat different in rats and mice from rabbits, since (1) trypan blue did not appear to enter rat and mouse yolk-sac fluid even when treatment was made on the 7th day of gestation, but (2) did collect in the yolk-sac epithelium within a day or less of its administration (Waddington and Carter 1953; Wilson, Beaudoin, and Free 1959; Nebel and Hamburgh 1966), continued to be deposited, and persisted until term. As mentioned before, Wilson, Beaudoin, and Free (1959) intimated that trypan blue was not found in the yolk-sac fluid of rats because it may be actively absorbed from the fluid by the visceral yolk-sac epithelium.

To sum up, the difference in this regard between rabbits on the one hand and rats and mice on the other is that trypan blue enters the yolk-sac fluid in the former and probably not in the latter, and that the yolk-sac epithelium probably does not take up the dye in early pregnancy in the first but does in the others. But, despite these differences, trypan blue is teratogenic in all 3 species, and therefore this distribution of the dye may be of no fundamental importance at all.

We return now to the question of why, after the 9th day, trypan blue is not teratogenic in rats, and why, on the 9th day, the permeability of rabbit blastocysts to trypan blue ceases. Wilson, Beaudoin, and Free (1959) believed that the abrupt end of the teratogenic action of trypan blue in rats during the 9th day of gestation is related to the near completion at this time of the encirclement of the embryo by the visceral layer of yolk sac, after which trypan blue no longer has access to the embryo and fetus and is merely absorbed by and immobilized in the yolk endoderm.

Turbow's (1966) recent in vitro study supports this interpretation. Rat embryos (5–14 somites, 10–11 days), surrounded by the amnion and yolk sac, were explanted to plasma clots and incubated for 18 to 48 hours. Before incubation the embryos were treated essentially in the following manner. Trypan blue was injected into the yolk sac and the embryos were then immersed in trypan blue, or they were immersed in the dye but not injected. At all but the highest concentration of trypan blue, a larger incidence of certain anomalies (edema, enlarged pericardium, subectodermal blisters, etc.) occurred in the injected than in the uninjected embryos. However, the uninjected specimens in all series had a greater incidence of abnormalities than glucose-treated controls. While Turbow (1966) anticipated the criticism (Beck and Lloyd 1966, p. 185) that followed his preliminary note (Turbow 1965), by showing that an irritant (carbon) did not have the same effects as trypan blue, he did not gainsay Beck and Lloyd's objection that "the method does not distinguish clearly between a teratogenic action directly on the embryo and an indirect effect produced by interference with the yolk sac." Thus, it is still premature to agree with Turbow's (1965) conclusion that his results show that "trypan blue has a direct teratogenic effect on the rat embryo."

Ferm (1956) offered 2 possible explanations for the situation in rabbits. The first is that during the 9th day the yolk-sac splanchnopleure develops selective and absorptive functions that permit the removal of foreign substances from the yolk-sac fluid. This possibility was not sustained, since after injection of the dye on the 10th and later days of pregnancy, the earliest it could be visually detected in the endoderm cells of the developing splanchnopleure, where the dye would accumulate if such an absorptive function were operating, was the 16th day of gestation. This possibility was therefore considered untenable.

The other explanation offered, but not substantiated, is that changes in permeability occur when the early histiotrophic phase of embryonic nutrition gives way to the definitive hemotrophic phase. This shift occurs in the rabbit on the 9th day of gestation when embryonic trophoblasts first make contact with maternal blood. Beginning at this time embryonic tissue may therefore be more selective of what it admits to its environment (Ferm 1956).

What is left unexplained is that rabbit blastocysts were also permeable to nonteratogenic azo dyes. After injection of the mother with Evans blue (Brambell and Hemmings 1949; Beaudoin and Ferm 1961) and Niagara blue 2B (Beaudoin and Ferm 1961) these dyes, too, were found in yolk-sac fluid. Nevertheless, the possibility must continue to be entertained that trypan blue is toxic, whereas these other dyes are not, despite their all being alike in approaching the embryo itself.

5

Ionizing Radiation

Introduction

Numerous experimental studies have been made of the effects of ionizing radiation on prenatal development of mammals. Beginning soon after the turn of the century with those of Hippel (1907) and Hippel and Pagenstecher (1907) on the rabbit eye, the experiments have continued to be of utmost interest and importance.

Most of the work done before the 1930's was poorly controlled, especially from the standpoints of dosimetry and timing of pregnancies. Thus, although the older efforts are of historical moment, they seldom contributed information that can be correlated with the data of more recent work. Furthermore, gross congenital malformations of the central nervous system were seldom seen in them. The comprehensive summary by L. B. Russell (1954) of the voluminous literature on the subject up to 1952 may be consulted for aspects that are not relevant here. Many early studies were also cited by Job, Leibold, and Fitzmaurice (1935).

In what may be the first experimental study in which congenital defects of the mammalian central nervous system were produced by irradiation, Hanson (1923), giving "the proper dosage" of X rays to female rats "in later stages of pregnancy," found one or more young with changes in the shape and reduction in size of the skull. Nobele and Lams (1927) irradiated rat and guinea pig embryos; some of the latter developed hydrocephalus postnatally. The studies of Kosaka, with mice (1927, 1928*a*), rats (1928*b*), guinea pigs (1928*c*), and rabbits (1928*d*), though careful and extensive, and apparently made for the purpose of defining prenatal susceptibility to radiation according to gestational stage, did not contribute much to the construction of such relations. Kosaka, in fact, according at least to the summaries in German following his Japanese papers (1928*a*, *b*, *c*, *d*), found no gross congenital malformation of the central nervous system, although histological damage of many organs, especially of the brain and spinal cord, occurred. The one possible exception was a case of microcephaly in rabbits (Kosaka 1928*d*).

General Survey
Rats

The story of X-ray teratogenesis starts with the work of Job, Leibold, and Fitzmaurice (1935) whose importance lies in the fact that they were apparently the first to realize the significance of knowing precisely what dose of X rays was being used and what age embryos were being irradiated. It is understandable, of course, that the earlier radiation workers should have had difficulty controlling dosage, but an even more serious shortcoming of their work was their not appreciating the importance of gestational stage and their consequent failure to time pregnancy carefully or, in some cases, at all.

Job, Leibold, and Fitzmaurice's (1935) animals (albino stock rats) were either unusually sensitive to the lethal effects of X rays, or to irradiation combined with being laparotomized twice during pregnancy, since doses greater than 95 r killed all offspring if administered during the first 18 days of pregnancy. In other series of experiments, females were exposed to single doses of less than 90 r on the 1st to 18th days of pregnancy. Only gross malformations were scored, and young with such defects were obtained only from females given 36 to 90 r on the 9th to 11th days of pregnancy; these had 175 offspring, of whom 75 were malformed. The females were allowed to deliver and the young to live to at least 40 days to ensure certainty of the diagnosis of defectiveness. Presumably, therefore, the offspring were not severely deformed, which is compatible with the relatively small doses of X rays they received. The abnormalities consisted of unspecified eye defects occurring alone or in combination with hydrocephalus and jaw defects. Hydrocephalus, which occurred in 17 cases, was apparently produced only by irradiation on the 9th day of pregnancy. No gross or microscopic description of any defect was given.

The next study with rats was that of Warkany and Schraffenberger (1947), who exposed Sprague–Dawley female rats to single doses of 190 to 950 r of X rays on the 10th to 16th days of gestation. In distinction to Job, Leibold, and Fitzmaurice's (1935) animals, which were all killed by doses greater than 95 r, and hence were apparently extraordinarily sensitive, those of Warkany and Schraffenberger (1947) were unusually resistant, since even as much (in 1 pregnancy) as 1120 r did not destroy all the young. This resistance may have been due, at least in part, to the females' receiving saline immediately after treatment.

Irradiation on the 10th day produced "defects of the skull and the skin of the head with partial protrusion of the brain," i.e., encephalocele, in 7/44 offspring (15.9%). This defect also occurred after treatment on the 12th and 13th days (16/54 = 29.6%, and 19/249 = 9.1%, respectively), but no externally recognizable defects of the central nervous system were found after irradiation on the 11th, 14th, 15th, or 16th day. Serial sections of an offspring with encephalocele showed deformity of the brainstem, atrophy of the cerebral cortex, and enlargement of the lateral ventricles, in addition to upward bulging of the brain through a hole in the top of the cranium against the thinned skin above it. A large number of affected offspring were cleared for visualization of the skeleton and many found with various degrees of defects of ossification of the skull. Most commonly involved were areas of the parietal, frontal, and interparietal bones.

Warkany and Schraffenberger (1947) did not usually relate the embryonic effects seen with the different doses of X rays used. L. B. Russell (1954) believed that the large doses given probably blurred the specificity of responses expected from treatment of different stages of gestation. But even so, the fact that the largest incidence of encephalocele occurred after treatment on the 12th day may indicate that this is a time of maximal susceptibility so far as development of certain structural attributes of the brain is concerned.

Wilson and coworkers irradiated pregnant Wistar rats on the 9th (Wilson, Brent, and Jordan 1953), 10th (Wilson, Jordan, and Brent 1953), 11th (Wilson and Karr 1951), and 12th (Wilson 1954*d*) days of pregnancy with single doses of 12.5 to 600 r of X rays. The pregnant females were laparotomized and 2 to 5 implantation sites in the same uterine horn were selected for irradiation. The other sites were lead-shielded and formed the nonirradiated controls. The females were killed at various 24-hour intervals after irradiation; the offspring were removed and thoroughly examined grossly and in serial sections for malformations. No malformations were found after irradiation on the 9th day with as much as 200 r (Wilson, Brent, and Jordan 1953), but following irradiation on the 10th or 11th day numerous defects occurred. Offspring irradiated on the 10th day of gestation (Wilson, Jordan, and Brent 1953) were examined 2 to 8 days after treatment and at term. A total of 40 instances (out of 166) of maldevelopment of the brain was seen in the groups given more that 25 r (50, 100, and 200 r), and the incidence was directly related to dosage (5.0, 27.4, and 77.8 %, respectively).

In the majority of cases (24/40) there was abnormal proximity or union of the brainwall and overlying ectoderm, with associated reduction or absence of the intervening mesoderm and vascular tissue. This abnormality was manifested as early as 2 days after irradiation. After this time the conjoined areas tended to become thinned and hypoplastic. By 5 days after irradiation abnormal areas bulged outward from the surface of the head, appearing, when the condition was localized in extent, as bubble-like elevations. When the defect involved a larger part of the brainwall the result was internal hydrocephalus, although histological examination usually revealed no obstruction at any point in the lumen of the neural tube. Many of the attenuated areas subsequently ruptured, and the fused portions of brain and ectoderm were everted to the exterior. Adjacent normal areas partook in this eversion and thus sometimes the process ended in the major part of the brain being herniated and in becoming distorted and undergoing degenerative changes. Had such affected offspring survived to term they would probably have had what is usually called anencephaly.

Although such defects were frequently found in fetuses, only 1/51 term offspring showed a brain abnormality ascribable to fusion of the brainwall with ectoderm, probably indicating that the majority of affected animals died prenatally. In the survivor the defect consisted of a localized, open lesion containing an elevated mass of disorganized brain tissue over the center of the cranium. Another term offspring showed a small elevated area on the head, dissection of which revealed apparently normal skin covering a localized protrusion of meninges and brain tissue through a skull defect, i.e., true meningoencephalocele. This defect apparently resulted from protrusion of a diverticulum of the brainwall toward the ectoderm; and in fact 5 embryos were observed in which this situation occurred, i.e., in which a localized area of the brainwall bulged outward from the general surface of the brain but remained separated from the ectoderm by mesodermal tissues of variable thickness. The encephaloceles found by Kaven (1938a), Warkany and Schraffenberger (1947), and Russell (1950) in their irradiated material were very likely the outcome of processes similar to those described by Wilson, Jordan, and Brent (1953).

Other abnormalities of the brain found (Wilson, Jordan, and Brent 1953) after irradiation on the 10th day were infrequent and less sharply defined than those described above. Such defects were the only types of malformation of the central nervous system produced by irradiating on the 11th day (Wilson and Karr 1951). Primarily they consisted of defects of the forebrain involving abnormalities of size, shape, and symmetry of the telencephalic lobes, and hypoplasia usually in localized regions of the forebrain, especially the telencephalon. As development progressed, these regions of deficient growth resulted in distortions of shape and size that affected not only the original site but adjacent portions of the brain as well (Wilson, Jordan, and Brent 1953).

Irradiation on the 10th day also produced malformations of the spinal cord (Wilson, Jordan, and Brent 1953). These defects were found in 23/101 embryos and fetuses examined, and like brain abnormalities their incidence increased with greater dosage ($1/32 = 3.1\%$ after 50 r, $16/60 = 26.7\%$ after 100 r, and $6/9 = 66.7\%$ after 200 r). But no animals so affected survived to term. All the spinal defects consisted of or appeared to result from anomalous outgrowths from the lateral wall of the cord, which varied in extent from mere circumscribed elevations to gross lateral displacements. In older embryos skeletal elements and spinal ganglia and nerves in the affected region were frequently deficient or distorted. No affected animal was found later than 6 days after irradiation, and hence the outcome of these anomalies is not known. Whether the spinal defects in mice reported by Russell (1950), Auerbach (1956), and Dagg (1963–64) resulted from such processes cannot be said.

Malformations of the central nervous system produced by irradiation on the 12th day (Wilson 1954*d*) consisted solely of eversion of the choroid plexuses and other minor distortions and did not occur after treatment with less than 200 r.

These investigations by Wilson, Karr, Brent, and Jordan, in which numerous malformations in addition to the ones discussed, such as those of the eye and cardiovascular and urogenital systems, etc., were induced by X irradiation, are the first in which exhaustive histological and embryological studies were made of the internal defects produced by this teratogen.

A survey of the effects of X irradiation on the development of the central nervous system of rats was made by Hicks (1953). Rats derived from Wistar and Sloniker stocks were given single doses of 100 to 400 r on the 1st to 21st days of pregnancy. Young were usually observed at term, but some fetuses were also examined. No developmental abnormalities were found in offspring irradiated during the first 9 days of pregnancy, thus confirming Russell's (1950) results from preimplantation irradiation of mice and Job, Leibold, and Fitzmaurice's (1935) and Wilson, Brent, and Jordan's (1953) studies of irradiation during early gestation in rats.

Hicks (1953) described the morphological effects of irradiation on the 10th and later days of pregnancy in some detail but usually neglected quantitative aspects. E.g., he seldom stated the number of females irradiated, the total number of offspring observed, and the doses that specific litters received, so that no incidences of malformations can be determined or relations drawn between dosage and severity or frequency of deformity.

Even for treatment on the 10th day, about which the most information was given, the data are incomplete. Seven litters were irradiated with 50, 100, or 150 r at this time in gestation. The members of one litter (number of young unstated), given 150 r and examined at term, all showed a severe deformity of the head, consisting of the components above the maxilla all being abortively formed or absent, i.e., "anencephaly." Those of a second litter (dosage administered not stated), removed on the 16th day of gestation, were also all (? number) anencephalic. A third litter, given 100 r, had lesser degrees of brain defect, and 4 other litters showed no defects of the brain. The dose given these last 4 litters was not stated, but it may have been 50 r. Hicks (1953) believed that the range of defects seen was caused by irradiating embryos of slightly different developmental stages, since the type and degree of malformation produced depends primarily on the radiosensitivity of the embryo, which waxes and wanes with increasing maturity. But since no statement to the contrary was made it may be that the unaffected and less affected young received one of the smaller doses of X rays used.

The specific doses given on later days of gestation and the number of young obtained after these treatments were also not usually stated, the report of these results being restricted to a general description of the defects produced. After irradiation on the 11th day there occurred severe defects of dorsal and anterior portions of the forebrain with corresponding failure of development of vertical portions of the parietal bones, the result being a degree of encephalocele. Irradiation on the 12th day caused hydrocephalus and narrowing of the aqueduct proximal to the 3rd ventricle, which were associated in 4 litters; but the total number of litters irradiated on this day and the number of young in which one, the other, or both of these abnormalities did not occur was not mentioned. In hydrocephalus, the lateral ventricles were especially affected, but the 3rd ventricle was also sometimes dilated. The cortex and underlying white matter were thinner than normal and the hippocampus, except most laterally and caudally, was virtually unformed; but the deficiency in substance of the hemispheres alone did not account for the dilated ventricles. There was no intrinsic malformation of the aqueduct. Sometimes the ependymal cells were closely approximated, but in other cases the iter was open.

The occasional association of hydrocephalus and narrow aqueduct seemed to indicate a causal relation. More recently, however, Hicks (1958) remarked that various degrees of hydrocephalus and narrow aqueduct may each occur in the absence of the other; hence the relation, if any, is unclear. The state of the 4th ventricle was not mentioned. Defects of the spinal column occurred in the sacral region, but gross defects of the cord itself were apparently not noted. In a later study (Hicks, Brown, and D'Amato 1957), the principal neural defect found after irradiation on the 12th day with 200 r was dorsal encephalocele or ventriculocele, which was due to outpocketing of the tela chorioidea at the junction of the 3rd and lateral ventricles. This defect and other abnormalities of the brain were described in detail.

Continuing with the results of the survey study (Hicks 1953), treatment on the 13th or later days apparently produced no externally observable defects of the central nervous system. Irradiation on the 13th day caused a much milder hydrocephalus than after the 12th day; the condition of the aqueduct in these cases was not mentioned. In addition there occurred different degrees of skin-covered encephalocele involving the posterior cerebral hemispheres. This defect resembled the markedly defective pattern produced in some animals by earlier treatment, but it was situated more caudally. Also produced by irradiation on the 13th day were various grades of distortion of the brain. The olfactory and frontal cortexes were jumbled. Periventricular regions, especially around the lateral ventricles, contained large rosettes, some of which had sizeable cavities, which occasionally connected with the main ventricle. This condition was called "porencephaly." Superiorly and anteriorly the hippocampus was almost completely absent. Absence of the corpus callosum resulted from treatment on any one of the 12th to 20th days, although irradiation at later times or with lower doses did not completely prevent the development of this part. Similarly, irradiation during the fetal period produced other, relatively nonspecific, types of brain damage. Defects of the brain caused by treatment on the 14th day consisted largely of severe malformations of the striatum, its junction with the medial cerebral cortex, and the hippocampus. These areas were the sites of numerous rosettes and completely jumbled architecture. With the corpus callosum absent, the striatum, anterodorsal hippocampal region, and cingular cortex formed a continuum of striatum-like cell masses with some fiber bundles. Anteriorly the result was fusion of hemispheric areas that are normally separate.

Similar patterns resulted from irradiation on the 15th and 16th days, but primarily involved the striatum, dorsal cerebrum, and hippocampus. Defects produced by treatment on the 17th day consisted more of architectural abnormalities and less of gross derangement of parts. Irradiation on the 18th to 22nd days produced damage of the cerebellum, of increasing degree as term was approached, being reflected chiefly in coarsening of the folia and deficiencies of the granular layers. Cortical and striatal damage toward term and after birth were less dramatic, but still severe when large doses of radiation were given.

Apparently being dissatisfied with the rather poor correlation between embryonic stage irradiated and resulting malformations, Hicks (1954a) attempted to devise a means of strengthening it. In order to know exactly what stage of development was irradiated, he removed some embryos at various times, beginning at about 4 hours after treatment on the 10th, 11th and 12th days of gestation. Making the tacit, and perhaps unwarranted, assumption that all littermates were at the same stage of development as those removed earliest, a timetable of susceptibility was constructed.

Hicks (1954a) believed the results firmly established the following relations. Anencephaly resulted from irradiation on the 10th day at a stage in the rat embryo immediately before somite formation, when the neural plate is just being formed anteriorly. Irradiation still during the 10th day, but of embryos with 1 or 2 somites, produced less severe malformations of the forebrain. Treatment of 11th-day, 4- to 7-somite embryos produced defects limited essentially to the eyes, despite widespread destruction of differentiating cells in neural tissue. Irradiation at the 8- to 10-somite stage, still on the 11th day, sometimes produced dorsal enlargement of the interventricular foramen at its junction with the 3rd ventricle, which increased after treatment of 14-somite young. This timetable, extended to include older stages, was summarized in a review article (Hicks 1958).

Even in the relatively few embryos examined, Hicks (1954a) found some variation in somite number from litter to litter of the same apparent chronological age, and even some overlap among embryos of different ages. This sort of variability was expected, of course, and his aim, by such a study, was to eliminate the confusion it causes. However, he neglected considering an equally prevalent and equally potent source of confusion: intralitter variability in somite number, i.e., variability of developmental age among embryos within the same uterus, which, as Allen and MacDowell (1940) showed for mice, may be quite great.

Detailed descriptions of the histological pattern of defects produced by irradiation with 150 to 200 r on the 12th and later days and of their histogenesis were reported (Hicks, D'Amato, and Lowe 1959). More recently, effects of irradiating middle and late fetal stages with relatively low doses (10–40 r) were studied (Hicks and D'Amato 1963a; D'Amato and Hicks 1965).

Murphy, Moro, and Lacon (1958) irradiated Wistar rats on the 13th day of pregnancy. The absolute dosages used were not specified, but it was established that 250 r of X rays were lethal to a majority of fetuses of 50 per cent of litters. Smaller doses produced encephalocele in 4/39 fetuses examined and greater doses produced the defect in all (14/14) examined. The defect occurred in various degrees of severity and was located in the occipital region. In skeletal preparations of young with encephalocele, gross skull abnormalities consisted of a circular defect involving parietal, interparietal, supraoccipital, and occipital bones. Bone anomalies often occurred in the absence of any detectable gross abnormality of the head. This was also true of Warkany and Schraffenberger's (1947) cleared specimens.

Anencephaly was produced in Wistar rats by X irradiating with 200 r on the 9th or 10th day and hydrocephalus by treating on the 12th day (Okano *et al.* 1957). Encephalocele was found after irradiation of Sprague–Dawley rats with 220 r on the 12th day of gestation (Murphree and Pace 1960). Hydrocephalus was the predominant defect (81 %) in offspring of Wistar rats exposed on the 12th day of pregnancy to 270 r from a radiocobalt source (Skalko 1965). The neuropathology of exencephaly induced in Wistar rats by X irradiation with 150 r on the 9th or 10th day of gestation was analyzed by means of electron microscopy (Roizin, Rugh, and Kaufman 1962).

Mice

One of the first radiation-teratology studies was made with mice, and already utilized one of the advantages mice possess—the existence of genetically homogeneous stocks of animals, i.e., inbred strains. Kaven's (1938a, b) studies were made with an inbred strain of albino mice obtained from Agnes Bluhm. Another novelty he practiced—the collection of a large control group—is still far from universally emulated.

One experiment (Kaven 1938a) consisted of a survey of the results of irradiating females on each day of the last two-thirds of pregnancy (8th–20th days) and the other (Kaven 1938b) was a more intense exploration of the effects of irradiating on the 8th or 9th day. In both studies pregnant females were exposed once to 200 r (178 r at the level of the embryo or fetus). In the first, all females delivered and the young were allowed to live; in the second, females were killed on the 14th to 20th days or allowed to deliver.

The survey study (Kaven 1938a) clearly revealed that different malformations are produced by irradiating at different times during pregnancy. Of the defects of interest here, meningocele and exencephaly (called "extrakranielle Dysencephalie") were produced by irradiation on the 9th day, "skull malformation" on the 11th day, and hydrocephalus on the 11th, 13th, and 14th days. Kaven failed to state the total number of offspring treated at particular times, so the incidence of the defects cannot be accurately determined; but the frequency of hydrocephalus was highest (about 10%) after irradiation on the 13th day. The hydrocephalus became apparent a few days after birth, and in animals reaching about 2 weeks of age symptoms of paralysis and disturbances of balance were displayed. Some histological investigations of this abnormality seem to have been made, as evidenced by the transverse section illustrated, but the hydrocephalus was only briefly and incompletely described.

In the study (Kaven 1938b) concentrating on the effects of irradiating on the 8th or 9th day, 2 types of malformation were produced—exencephaly and milder herniations (cranial meningocele and meningoencephalocele). The data scattered throughout this report on the incidence of these defects demonstrated several points. (1) 8th-day embryos are less susceptible to exencephaly than 9th-day ones, as determined by examination of young fetuses (12/72 = 16.7% vs. 4/81 = 4.9%). (2) But no exencephalic young were found at term, and it thus appeared that all with this defect died prenatally. (3) The incidence of milder herniations, on the contrary, usually increased with advancing pregnancy, so that a larger proportion of newborn showed these anomalies than did young fetuses. The difference in frequency of encephaloceles induced by irradiation on the 8th or 9th day was not great when observed in late fetal life (8th vs. 9th day: 9/51 = 17.3% vs. 32/117 = 19.7%), though a large difference was found at birth (8th vs. 9th day: 4/166 = 2.4% vs. 35/219 = 16.1%).

It appears that exencephaly was manifested early in pregnancy and then caused or was associated with death so that no young so affected were among those allowed to come to term. Meningocele and meningoencephalocele, on the other hand, first appeared relatively late in pregnancy (17th day), and then sometimes also decreased in frequency. Kaven considered the possibility that fewer animals with milder herniations and none with exencephaly were found among newborn young because they were eaten by the mothers—not an unusual fate for malformed mice.

In her definitive studies, Russell (1950), like Kaven, used genetically defined mice: C57BL strain females crossed to NB strain males; the irradiated young were thus F_1 hybrids and therefore both genetically uniform and vigorous. Females were exposed once to 100, 200, 300, or 400 r of X rays on the 1st to 16th days of pregnancy. In a pilot study, 200 r was found to give optimal results for a general survey of developmental sensitivity, since it did not greatly increase prenatal mortality and caused fairly specific gestation stage-related malformations. Most females were allowed to come to term; some were killed several days before delivery.

External and gross visceral malformations were scored. Only abnormalities or probable abnormalities of the central nervous system will be discussed here. There were not many different types of them. One was "dome-shaped" head, in which the profile showed an abrupt rise beginning anterior to the eye region to reach what was described as a vaulted cranium. The nasal region appeared short and slightly turned up. The underlying skeletal defects consisted of vaulting of the frontals and a variety of probably correlated changes. Whether the brain proper was also defective cannot be said, since no histological studies were made, but from the description of the external appearance of the head hydrocephalus may have been present. With 200 r domed head was produced only by 10th-day irradiation (18/33 = 54.5%). 300 r increased the frequency (8/10) when given on the 10th day and also induced the defect, but less often (3/22 = 13.6%), when given on the 11th day.

Another defect was "cranial blisters." These were slightly elevated areas, sometimes accompanied by hemorrhages in the immediately overlying or adjacent skin, occurring bilaterally, unilaterally, or centrally, in the frontal or parietal area. In all cases skeletal study revealed large median gaps in the roof of the cranium. The blisters thus probably represented localized herniations of the brain directly beneath the skin, i.e., small encephaloceles. This condition did not occur after irradiation with 200 r but was found in all offspring treated with 300 r on the 10th or 11th day (8/8 and 22/22, respectively).

One exencephaly (in 26 young) occurred after irradiation on the 8th day of gestation. The broadly protruding, naked brain resembled Kaven's cases of "extrakranielle Dysencephalie." The affected offspring was apparently accompanied by an excess of amniotic fluid, which was blood stained. Kaven produced this defect by irradiating with a similar dose also on the 8th day.

The final malformation of the central nervous system observed by Russell (1950) was spina bifida. It was produced by irradiating on the 10th day of gestation and occurred in 12/33 young (36.4%) with 200 r and 4/8 (50%) with 300 r (88% if based on skeletal diagnosis). In most cases it was in an occult form, being manifested only by a hole or cleft in the lumbosacral region of the vertebral column; but in 7/12 and 1/4 abnormal young from treatment with 200 r and 300 r respectively, the defect of the vertebral column was accompanied by spinal cord herniation, forming a round or slightly elongated subcutaneous hemorrhagic blister. The accompanying skeletal defects were described in a later publication (Russell 1956). Many of Russell's

(1950) results were extended and confirmed more recently (Russell, Badgett, and Saylors 1960); in the latter study, in which 10th-day, genetically heterogeneous embryos were exposed to about 200 r of X rays, the frequency of spina bifida (all occulta) was 25 per cent.

Auerbach (1956) studied the effect on spinal column development of X irradiation on the 10th day of gestation with 300 r given in single exposures or in 3 fractions each of 100 r at 30-minute intervals. He crossed strain 101 female mice to C3H males, and thus also irradiated F_1 hybrid, but genetically uniform, embryos. The offspring were examined 3 to 6 days after treatment. The spinal defect produced was located in the lumbosacral region and consisted of disorientation of the neural tube and somites resulting in neural arch malformation. To what extent, if any, the spinal cord was bifidous, either occult or apert, was not reported; the method of examination of the fetuses was not clearly indicated.

While the total incidence of spinal malformation was not affected by fractionation of the radiation (93/105 = 88.6% abnormal after single exposure vs. 68/80 = 85.0% after fractionated treatment), the proportion of severely affected offspring was increased by the multiple form of exposure (3/105 = 2.9% vs. 51/80 = 63.8%), severity being scored by length of anteroposterior axis affected. An increase in extent of deformity with fractionation also occurred for eye defects (coloboma, presumably of the iris).

Microscopic examination of the lumbosacral region at different stages (Auerbach 1955) indicated a close relation of abnormal development of ganglionic, cartilaginous, and muscular elements to somite disorientation, which, in turn, seemed causally related to malformation and degeneration of the neural tube.

The production of spina bifida in mice was briefly reported by Dagg (1963–64). C57BL/Ks mice, in which the defect occurs spontaneously only rarely, were irradiated on the 10th day of gestation. After 125 r, 4 per cent of surviving fetuses showed the abnormality, and after 175 r its incidence was 51 per cent. Grossly the defect appeared as a swelling in the sacral region. Microscopically it was revealed to be a myelomeningocele.

Various studies of the effects of irradiating inbred mouse embryos of the ddN strain were made in the laboratory of Murakami. In earlier studies (Murakami and Kameyama 1958; Kameyama 1959) mice were irradiated once with 25, 50, 100, or 150 r of X rays on the 8th day of pregnancy and examined, usually externally, on the 13th day. The malformations, whose frequency and severity were proportional to dosage, included several of the central nervous system: hydrocephalus, encephalocele, exencephaly, and spinal cord defects.

Hydrocephalus ranged from 26.2 per cent (37/141) and 26.1 per cent (35/134) after 150 and 100 r, respectively, to 5.4 per cent (8/147) and 1.4 per cent (2/138) after 50 and 25 r, respectively. In mice treated with the smaller doses the condition was slight and only detectable microscopically. The hydrocephalus was not described. In the group treated with 150 r there was, in addition, marked fusion of the bilateral telencephalon, resembling the types of defects found in later studies (Murakami *et al.* 1962), which are discussed below.

Encephalocele varied from 20.6 per cent (29/141) and 19.4 per cent (26/134) after 150 and 100 r, respectively, to 6.1 per cent (9/147) and 0 per cent (0/138) after 50 and 25 r, respectively. Various degrees of the condition occurred, but always in the region of the mesencephalon. Less marked lesions, seen in embryos that received 50 and 25 r, appeared as small elevations on top of the brain. In those treated with 150 and 100 r the mesencephalon bulged outwardly. When these maldevelopments were severe the brain burst outwards and sometimes was partly everted. Even in slight hernia, dilatation of ventricles and proliferation of ependymal elements were recognizable.

Exencephaly occurred only rarely (9/275 = 3.3%, after 150 or 100 r). The defect consisted of eversion of the brain in the region of the mesencephalon exposing its internal surface. The ependymal layer originally lining the ventricle was laden with rosette formations. Some other fetuses were microcephalic or oxycephalic. In most cases the telencephalon was asymmetric.

Various abnormalities of the spinal cord were noted. Among the less questionable of these were 2 small myeloceles in the lumbar region, in young given 150 r. This appears to contradict Russell's (1950) results, since she found spina bifida of any type in the mouse only after irradiation on the 10th day. Other spinal cord defects, such as curvature and distention, which were found quite frequently, may have been artifacts following postirradiation embryonic death. The development and transformation of these anomalies in later fetal life were investigated by Murakami, Kameyama, and Majima (1960), and further descriptions of some of these defects given by Majima (1961, 1962).

In a later study, Murakami *et al.* (1961) irradiated pregnant mice with 200 r on the 8th, 9th, 10th, or 11th day of gestation and examined the off-spring from the 13th to 19th days. Malformations of the central nervous system were found after irradiation at all 4 times, but considerable overlap occurred, i.e., similar defects were produced by treatment on different days. Exencephaly was produced by irradiation on the 8th and 9th days (4.5 and 2.0%, respectively), hydrocephalus on all 4 days (3.0, 4.0, 31.2, and 22.0%, respectively), and defects associated with univentricular telencephalon on the 9th to 11th days (31.6, 6.2, and 1.2% respectively). The latter will be discussed below. Other defects included abnormally-shaped head, due to encephalocele and rosette formation, microcephaly, and spinal cord defects, among which were spina bifida, diplomyelia, and other myelodysplasias. The same apparent nonspecificity of response was found in a subsequent study (Murakami, Kameyama, and Nogami 1963), in which several dosages were given on the 8th to 13th days.

Malformations associated with univentricular telencephalon were most frequent after irradiation on the 9th day (Murakami *et al.* 1961; Murakami, Kameyama, and Nogami 1963). For purposes of description, they were classified into 3 groups (Murakami *et al.* 1962). The first, comprising the most severe defects, was represented by an apparently univentricular telencephalon. The condition was externally diagnosable because of its association with a beaklike appearance of the snout. The position of the eyes was also unusual, since they were closer together than normal. One of the extreme cases had a rudimentary eye; the authors believed this to resemble cyclopia, but no true instance of the latter was found. The second group of malformations, thought to represent transitional conditions, was characterized by reduction of the cranium without severe effect on laterality of the ventricles. The abnormal shape of the telencephalon, appearing like a pair of cones with a common base, could be seen through the skin. The snout resembled that of the first group, but was less pointed. The eyes were also shifted toward the midline. In the third group the telencephalon appeared almost normal. The snout was like that of the second group, but in some cases the nostrils were fused. Abnormalities of the snout and nostrils were also found by Russell (1950), occurring most frequently after irradiation on the 9th day of pregnancy with 200 r.

In several cases (Murakami *et al.* 1962) chosen at random from the second and third groups for microscopic examination, the ventricles were found to be incompletely separated, being connected by bilateral interventricular foramens. These remained very broad even in later stages of fetal life. Part of the telencephalon sometimes contained a single cavity, suggesting a transitional state approaching the univentricular telencephalic defect. The authors believed these 3 types of defects resembled the cyclopia-arhinencephaly-otocephaly class of malformations occurring in human beings and other animals. Cyclocephalic defects and abnormalities of the rhinencephalon in mice after irradiation early in pregnancy were also reported, in brief communications, by Degenhardt (1963, and cited by Lund 1966), and Giroud *et al.* (1965, 1966).

Another survey experiment of the effects of X irradiating mice at different times during gestation was made by Kriegel, Langendorff, and Shibata (1962). Females of a local inbred strain of mice were given single whole body exposures of 200 r on the 6th to 16th days of pregnancy. Apparently, only externally visible abnormalities were studied. After treatment on the 6th day of gestation 2.7 per cent (5/183) abnormal young were found, the abnormalities being of the same types as some noted in control offspring, but the latter were somewhat less often affected (6/966 = 0.6%).

Various malformations of the central nervous system were produced by later irradiation. Treatment on the 7th day produced relatively small protruberances in the area of the forebrain in 2/188 (1.7%) offspring;

exposure on the 8th day resulted in various grades of encephalocele and mild exencephaly in 11/54 (20.4%), and severe exencephaly and sometimes almost total destruction of the entire head above the maxilla, called acrania and hemicrania, in 93/174 (53.4%); and irradiation on the 9th day caused noticeable "dysencephaly" (encephalocele, apparently) in 22/291 (7.6%). Minute elevations over the brain occurred after treatment on the 10th or 11th day in 17.4 and 44.9 per cent (12/69 and 62/138) of offspring, respectively. Irradiation on the 12th, 13th, or 14th day produced no external malformation of the central nervous system.

Pregnant mice were also X irradiated on the 6th or 9th day with a range of doses from 50 to 400 r (Kriegel, Langendorff, and Shibata 1962). Irradiation on the 6th day with 200 r or less did not increase the malformation rate over that found in controls. Larger doses produced exencephaly of various degrees, absence of much of the head above the tongue (hemicrania), and in one case (given 400 r) hydrocephalus. Anomalies of the spinal column were restricted to curvatures (kyphosis). Total abnormal offspring treated on the 6th day with 250 to 400 r comprised 37/248 (14.9%); 12 (4.8%) had abnormalities of the brain, and 6 (2.4%) abnormalities of the spinal column. Treatment on the 9th day was effective beginning with 100 r, producing 6/125 (4.8%) with encephalocele in the region of the forebrain. With 175 r rhinencephalic defects as well as brain hernias occurred (18/77 = 23.4%). Very few young survived 250 r and none 325 or 400 r. No defects of the spinal column were found after irradiation on the 9th day. The article by Kriegel, Langendorff, and Kunick (1962) appeared to contain nothing not already reported by Kriegel, Langendorff, and Shibata (1962).

Rugh and coworkers used exencephaly as the end-point in investigating the effects of fetal X irradiation. Female CF1 mice were exposed once to doses of 25 to 300 r at 12-hour intervals from the 7th to 10th days of pregnancy and killed near term (Rugh and Grupp 1959*a*). Exencephaly was induced, usually in low incidences, at each of these times except late on the 10th day and with all the different dose levels used except 25 r. Its frequency in surviving offspring cannot be determined, however, since the total number cited included resorptions, the incidence of which varies with gestation stage irradiated (Russell 1950), but in general it did not occur often. The overall impression gained from these data is one of little specificity of response, so far as this malformation is concerned, with regard to dosage or time irradiated. This impression is apparently strengthened by the results these authors obtained from irradiating preimplantation stages (Rugh and Grupp 1959*b*), a subject that will be explored in detail below.

Woollam and Millen (1958*b*) X irradiated Strong A female mice with 300 r on the 12th day of pregnancy. Defects of the central nervous system produced were hydrocephalus (frequency and description unstated) and meningocele. The latter occurred in 44/155 (28.4%) offspring. In a different study (Woollam, Pratt, and Fozzard 1957), in which hydrocephalus was produced in 3/81 irradiated young, the defect was associated with stenosis of the cerebral aqueduct. Birkner (1958) found disorganization of the brain, but apparently no gross malformations, in offspring of female mice given 200 r of X rays on the 7th day of gestation. Kraft (1959) gave "albino" mice single doses of 200 r on the 7th to 20th days of pregnancy. Surprisingly, only 2 grossly malformed offspring were produced by treatment during the first half of this period. Serial sections revealed brain damage after irradiation on the 13th day. Irradiation on the 14th day produced hydrocephalus in 4 offspring, 2 of which reached the age of 4 weeks. Tabuchi *et al.* (1962) using ddN mice found encephalocele and abnormal spine after irradiation on the 9th day with 200 rad. Ritter (1963) irradiated C57BL mice with 130 r of X rays on the 8th or 9th day and produced anencephaly and exencephaly. Kollath and Traut-mann (1965) gave mice of unstated origin 200 r of X or γ rays (Co^{60}) on the 10th day of pregnancy. "Dysencephaly" was produced by both types of irradiation in frequencies not significantly different from each other. Borden (1967) made a microscopic study of abnormalities of the otic primordia associated with developmental disturbances of the rhombencephalon in off-spring of F_1 female mice given 400 r of X rays on the 8th day of pregnancy. The defects consisted of closeness or union of the primordia and seemed to depend on rhombencephalic regression and underdevelopment.

Rabbits

Relatively few studies have been made of the effects of X irradiation on the prenatal development of rabbits. The work done before about 1952 was reviewed by L. B. Russell (1954). So fas as can be determined, in only 2 studies made before the 1950's were congenital malformations produced in rabbits by prenatal irradiation: defects of the eye (cataract, microphthalmia, and coloboma of the lid) by Hippel (1907), and microcephaly by Kosaka (1928*d*). Since then only a few experiments with this species have been reported. Various defects of the vertebral column and other parts, but apparently not of the central nervous system, were produced by Degenhardt and Grüter (1959) and Pobisch (1960).

More recent studies with rabbits yielded some malformations of the central nervous system. Females of commercially obtained mixed breeds were induced to ovulate and artificially inseminated, then irradiated once from a radiocobalt source with 250 or 400 r on the 7th to 22nd days of gestation (Chang, Hunt, and Harvey 1963). External malformations, scored in near-term young, were noted only in those irradiated on the 8th to 14th days. Defects of the central nervous system occurred rarely and defects of other parts were not frequent. An exencephaly and a "cranial blister" (out of 27) were produced by 250 r on the 8th day. All embryos exposed to 400 r on the 7th or 8th day died.

Female rabbits were acutely X irradiated with 12 r per day for the first 21 days of pregnancy, receiving a total, according to the author (Klosovskii 1963, p. 196), of 216 r. Young were examined before term and found to have micrencephaly and retarded development of the colliculi (no division into anterior and posterior colliculus) and cerebellum (no division into vermis and hemispheres).

Hamsters

Female golden hamsters were subjected to single exposures of 200 r from a radiocobalt source on the 1st to 12th days of pregnancy (Harvey and Chang 1962). Since all offspring irradiated with 200 r on the 7th day died and were resorbed, another group was given 100 r at this age. All young were examined on the 14th day, which is about 2 days before term.

Malformations of the central nervous system induced by postimplantation irradiation will be discussed here; defects found in offspring irradiated before implantation will be discussed below. Implantation occurs in this species at about $4\frac{1}{2}$ to $5\frac{1}{2}$ days after fertilization. Exencephaly occurred after treatment on the 8th day (5/33 = 15.2%). It also happened in 1/80 young irradiated on the 12th day, but it hardly seems possible that this occurrence was due to the treatment, since it was given after the time of closure of the head folds of the neural plate. Acrania, i.e., absence of much of the head above the maxilla, was seen in an animal irradiated on the 8th day. Cranial blister, described only as a blister-like distension on the top of the head and probably consisting of an encephalocele, occurred in low frequencies after treatment on many days (7th day, 3/29; 8th day, 1/33; 9th day, 2/79; 10th day, 1/67).

Spina bifida was produced by treatment on the 7th and 8th days (3/29 = 10.3%, and 4/33 = 12.1%, respectively). In a photograph of an affected specimen, this abnormality appeared as a small elevation in the lumbosacral area. In a photograph of a histological section through this defect, it could be seen that the spinal cord was duplicated into nearly equal-sized parts, one being on the midline, the other lying ventrolateral to the first. No vertebrae appeared to be present; one large ganglion occurred ventral to the lateral spinal half. The cord was covered by thin skin and hence the defect was occult.

In another survey study with golden hamsters (Jensh and Magalhaes 1962), 20, 100, or 200 r of X irradiation was given once on the 1st to 11th days of pregnancy and young were examined on the 14th day. Defects occurred only after irradiation on the 8th, 9th, or 10th day. Abnormalities included encephalocele, exencephaly, and hydrocephalus. In a different study (Kowalczyk 1964), irradiation of female golden hamsters with 30 to 70 r of X rays on the 7th or 8th day of pregnancy resulted in some instances of encephalocele, typical exencephaly, certain histological brain defects, and spina bifida. Chromosomal aberrations were found in irradiated late fetuses.

Other Animals

A study was made of the effects of prenatal irradiation of goats (O'Brien *et al.*
1963, 1964). A Spanish goat was irradiated with 300 r (100 r/hour) of γ rays
from a cobalt-60 source on the 30th day of pregnancy (O'Brien *et al.* 1963).
A kid with numerous defects was born, among which was microcephaly.
Six days after birth, it was able to hold its head erect and a few days later
was able to rise on its hind legs, but could not do both simultaneously. At
no time did it have coordinated muscular control. The kid died from pneu-
monia on the 34th day of life, but apparently no dissection was made of its
nervous system.

Cattle, sheep, and swine were exposed (Erickson and Murphree 1964;
McFee, Murphree, and Reynolds 1965) to single doses of 100 to 400 r of
γ irradiation from a cobalt-60 source. Cattle were irradiated during the 27th
to 34th days of gestation, sheep during the 20th to 29th days, and swine
during the 15th to 27th days. Skeletal defects of limbs occurred, but no central
nervous system defects were mentioned.

Much of the Soviet experimental work on the effects of radiation on
pregnancy and prenatal development was summarized by Pobedinskiy (1961).

Radioisotope Studies

Very few experiments have been made of the effects of radioisotopes on prenatal mammalian development. The earliest ones, in which no or only slight
effects were reported, were reviewed by L. B. Russell (1954) and Kalter and
Warkany (1959*a*). Other studies were made more recently. Wistar rats were
injected (Sikov and Noonan 1958) intraperitoneally on the 7th, 9th, 10th, or
11th day of gestation with doses of 0.3 to 2.0 millicuries (mc) of an inorganic
phosphorus-32 solution of high specific activity. In general, the incidence and
severity of malformations, scored in embryos and young fetuses, increased as
larger doses were given. Although the frequency and type of malformations
were somewhat dependent on the day of gestation on which injection was
made, the differences were not nearly so marked as those sometimes found
after X irradiation at different times.

The effects on the development of the central nervous system were few
and slight. Several cases of telencephalic bulbs of unequal size were found after
injection on the 7th, 9th, or 10th, but not the 11th day. The only other neural
defect noted was lateral displacement of a wall of the spinal cord, resembling
the anomaly produced by irradiation on the 10th day by Wilson, Jordan,
and Brent (1953). This occurred in 2 specimens from females treated on the
9th day with 0.5 or 0.6 mc.

Since Wilson (1954*d*), Hicks (1953), and others were unable to produce
malformations by irradiating rats before the 10th day, Sikov and Noonan's
(1958) results are not easy to interpret. The authors felt that they could not be
entirely explained by persistence of radiation into the susceptible period,

since the residual radioactivity was too little to cause the amount of damage found. It may be that, if pursued, the finding of Sikov and Lofstrom (1961) that X irradiation on the 7th day, which by itself did not produce malformations, potentiated the teratogenic effects of irradiation on the 10th day, will provide some explanation for this apparent inconsistency.

Fifty mc of phosphorus-32, given (Arnikar, Singh, and Udupa 1963) to a female rat on about the 9th day of pregnancy, produced offspring with gross limb defects. Strontium-90 resulted in defects largely of the skeleton and none of the central nervous system when administered to mice (Hiraoka 1961). Long–Evans females were injected (Hopkins and Casarett 1964) with 181 or 382 mc of strontium-90 on the 2nd or 10th day of gestation and the offspring examined near term. Only one malformation (an absent tail) occurred in offspring exposed on the 2nd day, and while various defects (especially of eye and skeleton) were produced by 10th-day treatment, no malformations of the central nervous system were noted.

A study was made in which a radioisotope was administered chronically (McClellan, Kerr, and Bustad 1963). Pitman–Moore miniature swine were fed strontium-90 daily beginning about half a month before conception and throughout pregnancy at levels of 1 to 31 mc per day. Apparently, no congenital malformations were found. However, because strontium-90 is largely sequestered by the maternal skeleton, the fetuses were exposed to a far smaller dosage of radiation than was administered, as evidenced by about one-eighth as much strontium-90 relative to calcium being found in fetal bone as in adults.

Postnatal Studies

A number of studies were made of brain abnormalities present in postnatal animals that were irradiated in utero at various times during pregnancy, especially the last third of pregnancy, i.e., in the period of the fetus. The first such study was made by Bagg (1922), who exposed rats to γ rays (radium source) 3 to 4 days before term. In survivors autopsied at about one year of age Bagg found that the cerebral hemispheres, especially the neopallia, were greatly reduced in size and that in several cases little or no cortical material remained. Correlated with the brain disturbances were skull defects, such as asymmetries and distortions of shape and thickness. Cowen and Geller (1960) called attention to the oddity that in Bagg's study there was damage of the cerebral cortex but not of the cerebellum, whereas recent studies have shown that irradiation late in gestation produces just the reverse type of damage. However, Cowen and Geller (1960) believed that a drawing presented by Bagg (1922) showed some cerebellar changes.

In an apparently unpublished study, Grobman (cited by L. B. Russell 1954, pp. 896–97) examined young mice (37–49 days old) that were X irradiated with 300 r on the 15th or 16th day of gestation and found absence of the corpus callosum. In otherwise unpublished work, Russell and Russell (1952) noted that mice irradiated in the fetal period developed hydrocephalus and behavior disturbances a few weeks after birth.

Hicks (1950) X irradiated rats and mice with 150 or 200 r during the third week of pregnancy. The offspring were studied from the ages of a few days to 3 weeks after birth. Detailed histological studies were not made, but the abnormalities noted included virtual absence of the corpus callosum associated with cortical and hippocampal defects, incompletely formed striatum, irregular, malformed, and dilated ventricles, and cerebellar defects. No attempt was made to relate the type or severity of defect with time of irradiation during gestation. In a number of other publications, Hicks (1952, 1954b) and Hicks, D'Amato, and Lowe (1959) mentioned and provided illustrations of abnormalities found in some animals permitted to live a year or more after having been irradiated at various stages of gestation. Among them were hydrocephalic animals treated with 200 r on the 11th day. In most cases the hydrocephalus increased greatly postnatally and the animals lived only a few weeks; at autopsy the cortex was paper thin. One apparently nonhydrocephalic littermate lived a year and a half, but when autopsied its dorsal cortex was thinned and the lateral and 3rd ventricles were enlarged (Hicks and D'Amato 1961).

Riggs, McGrath, and Schwartz (1956) treated pregnant Wistar rats 5 to 9 days before delivery with single exposures of 150 r of X rays. The offspring were killed at 60 days of age, but some much younger ones were also examined. Although not specifically mentioned, it is obvious from the photograph of whole brains presented that micrencephaly occurred. The only malformations stated to have been found formed a pattern of related structural deformities of the telencephalon, the basic features of which were established by the time of birth. This pattern occurred in 88.6 per cent (117/132) of the specimens examined. Its basis appeared to be dystrophic development of the neocortex. The defects varied in severity and extent, but these differences were apparently not closely related to the fetal age at exposure, since many degrees of defects occurred after treatment at all gestational times irradiated.

Alexandrovskaya (1959) irradiated rats on the 12th day of pregnancy with 150 to 200 r of X rays. The brains of irradiated offspring were examined at 16 months of age. Macroscopically, pronounced hypoplasia of the cerebral cortex was found, expressed by the fact that the cerebrum did not cover the colliculi and in some cases not even posterior portions of the diencephalon. In addition, subcortical structures were reduced in size, owing to hypoplasia or complete absence of the corpus callosum and hypoplasia of Ammon's horn. Severe hydrocephalus occurred in 4 animals with pronounced atrophy of the cerebral cortex and atrophy of subcortical ganglia. Detailed descriptions were given of cytological changes and other microscopic findings.

Cowen and Geller (1960) exposed female Sherman rats to single doses of 250 r of X rays on all days of gestation from the 1st to 23rd. No malformations were noted in offspring irradiated during the first 9 days of gestation. Treatment from the 10th to 15th days often (no number given) produced severe congenital malformations, including encephalocele and exencephaly. Young exposed at these times were all dead at birth or died soon after, and no adult survivors were obtained.

The offspring of females irradiated on the 16th to 23rd days of gestation were examined at the time of death (3–19½ months, the majority 6–16 months). They were found to have a variety of gross and microscopic developmental malformations, the type, severity, and frequency of which were related to the time of irradiation. Exposure on the 16th or 17th day was followed by the most severe forebrain defects, including marked reduction in size of the cerebral hemispheres and skull (micrencephaly and microcephaly), structural defects of the neocortex, multiple heterotopias in the ventricular walls and cortex, and agenesis of the corpus callosum. Some of these abnormalities also occurred after 18th-day irradiation, but were less severe and less common than after earlier treatment. Total callosal agenesis was produced only by exposure on the 16th to 18th days. Various gross and microscopic defects of the cerebellum were found after treatment on as early as the 17th day but were much more severe after irradiation on the 19th and later days. A few examples of microcephaly and microscopic cortical defects occurred after irradiation on as late as the 22nd day.

These malformations evidently represented outcome of damage to the neural parenchyma that occurred fairly soon after exposure to irradiation, since malformations of the same type were present in animals that died at or were killed shortly after birth.

It should be stated that a source of some confusion has crept into this otherwise excellent paper (Cowen and Geller 1960). The authors chose, as others have, to call the day on which sperm were found in the vaginal smear day 0, the day following day 1, and so on. Although I believe another system to be preferable, so long as consistency is followed any method is acceptable. The authors, however, used ordinal and cardinal designations synonymously, e.g., using the terms day 15 and 15th day interchangeably. But if day 0 designates the 1st day of pregnancy, then obviously day 9, e.g., is not the 9th day but the 10th. Therefore, in the above discussion of this paper I have rectified the authors' inconsistencies for the sake of clarity and uniformity.

Brizee, Jacobs, and Kharetchko (1961) irradiated pregnant rats with 60 r of X rays per day for 5 days from the 10th through 14th days of gestation, for a total of 300 r. The offspring were allowed to be born and were killed from the day of birth to 20 days of age. Brain weight and cerebral cortical thickness were reduced at all postnatal stages. Although the total number of cells in the cortex was greatly reduced by prenatal irradiation the surviving cells tended to follow normal growth patterns and to establish normal spatial integrity. In comparing their results with those of others, the authors noted that fractionated doses of X rays caused far milder damage to the cerebral cortex than was produced by single large doses.

In 90-day-old Long–Evans rats X irradiated with 150 r on the 14th day of pregnancy, Ershoff, Steers, and Kruger (1962) found reduction in brain weight and distinct change in gross morphology of the cerebral hemispheres. The most severe change was evident in the posterior medial portion of cerebral cortex, where the superior colliculus was exposed rather than being overlapped by the caudal pole of the cortex.

Offspring of Wistar rats X irradiated on the 18th day of pregnancy with 270 r were examined for tumors and malformations when they died (Wegner, Stutz, and Büchner 1961). The brains of 145 animals were studied and 133 (91.7%) found defective, including those with small and abnormal forebrain, partial or complete absence of the corpus callosum, etc.

Several offspring of Wistar rats X irradiated with 100 r on the 10th day of gestation survived with hydrocephalus for various times after birth, one for as long as 6 months (Rugh *et al.* 1963). Electroencephalographs of the animals showed no obvious disturbances that could be specifically attributed to the brain abnormalities. Electroencephalographic studies were also done (Berry, Clendinnen, and Eayrs 1963) in 30-day-old offspring of a stock of Birmingham albino rats X irradiated with 200 r on the 17th, 19th, or 21st day of pregnancy. Total absence of the corpus callosum was found after treatment on the first and second of these days and partial absence (rostal extremities were present) after the last. Severe hydrocephalus ("in cerebral hemispheres") occurred in offspring treated on the 17th day and markedly disorganized cortical structures and thinning of the cortex were found in those treated on all these days. The abnormalities were associated with changes in electrocortical activity, which to some extent were related to the severity of the structural disorganization.

Sprague–Dawley-derived rats were irradiated continuously during the first 20 days of pregnancy with a total of 1000 r of gamma rays (Coppenger and Brown 1965). The offspring were examined at 350 days of age and all found to have reduced brain size, especially of the cerebrum. Surprisingly, no agenesis of the corpus callosum was found. Wistar rats were given 100 r doses of X rays on the 9th day of pregnancy (Wegner and Damminger 1963). Of 92 viable offspring, 37, which lived 8 or less weeks, had macroscopically recognizable abnormalities of skull shape. Sections of these animals revealed severe grades of internal hydrocephalus of lateral ventricles. Mild to moderate grades of hydrocephalus, affecting lateral and 3rd ventricles, were found in others that survived to a mean age of 18 months.

The locomotor behavior of offspring of female rats X irradiated with 200 r on the 17th day of gestation or 1 or 3 days postnatally was tested when the animals were about 90 days old (Lipton 1966). The animals were killed at about 90 or 120 days of age and their brains studied. Irradiation, especially prenatal, produced deficits in locomotor skills, which were sometimes, but not always, clearly related to the cerebellar defects caused by the X rays.

Finally, a rhesus monkey exposed (Rugh *et al.* 1966) to 300 r of X rays at about 60 days of pregnancy was severely stunted and had persistent microcephaly, at 32 weeks of age. Periodic electroencephalograms indicated central nervous system damage (Rugh 1965).

Malformations after Preimplantation Irradiation

Several studies have been made in which a few malformed offspring were obtained from females irradiated early in pregnancy, during the preimplantation period. A number of mice with skeletal and visceral defects were found by Russell and her associates (summary in Russell 1965). After irradiation on the 1st to 5th days of pregnancy with single exposures of 100 or 200 r, 10/70 (14.3%) offspring had skeletal deviations (vs. 7/137 = 5.1% in controls), 4 of which were similar to types found in controls, the other 6 resembling types found with high frequency after postimplantation irradiation (Russell 1950, 1956). In addition, 200 r at these early times resulted in 3/397 young with external defects (vs. 1/756 in controls), comprising one skull malformation, similar to the control abnormality, one microphthalmia, and one otocephaly (Russell and Russell 1950, 1954*a*; Russell and Montgomery 1965).

Treating unpedigreed mice with single doses of 50 or 200 r on the 1st to 10th days of pregnancy, Rugh and Grupp (1959*b*) found low numbers of exencephalic near-term offspring among those irradiated at several preimplantation ages. Even doses as low as 15 r given on the 1st or 2nd day seemed to induce the defect in a small number (Rugh and Grupp 1959*c*). Exencephaly was not found in 591 control fetuses (Rugh and Grupp 1960*a*); for a further discussion of abnormalities in controls, see below. The mechanism invoked to explain the production of the defect by preimplantation irradiation was chromosomal damage, but no cytological or cytogenetic studies were made to support this contention.

In a recent study, Ohzu and Makino (1964) and Ohzu (1965) found that preimplantation exposure (1st or 2nd day) of pregnant mice with relatively low doses of X irradiation (5–25 r) resulted in some malformed offspring, including several with exencephaly (8/724 or 8/695 living offspring; a slight discrepancy in total offspring was reported in these 2 publications, which otherwise appear to deal with the same study).

Evidence of malformations induced by irradiation prior to or at the time of implantation was obtained in a study (Harvey and Chang 1962) utilizing hamsters. The defects consisted of cranial blister, which occurred in 1/74 irradiated on the 1st day and in 2/84 irradiated on the 6th day of pregnancy; and of certain other anomalies, such as eye defects, umbilical hernia, and digital abnormality, which were also infrequent. A total of 5/266 (1.9%) or 9/350

(2.6%) abnormal offspring irradiated on the 5th or 6th day, respectively, and earlier were found. Harvey and Chang (1964a) also irradiated hamster ovarian ova with several doses of X rays and noted abnormalities in 8/350 viable young. Seen were one offspring with anophthalmia and cranial blister and another with syndactyly; the remainder were not described. One abnormal offspring was also found among 134 controls.

In contrast to Rugh and Grupp (1959b), who reported only one type of defect, exencephaly, and to Ohzu and Makino (1964), who saw only exencephaly and polydactyly (of questionable significance), after early treatment, Russell (1965) and Harvey and Chang (1962, 1964a) got no uniformity of abnormal response. Lack of specificity and absence of exencephaly in the early-treated hamsters appear to cast some doubt on Rugh and Grupp's (1960a) contention that production of this defect by irradiation at any time over a long span of prenatal development as well as its production by various other techniques means that exencephaly is a nonspecific indicator of the sensitivity of the developing organism to any interfering agent, not merely to radiation.

This sort of argument has been current for many years, more generally being cast as a blanket statement (e.g., Gentry 1962) that no relation exists between any particular agent used and the type of defect produced, since the same (or what appears to be the same) abnormality may be produced in so many different ways. It is fair to say that those who make this claim loudest seem to be least acquainted with the modern mammalian teratologic literature.

The studies mentioned above contradict a number of others in which preimplantation irradiation never or only rarely was associated with malformations. Job, Leibold, and Fitzmaurice (1935) found that irradiation during the first 6 days of pregnancy either killed rat embryos or had no apparent detrimental effect. Hicks (1953) and Cowen and Geller (1960) produced no developmental anomalies in rats by irradiating on any of the first 9 days of pregnancy.

Negative results were also obtained in rats after irradiation on the 4th (Kalinina 1957), 5th (Miklashevskiy and Gol'dberg 1961), 6th (Sikov and Lofstrom 1961), and 9th days (Wilson, Brent, and Jordan 1953; Lengerová 1957; Brent, Franklin, and Bolden 1963); in mice after irradiation on the 1st (Sato 1963) and 5th days (Tabuchi et al. 1962); in rabbits after irradiation at several different times before implantation (Chang and Hunt 1960; Chang, Hunt, and Harvey 1963; Inman and Markivee 1963); and in hamsters after irradiation on the first 7 days of pregnancy (Jensh and Magalhaes 1962). Other such negative results in various species were reviewed by L. B. Russell (1954).

Studies by Chang, Hunt, and Romanoff (1958) and Chang and Hunt (1960) provided additional negative data. Fertilized and unfertilized rabbit ova were irradiated in vitro, transplanted into recipient animals, and examined

22 to 28 days later. Congenital malformations were found in no surviving fetus, and, further, there was no evidence of differential radiosensitivity at the various preimplantational stages irradiated. Cytological study of irradiated blastocysts revealed no chromosomal breakage immediately after treatment; abnormalities such as fragmentation and condensation showed up later during culture of irradiated blastocysts (Chang and Hunt 1960).

No gross abnormalities were detected in surviving mouse fetuses that had been irradiated in vivo or in vitro as unfertilized oocytes and transferred to irradiated or unirradiated uteri (Glass and McClure 1964); nor was there an association between visible chromosome damage and preimplantation death caused by in vitro irradiation of unfertilized mouse oocytes (Lin and Glass 1963).

In the face of the numerous studies in which congenital malformations were not induced by X irradiation at gestational stages prior to implantation, the reports of Russell (1965), Rugh and Grupp (1959b, c), Ohzu (1965), and Harvey and Chang (1962, 1964a), in which such effects apparently occurred, call for special attention. The incidence of malformed young in the studies of Russell and coworkers (Russell 1965) is only slightly different from the control value; which is also true of the results of Harvey and Chang (1962, 1964a) and Ohzu (1965). Results obtained in Rugh's laboratory, however, may be highly significant.

Rugh (1962) claimed that the negative results of most other workers were due to their using large doses of X rays, which kill abnormal offspring and thus permit only unaffected ones to survive. Let us explore this possibility by examining, e.g., some of Russell's (1950) data. It is true that in her study the mean litter size from females irradiated with 200 r before implantation (1st–5th days) was significantly smaller than the mean control litter size. But how the sparsity of gross anomalies among these irradiated young can be interpreted by Rugh as due to the dose of 200 r having been used is hard to understand, since this is the quantity that Rugh and Grupp (1959b) themselves used in early pregnancy (1st–5th days); and by which they produced exencephaly in merely (as near as can be calculated from the data presented) 2.7 per cent (6/221) of survivors. Incidentally, as Russell (1965) pointed out, Rugh (1962) erroneously quoted the Oak Ridge Laboratory workers as stating that all embryos surviving preimplantation irradiation were normal.

Let us for a moment consider a different, but highly pertinent subject, the question of controls—what their purpose is and how they are collected. Put most simply, the control provides a standard against which comparison is made in order to determine whether or not the experimenter's intervention has had an effect. For the comparison to be valid, the control and experimental groups must be as alike as possible in all relevant characteristics of which one is aware and must be manipulated in exactly the same manner but for the one situation, and that one alone, whose possible influence is being tested.

The method of forming the control must therefore be as well thought out as are the questions involving the experimental group. These topics were well discussed by Fraser (1964).

In the case of teratological studies in which the incidence of defects may be low but of some special significance, the crucial considerations are size and diagnosis: the number of control subjects should be not less but perhaps far larger than the number of experimental subjects, and the controls should be examined not less but at least as diligently and exhaustively for the pertinent phenomena. And, of equal importance, a new control group should be obtained for each new experimental group, since a past control cannot be a reliable index of the effectiveness of a present manipulation, as was dramatically shown in a study of mine (Kalter 1959a). We sympathize with Brent (1964a) in his remark that "it is disconcerting to read reports which describe no malformations in the controls. In many instances this indicates that there were too few controls or they were not examined."

Now let us return to the studies discussed above. Rugh and Grupp (1959b) found no control offspring with exencephaly but failed to state the total number examined. In several subsequent publications one and the same number of controls (viz., 519) was cited (Rugh and Grupp 1959a, c, 1960a, 1961; Rugh 1962). In other words, one set of control data was used for comparison with several noncontemporaneous sets of experiments.

Later, exencephaly was noted (Rugh and Wohlfromm 1962) in 0.25 per cent of controls. But this percentage is ambiguous, since it is not entirely clear whether it is based on the 2258 implantations or the 84 per cent survivors; if, as seems likely, it refers to the former, the incidence of exencephaly among the surviving control offspring was about 0.32 per cent (6/1897).

Summarizing: 3 studies were made (Rugh and Grupp 1959b, c; Rugh and Wohlfromm 1962) in which single doses of X rays of from 5 to 300 r were administered to CF1 female mice on the 1st to 5th days of pregnancy, and exencephaly was found in a total of 24/2400 (1.0%) surviving offspring. But the control value given above should not be compared with this total frequency but only with the experimental results obtained during the time these controls were collected (Rugh and Wohlfromm 1962), when exencephaly was noted in 8/661 (1.21%) offspring. I found this frequency to be statistically significantly different from the control value ($\chi^2 = 5.65$, P = 0.01–0.02). Thus, it appears that a small increase over the spontaneous incidence of this defect occurred after preimplantation irradiation. It should be noted, however, that in the 3 studies cited no discernible pattern of susceptibility related to dosage or day of treatment emerged, as commonly occurs after exposure later in pregnancy. Furthermore, the results are still to be regarded cautiously because, as Russell (1965, p. 234) remarked, "there is no indication they [the controls] were comparable genetically (no standard inbred strain was used), in age, and in parity. They were apparently not sham-irradiated."

A small number of offspring with exencephaly were also found by Ohzu (1965). First generation hybrid female mice (dd/Mk × CBA/Mk) were bred and X irradiated with 5, 15, or 25 r on the 1st or 2nd day of pregnancy. Exencephaly was found in 8/695 living offspring but was not observed in the control mice, only 188 of which were collected, however. Polydactyly of the hindfoot was found in 2 experimental offspring (and in no controls), and of the forefoot in 25 per cent of irradiated offspring and 14 per cent of controls. The increased incidence of the latter was considered to have resulted from enhancement of the spontaneous occurrence.

Harvey and Chang's (1962) claim that preimplantation irradiation produced malformations in their hamsters must be regarded skeptically for several reasons. For example, their control was far too small to give an accurate indication of the rate of spontaneous defect; the abnormal animal occurring in the experimental group after irradiation at a time when the treatment could hardly be held responsible for it may indicate that spontaneous anomalies occur in these animals. In the more recent report (Harvey and Chang 1964a), in fact, there was an abnormal control offspring.

Despite these remarks, the infrequent occurrence of malformed offspring may be a real outcome of preimplantation irradiation, since in all the experiments discussed there was, or may have been, a slight excess of abnormals. Most of the studies also agreed that no specific pattern of defects was induced and that no temporal gradient of teratologic susceptibility exists during the preimplantation period. These results no doubt indicate that irradiation before implantation produces malformations in a different manner from irradiation after implantation, and that the former may not even work through direct action on the ovum.

Preconception Irradiation and Defects in First-Generation Offspring

In studies done before the Second World War, so far as I am aware, only one malformed young was found (Snell and Ames 1939) among the offspring of animals irradiated before conception. In this case the animal, a female mouse, was irradiated, mated $1\frac{1}{2}$ days later, and killed 12 days after mating. Among her 9 living embryos there was one with an anteriorly-open neural groove.

More recently there have been several additional reports of the occurrence of congenital malformations of the central nervous system in offspring of parents thus irradiated. In a study (Pozhidayev 1961) in which female rats were X irradiated with 600 r, some offspring with hydrocephalus were discovered at examination on the 17th day of pregnancy. Another such report (Wachsmann, Utreras, and Schreiner 1963) is of an experiment in which NMRI female, male, or female and male mice were irradiated with 200, 400, or 600 r of X rays at different times before conception. Among 1388 near-term offspring, 5 were found with exencephaly. The abnormalities were considered to be the result of true radiation-induced mutations, a statement whose ambiguity shelters it from criticism.

In several studies malformations occurred, or possibly occurred, in first and later generation offspring of X irradiated animals. In one report (Rugh and Grupp 1960*a*) it was merely stated in a footnote that "100 r to the ovary [of mice] produced exencephalia for three generations." Further details of these results have not been published. Young rats were irradiated with 500 r and given an intraperitoneal injection of AET (Léonard, Maisin, and Malfait 1964). A quarter of them had offspring 5 per cent of which were microcephalic or anencephalic. The authors failed to make it entirely clear whether the abnormal young occurred in the first, second, or third generation descendants of the irradiated individuals, or in all 3.

Similar results were obtained by Osipovskiy and Kunicheva (1959) and Osipovskiy *et al.* (1963). A month before breeding, male and female guinea pigs were irradiated from a radiocobalt source with 225 or 450 r. Anomalies of the eye occurred in several of their offspring. In second and third generation offspring other abnormalities were also found, such as those of skeleton, teeth, and central nervous system, the total incidence of defective offspring increasing with each generation, being 7.6, 36.2, and 55.7 per cent, respectively, in the 3 generations. Abnormalities of the central nervous system consisted of a case of exencephaly and one of possible congenital hydrocephalus, both of which occurred in the second generation, and several instances of less marked changes (Osipovskiy and Kunicheva 1959). In a second study, (Osipovskiy *et al.* 1963), utilizing the same species and apparently the same procedures, a low incidence of hydrocephalus and other malformations was found in the offspring of irradiated animals and in those of 3 further generations. The hydrocephalus was not described.

Malformations Caused by Radiation-Induced Chromosomal Aberrations

In various other studies in which mice were irradiated before being mated, embryonic maldevelopment occurred only in second and later generation offspring.

It was noticed that some of the viable F_1 offspring sired by irradiated males during the presterile period consistently produced small litters when crossed to normal individuals (see references in W. L. Russell 1954). Such F_1 animals are termed semisterile or partially sterile, and the condition partial sterility is a quasi-dominant trait, with about half the viable offspring of partially sterile animals also showing this characteristic. It was found (Snell, Bodemann, and Hollander 1934; Snell 1935) that the decreased litter size resulted from the death in utero of a certain proportion of embryos; and Snell (1935) pointed out that the results fitted the interpretation that partially sterile animals were heterozygous for a reciprocal chromosomal translocation, a conjecture that was later confirmed, genetically and cytologically (Koller and Auerbach 1941; Koller 1944; Snell 1946).

In cytogenetics, a translocation is the exchange of parts between two nonhomologous chromosomes. Individuals heterozygous for a translocation produce several kinds of gametes, so far as chromosome structure is concerned (Griffen 1966). Some gametes contain all normal chromosomes, and these, of course, give rise to normally fertile offspring. Other gametes contain the normal complement of genes but have exchanged chromosomal parts. These, combined with a normal gamete, produce individuals heterozygous for the translocation and that are, therefore, partially sterile like one of the parents. Finally, some gametes contain unbalanced sets of chromosomes, i.e., containing deficiencies and duplications of chromosomal segments, and these may give rise to inviable and abnormal embryos.

In the first radiation-induced translocation analyzed, Snell, Bodemann, and Hollander (1934) found that most of the embryos carrying unbalanced chromosomal combinations died shortly after implantation. A few, however, developed beyond this stage, and these had gross abnormalities of the brain owing to failure of the neural groove to close anteriorly, i.e., exencephaly. A small number of such animals even survived to term, but were always dead when first examined. Several abnormal mice of this sort had been noted by Little and Bagg (1923) in the descendants of X irradiated mice. Snell and Ames (1939) considered Little and Bagg's malformed animals as probably due to an induced translocation, which was thus the first such induced change recorded.

Two groups of litters conceived by a partially sterile parent were obtained (Snell, Bodemann, and Hollander 1934). One was allowed to come to term and had 9/361 (2.5%) exencephalic offspring. The second group was examined 10 to 13 days after mating, and yielded 10/162 (6.2%) with a cranial defect. The defects in the fetuses were of 2 clearly distinguishable types, 5 having the cleft in the area of the rhombencephalon, and the other 5 in the area of the diencephalon. Nine other embryos (5.5%) had a distended central nervous system in which the brain, spinal tube, or both were kinked and folded to accommodate to the available space. Cross sections of the cord showed distention of the central canal. Since a small number (1.8%) of control embryos also had this feature, it may not have resulted from the induced chromosomal change. Fifty per cent of the embryos were resorbed, thus indicating massive early embryonic death.

Investigation of a second induced translocation (Snell and Picken 1935) revealed a far smaller incidence of prenatal death than was produced by the first one, and also that death seldom if ever occurred in early stages of development. It was therefore believed that this translocation would provide greater opportunity for studying the abnormal morphology of embryos carrying unbalanced chromosome combinations. The rate of malformed offspring was not greater than with the first translocation, however. The incidence of exencephaly in newborn offspring was again lower (1.5%) than among fetuses (13/282 = 4.6%) examined from the 12th to 15th days after mating (Snell and Picken 1935).

Many of the abnormal fetuses were individually described in great detail. In all 13 the basic defect was failure of the neural groove to close in a part of its anterior end. But in distinction to the abnormalities found in the earlier study (Snell, Bodemann, and Hollander 1934), the areas of the brain that were affected did not fall into different, clearly definable types. Instead, large regions were usually involved and great variability in extensiveness of the defect occurred (Snell and Picken 1935).

Although it seemed probable that the different anomalies (cleft diencephalon, cleft rhombencephalon, distended central nervous system, and different types of resorption) in the earlier study (Snell, Bodemann, and Hollander 1934) may each have resulted from a different form of chromosomal imbalance, no evidence for this possibility was forthcoming in the later study (Snell and Picken 1935), in which it appeared that all unbalanced zygotes, whether carrying deficiencies or duplications of chromosomal material, developed into embryos with essentially similar malformations. This conclusion was further supported by apparently unpublished studies of Bodemann (cited by Snell and Picken 1935), in which at least 8 out of 10 translocations were associated with brain anomalies similar to those described above. Since these translocations probably affected different chromosomes, it appeared to Snell and Picken (1935) that imbalance for almost any chromosomal region may have similar effects on embryonic development. Still, numerous differences occurred in the abnormal embryos, and it even seemed likely that some genetically unbalanced ones may have developed entirely normally. These variations were explained as due to the existence of modifying and protective intrauterine conditions, some hereditary, others not.

In a study of the descendants of females irradiated before mating (Snell and Ames 1939), a few abnormal offspring were found, but several of these came from mice that may not have been partially sterile.

In studies of a number of translocation-bearing lines, Hertwig (1940) noted some 8th- to 9th-day embryos that were small and developmentally retarded. In several cases neural tube closure was arrested. These small, retarded, and malformed embryos were considered to be aneuploids, i.e., to have unbalanced chromosomal constitutions.

In the postwar period, Otis (1953) examined the effects of prenatal development of 17 different radiation-induced translocations in mice. As in earlier studies, the greatest effect of chromosomal imbalance was usually on the implanting and early embryo with an overall 88 per cent embryonic loss in the first 9 days of pregnancy. Some deaths also occurred later in pregnancy, with 12 per cent dying after the 13th day or surviving to term.

Among the embryos surviving the 9th day of pregnancy, a small number were found with open anterior neural groove. Such abnormalities were associated with 8 of the 17 translocations. The defect varied from a narrow to a wide open condition of some part of, or the entire, anterior central nervous system.

In one line the condition resembled that termed cleft rhombencephalon by Snell, Bodemann, and Hollander (1934). The pattern of abnormalities seen on the 11th, 12th, and 13th days of gestation was almost uniform in 10/11 embryos examined microscopically. The myelencephalic region consisted of a thickened floor, no roof, and lateral components that had grown outward to fit down closely over the surface of the head. The entire lumen of the brain was decreased and the walls had abnormal deflections. Abnormal 13th- and 14th-day fetuses were observed but not older ones.

Possible abnormalities, such as narrow neural canal in the hindbrain region and thinness of the roof of the hindbrain, were associated with 2 other translocations. No malformations of the central nervous system occurred in 7 translocations, but death of embryos carrying unbalanced combinations of the relevant chromosomes occurred between the time of implantation and the 9th day of gestation. Even in this material it was possible to detect an early-appearing anatomical anomaly—failure of the allantois to take part in the formation of the placenta. But, obviously, death occurring even earlier than this event normally takes place must have a still more primary cause, perhaps a general failure of mesodermal expansion and specialization, as Otis (1953) suggested. However, evidence of a single, initial, abnormal effect of chromosomal imbalance was totally lacking.

As mentioned above, Snell, Bodemann, and Hollander (1934) postulated that since nearly all translocations appeared to produce similar abnormalities in embryos, the effect is due to chromosomal imbalance per se rather than to the action of more specific factors. But Otis (1953) found it difficult to understand why such imbalance should have what appeared to be an almost selective effect on the development of the nervous system, since numerous other systems rapidly differentiating during the period of organogenesis would surely also be influenced by the biochemical effects of a generalized upset in the supply of substrates produced by translocations.

In fact, it was possible, she believed, that this selectivity was only apparent, and was caused by abnormalities of the nervous system being far more easily detectable in late embryos than failure of development of, say, the circulatory or urinary system.

A syndrome of abnormalities, presumably due to a radiation-induced chromosomal aberration, was described by Hertwig (1955) in the Hydrops line of mice. In addition to hydropic specimens, which died soon after birth, other lethal types occurred. These included offspring with exencephaly, and, in some young surviving for a short time, degeneration of the flocculus cerebri associated with a characteristic abnormality of gait. Exencephaly was found in 9/174 (5.2%) surviving late embryos and fetuses from females of a normal stock crossed to Hydrops-line males, and in 5/27 (18.5%) from Hydrops-line animals crossed *inter se*. The line was characterized by small litter sizes caused by high prenatal mortality, contributed to, no doubt, by the death of exencephalic specimens.

The line was descended from a male whose sire received 1500 r of X rays. The irradiated male was mated to unrelated females 7 months after exposure, following a long period of sterility, and hence the originator of the line came from an irradiated spermatogonium. About half the offspring of partially sterile parents were also partially sterile. This characteristic was, therefore, probably due to heterozygosity for a reciprocal chromosomal translocation; and the malformed and defective offspring were probably carriers of unbalanced chromosomal complements. Whether the different sorts of abnormalities were caused by different kinds of chromosomal aberrations is unanswerable, but Grüneberg (1956a) considered that in part, at least, they may have represented different unbalanced genotypes.

Rugh and Grupp (1959a) crossed irradiated C57BL male mice to CF1 females. F_1 offspring of this cross were bred to CF1 mice, and 145 litters containing 1292 near-term fetuses were obtained, among which occurred 5 (0.39%) with exencephaly. The authors failed to state (1) the sex of hybrid parents of abnormal offspring, (2) whether these F_1 parents were rebred to determine if they continued to have deformed young, (3) whether litters produced by these parents were reduced in size, or (4) whether cytological studies were made to detect possible chromosomal aberrations.

An apparently spontaneous translocation occurred in rats (Waletzky and Owen 1942; Tyler and Chapman 1948). The condition was first detected in a partially sterile hooded male that sired abnormally small litters, and was inherited by about half his viable offspring. A few 14th- to 17th-day embryos with anteriorly open neural tubes were found (Waletzky and Owen 1942), but no such gross abnormalities were noted in a detailed embryological analysis (Bouricius 1948) of deaths induced by the translocation.

Strain Differences and Genetical Studies

The genetic influence on the effects of prenatal irradiation has been little investigated. Few reports have appeared of differences among strains and stocks in this regard, and no satisfactorily thorough examination of the genetic bases of these differences has been made.

Russell and Russell (1954a) studied the role of genetic constitution in radiosensitivity to the induction of homeotic shifts in vertebral (thoracolumbar) borders and related changes in the thorax, as expressed by the incidence of sides of animals having fewer than 13, 13, and more than 13 ribs. The most sensitive stage for production of an anterior shift (resulting in more than

13 ribs) came before that for a posterior shift (resulting in less than 13 ribs). Mice of 3 genotypes had different types and degrees of alteration in rib number in response to irradiation; which, however, were considered not necessarily to have been due to genetic differences in sensitivity to primary radiation damage, but as possible expressions of differences in a continuous array of variation in an underlying process with developmental thresholds at particular levels (cf. the quasi-continuous variation concept of Grüneberg 1952*a*).

Russell, Badgett, and Saylors (1960) noted certain malformations in offspring irradiated on the 8th day of pregnancy that in earlier studies, with mice of a different genotype, had occurred after irradiation on the 9th day. The cause of this inconsistency was probably not genetic but perhaps that the embryos were similar in developmental attainment, although of different chronological ages. Callas and Walker (1953) exposed C57BL and A/J mice to about 300 r of X rays on the 12th day of pregnancy, and produced cleft palate in 73.1 and 99.5 per cent of their offspring, respectively. Differences in palate morphology also occurred. Various other malformations were observed, but whether strain differences also occurred in the rate or severity of these defects was not mentioned. Further study of this possibly genetic difference has not been reported.

Rugh, Grupp, and Wohlfromm (1961) and Rugh and Wohlfromm (1963*a*) irradiated CF1 and C57BL/6 mice and certain of their hybrids with 200 r of X rays on the 9th day of pregnancy. The resorption (fetal death) and malformation data will be discussed separately. The incidence of resorption was about 35 per cent in CF1 mice and about 90 per cent in C57BL's. A strain difference in radiosensitivity was thus found, so far as fetal death is concerned. Treatment of CF1 females crossed to C57BL males, thereby exposing F_1 hybrid embryos, resulted (Rugh, Grupp, and Wohlfromm 1961) in 31.4 per cent resorption, which was similar to that for pure CF1 mice. Therefore F_1 hybrids were not more resistant to the lethal effects of radiation than CF1 mice, despite Rugh, Grupp, and Wohlfromm's (1961) contention that heterosis (i.e., hybrid vigor) was demonstrated by the data.

Backcrosses were made of F_1 hybrid females to parent type males (Rugh and Wohlfromm 1963*a*); when made to CF1 males the resorption rate was lower (22.0%) than when made to C57BL males (38.2%), which indicates that radiation-induced death may have been, at least in part, controlled by the fetal genotype. But since the reciprocal cross between the parent types, viz., C57BL females to CF1 males, was not made, it is not possible to state whether a maternal (i.e., physiological) attribute also played a part in this response to X rays. Whether developmental factors, such as possible advanced maturity of some embryos relative to their chronological age, may also have been responsible for any of these differences in lethality was not determined or discussed.

As for malformations, in the earlier study (Rugh, Grupp, and Wohl-fromm 1961) no data for individual anomalies were given, only the total frequency of defective offspring being reported. In the CF1 mice there were defects in 127/430 (29.5 %) surviving offspring, in the C57BL's 10/48 (20.1 %), and in the (CF1 × C57BL) F₁ hybrids 51/210 (24.3 %). The figures for the pure types are not statistically significantly different from each other (thus no strain difference in this regard was demonstrated); nor is the hybrid incidence significantly different from those of the pure types.

It may be argued, as the authors did (Rugh and Wohlfromm 1963a), that relatively few malformed C57BL offspring occurred because most of them were lost owing to the high resorption rate of this strain, and that among those lost were probably many that, had they survived, might have exhibited anomalies. Although evidence has been found (Beck and Lloyd 1963b) for a relation between fetal death and fetal malformation such a relation cannot be taken for granted in all cases and for all teratogens, since other findings (Wilson 1964; Kalter 1965a; Brent 1966a) suggested that mortality and teratogenicity are separate effects and not merely different degrees of expression of the same reaction to injury on the part of the embryo. Most relevant here are Dagg's (1964) results. He found no clear indication of a relation between incidence of death and deformed offspring in C57BL mice exposed on 12th day of gestation to X rays over the range of 100 to 175 r.

In the later study (Rugh and Wohlfromm 1963a), the data for different types of defects were somewhat more explicitly presented, those of the tail, eye, and central nervous system being individually cited. Malformations of the central nervous system, which consisted of microcephaly and various grades of exencephaly, occurred in 33/159 (20.8 %) CF1's and in 0/21 C57BL's. That the absence of central nervous system defects in the C57BL mice was not necessarily due to their high mortality rate was shown by the results of the backcrosses, since although the fetal resorption rate (see above) of F₁ hybrid females crossed to C57BL males was not extremely high, the frequency in their offspring of defects of the central nervous system was still lower than in those of F₁ hybrid females crossed to CF1 males (2/157 = 1.3 % vs. 20/206 = 9.7 %). These results indicate that C57BL genes contributed to the resistance of fetuses to the induction of such defects by irradiation. Again, however, it is not possible to say whether the basis of this greater resistance was intrinsic or rested on developmental precocity induced by a greater proportion of C57BL genes.

Dagg (1964) exposed mice of the BALB/cGn, C57BL/Ks, and 129/Rr strains and F₁ hybrids of reciprocal crosses between BALB/c and C57BL mice to a range of doses of X rays at different times in pregnancy. The mortality rate of BALB/c embryos following irradiation on the 12th day increased with dose (100–175 r), but no clear indication of such a relation occurred in C57BL embryos. A trend of this sort existed in both these strains after treatment on the 11th day, but in 129 mice the mortality rate was only slightly elevated even with 200 r.

Of the 4 external features examined—cleft palate and abnormalities of the tail, hindfeet, and forefeet—the C57BL strain, after treatment on the 12th day, had a higher incidence than the BALB/c only of defects of the forefeet. Both types of embryos had high frequencies of tail defects, but somewhat higher doses were usually required to produce comparable rates of the defect in C57BL animals than in BALB/c. Despite a low spontaneous occurrence of abnormality of hind digits in C57BL mice, irradiated offspring of this strain had a lower frequency of this defect than BALB/c young. The latter strain was also more susceptible to the production of cleft palate; to which both strains showed a clear threshold, but that for the BALB/c was somewhat (approximately 25 r) lower than for the C57BL.

Measurements of the sizes of unirradiated embryos on the 11th to 13th days disclosed that C57BL's had a larger mean crown-rump length than BALB/c mice, equivalent to being about 12 hours older. This fact suggested that the differences in susceptibility to radiation-induced damage may have been due to differences in relative developmental stages treated rather than to inherent dissimilarities in response to X rays. In addition, measurements of reciprocal F_1 hybrid embryos showed that those with C57BL mothers were larger than those with BALB/c mothers, larger, in fact, than homozygous C57BL embryos, and that those with BALB/c mothers were intermediate in size to the pure strain embryos. In order to adjust for this differential in developmental maturity, another experimental series was undertaken (Dagg 1964) in which BALB/c mice were irradiated 12 hours later than C57BL's on the 11th day of gestation. When thus treated at comparable developmental stages, these strains responded quite similarly.

Discrepancies concerning this size-susceptibility relation should be noted, however. C57BL offspring had a larger frequency of cleft palate than (C57BL ♀ × BALB/c ♂) F_1's, when both were treated at the same stage, despite being approximately the same size; and the percentage of cleft palate was higher in (C57BL ♀ × BALB/c ♂) F_1 offspring than in those of the reciprocal cross, despite the former being larger. The first discrepancy may indicate that "susceptibility" to the effects of radiation is not merely a function of degree of maturity attained, but may in some measure be determined by intrinsic factors. The second discrepancy, which indicates the operation of maternal factors, may also be taken as underscoring another curiosity displayed by the results: viz., a switch that appears to have occurred in the relative susceptibility to cleft palate of the C57BL and BALB/c strains, the former being less susceptible when irradiated on the 12th day and more on the 11th day than the BALB/c strain. The fact that after treatment on the 11th day (C57BL ♀ × BALB/c ♂) F_1 offspring had a greater frequency of cleft palate than did the reciprocal cross offspring is inexplicable in the context of the 12th-day results for the pure strain mice, but is not meaningless if considered as strengthening the supposition that a reversal of susceptibility of the pure strains did in fact occur.

This switch may somehow be related to the interesting discovery that there appear to be 2 discrete embryonic periods in mice of susceptibility to radiation-induced cleft palate separated by a phase, the 10th day of pregnancy, of relative or complete resistance to the induction of this defect (Russell and Russell 1954a; Heitz and Martinet 1961).

Several investigators have among them used various strains and types of mice, and, although dangerous, a quantitative comparison of their results might be made. One example will suffice. In 4 studies spina bifida was produced in mice by irradiating on the 10th day of pregnancy. Russell (1950) treated (C57BL × NB) F_1 hybrid embryos and found 36 per cent abnormal after 200 r and 88 per cent abnormal after 300 r. Auerbach (1956) used (101 × C3H) F_1 young and produced the defect in 89 per cent with 300 r. Russell, Badgett, and Saylors (1960) gave about 200 r to (101 × C3H) F_1 females mated to males of the same type; the incidence of the defect in their offspring was 25 per cent. Dagg (1963–64) irradiated C57BL mice and produced the malformation in 4 per cent of offspring with 125 r and in 51 per cent with 175 r. The dose-response relation was thus excellent, despite hybrid embryos being used in 2 of the studies, and genetically heterogeneous offspring in another.

In a study (Jensh and Magalhaes 1962) made with 2 inbred hamster strains, one with the usual golden fur and the other a mutant cream strain, the former was apparently more susceptible to the teratogenic effects of X irradiating on the 8th or 9th day of pregnancy.

Modification of the Fetal Effects of Radiation

I should like to discuss the few studies that have dealt with modification of the teratogenic effects of radiation.

Hypoxia

To my knowledge, the first study of this sort was that of Russell, Russell, and Major (1951), whose results were presented in greater detail by L. B. Russell (1954). Pregnant mice were X rayed (0, 100, 200, 300, or 400 r) on the 12th day of gestation after 10 minutes in a 5 or 21 per cent oxygen-containing atmosphere. The offspring were examined at birth for 6 characteristics— birth weight, viability (i.e., % alive), tail length and shape, and forefoot and hindfoot abnormality. For all these "end points" the hypoxic condition reduced the frequency or degree of damage done by irradiation, so that in effect irradiation in a lowered percentage of oxygen was equivalent to treatment with a smaller dose of X rays. Further, it was demonstrated that the magnitude of protection was approximately the same for all the characteristics studied. No statistical evaluation of these results can be made, however, since even in the more detailed report (L. B. Russell 1954) no absolute numbers were given. Since it was shown by various investigators that hypoxia protects against different types of radiation damage, such as chromosome breakage and sex-linked lethal mutation, it was suggested (L. B. Russell 1954) that the protection provided by hypoxia against the prenatal effects of radiation may have been exerted at the intracellular level. But the results provided no evidence in favor of any particular type of intracellular damage being involved.

Another study of the protective effects of hypoxia in mammals was made by Rugh and Grupp (1960*b*). CF1 mice were exposed to 6 per cent oxygen for 8 to 13 minutes prior to X irradiation with 200 r on the 9th day of pregnancy. Near-term offspring were scored for exencephaly and other conditions and characteristics. Of 109 full-grown young treated with X rays alone, 34 (31.2%) had exencephaly, whereas 19/119 (16.0%) given the combined treatment had exencephaly. The resorption rate was also smaller in the litters exposed to combined treatment than in those only irradiated (22/141 = 15.6% vs. 56/165 = 33.9%). Again, therefore, hypoxia apparently proved efficacious in reducing the harmful prenatal effects of radiation.

Runner's (1965) investigation of the interaction of X irradiation and hypoxia revealed new features. When a single dose of 100 r was given to female mice early in pregnancy at the onset of 4 hours of exposure to a 7 per cent oxygen atmosphere, certain anomalies (axial skeletal defects and exencephaly) were not influenced, while the frequency of other skeletal abnormalities was potentiated. X irradiation given at the end of the hypoxic period, however, greatly reduced the malformation rate so far as 5 morphological criteria were concerned. Runner's conclusion also introduced something new: "It is concluded that irradiation has protected from or reduced the teratogenic risk from treatment with anoxia."

Chemicals

The protective effect of a chemical substance against the teratogenic action of radiation was first demonstrated by Wolff and Kirrmann (1954), who found that the simple sulfhydryl compound, cysteamine (2-aminoethanethiol, or β-mercaptoethylamine), mitigated the cephalic anomalies produced by X rays in chick embryos. The influence of this substance on the developing mammal was studied by Maisin *et al.* (1955) and Rugh and Clugston (1955), who reported that protection occurred so far as postnatal weight, survival, and growth of prenatally irradiated mice and rats were concerned.

Protection by cysteamine against mammalian maldevelopment was investigated by Woollam and Millen (1958*b*). On the 12th day of pregnancy Strong A mice were X irradiated with 300 r or were given an intraperitoneal injection of 4 mg cysteamine and irradiated 2 to 5 minutes later. Term offspring had several types of malformations, including syndactyly, micromelia, anophthalmia, hydrocephalus, meningocele, and cleft palate. The frequency of meningocele was sharply reduced in the drug-treated group (4/163 = 2.4% vs. 44/155 = 28.4%), while that of cleft palate was only moderately reduced (144/163 = 88.3% vs. 149/155 = 96.1%). Data concerning the other defects were not given.

Rugh and Grupp (1960b) found that cysteamine, as well as another sulfhydryl compound, cystamine [2,2'-dithiobis(ethylamine)], lessened the teratogenic and embryocidal effects of X rays in CF1 mice. Three mg cysteamine or cystamine given intraperitoneally 30 minutes before X irradiation with 200 r on the 9th day of pregnancy decreased the X-ray-induced frequency of exencephaly (34/109 = 31.2% vs. 48/283 = 17.0% and 16/187 = 8.6%, respectively). Curiously, AET (S,2-aminoethylisothiuronium.Br.HBr), another sulfur-containing radioprotective agent (Shapira, Doherty, and Burnett 1957), was entirely without protective effect against radiation-induced exencephaly (Rugh and Grupp 1960b).

Ershoff, Steers, and Kruger (1962), on the other hand, reported that AET diminished some of the effects of prenatal irradiation. Long–Evans female rats were exposed to single doses of 150 r of X rays on about the 14th day of pregnancy or irradiated 20 minutes after intraperitoneal injection with 100 mg/kg cysteamine, AET, or MEG (2-mercaptoethylguanide.HBr, into which AET is transformed by intratransguanylation when injected into animals; it is thus the actual protective agent). The females were allowed to deliver and most of the surviving offspring were raised. The abnormalities noted at weaning were oligodactyly, clubhand and clubfoot, other paw defects, and abnormalities of gait.

In general, abnormalities of the forefoot occurred more frequently than those of the hindfoot, but the latter were usually more severe. In the group only irradiated, 69.8 per cent (44/63) of the young examined had defects of the forefoot, whereas in the groups given the 3 different combined treatments, as listed above, the incidence was reduced to 25.5 (13/51), 32.6 (33/49), and 16.1 per cent (10/62), respectively. The incidences of hindfoot defects in these 4 groups were 34.9 (22/63), 9.8 (5/51), 24.5* (12/49), and 3.2 per cent (2/62), respectively. The frequencies after combined treatment are all significantly different statistically from that produced by irradiation alone, with the exception of the one starred. Hence, there occurred a marked degree of radioprotection by these compounds, so far as these anomalies are concerned.

The gait defect, which was restricted to the hindlimbs, consisted of a hopping motion and contained both sensory and motor components. It occurred in 23.8 per cent (15/63) of the young only irradiated and in 0 (0/51), 12.2* (6/49), and 1.6 per cent (1/62) of those treated additionally with the substances named above, respectively. Again the frequencies in the young given the combined treatments are statistically significantly different from that occurring after irradiation alone, with the exception of the one starred. It should be noted that both nonsignificant differences were due to AET, and hence it appears that this substance was not as uniformly good a radioprotector as cysteamine or MEG. The gait defect was apparently not correlated with foot deformities, since in some cases each of these abnormalities occurred in the absence of the other.

In addition to foot and gait defects, radiation produced microcephaly and micrencephaly, i.e., decrease in brain weight, in both males and females examined at 90 days of age. The radioprotective agents were without significant effect in diminishing the incidence of these phenomena. In the group irradiated only, in addition to overall decrease in brain size, there was also apparent differential reduction in dimensions of the cerebral hemispheres. This change was most obvious in the posterior medial portion of the cerebral cortex, where the superior colliculus was exposed instead of being overlaid by the caudal margin of the cortex. A milder degree of this abnormality occurred in young subjected to the radioprotective drugs. No significant differences in the gross or microscopic appearance of the brain were noted between young with or without gait defects.

It was also observed (Ershoff and Bajwa 1963) that MEG and cysteamine markedly reduced the testicular damage done by irradiating rat fetuses on the 18th day of gestation, but that MEG did not diminish the incidence of eye defects or influence the increased caries susceptibility of rats irradiated on the 10th day of pregnancy. In another study (Loawhakasetr 1965), AET and MEA (2-mercaptoethylamine.HCl), separately or, more effectively, when combined, reduced the resorption rate and incidence of eye defects in irradiated rats.

The mechanism of action of these radioprotective chemicals was discussed by Bacq and Alexander (1961, pp. 465–77). A number of theories explaining their properties have been proposed, but none of them is completely satisfactory even so far as radioprotection during postnatal life is concerned.

The lethal effects of preimplantation irradiation were reduced by prior administration of acetylcholine (Kalinina 1961). Other Soviet studies of radioprotection were also mentioned by this author. In further studies, Kalinina (1964) administered phenatin (a product of the condensation of amphetamine and nicotinic acid), magnesium sulfate, chlorpromazine, or mercaptamine. Rats were X irradiated with 200 to 300 r on the 11th day of pregnancy, several minutes before or after receiving these substances. When examined on the 22nd day of pregnancy, the frequency of dead or malformed offspring was somewhat diminished in groups given combined treatments.

Cortisone

Wistar rats were X irradiated with 258 r on the 11th day of pregnancy or irradiated and given subcutaneous injections of 20 mg cortisone acetate per day from the 9th to 12th days (Woollam, Millen, and Fozzard 1959). The offspring were removed near term, serially sectioned, and examined for eye abnormalities. While radiation alone produced but few cases of deformity $(4/77 = 5.2\%)$, the combined treatment appeared to augment the incidence $(13/68 = 18.8\%)$.

Vitamins

In another study from the same laboratory (Woollam, Pratt, and Fozzard 1957), apparent intensification of radiation-induced teratogenesis was also produced by feeding vitamins. In this experiment, female Wistar rats were X irradiated on the 11th day of pregnancy (see p. 4) or irradiated and given single parenteral injections of a mixture of vitamins. Near-term young were scored for eye defects (microphthalmia and anophthalmia) and hydrocephalus. Unfortunately the results were presented in the form of number of abnormal eyes rather than of number of offspring with abnormal eyes. Thus, although there was more anophthalmia in the group that received the combined treatment than in the group exposed to X rays only, the data cannot be easily evaluated statistically. So far as the other malformations are concerned, the difference in the number of microphthalmic eyes between the 2 groups was not large, nor was the difference in frequency of hydrocephalus statistically significant $(3/81 = 3.7\%$ vs. $8/88 = 9.17\%, \chi^2 = 1.2, P = 0.2–0.3)$.

Miscellaneous Substances

Pantelouris (1958) noted a decreased resorption rate after injection with macerated fetal liver. Ershoff, Steers, and Kruger (1962) significantly increased the frequency of foot deformities and gait defects with saline, and of hindfoot abnormalities with a phosphate buffer solution.

In addition to investigating the radioprotective properties of hypoxia and sulfhydryl drugs, as discussed above, Rugh and Grupp (1960*b*) tested the effects of other substances. As measured by frequency of exencephaly, most of them (dextrose, insulin, alcohol, distilled water, hypertonic saline) and spleen, bone marrow, and brain homogenates had no influence on the results of X rays. Two (physiological saline and a liver homogenate) apparently reduced the proportion of exencephalic near-term offspring $(34/109 = 31.2\%$ vs. $44/261 = 16.8\%$ and $12/76 = 15.8\%$, respectively), but did not lower the resorption rate.

It must be remarked that Rugh and Grupp (1960*b*) computed the rate of exencephaly on the basis of number of implantations rather than on the near-term survivors. Thus the females exposed to X rays alone had 165 implantations, 56 resorbed sites, and 34 exencephalic offspring; the last therefore constituted 20.6 per cent of implantation sites and 31.2 per cent of the young seen near term. In above discussions of the studies of these authors (pp. 121–22), all frequencies of abnormality mentioned were recalculated and are based on surviving offspring.

Their method of reckoning percentage of abnormality seems to have been used because their main criterion of radioprotection apparently was proportion of implantations giving rise to living, normal, full-grown offspring. By overemphasizing this formula, and by ostensibly believing that resorbed young must have been abnormal, they were led to overlook data of possible significance. First it seems not to have been recognized that several different gauges of radioprotection may exist and that reduced frequency of a specific malformation may be as valid a standard, or even more so, than one as general (and vague) as "normality." They thus disregarded the possible protection afforded by physiological saline and liver homogenate simply because these substances did not increase the proportion of surviving offspring.

As shown by the studies of Ershoff, Steers, and Kruger (1962) and Ershoff and Bajwa (1963), already discussed, the radioprotective agents do not give blanket and equal protection to even the few measures of fetal damage so far investigated. As Ershoff, Steers, and Kruger (1962) mentioned, this fact may be due simply to different organs' requiring different doses of these agents for protection to be provided. It may also be that the sort of radiation damage leading to certain aberrations cannot be remedied by the type of agents so far tried.

Uterine Clamping

An entirely different method of radioprotection was used by Brent, Franklin, and Bolden (1963) in rats. On the 9th or 10th day of pregnancy, the cervical and ovarian ends of one uterine horn were clamped for 45 minutes, the horn thus being completely isolated from the maternal circulation. The embryos in both horns were irradiated with one of several doses of X rays just before the clamps were removed. This procedure apparently decreased the mortality rate and growth retardation of near-term fetuses in the clamped as compared with those in the unclamped horn. While clamping did not lower the incidence of malformations produced by 100 or 150 r on the 10th day, it may have reduced their severity.

Maternal Factors

The role of maternal age in the induction of fetal death and deformity by prenatal irradiation was investigated in CF1 mice by Rugh and Wohlfromm (1963b). The animals used were 2-month-old primiparae and 10- to 12-month-old multiparae. Only the results for X irradiation on the 9th day with 100 or 200 r will be discussed because all but one of the instances of congenital malformation of the central nervous system noted occurred under these conditions. The abnormalities included hydrocephalus, microcephaly, exencephaly, and anencephaly. There was no significant difference between the offspring of young and old females in frequency of defects after 100 r; but after 200 r there was such a difference, 14.0 per cent of the offspring of young mothers showing defects of the central nervous system, while but 5.3 per cent of the offspring of old mothers had such defects.

As is usual with reports from Rugh's laboratory, these percentages were based not on surviving young, but on number implanted. It seems to me that this method is less legitimate, especially in this experiment, than basing the incidence figures on surviving fetuses, and that, in fact, it introduces a definite bias. The fetal resorption rate in young control females was somewhat lower than in old ones (12.7 vs. 16.8%) and the 200 r-induced rate was much lower in young than old females (32.3 vs. 65.5%). Litter size, as is well known, decreases with advancing maternal age and after about the fourth litter (E. S. Russell 1954; Finn 1962; Talbert and Krohn 1966). In addition to a generalized decrease in ability of old females to carry fetuses to term, there may be preferential prenatal destruction of abnormal conceptuses, so that fewer of their offspring would be malformed. Intrauterine competition in polytocous mammals has been postulated to account for the decreased frequency of congenital malformations in the offspring of old mice (Bodmer 1961; Parsons 1963).

The influence of these possible phenomena associated with ageing can be offset by basing the frequency of congenital malformations on live offspring. If this method is employed for the data of the study under discussion (Rugh and Wohlfromm 1963b), the results are as follows. Young females given 200 r still had a higher proportion of abnormal offspring than old ones ($33/130 = 25.4\%$ vs. $11/54 = 20.4\%$), but the difference is not statistically significant ($\chi^2 = 0.29$, $P = 0.6$). Hence a maternal age influence was not demonstrated.

A similar study was made (Rugh and Wohlfromm 1966) using primiparous and multiparous CF1 mice that were all 7 to 9 months old, which were given 150 r of X rays at 8 days after mating. Omitting "stunted" offspring, which were counted as anomalous, primiparae again had a higher level than multiparae of surviving malformed young ($180/440 = 40.9\%$ vs. $165/454 = 36.3\%$), but this difference is not statistically significant either ($\chi^2 = 1.78$, $P \doteqdot 0.2$). The difference between the 2 groups with respect to frequency of malformations of the central nervous system is even smaller ($145/440 = 33.0\%$ vs. $134/454 = 29.5\%$, $\chi^2 = 1.08$, $P \doteqdot 0.3$).

Fractionated and Chronic Irradiation

Comparison of the effect on embryonic development of fractionated, chronic, and acute irradiation has been made in a number of laboratories. Auerbach (1956) did not produce a different total incidence of malformations by X irradiating 10th-day mouse embryos with 300 r in 3 fractions of 100 r than with single 300 r doses, but the former did increase the proportion of more severely affected offspring.

Brizee, Jacobs, and Kharetchko (1961), comparing the results they obtained using fractionated doses applied during the 10th to 14th days, inclusive, with those gotten by Hicks (1950) and Hicks, D'Amato and Lowe (1959) after single doses, found that divided doses produced much less severe cerebral cortical damage in rats than single applications. More recently, Brizee (1964) noted that a total of 150 r of X rays given in 5 equal fractions over 12 hours on the 16th day of gestation did not have significantly different effects on postnatal brain growth from that produced by the same total dose given once, though there was some indication that fractionated doses had a less severe growth-retarding effect on the prosencephalon and cerebellum than single doses. The same effect of fractionated versus single doses occurred after irradiation of rats on the 14th day of pregnancy (Jacobs and Brizee 1966). It could not be determined whether fractionated doses were less effective because of cell recovery or because of other factors, such as a relatively weaker effect of lesser doses. Slightly reduced incidences of exencephaly, but not of resorption, were produced (Rugh and Grupp 1960a) by 25 r of X rays given twice from 1 to 8 days apart beginning the 1st day of pregnancy, compared with that produced by single doses of 50 r given during this time in gestation.

Harvey and Chang (1964b) X irradiated female hamsters on the 7th or 8th day of gestation with single doses of 50 to 200 r or with repeated 25 r doses at 30- or 60-minute intervals totalling these same quantities and found no consistent differences in frequency of central nervous system malformations (spina bifida, exencephaly, cranial blister) between the groups exposed to single or fractionated doses. Harvey and Chang (1964a) also irradiated hamster ovarian ova with several amounts of X rays and examined the pregnant females about $1\frac{1}{2}$ days later or on the 14th day of gestation. Among the doses used were single ones of 50 r and 2 of 25 r each 5 or 60 minutes apart. There were no defects in the 63 fetuses irradiated with single doses and there were 6 abnormal ones among the 205 given fractionated treatment. Since an abnormal offspring occurred in the control group of 134, and because the data are limited, it is difficult to interpret these results. There were no significant differences in resorption rate or in fraction of degenerating ova between the groups treated with fractionated and single doses.

Russell, Badgett, and Saylors (1960) exposed mice to daily acute doses of 12.8 r of γ radiation for the first 15 days of pregnancy, the total accumulated dose therefore being 191.4 r. The newborn offspring of these females were compared morphologically with those that were irradiated continuously with the same total dose during the same period in pregnancy. Both groups of offspring showed little, if any, effect of the treatments. They also compared the effects of a total of about 200 r of gamma rays given continuously from the 1st to 14th days of pregnancy with those of approximately the same dose of X rays administered in single doses on any of several days of gestation.

The offspring were examined at birth. Most of the young acutely irradiated on the 8th, 10th, or 12th day were severely malformed, with defects generally similar to those found in earlier studies (Russell 1950). The chronically irradiated offspring, however, were again found to be virtually normal.

Kriegel and Langendorff (1964) X irradiated inbred mice with acute daily doses of 2.5, 5, 10, 20, 40, 60, or 80 r from the 1st to 18th days of pregnancy for a total of 45 to 1440 r. The 80 r dose level interrupted all pregnancies. Daily doses of 10 r or less had no effect on the resorption rate or on embryonic development. A small increase in the frequency of resorption and of maldevelopment was produced by 20 r, and larger increases were caused by 40 and 60 r (the malformation rates were: control, $7/1523 = 0.4\%$; 20 r, $16/515 = 3.1\%$; 40 r, $77/350 = 22.0\%$; 60 r, $70/126 = 55.6\%$). The frequency of malformations of the brain produced by 20, 40, and 60 r were 0.6, 6.8, and 5.6 per cent, respectively, and the defects consisted of encephalocele, hydrocephalus, exencephaly, and hemicrania. There appeared to be no particular relation between the amount of radiation used and the type or degree of defect, most of the different malformations being produced by all the teratogenic dose levels. Unfortunately, the authors did not compare their results with what may have been produced by continuous irradiation with the same total doses.

Female Holtzman rats were subjected (Coppenger 1964) to chronic gamma irradiation (50 r/20 hr. day) from the 1st day of pregnancy, and the offspring were examined at different times between the 10th gestation day and birth. Gross defects observed in late fetuses and newborn young were microcephaly, micrencephaly, eye defects, etc. In offspring examined (Coppenger and Brown 1965) after a period of postnatal growth there was generalized reduction of cerebral size with a lesser effect on the cerebellum and brainstem.

In similar studies (Brown, Krise, and Pace 1963), female Holtzman rats were continuously exposed throughout their reproductive lifetime to gamma irradiation at levels of 2, 5, 10, or 20 r per day beginning with the onset of the first pregnancy. No significant alteration in litter size of the first 6 litters resulted from the 10 r or smaller doses; at 20 r only one offspring was born in the fifth litter and none in the sixth. No malformations were observed at any level of radiation used.

The relative teratogenic effects of gamma and X rays and the influence of dose rate were studied by Sikov and Lofstrom (1962). Holtzman rats were given acute or protracted doses of 110 to 450 r of X rays or gamma rays on the 10th or 11th day of pregnancy. The same array of malformations was found at examination of the fetuses on the 15th day of gestation after both types of rays, namely defects of the eye, maxilla, mandible, hindlimbs, and tail. Apparently no malformations of the central nervous system occurred. But in almost every instance X rays produced a higher, and often a substantially higher, frequency of malformation (and fetal death) than did physically equivalent doses of gamma rays applied at the same time in gestation. The greatest differential occurred at low doses. In addition, in most cases protracted treatment was less effective than acute exposure.

To sum up, in almost every study in which comparison was made, fractioned and chronic irradiation were less teratogenic than acute irradiation. The exceptions were a study (Harvey and Chang 1964b) in which no differences were noted; and one (Auerbach 1956) in which fractioned doses produced more severe but not more frequent anomalies. Russell, Badgett, and Saylors (1960) stated that the intensification seen by Auerbach may have been due to the cyclic recurrence of a susceptible phase. The more usual result—reduced effectiveness of fractionation and chronicity—can possibly be explained as resulting from either smaller doses accumulating during a sensitive stage, or repair (whatever it may consist of) occurring in the intervals between exposures or during low-level protracted exposure.

The Mechanisms of the Teratogenic Effects of Radiation

It was long assumed that the effects of irradiation on prenatal development are due to direct action upon the ovum, embryo, and fetus. But it was not until the early 1950's that this supposition was put on a firm footing by the studies of Wilson and his colleagues (Wilson and Karr 1951; Wilson, Brent, and Jordon 1953; Wilson, Jordon, and Brent 1953; Wilson 1954d), in which selected individual implantation sites were exposed, and only those exposed made malformed. More recently, Brent and McLaughlin (1960) partly reversed this procedure, i.e., irradiated pregnant rats while shielding embryos, and failed to produce congenital malformations. Nor did malformations result when only the placenta was irradiated (Brent 1960).

In addition, various bits of circumstantial evidence support the belief of the unimportance of intermediate maternal effects in the origin of most abnormalities; these are the shortness of the critical periods in radiation-induced teratogenesis (Russell 1950) and the rapidity of detectable response to radiation in embryonic tissues (Kosaka 1927; Hicks 1950; D'Agostino and Brizee 1966).

Nevertheless, irradiation of the pregnant maternal organism has sometimes been not entirely without effect, at any rate so far as the lethal action of irradiation is concerned. Chang and Hunt (1960), e.g., using rabbits, showed that unirradiated 6-day ova transplanted to irradiated recipients resulted in fewer survivors than did the reverse situation. The same appeared to be true for rats (Ketchel and Banik 1964). Additive effects were found in rabbits when ova irradiated in vitro were transferred to irradiated uteri (Hunt 1964). Evidence of a maternal role in offspring death was also obtained by irradiating during a fetal stage (Duplan and Monnot 1965). On the other hand, egg-transplantation studies in mice indicated that death resulted from damage to oocytes rather than to the maternal organism (Glass and Lin 1963; Glass and McClure 1964). Russell and Russell (1954*a, b*) also conceded that an intermediary role of the mother is possible in the case of embryonic death manifested in prenatal loss of whole litters, especially that caused by irradiation during preimplantation stages. But recent studies (Russell and Montgomery 1965) made it seem doubtful that maternal factors play a great role in radiation-induced prenatal mortality.

If, as now seems certain, the *teratogenic* effects of ionizing radiation are due to direct action upon the embryo, we must inquire what this action consists of. Russell and Russell (1954*a*) held that the basis of radiation-induced embryonic maldevelopment is cell death caused by mitotic failure resulting from chromosomal aberrations. They believed that a threshold proportion of cells must be affected in a precursor in order to produce an abnormality, and that the number of cells affected above this threshold determines the degree of abnormality. The particular precursor affected and the manner in which it responds depend on (1) differential rates of activity, e.g., uneven distribution of relative proportions of cells in mitosis in various regions (L. B. Russell 1954); and (2) differential degrees of regulatory ability. Thus, selective initial damage and characteristic power of recovery, as well as secondary events interacting with the primary ones, determine the form of the prenatal effect.

So far as distribution of mitosis is concerned, Wilson (1954*d*) found the same uniform distribution in teratogenically resistant 9th-day rat embryos as in susceptible 10th-day ones; further, although mitotic activity became more localized in regions of active organogenesis on the 11th and 12th days of gestation, the reactions of embryos of these ages were only quantitatively different from those of 10th-day embryos. He concluded, therefore, that there was nothing to indicate that either the rate or distribution of mitosis was responsible for the type of response of the embryo. Škreb, Bijelić and Luković (1963) also excluded greater mitotic activity as the main reason for increased radiosensitivity. Thus, being unable to see how all the effects of radiation can be attributed simply to cell death or slowed mitotic rates, Wilson suggested (Wilson and Karr 1951; Wilson, Brent, and Jordon 1953; Wilson, Jordon, and Brent 1953; Wilson 1954*d*) that radiation produces congenital defects by inducing somatic mutations.

Addressing themselves to this suggestion, Russell and Russell (1954*a*) stated that somatic mutation may be ruled out because in order to account for consistency of response, it would be necessary to assume either directed mutations or a high rate of gene changes with dominant cell-lethal effects. The former assumption is contradictory to the findings of radiation genetics; and the latter was rejected because the radiation-induced somatic mutation rate is far below (Russell and Major 1957) that needed to account for observed frequencies of embryonic malformations.

The specific action of radiation on cells of the developing mammalian nervous system will now be discussed briefly, for the light it may shed on the problem of the mechanism of the teratogenic action of X rays. Hicks (1950) noted that irradiation of pregnant rats and mice resulted in acute necrosis of rapidly growing parts of the fetal brain, spinal cord, and retina, which appeared within a few hours and seemed to be highly selective for the central nervous system; in fact, the developing brain was the most radiosensitive tissue in the fetus in the latter half of gestation. Although Hicks (1950) could not explain this great sensitivity, he noted that cells in the areas affected were not only rapidly multiplying but also rapidly growing and differentiating.

On the other hand (Hicks 1953, 1954b), malformations of the central nervous system were also associated with or initiated by destruction of differentiating, but nonmitotic, primitive neuroblasts and spongioblasts (cells later giving rise to neurons and glia, respectively), which were selectively killed by even low doses of radiation. But it appeared (Hicks 1954a) that despite extensive necrosis of differentiating neural cells, complete or nearly complete repair can occur in many zones, stemming from primitive mitotic cells, such as neurectoderm and some primitive mesenchyme cells, which are relatively radioresistant. Thus, it was concluded that malformations are the end product of a balance between radiation damage and the capacity to undergo repair in any given anlagen or area.

These observations were refined by studies (Fujita *et al.* 1964) employing the technique of tritiated thymidine autoradiography, in which it was found that 200 r of X rays administered to mice early on the 11th day of pregnancy damaged neural matrix cells (i.e., spongioblasts or primitive ependymal cells) but not neuroblasts. Radiation induced a temporary block in the flow of matrix cells at the t_2 period of the mitotic cycle, i.e., just before prophase, so that subsequently the number of cells undergoing division decreased. It thus appeared that teratogenic doses of X rays suppressed the proliferative activities of matrix cells and hence partially depopulated them. On the other hand no such cytokinetic changes were induced by the radiomimetic alkylating agent, thio-TEPA (Fujita *et al.* 1964), a substance not found to induce congenital malformations of the central nervous system in mice (Tanimura and Nishimura 1962), but which produced a low incidence of cranial defects in studies with rats (Thiersch 1957a; Murphy, Moro, and Lacon 1958).

Patterns of cell death and regeneration in the central nervous system of 11th- to 20th-day rat embryos and fetuses were described in detail by Hicks, Brown, and D'Amato (1957), Hicks, D'Amato, and Lowe (1959), Berry and Eayrs (1966), D'Agostino and Brizee (1966), and Hicks and D'Amato (1966).

Similar patterns of radiation-induced destruction and repair were noted in fetal mouse and rat eyes (Rugh and Wolff 1955a, b; Hicks and D'Amato 1963b). Four hours after exposure of 14th-day CF1 fetal mice to 300 r of X rays (Rugh and Wolff 1955a), the presumptive retina showed extreme cellular damage, despite the general contours of the retina remaining intact. This damage persisted at 24 hours after irradiation, but some of it had been removed by phagocytosis. By 72 hours, however, the retina was usually free of dead cells but was retarded in development, and the eye as a whole was smaller than normal. In addition, a few fetal eyes showed residual damage in the form of rosettes at this stage. Nevertheless, at birth (6–7 days after treatment), all eyes appeared normal in size and structure. The most severely damaged cells were discarded, by sloughing off into the vitreous body and the space between the sensory and pigmented layers, with reconstitution of the retinal cell population originating from the undamaged primitive neurectoderm. The lens, its epithelium and vascular tunic, and the pigmented layer were apparently unaffected. More or less the same events occurred in irradiated fetal rat eyes (Hicks and D'Amato 1963*b*).

Fetal eyes treated one day earlier had a somewhat different fate. Pregnant CF1 mice (Rugh and Wolff 1955*b*) were X irradiated on the 13th day with 50, 150, 250, or 300 r and examined 4, 24, and 72 hours, and 6 days (at birth) later. At the stage irradiated the presumptive retina consists of neurectoderm cells that are in the process of multiplying and differentiating into neuroblasts. The 50 r dose had no discernable effect, but the larger doses all produced extensive necrosis of the retina. While exposed eyes seemed fully recovered by 72 hours, they all showed persistent damage in the form of microphthalmia at birth.

Val'shtrem (1960) provided statistical evidence that repair processes occur after embryonic irradiation. He X rayed rats with 130 or 240 r on the 10th day of pregnancy and examined the offspring at daily intervals from the 11th to 17th days of pregnancy. After 130 r the frequency of living anomalous young (with underdeveloped brain, eye, etc.) rose slowly from 2.8% on the 11th day, reached a peak of 75.5% on the 13th day, and declined thereafter to levels of about 40 per cent. Since the mortality rate at the end of this period did not appear to rise in correspondence with the fall in frequency of anomalous fetuses, the author felt that repair of radiation-induced injury may have been partly responsible for the decrease. A similar decrease in anomalous offspring after 240 r, on the contrary, could be explained by the accompanying increase in fetal death. Supporting the belief that repair occurred is the finding (Val'shtrem 1961) that the percentage of dividing cerebral ependymal cells was greatly reduced for 3 days after irradiation on the 10th day, but that thereafter the frequency of mitosis returned to the control level.

The role of the state or degree of differentiation of the embryo in susceptibility to radiation-induced teratogenesis was discussed by Wilson, Brent, and Jordon (1953) and Wilson (1954*d*). Susceptibility of cells to irradiation is usually considered to be inversely related to their degree of differentiation. But this generalization refers to adults, even in which numerous exceptions exist (Patt and Brues 1954). Wilson and coworkers, in fact, found that the

less differentiated 9th-day rat embryo did not develop congenital malformations after irradiation and did not show a graded increase in mortality with
increase in dosage of radiation; whereas the more differentiated 10th- to
12th-day embryos were susceptible to the induction of congenital malformations, and their mortality rate, growth retardation, and malformation frequency increased with dosage. Therefore, so far as this difference between
9th-day and the 10th- to 12th-day embryos was concerned, the generalization
regarding the inverse relation of differentiation and susceptibility broke down.

Within the susceptible period, on the other hand, the generalization
seemed to hold, since the more differentiated, i.e., the older, the embryo the
less susceptible it was, taking more radiation to produce the same amount
of effect. Thus in rats a qualitative change occurs between the 9th and 10th
days of gestation and a quantitative one from the 10th through 12th days,
insofar as the teratogenic response to radiation is concerned.

Interpreting these observations, Wilson, Brent, and Jordon (1953) and
Wilson (1954*d*) proposed that in relatively undifferentiated 9th-day rat embryos a given dose of radiation destroys or disturbs a certain number of
blastomeres, and that if those destroyed comprise fewer than a certain number the result is a slowdown in the developmental schedule equivalent to the
time needed to replace the missing or aberrant cells, with the outcome an
inapparent one or merely a generalized growth retardation. Of course, cell
destruction beyond a tolerable point would be expected to cause embryonic
death (a sentence which, though pleonastic, I favor retaining for completeness).

The effects of irradiating during the period of teratogenic susceptibility
are decided by the degree of differentiation of the embryo. I.e., since different
groups of cells have by then acquired various developmental potentialities as
well as variable radiosensitivity, cell loss is tissue- or organ-localized and
hence less able to be recovered. The result is dose-graded mortality or specific
congenital defects, requiring larger doses to elicit comparable effects as the
embryo ages, i.e., as it consists of ever greater proportions of cells with restricted developmental potentialities.

Let me summarize these facts and points of view. Prenatal irradiation
produces death, decreased size, and congenital malformations. Preimplantation, preorganogenetic, and undifferentiated embryos are killed or retarded in
growth, but not usually malformed, whereas those undergoing differentiation
or organogenesis are malformed as well as stunted and killed. The difference
in teratologic response between very young and older embryos is probably
not based on rates or distribution of mitosis *per se*. In fact, whether a cell is
in mitosis or not may be less indicative of its radiosensitivity than whether it
has attained a particular degree or type of differentiation. Thus mitotic
neurectodermal cells are radioresistant, whereas cells they give rise to, the
nonmitotic neuroblasts, are extremely radiosensitive, and the cells they in
turn give rise to, the nonmitotic neurons, are again radioresistant.

The embryonic effects of radiation are ultimately due to cell death, the number of cells killed being related to dose, all other things being equal. Since the very young embryo is almost entirely composed of undifferentiated, totipotent cells, death of such cells below a critical proportion is compensated for by their replacement and is therefore almost entirely without effect on morphogenesis, beyond a possible overall reduction in size, which may or may not be persistent. Embryonic death will result if the number of cells destroyed is greater than can be replaced before their presence is required for continued development.

As cellular totipotency gives way to pluripotency and in turn to ever more contracted developmental potentialities during advancing embryonic life, the number and type of cells destroyed by a given dose of radiation becomes increasingly limited by 2 factors; the emergence of (1) variable sensitivity of different cells and cell aggregations, and of (2) variable powers of restoration of lost cells through proliferation of less differentiated precursor lines. It is thus through these mechanisms, and interactions with them of secondary events, that specific types and frequencies of congenital malformations are produced by irradiation with particular doses of X rays at certain times in gestation.

Can incomplete or delayed restitution of cell loss explain all X ray-induced embryonic malformation? As Gruenwald (1954) has noted, even abnormal cellular differentiation is not involved for certain, since, e.g., in the case of fused kidney, the tissues are still normal kidney tissues, and hence what is possibly at work are abnormal growth patterns. On the other hand, the kidney malformation may be the relatively remote consequence of a situation (cell loss or abnormal differentiation or disturbed growth pattern) in a surrounding or antecedent structure that no longer exists or manifests the primary abnormality.

Such a discussion may continue for hours and pages; but essentially the argument may be set forth as follows. While some abnormalities, such as microphthalmia and reduced thickness of the cerebral cortex, may sometimes be conveniently explicable on the basis of failure to make up for cell destruction, others, such as hydrocephalus and atresia of the anus, are not so easily explained in this manner. It is, of course, not possible to deny that so wide-sweeping and all-embracing a postulation as cell loss or damage and all its infinite theoretical ramifications can be invoked as responsible for any and all developmental abnormalities, not only induced by radiation but by every teratogen. I feel, however, that it would be unwise to do so for 2 reasons. First, the theory is still so vague that it really says nothing, but sounds so logical that it engenders complacence; and second, it closes the mind to alternatives, of which we must always be prepared to conceive.

6

Other Teratogenic Substances

Alkylating Agents

Nitrogen Mustard

Nitrogen mustard [2,2'-dichloro-N-methyldiethylamine N-oxide hydrochloride, or methyl-bis(β-chloroethyl)amine hydrochloride] was one of the earliest chemical teratogens discovered (Haskin 1948). It has been given to pregnant rats (Haskin 1948; Murphy and Karnofsky 1956; Murphy, Moro, and Lacon 1958; Okano *et al.* 1958; Brock and Kreybig 1964; Müller and Škreb 1964; Müller 1966) and mice (Danforth and Center 1954; Thalhammer and Heller-Szöllösy 1955; Nishimura and Takagaki 1959*a*; Jurand 1961). The commonest defects produced were those of the skeleton, but malformations of the central nervous system also occurred in most studies. An unusual feature of many of the experiments is that exencephaly was induced by treatment given relatively late in pregnancy, at times when the neural tube is apparently already normally closed.

In rats, Haskin (1948) produced exencephaly confined to the occiput with injection on the 13th or 14th day of pregnancy; Murphy, Moro, and Lacon (1958) obtained minimal encephalocele in a small number of offspring after treatment on the 13th day; and Müller and Škreb (1964) got exencephaly with treatment on the 12th or 14th day. Okano *et al.* (1958) also noted this defect. Hayashi, Yama, and Fujii (1957) caused no congenital malformations in rats with treatment on the 8th day of pregnancy. In mice, Danforth and Center (1954) produced exencephaly by intraperitoneal injection on the 10th to 12th days; and Nishimura and Takagaki (1959*a*) one case after injection on the 12th day. In addition, hydrocephalus was found by Danforth and Center (1954).

Jurand (1961) gave pregnant mice nitrogen mustard and 2 of its derivatives during early embryogenesis, and produced histological changes in the neural tube, as seen at early and middle fetal stages. Embryos the closure of whose neural plate was prevented or retarded died before the 13th day of pregnancy.

Müller (1966) gave intrauterine injections of water-soluble nitrogen mustard on the 14th day of pregnancy in rats and produced malformations typical of the teratogen in about half the offspring in treated horns, but did not damage offspring in untreated horns of the same females; thus apparently demonstrating that the compound's teratogenic effects result from direct action upon fetuses.

Triethylene Melamine

Triethylene melamine (TEM) was used by Sobin (1955), Thiersch (1957*a*), Murphy, Moro, and Lacon (1958), Tuchmann-Duplessis and Mercier-Parot (1958*a*), Jurand (1959), Kageyama (1961), and Kageyama and Nishimura (1961). In rats, Thiersch (1957*a*) obtained a few cases of cranial defects, such as exencephaly and encephalocele; and Murphy, Moro, and Lacon (1958) produced encephalocele in 11/60 (18.3%) offspring. In mice, Jurand (1959) noted kinking of vertebrae and spinal cord with fusion of spinal ganglia in 28.5 per cent, 3 cases of exencephaly, and one of craniorachischisis, in offspring examined on the 15th day of gestation and at term; and in one strain used, Kageyama (1961) and Kageyama and Nishimura (1961) recorded bulging of the crown region consisting of a prominent localized protrusion. This defect was not further described but may have been encephalocele.

Triethylene Thiophosphoramide

Triethylene thiophosphoramide (thio-TEPA) and a variant (TEPA) both produced low incidences of cranial defects in rats (Thiersch 1957*a*; Murphy, Moro, and Lacon 1958; Okano *et al.* 1959). In mice, only skeletal defects were induced by thio-TEPA (Tanimura and Nishimura 1962; Nanjo 1964; Nishikawa 1964; Takano, Tanimura, and Nishimura 1965).

Busulfan

Busulfan (1,4-dimethanesulfonyloxybutane), or myleran, did not induce congenital malformations of the central nervous system in rats in some studies (Murphy, Moro, and Lacon 1958; Hemsworth and Jackson 1963*a, b*), but did so in others (Alexandrov 1964, 1965, 1966) after treatment on the 8th or 9th day of pregnancy. The nature of the lethal effect of a large dose of busulfan was studied by Alexandrov (1966), who found evidence for its basis being failure of the allantois to join with the ectoplacenta in forming the definitive placenta; it thus appeared that embryonic mortality was unrelated to the other teratogenic effects of the drug at the stage given.

Chlorambucil

Chlorambucil [p-(N,N-di-2-chloroethyl)aminophenylbutyric acid] was used by Didcock, Jackson, and Robson (1956), Murphy, Moro, and Lacon (1958), Monie (1961), and Tuchmann-Duplessis and Mercier-Parot (1964*a*), all working with rats. Murphy, Moro, and Lacon (1958) produced a high incidence of encephalocele (66/106 = 62.3%), and Monie (1961), although finding no externally visible defects of the central nervous system, noted anterior spina bifida in 4/5 sectioned offspring. Tuchmann-Duplessis and Mercier-Parot (1964*a*), beginning treatment on the 6th or 7th day of pregnancy, found exencephaly, spina bifida, and craniorachischisis.

Cyclophosphamide

Cyclophosphamide [1-bis(2-chloroethyl)-amino-1-oxo-2-aza-5-oxaphosphoridin], or cytoxan, a powerful teratogen in rats (Murphy 1962), produced severe exencephaly, otocephaly, and hydrocephalus when administered on the 13th day of pregnancy. It also caused malformations of the central nervous system in 3 stocks of rats after single administrations (Brock and Kreybig 1964) of 40 mg/kg at the remarkably early time of the 4th day of pregnancy. When this dose was divided and 5 mg/kg given daily from the 8th to the 15th days of gestation, skeletal defects were induced. Kreybig (1965*a, b*) noted a variety of partly phase-specific defects, including microcephaly, encephalocele, and exencephaly, after single treatment in rats on the 12th, 13th, or 14th day of pregnancy. These results were compared with the defects produced in 2 strains of mice by treating with cyclophosphamide on the 10th, 11th, or 12th day of pregnancy (Hackenberger and Kreybig 1965). Injection on the 10th day resulted in microcephaly and hydrocephalus; on the 11th day, in encephalocele and exencephaly; and on the 12th day, in microcephaly and encephalocele. Some possible strain differences were encountered. Wilson (1964) found the action of cyclophosphamide to be potentiated by sub- and suprathreshold doses of 5-fluorouracil and by actinomycin D. Cyclophosphamide was also teratogenic in rabbits (Gerlinger 1964; Gerlinger and Clavert 1965), but, as employed, it did not produce defects of the central nervous system.

Apholate

A ewe on a chronic toxicity experiment utilizing apholate [2,2,4,4,6,6-hexahydro-2,2,4,4,6,6-hexakis-(1-aziridinyl)-1,3,5,2,4,6-triazaphosphorine], an ethylenimine-type polyfunctional alkylating agent, used as an insect chemosterilant, delivered a lamb with congenital anomalies (Younger 1965). Among the defects were small and misshapen cranium, absent optic nerves and optic chiasm, and cerebral agyria.

Metepa

Another chemosterilant, metepa (tris[1-2(2-methylaziridinyl)]phosphine oxide), proved teratogenic in Sherman rats (Gaines and Kimbrough 1966);

intraperitoneal injection of 30 mg/kg on the 12th day of pregnancy produced malformation in all survivors, including one with hydrocephalus and 4 with meningocele.

Purine and Pyrimidine Antimetabolites

A large number of antimetabolites of purines and pyrimidines have been tested for their teratologic and antifertility properties. Some of these substances resulted in congenital malformations, but the defects have only rarely been fully described.

Purine Antimetabolites

6-Mercaptopurine induced some malformations (Thiersch 1954*b*; Zunin and Borrone 1955; Didcock, Jackson, and Robson 1956; Tuchmann-Duplessis and Mercier-Parot 1958*a*, 1966; Adams, Hay, and Lutwak-Mann 1961; Murphy 1962; Bragonier, Roesky, and Carver 1964) but those of the central nervous system were usually few. Using rats, Zunin and Borrone (1955) found hydrocephalus, which was not described, in 55 per cent of offspring. Murphy (1962) produced encephalocele after treating Wistar rats on the 12th day of pregnancy. Tuchmann-Duplessis (1960) stated that treatment started earlier produced more malformations of the nervous system. An exencephaly occurred after treatment with 2-amino-6(1'-methyl-4'-nitro-5'-imidazolyl)mercaptopurine (Thiersch 1960, p. 268); but further studies with this compound failed to give malformations (Thiersch 1962*a*). Rabbits treated on the 6th to 9th days of gestation had 55 per cent malformed surviving young, and the defects included spina bifida aperta and encephalocele (Tuchmann-Duplessis and Mercier-Parot 1966).

Numerous other purine antimetabolites were also used (Thiersch 1957*b*, 1962*a*, *b*; Tuchmann-Duplessis and Mercier-Parot 1959*b*). In rats cranial defects with and without hydrocephalus were seen after 2,6-diaminopurine, 6-chloropurine, and thioguanine (Thiersch 1957*b*), and exencephaly after azaguanine (Thiersch 1960, p. 111). Mice, rats, and rabbits were injected with azathioprine [6(1'-methyl-4'-nitro-5'-imidazolyl)mercaptopurine] (Thiersch 1962*a*; Tuchmann-Duplessis and Mercier-Parot 1964*b*, *c*; Githens, Rosenkrantz, and Tunnock 1965; Rosenkrantz *et al.* 1967). The effects were somewhat conflicting, but in any case, central nervous system defects may have occurred only in a few mice (Githens, Rosenkrantz and Tunnock 1965; Rosenkrantz *et al.* 1967).

Pyrimidine Antimetabolites

About a dozen halogenated pyrimidines are teratogenic in rats, mice, and hamsters (Karnofsky, Murphy, and Lacon 1958; Dagg 1960, 1963; Murphy 1960, 1962, 1965; Murphy, Dagg, and Runner 1961; Dagg and Kallio 1962; DiPaolo 1964; Ruffolo and Ferm 1965*a*, *b*). Only some have caused congenital malformations of the central nervous system. Murphy (1960, 1962) found marked degrees of exencephaly in Wistar rats after treatment with 5-fluorodeoxyuridine on the 10th day of pregnancy; and produced (Murphy 1965) encephalocele with 5-fluorodeoxycytidine, 5-chlorodeoxyuridine, and 5-bromodeoxyuridine, by treating on the 13th day of pregnancy. Pregnant Syrian hamsters were given intravenous injections of 5-bromodeoxyuridine on the 6th, 7th, or 8th day of gestation (Ruffolo and Ferm 1965*a*, *b*). Single doses of 400 mg/kg caused malformations in 82 per cent of survivors after treatment on the 8th day. Most frequently encountered was exencephaly, ranging from a slight knobby protruberance of brain tissue to complete cerebral herniation Spina bifida occurred in one surviving offspring after 7th-day treatment; no malformations were seen after 6th-day treatment.

The teratogenic properties of 5-chlorodeoxyuridine in Wistar rats were studied in detail by Chaube and Murphy (1964). Although treatment on the 12th day led to various defects, those of the central nervous system were apparently not found. Treatment on the 13th day was made with doses ranging from 62 to 1000 mg/kg, but only with the largest dose was a malformation of the central nervous system, encephalocele (called exencephaly), produced (22/35 = 63%). A minimal dose of 125 mg/kg thymidine was required to provide complete protection of fetuses against 500 mg/kg 5-chlorodeoxyuridine. The protection afforded decreased with the amount of time between administration of the 2 compounds, whether the thymidine was given before or after the 5-chlorodeoxyuridine. Thymidine was also somewhat protective in mice (Dagg and Kallio 1962).

The teratogenic action of 5-fluorouracil was strongly potentiated by trypan blue, 6-mercaptopurine, actinomycin D, and cyclophosphamide (Wilson 1964).

Glutamine Antimetabolites

Two compounds of this sort have been used, o-diazoacetyl-l-serine or azaserine (Murphy and Karnofsky 1956; Friedman 1957; Thiersch 1957*c*), and 6-diazo-5-oxo-l-norleucine or DON (Thiersch 1957*d*; Murphy 1960; the latter also mentioned the use of this compound by Friedman 1959). Malformations produced with both substances were mostly of the skeleton. Certain schedules of treatment with azaserine in rats induced hydrocephalus and "malformed heads" (Thiersch 1957*c*). No congenital malformations were reported in mice surviving treatment with DON (Jackson, Robson, and Wander 1959).

Alkaloids

Colchicine

Several abnormal offspring resulted from artificially inseminating female rabbits with sperm suspended in a solution of colchicine (Chang 1944). The abnormalities included unclosed anterior fontanelle, otocephaly, and microcephaly. According to the author the malformations may have been the result of: polyploidy induced in the sperm, a disturbance in nuclear mechanism or organizer system, some substance carried into the ovum, or the presence of some substance in the environment of the egg that affected it at a later stage of gestation. These results have not been confirmed.

Total litter destruction was usually produced by administering colchicine or certain of its derivatives to pregnant mice (Kerr 1947; Didcock, Jackson, and Robson 1956; Wiesner, Wolfe, and Yudkin 1958), rats (Conaway 1955; Thiersch 1958; Tuchmann-Duplessis and Mercier-Parot 1958*a*), and rabbits (Didcock, Jackson, and Robson 1956). In only one of these studies (Wiesner, Wolfe, and Yudkin 1958) were congenital malformations noted; various defects apparently occurred, but only those of the tail were mentioned. In another study (Van Dyke and Ritchey 1947), several abnormal rat offspring, including one with diencephalic hydrocephalus, occurred after treatment on the 10th day of pregnancy. Three malformed rabbits (2 spina bifida, 1 spina bifida and hydrocephalus) were produced by colcemid administration, but no fetal effects of this agent were noted in macaque monkeys (Morris *et al.* 1967*a*).

Recent studies with mice were somewhat more productive. Shoji and Makino (1966) gave female dd type mice single subcutaneous injections of 0.5, 1.0, or 2.5 mg/kg colchicine on the 2nd to 14th days of pregnancy. The fetal mortality rate was significantly increased only by the largest dose, but malformations occurred after all 3 doses. Exencephaly, the only nervous system anomaly produced, was seen in just a few cases. Vankin and Grass (1966) gave C57BL females crossed to BALB males single intraperitoneal injections of 1.8 mg/kg colcemid early on the 9th day of gestation. Among the 166 survivors on the 17th day 38 were grossly abnormal, 22 (13.2%) with exencephaly, which again was the only defect of the nervous system noted.

Congenital malformations were reported (Ferm 1963*a*) in offspring of pregnant golden hamsters treated intravenously with colchicine on the 8th day of gestation. Surviving young exhibited various anomalies including exencephaly of various degrees. Incipient hydrocephalus was noted in embryos recovered 24 hours after treatment (Ferm 1965*a*).

Veratrum

A congenital cyclopean type of malformation occurred in 1 to 25 per cent of lambs in flocks that grazed on certain alpine meadows in southwestern Idaho (Binns *et al.* 1959). The abnormalities were confined to the head and consisted of severe cases of distortion or absence of some bones of the face, cyclopean deformity of the eyes, fusion of the cerebral hemispheres, and hydrocephalus. The lambs were usually born alive but died immediately after birth owing to suffocation. Milder cases, whose only outward defect was short upper jaw, sometimes survived, but had difficulty nursing because of the jaw condition.

One hundred and sixteen malformed lambs were examined over a 4-year period (Binns, Anderson, and Sullivan 1960). The most extreme outward abnormality was single median cyclopean eye, but lesser degrees of ocular defect also occurred. The formation of the cerebrum varied from a small, rudimentary, unsegmented structure to apparently normally-divided hemispheres. In most lambs with extensive facial deformities the cerebral hemispheres were fused and cystic, there were no olfactory bulbs, only a single optic nerve was present, and the pituitary was missing.

Four lambs were selected as representative of the various degrees of malformation encountered and were described in detail. In the least deformed specimen, in which the eyes were normally placed, but the upper jaw was slightly short, no abnormalities of the brain could be found. In the second animal, with slight orbital and various facial defects, the olfactory bulbs were absent and the cerebral hemispheres were small and fused. There were no convolutions and the lateral ventricles were represented by a single, large, fluid-filled cavity. The pituitary was absent, but the brainstem and cerebellum were normal in shape and size. A single median optic nerve was present, but the optic chiasm was absent.

The third animal, which had a single eye and more severe facial abnormalities, also lacked the olfactory brain and had a median optic nerve. The cerebral hemispheres were fused and the tissues were indistinct. Internally the hemispheres consisted of a large fluid-filled space, which was lined by a thin layer of cortical tissue compressed against the cranial wall. Again no changes were found in the brainstem and cerebellum, but the pituitary was absent. In the last specimen, one with a severely misshapen head and single median eye, the brain was so anomalous it could not be removed intact. It was obvious, however, that the forebrain consisted of a fluid-filled vesicle. The amount of fluid was so great it forced cerebral tissue through the top of the cranium, resulting in a large circular defect in the skull. Again no pituitary was found.

"Carrier" ewes bred to their sons failed to have cyclopic offspring, thus eliminating the possibility that the condition was hereditary (Binns *et al.* 1959). And so, at this time the investigators suspected anoxia, nutritional imbalance, or a toxic plant or mineral substance ingested in early pregnancy (Evans, Ingalls, and Binns 1966).

In searching for the responsible agent, it was noted (Binns *et al.* 1962) that the grazing areas associated with defective lambs had 2 characteristics in common: they were above 6,000 feet in elevation, and they contained wet, seepage meadows in which the plant *Veratrum californicum* was present and eaten by the sheep during the breeding season. In addition to these observations, the suspected etiologic relation of the plant to the cyclopean malformation was confirmed by the production of the anomaly in extensive feeding trials with Veratrum.

Field studies showed (Babbott, Binns, and Ingalls 1962) that the critical gestation stage for production of the malformation was the second and third weeks after conception. This was later verified by feeding fresh Veratrum early in pregnancy. Animals fed the plant for the first 5 to 10 days of pregnancy all delivered normal lambs, while those on Veratrum for 15, 20, or 30 days after breeding had malformed lambs (Babbott, Binns, and Ingalls 1962; Binns *et al.* 1963). It thus appeared that the teratogenic action of the plant was exercised between the 10th and the 15th days of pregnancy. It was also learned that plants obtained from different range areas varied widely in toxicity and teratogenicity (Binns *et al.* 1963; Binns, James, and Shupe 1964).

The time of action of the plant was further delimited by feeding (Binns *et al.* 1965) the plant on single days from the 11th to 16th after breeding; which resulted in defects only when it was given on the 14th day, at a time when sheep embryos are $12\frac{1}{2}$ to 13 days old, and have no somites. Further proof of the limited time of action of the plant was furnished by feeding dyed material, which left the rumen within 24 hours. *Veratrum californicum* was also fed to rabbits, mice, rats, guinea pigs, and swine, but did not produce the cyclopean defect (Binns 1965).

By ethanol extraction (Keeler and Binns 1964), a teratogenic substance was obtained from all parts of dried Veratrum plants. The material was believed to contain at least 2 or 3 alkaloids of the veratrum series, any one or possibly all of which may be the teratogen responsible for the cyclopean-type malformation. Further efforts along these lines succeeded in isolating and identifying 4 known alkaloids and 2 previously unreported ones (Keeler and Binns 1966*a*), and in demonstrating that certain fractions as well as glycosidic and parent alkamine alkaloid preparations derived from the plant were teratogenic (Keeler and Binns 1966*b*). The malformation produced, however, was not cyclopia, but an entirely different and unexpected condition, bowing of legs (Keeler and Binns 1966*c*).

Vinca Alkaloids

The chemotherapeutic alkaloids, vincaleukoblastine (or vinblastine) and vincristine, derived from the common periwinkle plant *Vinca rosea* L. are teratogenic in hamsters, rats, rabbits, and monkeys. Ferm (1963*b*) gave golden hamsters these substances intravenously on the 8th day of pregnancy. The highest incidence of anomalies in surviving offspring was obtained with injections of 0.25 mg/kg vinblastine (28.6%) and 0.1 mg/kg vincristine (15.4%). Among the defects produced by the former was spina bifida and by the latter, mild exencephaly.

DeMyer (1964) gave single intramuscular injections of 0.025 mg vinblastine to Long–Evans and Holtzman rats on about the 9th day of pregnancy and induced malformations, including microcephaly, other brain defects, and spinal defects in 44.5 per cent of surviving offspring. Sections of one offspring revealed a holistic prosencephalon, i.e., one not divided into cerebral hemispheres; olfactory bulbs were also lacking.

In a study with vincristine sulfate (DeMyer 1965*b*), rats of the same stocks given single intramuscular injections of 0.05 to 0.075 mg on the 9th day of pregnancy had offspring 83.4 per cent (222/266) of which were malformed when examined about a week before term. Sixty-one of the animals had microcephaly, 14 encephalocele, and 59 exencephaly or anencephaly. In addition, 6 animals were aprosopic, 19 had otocephaly, many had clefts of various facial structures, and 30 had spinal dysraphism, the last of which was not described. Another large number (53) had median defects of the upper lip and jaw, and most of them had microcephaly associated with incomplete development of the prosencephalon. Microscopic study of some of these fetuses showed the cerebrum to be undivided into hemispheres and the olfactory bulbs and tracts to be absent.

Cohlan and Kitay (1965) gave 0.1 to 0.5 mg/kg vinblastine, intraperitoneally, to Wistar rats, daily from the 7th to 12th days of pregnancy. The highest incidence of malformations (9.4%) was obtained with a dose level of 0.25 mg/kg. Sixty per cent of the abnormal offspring had a characteristic constellation of defects, which included exencephaly, iniencephaly, and spina bifida. A few malformed rabbits (including 1 hydrocephalus and 1 exencephaly) were caused by vinblastine (Morris *et al.* 1967*a*).

Ohzu and Shoji (1965) gave daily subcutaneous injections of 2.5 mg/kg vinblastine sulfate to pregnant mice of 2 strains on the 11th to 14th days of gestation. The only central nervous system defect noted, in near-term young, was exencephaly, which occurred exclusively in one of the strains (MT) and not the other (dd). However, this defect also occurred in saline-treated MT offspring, and the incidence in both groups was relatively high.

Presumptive evidence that vincristine and vinblastine enter rat embryos was obtained by DeMyer (1965*a*), who noted an accumulation of cells arrested in metaphase in embryos taken soon after treatment of pregnant rats with teratogenic doses of these drugs.

Two of 4 monkeys (*Macaca mulatta*) given single doses of vincristine sulfate (0.15–0.2 mg/kg) on the 25th to 36th days of pregnancy had malformed offspring (Courtney and Valerio 1967). One abnormal baby, whose mother received 0.175 mg/kg of the drug on the 28th day, had an encephalocele; the other had syndactyly.

Rauvolfia Alkaloids

Deserpidine (11-desmethoxyreserpine), obtained from *Rauvolfia canescens* L., produced skeletal and tail defects in rats, but not defects of the central nervous system (Tuchmann-Duplessis and Mercier-Parot 1961*a*). Another Rauvolfia alkaloid, reserpine (derived from *Rauvolfia serpentina* L.), prevented implantation and caused embryonic death in rabbits and rats (Kehl *et al.* 1956;

Tuchmann-Duplessis, Gershon, and Mercier-Parot 1957; Bovet-Nitti and Bovet 1959). When Sprague-Dawley rats were given single intramuscular injections of reserpine (0.1–2.0 mg/kg) on the 9th or 10th day of pregnancy, a total of 30/735 deformed offspring resulted, including one with exencephaly and 2 with encephalocele (Goldman and Yakovac 1965).

Heliotrine

The pyrrolizidine alkaloid heliotrine, a class of compound found in 3 important plant families (Senecio, Crotalaria, and Heliotropium), caused skeletal malformations in rats, but defects of the central nervous system were not noted (Green and Christie 1961).

Hypoglycemic Agents

Insulin

Administration of insulin to pregnant rats has only rarely been reported to induce congenital malformations. Chronic treatment with 20 to 40 units (U)/kg daily from weaning (Ferrill 1943) was not teratogenic. Injection of 7 or 8 U per day throughout pregnancy (Lichtenstein, Guest, and Warkany 1951), of 0.5 U per 12 hours during the last one or 2 weeks of pregnancy (Love, Kinch, and Stevenson 1964), and of 8 U per day for 4 days during the middle of pregnancy (Tuchmann-Duplessis and Mercier-Parot 1958b), produced no malformations. In rats made diabetic by administration of alloxan before conception and in which the diabetes was controlled by injections of insulin (5 or 10 U/day) during pregnancy, offspring had no congenital malformations (Kim *et al.* 1960; Wells, Kim, and Lazarow 1960).

Scaglione (1962) used rats of unspecified origin and administered, by an unstated route, 0.5 U insulin per 12 hours from the 8th to the 14th or 19th days of pregnancy. No gross defects were produced. Survivors of the longer treatment were also microscopically normal, but abnormalities were noted in those from the shorter course of treatment. The defects consisted of dilatation of the 4th ventricle and thoracic portions of the central spinal canal. There was also evidence of diplomyelic changes at this level of the cord.

Mice were used in studies by Smithberg, Sanchez, and Runner (1956) and Smithberg and Runner (1963). Prepubertal strain 129 mice, induced to ovulate and given 0.1 U protamine zinc insulin on the 9th day of pregnancy (Smithberg, Sanchez, and Runner 1956), produced offspring 63 per cent of which had exencephaly or other abnormalities. Control mice, injected with distilled water, had 5 per cent malformed offspring. The effects of insulin or tolbutamide, alone or in conjunction with nicotinamide, were compared in 2 inbred strains, 129 and BALB/c (Smithberg and Runner 1963). Females received single intraperitoneal injections of 0.1 U protamine zinc insulin on the 10th day of gestation. As in the previous experiment, food was withheld for 6 hours after injection. The 2 strains responded quite differently from each other.

In the 129 strain, the total rate of congenital malformation produced by insulin (62%) was similar to that produced by tolbutamide (56%). The incidence of particular defects, however, was different after these 2 treatments, exencephaly being commoner after insulin (30%) than after tolbutamide (18%). Furthermore, concurrent treatment of strain 129 mice with insulin and nicotinamide produced a picture (all defects 58%, exencephaly 33%) similar to that done by insulin alone (62 and 30%, respectively).

In the BALB/c offspring, however, only 3 per cent were defective after insulin treatment, whereas 44 per cent were defective after tolbutamide; and while in the 129 strain no potentiation of the effects of insulin occurred after concurrent treatment with nicotamide, intensification was seen in the BALB/c mice—49 per cent defective offspring resulted after concurrent administration of the 2 compounds (but only 3% had exencephaly).

The rabbit also proved to be a choice animal for demonstrating the teratogenic effects of insulin. Chomette (1955) used rabbits of several breeds and gave (route unspecified) 20 to 22 U on the 6th, 7th, 9th, or 11th day of pregnancy or 20 to 22 U on the 6th or 9th day followed by half that dose on the next day. Females injected once had macroscopically normal offspring, but those treated on 2 successive days produced several abnormal young. The malformations consisted of microcephaly and ectopia cordis. Brinsmade (1957) and Brinsmade, Büchner, and Rübsaamen (1956), also using various breeds of rabbits, administered 20 to 22 U of insulin intravenously on the 6th to 13th days of pregnancy. Among the survivors, removed on the 15th day, were many with external and microscopic abnormalities, including microcephaly, atypical head, spinal cord asymmetries and irregularities, diplomyelia, and spina bifida occulta and aperta in the caudal region.

A protective effect of insulin on teratogenesis produced by other substances was noted by Millen and Woollam (1958b) and Woollam and Millen (1960), but these results were not confirmed in extensive studies by Cohlan and Stone (1961).

Sulfonylurea Drugs

A number of sulfonylurea drugs are teratogenic in animals. Most of the abnormalities produced in rats were of the eye (Tuchmann-Duplessis and Mercier-Parot 1958b, c; Meyer and Isaac-Mathy 1958), but occasional malformations of the central nervous system were also noted. Tuchmann-Duplessis and Mercier-Parot (1959c) found about 5 per cent exencephaly and spina bifida after treatment with carbutamide (1-butyl-3-sulfanilylurea). Meyer (1961) induced hydrocephalus in a small number of offspring; the condition consisted of dilatation of the lateral and 3rd ventricles with great thinning of the surrounding cerebral tissues. Barilyak (1965) produced encephalocele and hydrocephalus, as well as eye defects. Another hypoglycemic drug, 1,1-dimethylbiguanide hydrochloride, used in rats, caused rare instances of craniorachischisis and duplication of head and body (Tuchmann-Duplessis and Mercier-Parot 1961*b*; Roux 1962).

Tolbutamide [1-butyl-3-(p-tolylsulfonyl)urea], given to rats, was found to be much less teratogenic than carbutamide (Tuchmann-Duplessis and Mercier-Parot 1958*c*; Meyer 1961); to cause minor skeletal modification only (Dawson 1964; McColl, Globus, and Robinson 1965); or not to be teratogenic at all (Bänder 1963, cited by Lazarus and Volk 1963). Chlorpropamide [1-propyl-3-(p-chlorobenzenesulfonyl)urea], was not teratogenic in rats in one study (Tuchmann-Duplessis and Mercier-Parot 1959*d*), but induced eye defects in another (Meyer 1961). Glybuthiazole [N'-(5-tert.-butyl-1,3,4-thiadiozol-z-yl)-sulfanilamide] (Tuchmann-Duplessis and Mercier-Parot 1958*c*) and acetohexamide [N-p-acetylphenylsulfonyl)-N'-cyclohexylurea] (Barilyak 1965) were not teratogenic.

Such agents are also teratogenic in mice. Smithberg (1961) and Smithberg and Runner (1963) administered tolbutamide (1 mg/g) intraperitoneally, on the 10th day of gestation, to female mice of 3 inbred strains, 129, BALB/c, and C57BL/6, and induced vertebral and rib defects and exencephaly. The total incidence of malformed offspring in the strains was 56, 44, and 13 per cent, respectively; and of exencephaly was 18, 1, and 0 per cent, respectively. Quantitative strain differences were thus demonstrated.

The effect of concurrent administration of tolbutamide and nicotinamide was also investigated by these authors. Whereas an augmenting influence of nicotinamide occurred in 129 and C57BL/6 mice (total incidence of defects, 84 and 42%, respectively; of exencephaly, 36 and 11%, respectively), no such interaction took place in BALB/c mice (total incidence, 42%; exencephaly, 3%).

Carbutamide in mice produced eye defects and one case of exencephaly, and in rabbits eye defects only (Tuchmann-Duplessis and Mercier-Parot 1963*a*), while tolbutamide caused no defects, gross or microscopic, in rabbits (Lazarus and Volk 1963).

Alloxan

This section will deal mostly with the effects on prenatal development of alloxan administered during pregnancy and, with one exception (Endo 1966), will not consider the question of the effects on pregnancy of maternal diabetes induced by alloxan given before conception, since gross developmental defects almost never resulted from such treatment. The latter subject was exhaustively reviewed by Angervall (1959) and Koskenoja (1961).

Alloxan [2,4,5,6(1,3)-pyrimidinetetrone] was given to pregnant rats by several investigators (Bartelheimer and Kloos 1952; Kreshover, Clough, and Bear 1953; Angervall 1959; Solomon 1959; Lazarow, Kim, and Wells 1960), but except for one tail and one eye defect (Bartelheimer and Kloos 1952) no gross congenital malformations were reported. Some histological abnormalities of dental tissues were noted (Kreshover, Clough, and Bear 1953), and morphological changes occurred in the chorioallantoic placenta (Mohr, Althoff, and Wrba 1964).

Mice are apparently more susceptible to the teratogenic effects of alloxan, since in all experiments made with this species congenital malformation was reported. Ross and Spector (1952) gave "white" mice 100 to 150 mg/kg alloxan, subcutaneously, on 3 successive (but unspecified) days of gestation. In 5 of 24 litters some of the offspring had a "head defect which suggested myeloencephalocele." Watanabe and Ingalls (1963) and Takano, Tanimura, and Nishimura (1965) produced orofacial and skeletal defects, but no abnormalities of the central nervous system, after single administrations on the 9th to 14th days of pregnancy. Horii (1964) also produced oral defects (25/369 = 6.8% cleft palate), which were prevented by insulin injections. Koskenoja (1961) found a significant incidence of lens anomalies in offspring of females given alloxan between the 12th and 15th days of pregnancy.

Treatment early in pregnancy induced congenital malformations of the central nervous system. Horii, Watanabe, and Ingalls (1966) gave alloxan monohydrate (80 mg/kg) intravenously on the 4th day of pregnancy to stock colony mice. This treatment produced 22/437 malformed offspring; 7 of the defective young had craniorachischisis, one had exencephaly, one spina bifida, and one spina bifida occulta. Pregnant females treated additionally with lente insulin hypodermically (0.4 U/12 hours beginning 30–36 hours after alloxan, continuing until the 16th day of gestation) had only 1/472 malformed offspring (cleft palate).

Endo (1966) gave single intravenous injections of 50 mg/kg alloxan to young CF1 mice, which were bred 3 days later. Of 100 treated females that became pregnant, 37 bore malformed offspring; in all 100 females, 67/858 (7.8%) surviving late fetuses were defective. Two defective offspring (1 with exencephaly, 1 with agnathia) were found among 974 living control fetuses. Various types of defects occurred in the experimental group, the most frequent of which was agnathia; defects of the central nervous system consisted of exencephaly (12 cases), craniorachischisis (8 cases), microcephaly (3 cases), and spina bifida (2 cases). All but 10 defective fetuses had single malformations.

Klosovskii (1963, pp. 174–83) reported studies done with rabbits. Females that received 100 to 180 mg/kg alloxan on the 2nd or 3rd day of pregnancy had offspring with marked decrease in size of all parts of the brain, especially the cerebellum, which had a reduced number of laminae in the vermis. In addition, 4 offspring had gross defects, including cyclopia and curvature of the spine. Alloxan treatment on the 9th day of pregnancy resulted in one offspring, from a severely diabetic female given insulin, with marked internal hydrocephalus, in which the walls of the cerebral hemispheres were very thin; in addition there was almost complete absence of the cerebellum. Details of this study can be found in Barashnev (1964).

A paper in Japanese (Fujimoto *et al.* 1958), cited by Takano, Tanimura, and Nishimura (1965), reported the production of malformations, mostly of the central nervous system, in 10/93 liveborn offspring from alloxan-diabetic rabbits. The latter authors did not make clear whether the rabbits were treated before or during pregnancy.

Thyroid Factors

The effects on reproduction and prenatal development of maternal hypo-thyroidism produced by thyroidectomy and goitrogens have often been investigated (see Krementz, Hooper, and Kempson 1957; Kalter and Warkany 1959*a*; Parrott, Johnston, and Durbin 1960; Stempak 1962; and Hamburgh, Lynn, and Weiss 1964, for reviews and citations of the literature). The usual results were fewer conceptions, increased resorption rate, retarded growth, and lowered offspring weight.

In only few cases were congenital malformations believed to be induced. Eye defects and other abnormalities were noted in offspring of female rats partially thyroidectomized at certain times before conception. and similar eye defects were produced by giving methylthiouracil starting before concep-tion (Langman and Faassen 1955). However, ocular defects were also noted in controls (Faassen 1957). Other studies (Stempak 1962; Christie 1966) failed to confirm that maternal thyroidectomy is teratogenic. Thyroxin was reported (Giroud and Rothschild 1951) to produce cataract (and a case of exencephaly) in rats; but in an earlier study (Bodansky and Duff 1936) in which thyroxin was given to pregnant rats, no deformities occurred.

Young from chinchillas treated with methylthiouracil (Klosovskii 1963, pp. 161–67) had cardiovascular anomalies and reduced brain. Some offspring had hydrocephalus and considerable cerebellar aplasia without differentiation into vermis and hemispheres. Offspring of females treated with thyroxin for 10 days before conception and during pregnancy had cardiovascular defects, aplasia of brainstem, cerebellum, and frontal and occipital lobes, and marked hydrocephalus, the last in 2 cases.

Thyrotropin started the 11th day of pregnancy in rats caused fetal death, but no defects were mentioned (Tobin 1941). In a recent study (Beaudoin and Roberts 1966), a total of 20 USP units thyrotropin given intraperitoneally from the 8th to 11th days of pregnancy to rats produced congenital malfor-mations in 25 per cent of surviving fetuses. The abnormalities included hydrocephalus and exencephaly. When, in addition to TSH, a nonteratogenic dose of trypan blue was given on the 9th day, the incidence of defects was increased to 60 per cent. In some respects the syndrome produced by the combined treatment more closely resembled that due to TSH alone than to teratogenic doses of trypan blue.

Salicylates

The teratogenic action of salicylates was discovered by Warkany and Takacs (1959). Female rats of commercial origin were given single subcutaneous injections of 0.1 to 0.5 ml methyl salicylate or 60 to 180 mg sodium salicylate on the 9th, 10th, or 11th day of pregnancy. At least 40 per cent of the offspring of methyl salicylate-treated females and at least 26 per cent of the offspring of sodium salicylate-treated females had gross external and skeletal malformations.

Several types of abnormalities of the central nervous system occurred. These were craniorachischisis (fig. 15), exencephaly, and hydrocephalus of the lateral and 3rd ventricles associated with occlusion of the cerebral aqueduct. Probably related to some of these defects were abnormalities of the axial skeleton seen in cleared specimens. For descriptions of these and other malformations, which were made in great detail, the reader is referred to the original paper (Warkany and Takacs 1959).

Similar malformations in rats were also produced with salicylates by Gulienetti, Kalter, and Davis (1962), Goldman and Yakovac (1963), Bertone and Monie (1965), Lorke (1965), McColl, Globus, and Robinson (1965), and Nagahama, Akiyama, and Miki (1965). In addition to such defects, Goldman and Yakovac (1963) also noted small occipitoparietal encephalocele and spina bifida without gross brain involvement. So far as dose-response relations are concerned (Goldman and Yakovac 1963), treatment on the 10th day of pregnancy with 300 mg/kg or less sodium salicylate was not teratogenic, while 400 mg/kg produced 5.4 per cent malformed young (2.3% central nervous system defects) and 500 mg/kg 14.9 per cent (7.9% central nervous system).

Brown and West (1964) gave hooded Lister rats 50 to 500 mg/kg/day acetylsalicylic acid mixed with the diet throughout pregnancy. Even the lowest quantity (equivalent to a large clinical dose) caused fetal death and possibly some congenital defect, as seen in the (poor) photograph included in the paper. All fetuses were killed by treatment of rats with 600 mg/kg/day acetylsalicylic acid from the 6th to the last day of pregnancy (Obbink and Dalderup 1964). McColl, Globus, and Robinson (1963) produced skeletal defects, including inhibition of ossification of the skull, in rats, with 250 mg/kg acetylsalicylic acid.

Mice were used in several studies. Larsson, Boström, and Ericson (1963), Larsson and Boström (1965), and Larsson and Eriksson (1966) injected inbred mice with single intramuscular doses of 10 mg sodium salicylate on various days of pregnancy. Skeletal defects and hematomata at extremities predominated, but several cases of exencephaly were also seen. Obbink and Dalderup (1964) saw no malformations in the few surviving offspring given 1.2 g/kg acetylsalicylic acid daily from the 6th to the last day of pregnancy. Trasler (1965) administered 2 or 3 doses of a mixture of about 15 or 25 mg acetylsalicylic acid and a trace of Tween 80 in distilled water to A/J and C57BL/6 mice by stomach tube on the 9th and 10th or 10th and 11th days of pregnancy. Numerous congenital malformations were produced in off-spring of both strains, including exencephaly, microcephaly, and spina bifida.

Lapointe and Harvey (1964) gave salicylamide (o-hydroxybenzamide) orally to golden hamsters. Four doses of 0.5 grain each were administered at 12-hour intervals beginning on the 7th or 10th day of pregnancy. The earlier-beginning treatment caused 39 per cent abnormality, including 16 per cent "cranial blister" (probably encephalocele); and the later-beginning treatment 68 per cent abnormality, including 30 per cent cranial blister. The volume of amniotic fluid of craniorachischitic offspring of sodium salicylate-treated pregnant rats was twice as great as the control value (Gulienetti, Kalter, and Davis 1962).

In several studies (Goldman and Yakovac 1963, 1964a, b, 1965), attempts were made to modify the teratogenic effects of sodium salicylate. Various procedures were used, some of which were claimed to be successful in altering the incidence of malformed offspring. Salicylate-treated females receiving sodium carbonate or sodium chloride in drinking water had no abnormal offspring, while those drinking ammonium chloride had a higher percentage of malformed offspring than females receiving salicylate alone. Ammonium chloride by itself was not teratogenic (Goldman and Yakovac 1964a).

Salicylate combined with maternal adrenalectomy did not affect the rate of abnormality produced by salicylate alone, while the effects produced by salicylate plus cortisone were equivocal (Goldman and Yakovac 1964a). Immobilization of pregnant females appeared to raise the incidence of malformed offspring produced by salicylate (Goldman and Yakovac 1963), and this potentiation may have been reversed by the central nervous system depressant drugs sodium pentobarbital and chlorpromazine (Goldman and Yakovac 1964b). But another depressant, reserpine, seemed, on the contrary, to increase the teratogenicity of sodium salicylate in both immobilized and unimmobilized rats (Goldman and Yakovac 1965).

I must confess to not understanding the audacity that can draw unequi-vocal conclusions on the basis of pitifully small numbers of surviving offspring such as were observed by these authors.

Bertone and Monie (1965) stated that the teratogenic effects of methyl salicylate combined with hypoxia were additive, the defects produced by both together being similar to those found after either procedure used alone. The defects caused by hypoxia, however, were not named; if defects occurred, this study represents one of the very few claiming that hypoxia is teratogenic in rats.

Antibiotics

The above heading is given to this section because, although the substances discussed here are not all used therapeutically as antibiotics, they all conform with the generally accepted definition of the word (Mandel 1967).

Tetracycline produced skeletal defects in rats in one study (Filippi and Mela 1957*a*), but this result was not confirmed (Bevelander and Cohlan 1962; Carey 1962; Hurley and Tuchmann-Duplessis 1963). Abortion was induced in rats by treatment on the 14th day of pregnancy (Steiner, Bradford, and Craig 1965). No congenital defects occurred after treatment of pregnant mice with this antibiotic during the last half of gestation (Boucher and Carteret 1965).

Combined administration of penicillin and streptomycin caused skeletal defects in rats (Filippi and Mela 1957*b*), but treatment of pregnant mice with streptomycin alone (Ericson-Strandvik and Gyllensten 1963; Boucher and Delost 1964*a*) or penicillin alone (Boucher and Delost 1964*b*) failed to produce gross or microscopic abnormalities in the offspring. Nor was kanamycin teratogenic in rats (Bevelander and Cohlan 1962).

Hadacidin (N-formyl hydroxyaminoacetic acid), given in doses toxic to the pregnant organism, produced malformations in rats (Chaube and Murphy 1963; Murphy 1965). Exencephaly occurred in 97 per cent of surviving off-spring treated on the 11th day of pregnancy with 5.0 mg/kg, and in 9 per cent with 2.5 mg/kg. Treatment of rats on the 12th or 13th day produced cleft lip and palate, but apparently no external defects of the central nervous system (Lejour-Jeanty 1966). However, observations of early fetuses revealed that this defect was apparently an outcome of a primary injury to the anterior extremity of the telencephalon.

The teratogenic effects of actinomycin D were discovered by Tuchmann-Duplessis and Mercier-Parot (1958*d*). Wistar rats were injected intraperitoneally with 25 to 100 µg/kg/day for 2 or 3 days during the first half of pregnancy (Tuchmann-Duplessis and Mercier-Parot 1958*d*, 1959*e*, 1960*a*). No congenital malformations were seen in surviving fetuses treated before implantation or on the 10th and later days of gestation; but they did occur after administration of daily doses of 50 to 100 µg/kg during the 7th to 9th days, ranging in total incidence from 14 to 56 per cent.

Among the commonest defects were those of the central nervous system, which comprised exencephaly of various degrees, encephalocele, spina bifida, and, more rarely, craniorachischisis. Complex malformations of the face were sometimes produced by the highest dose; included were unusual mandibular malformations and low-set, fused external ears, which may have been parts of an otocephaly-like condition.

Wilson (1965), using rats of Wistar descent, gave single intraperitoneal injections of 100, 200, or 300 µg/kg actinomycin D on the 7th to 12th days of pregnancy. Malformations of virtually every organ system in the body were produced by the larger doses. But the only defect of the central nervous system mentioned was hydrocephalus, induced by 200 µg/kg on the 9th or 10th day and 300 μg/kg on the 8th day. When the antibiotic was administered (Wilson 1964) in conjunction with cyclophosphamide, 5-fluorouracil, or both, pronounced potentiation of the teratogenic effect occurred.

Rabbits treated (Tuchmann-Duplessis and Mercier-Parot 1960b) with 150 or 200 μg per day during the 8th to 10th days of gestation had some deformed offspring, including those with encephalocele and small lumbosacral spina bifida.

Several other aspects of actinomycin D-teratogenesis merit attention. First, both Tuchmann-Duplessis and Mercier-Parot (1960a) and Wilson (1966) found that treatment of rats started after the 10th or 11th day of gestation produced no malformations, contrary to the action of many teratogens, which still cause maldevelopment during this period of embryogenesis. Second, while the former authors, using multiple-day treatments, saw no malformations after preimplantation treatment, Wilson (1966), using single injections, did cause defects by injecting just before and around the time of implantation. And, last, while Tuchmann-Duplessis and Mercier-Parot (1959e) noted that 2-day treatments were far more teratogenic than 3-day treatments with the same daily dose, Wilson (1966) found that a period of chronic pretreatment accentuated the teratogenic effect of large, single doses.

Winfield (1966) treated "Black Spot" mice early on the 7th day of pregnancy with 100 μg/kg actinomycin D. Offspring were examined 1, 2, or 3 days later and all found abnormal. Some of the defects noted in 9th- and 10th-day-old embryos were disorganization or degeneration of the neural tube, nonclosure of the neural tube, and hydrocephalus. (The last is difficult to diagnose in embryos and even in young fetuses.) Because the abnormalities were similar to conditions found in embryos homozygous for certain T alleles (see pp. 216–22) causing early embryonic death, the possible synergistic action of actinomycin D and the Brachyury gene (symbol T), which produces death in homozygotes, was investigated. When mice lacking this allele were bred ($+/+ \times +/+$), and given 70 μg/kg actinomycin D, no abnormal embryos were seen, while 37 per cent of embryos similarly treated but obtained from $T/+ \times +/+$ matings were abnormal, a result taken to indicate that a synergism between gene and teratogen occurred, i.e., phenocopies were produced (see p. 9). Interestingly, abnormal embryos did not differ from normal littermates in RNA content, although actinomycin D is known to combine with chromosomal DNA and thus to inhibit the synthesis of messenger RNA.

Mitomycin C caused skeletal and other noncentral nervous system defects in different frequencies according to the inbred mouse strain used (Nishimura 1963). Pregnant rats were injected subcutaneously on the 6th to 10th days of gestation with actinomycin C, mitomycin C, sarkomycin, carzinophilin, or chromomycin A3 (Takaya 1963). All were teratogenic, but the most potent were actinomycin C and mitomycin C. Among the defects found were exencephaly and spina bifida.

Unusual congenital malformations of the central nervous system were produced in rats by streptonigrin (Warkany and Takacs 1965). Single intraperitoneal injections of 250 μg/kg given on the 9th, 10th, or 11th day of pregnancy led to 48, 96, and 75 per cent malformation, respectively. Externally recognizable abnormalities of the central nervous system, and their frequencies after treatment on these days, were: exencephaly (4, 31, and 1%), meningocele (3, 4, and 0%), hydrocephalus (14, 8, and 2%), iniencephaly (2, 0, and 0%), and spina bifida (1, 3, and 0%). There also occurred a condition called "short trunk" (7, 64, and 16%), which upon microscopic examination was found to consist of complete absence of the lumbosacral axial skeleton and various forms and grades of myelodysplasia, including absence of the spinal cord.

Exencephaly and meningocele varied in degree and type. The hydrocephalus involved enlargement of the lateral and 3rd ventricles and was associated with occlusion of the aqueduct. Spina bifida with persistence of the open neural plate was found. Spinal and autonomic ganglia were often deformed and misplaced. Iniencephaly consisted of marked retroflexion of the head and exaggerated lordosis of the spine. The head appeared large and was bent backward on the spine, so that it faced upward. The neck was absent and the skin of the face was continuous with the skin of the chest, and scalp with the skin of the lower back. The occiput was defective and the foramen magnum was greatly enlarged. Large parts of the brain and cerebellum protruded through this enlargement and were abnormally folded. For detailed descriptions of these defects, see the original paper (Warkany and Takacs 1965).

Antihistamines

Cyclizine hydrochloride (1-diphenylmethyl-4-methylpiperazine hydrochloride) caused eye defects in mice, rats, and rabbits, one rat offspring with craniorachischisis, and rabbit offspring with spina bifida, encephalocele, microcephaly, and tail and limb defects (Tuchmann-Duplessis and Mercier-Parot 1963b). Treatment of rats with cyclizine at later stages of pregnancy produced orofacial and eye abnormalities, but none of the central nervous system (King, Weaver, and Narrod 1965). Chlorcyclizine had similar effects, but a much smaller dose was required. Defects were also induced in mice by the latter substance (King and Howell 1966).

Meclizine hydrochloride [1-(p-chloro-α-phenylbenzyl)-4-(m-methylbenzyl)piperazine hydrochloride] given to pregnant rats produced orofacial and other skeletal defects (King 1963; Kendrick and King 1964) and hydramnios (Kendrick and Weaver 1963), but not defects of the central nervous system. In a different laboratory, using a somewhat smaller dose of meclizine, no defects were seen (Bovet-Nitti, Bignami, and Bovet 1963).

Giurgea and Puigdevall (1966) compared the effects of meclizine in 4 species. NMRI mice, a local variety of rabbits, and pigs of the Pietrain and

VDL stocks were resistant to the teratogenic effects. Wistar rats, on the other hand, were susceptible, and showed high incidences of skeletal defects and cleft palate.

Study of the metabolism of meclizine in rats (Narrod, Wilk, and King 1965) revealed it to be transformed into norchlorcyclizine, with only the latter substance being found in fetuses. Norchlorcyclizine was tested for teratogenicity and found to induce exactly the same malformations as meclizine and chlorcyclizine, but to be effective in smaller doses than either of the latter related antihistamines (King, Weaver, and Narrod 1965). Thus meclizine— and chlorcyclizine (Burns, cited by Narrod, Wilk, and King 1965)—is metabolized to norchlorcyclizine, traverses the placenta, and is apparently the actual teratogen.

Pyrilamine (2-[(2-dimethylaminomethyl) (p-methoxybenzyl)amino]pyridine) maleate apparently produced no congenital malformations in mice (Goldstein and Hazel 1955) and rats (Bovet-Nitti, Bignami, and Bovet 1963), although in another study (Bovet-Nitti and Bovet 1959) malformed rat fetuses (not further described) were found after pyrilamine administration at about the time of implantation.

Other antihistaminic substances were administered during pregnancy without causing anomalies in surviving offspring (Shelesnyak and Davies 1955; Kameswaran, Pennefather, and West 1962; King, Weaver, and Narrod 1965). Presumably, therefore, it is not the antihistaminic properties of the teratogenic antihistamines that are responsible for embryonic maldevelopment.

Thalidomide

The discovery of the prenatal danger of thalidomide for children (Lenz 1961; McBride 1961) led in a few years to a large number of experimental studies of the teratogenic properties of the drug. Of the species commonly used in such experiments, rabbits proved to be the most susceptible, mice far less so, and rats least susceptible of all, to the overall prenatal effects of thalidomide. Judging from the usual brief reference to malformations of the central nervous system, interspecific differences in susceptibility to such abnormalities followed those of teratologic susceptibility in general.

The following central nervous system defects occurred in rabbits. Abnormalities in embryonic closure of the brain (exencephaly and encephalocele) were found by Giroud, Tuchmann-Duplessis, and Mercier-Parot (1962a, b), Bough et al. (1963), Felisati and Nodari (1963), Dekker and Mehrizi (1964), Fabro et al. (1964a), Hay (1964), Loustalot (1964), Drobeck, Coulston, and Cornelius (1965), Ikeda et al. (1965), Roux, Cahen, and Dupuis (1965), Sawin et al. (1965), Heine and Stüwe (1966), Fabro and Smith (1966), and McColl (1966). Spina bifida was found by Hay (1964) and Sawin et al. (1964, 1965). Hydrocephalus was noted by Felisati (1962), Felisati and Nodari (1963), Drobeck, Coulston, and Cornelius (1964), Erfurth (1965), Fratta,

Sigg, and Maiorana (1965), Ikeda *et al.* (1965), Fabro and Smith (1966), Pearn and Vickers (1966), McColl, Robinson, and Globus (1967), and Vickers (1967). The last author, however, found about the same incidence of hydrocephalus in controls as in the drug-treated offspring. Encephalocele was noted by Giurgea and Puigdevall (1966) in experimental offspring, but an instance of the same defect also occurred in control young. Strain differences were recorded in detail by Sawin *et al.* (1965). The toxic and teratogenic effects of thalidomide in rabbits appeared to be intensified by pantothenic acid deficiency (Fratta, Sigg, and Maiorana 1965) and by injection of carbon tetrachloride (Heine *et al.* 1965) and dimethyl sulfoxide (Schumacher and Gillette 1966).

Descriptions of these defects were given only rarely. Felisati and Nodari (1963) mentioned that the hydrocephalus in their animals affected the lateral ventricles and that in some cases it was of a degree of severity that reduced the cortex to a thin layer. Incidence of such defects was also usually neglected. Mention of the frequency of an abnormality of the central nervous system occurred in a table (Fabro *et al.* 1964*a*), from which it was gleaned that exencephaly and limb defects were found in 16/43 offspring from females treated orally with 150 mg/kg thalidomide daily from the 8th to 13th days of pregnancy. Encephalocele occurred in 6/77 (7.8%) offspring of rabbits given (Roux, Cahen, and Dupuis 1965) 150 mg/kg daily from the 6th to 14th days of pregnancy, and hydrocephalus in 3/121 (2.5%) young from females that received 150 or 300 mg/kg daily from the 8th to 14th days of pregnancy. In offspring of females of a mixed albino and Dutch black strain given 300 mg/kg/day, orally, from the 8th to 16th days of pregnancy, encephalocele was found in 25 per cent of those examined on the 29th day and in 5 per cent of term young (McColl, Robinson, and Globus 1967). In other cases incidences, when stated, were usually lower.

Similar defects also occurred in mice. Exencephaly was reported by Giroud, Tuchmann-Duplessis, and Mercier-Parot (1962*b*, *c*), Knoche and König (1964), and Silvestrini and Garau (1964); and hydrocephalus by Brown (1963, and private communication) and DiPaolo (1963). Although not specifically mentioned in the text, photographs of the skeletons of 2 offspring presented by DiPaolo, Gatzek, and Pickren (1964) had legends stating them to have exencephaly, and exencephaly and spina bifida, respectively. The skeletal preparations were poor, however, and these defects were not discernable. Porencephaly of the 3rd ventricle was found in 3/217 sectioned 12th-day mouse embryos from females given 10 mg/kg thalidomide subcutaneously on the 6th day of pregnancy (Sinclair and Abreu 1965).

In rats, exencephaly was found by Bignami *et al.* (1962) and Bignami, Bovet-Nitti, and Rosnati (1963); and hydrocephalus by Heine and Kirchmair (1962), who diagnosed the condition by head shape, and by Moore, Dwornik, and Dalton (1964), who were unable, however, to confirm its presence in cleared specimens, nor apparently to reproduce it in further studies (Dwornik and Moore 1965). Hydrocephalus was said, in a preliminary communication (Rogers, Lloyd, and Fowler 1965), to have been produced in an unstated rat stock by thalidomide, and the incidence apparently to have been increased by a concomitant mild riboflavin deficiency. Until this study is more fully reported it is better to remain unconvinced.

Cynomolgus monkeys were given 10 mg/kg thalidomide daily for 6 to 10 days from the 32nd to 42nd days of pregnancy (Delahunt and Lassen 1964). Several malformed offspring resulted. One, aborted at the 5th month, had a greatly enlarged head, which was most likely due to an internal hydrocephalus associated with a defective foramen magnum similar to that occurring in the Arnold–Chiari malformation. No live births were obtained from 32 rhesus monkeys given 50 or 200 mg thalidomide daily in drinking water during early pregnancy (Lucey and Behrman 1963). It was believed that under these conditions the embryos died prior to implantation. Malformations of various types were induced (Hendrickx, Axelrod, and Clayborn 1966) in baboons of undesignated species by 5 mg/kg thalidomide daily for 12 to 22 days beginning the 12th to 22nd days of pregnancy. One of the abnormal specimens had a spina bifida (called "cystica") in the lumbosacral region. Treatment of one female beginning at conception did not prevent implantation.

In a study in which several inbred strains and a randombred line of golden hamsters were used (Homburger *et al.* 1965), a low incidence of congenital malformations, including exencephaly, resulted. Pregnant dogs of various breeds were given thalidomide (Weidman, Young, and Zollman 1963; Delatour, Dams, and Favre-Tissot 1965). Several types of defects were found, but those of the central nervous system were induced only by the latter workers, who noted one offspring with encephalocele and 2 with exencephaly among 37 examined. Large doses of thalidomide failed to deform guinea pig embryos (Arbab-Zadeh 1966).

In studies (Lutwak-Mann 1964; Lutwak-Mann, Schmid, and Keberle 1967) in which thalidomide was fed to male rabbits, effects on the offspring were obtained, such as prenatal and postnatal death and congenital malformations in 6 cases (including 1 spina bifida and 1 cranial blister). The colony from which the animals came had a spontaneous malformation rate of less than 1 per cent. Studies with radioactive thalidomide revealed the presence of the drug in semen soon after its ingestion.

Intensive chemical studies of thalidomide were begun as soon as its teratologic properties became known. In fact, no other teratogen has been under such close biochemical scrutiny. Certainly, it is not hard to understand why concentrated attention was and is being given this compound. Of course, it was paradoxical and needed clarification why a substance usually harmless for adults should be so destructive to embryos. But far more compelling was the fact that our species was struck, and might be again, unless a great deal was learned about the drug that did it, and thereby possibly about teratogenesis in general.

Thalidomide [3'-phthalimidoglutarimide or 1,3-dioxo-2-(2',6'-dioxopiperidin-3'-yl)isoindoline] is spontaneously hydrolyzed in vivo to form a relatively large number of metabolites (Faigle *et al.* 1962; Williams *et al.* 1965). The question that thus immediately presented itself was whether the teratogen is thalidomide or one or more of its many metabolites. And although the metabolic products were found nonteratogenic, or practically so, in various studies (Fabro *et al.* 1964a, 1965; Hay 1964; Fratta and Sigg 1965; Fritz 1966; Heine 1966), it was felt that the problem still remained.

Two experiments explored the question further by studying the distribution of radioactive thalidomide after its administration to pregnant rabbits. Fabro *et al.* (1964b) found that rabbit embryos contained radioactivity the major component (*ca.* 70%) of which was represented by thalidomide; the largest part (*ca.* 12%) of the remainder was α-(o-carboxybenzamido)glutarimide, a primary hydrolysis product of thalidomide. However, since all the metabolites of thalidomide are polar compounds and thus do not cross membranes as readily as thalidomide, which is nonpolar and hence more lipid soluble than its hydrolysis products (Williams *et al.* 1965), it is likely that the metabolites found in the embryos were largely formed by the intraembryonic degradation of thalidomide. This possibility was supported by the findings of Keberle *et al.* (1965), who gave radioactive thalidomide and 2 of its metabolites in radioactive form to female rabbits at 3 different early stages of pregnancy, and determined that at the earliest stage far more thalidomide entered the embryo than did the metabolites.

In sum, therefore, it appears that it is thalidomide that enters embryos, persists there for an appreciable time (Fabro, Smith, and Williams 1965), and is there converted to its hydrolysis products, which accumulate, being unable to leave cells once formed. Thus, as Williams *et al.* (1965, p. 179) put it, "it is therefore not possible at present to decide whether it is thalidomide or one of its breakdown products which is the direct teratogen. However, it can be said that thalidomide itself is the carrier of the teratogenic material into the embryo."

Needless to say, uncertainty also remains as to the mode of entry of thalidomide into the embryo, what it does once there that produces its specific pathological effects, and numerous other points.

Urethan

Urethan (ethyl carbamate) has been given to pregnant mice (Sinclair 1950; Höglund 1952; Nishimura and Kuginuki 1958; Kauffman 1964; Tsuchikawa and Akabori 1964, 1965), rats (Hall 1953; Tuchmann-Duplessis and Mercier-Parot 1958a; Murphy and Chaube 1964; Kreybig 1965c; Chaube and Murphy 1966; Takaori, Tanabe, and Shimamoto 1966), and hamsters (Ferm 1966a).

Sinclair (1950) gave 15 mg urethan subcutaneously to CF albino mice, beginning the 7th or 8th day of pregnancy. When treatment was begun on the 7th day, offspring were found with the entire brain exposed (exencephaly), the lateral ventricles spread open just above the eye, and the skin continuous with the choroid plexus of the 4th ventricle. Treatment begun on the 8th day caused an abnormality involving degeneration of the basal plate of the brain and of the incipient motor cells of the entire central nervous system. Nishimura and Kuginuki (1958) injected mice intraperitoneally with 1.5 mg/kg urethan during the 3rd to 16th days of pregnancy. Malformations were produced only by treatment beginning the 9th to 12th days. The defects were mainly skeletal, but some exencephaly was also seen. Kauffman (1964) injected pregnant mice on the 10th day of gestation with 0.5 to 1.0 mg/kg urethan. The pregnant animals were killed at intervals over the 24 hours following treatment. An absolute decrease in mitosis and abnormal mitosis was seen in the neural tube, but by 24 hours adequate regeneration was occurring to maintain the structural integrity of the neural tube. Tsuchikawa and Akabori (1964, 1965) treated several inbred mouse strains intraperitoneally with 1.5 g/kg ethylurethan on the 7th to 13th days of pregnancy, and noted strain differences in teratogenic susceptibility. Treatment on the 9th day of pregnancy, e.g., caused exencephaly in 30 per cent of C3HeB/Fe offspring, but in none of the CBA young. Reciprocal crosses between the strains demonstrated a maternal influence over the expression of the malformation: CBA females crossed to C3H males had no exencephalic offspring, while C3H females mated to CBA males had 12 per cent exencephalics. Blood studies showed no strain differences in level of ethylurethan.

Studies with rats were less productive. Hall (1953) noted some eye defects after injection of urethan during the middle of pregnancy. Tuchmann-Duplessis and Mercier-Parot (1958a) found one offspring with clubfoot. Murphy and Chaube (1964) and Chaube and Murphy (1966) produced no defects with urethan but did find hydroxyurethan teratogenic. Kreybig (1965c) had no defects with either urethan or methylnitroso-urethan. Defects occurred in Wistar rats (Takaori, Tanake, and Shimamoto 1966) after daily oral doses of 1 g/kg ethylurethan during the second trimester. The most common abnormalities were skeletal, but there were 3 cases of exencephaly.

Ferm (1966a) gave 25 to 100 mg urethan intravenously or intraperitoneally, on the 8th day of pregnancy to golden hamsters. The embryos were examined macroscopically 1, 2, or 3 days later and found to have various malformations including exencephaly, spina bifida, and marked degeneration of the anterior neural tube with nonclosure of the neural folds. Urethan given intravenously was apparently more teratogenic than when administered intraperitoneally.

Hydroxyurea

Single or multiple intraperitoneal injections of hydroxyurea were given in a wide range of doses to Wistar rats on the 10th to 13th days of gestation (Murphy and Chaube 1964; Murphy 1965; Chaube and Murphy 1966). Various skeletal malformations were produced but the only central nervous system malformations noted in near-term offspring were exencephaly and encephalocele. The former occurred only when the time of treatment included the 10th day of pregnancy, while the latter resulted only after injections on the 12th or 13th day or both. The minimum teratogenic dose increased with each successive day of pregnancy; single doses of 185 mg/kg on the 10th day produced 16/30 young with exencephaly; whereas on the 13th day single treatments with 750 mg/kg were needed, and caused 29/30 with encephalocele. In general, the rate and severity of the defects increased with dose. Thus, in exencephaly produced by single doses of 375 mg/kg on the 10th day, the brain and cranium were apparently absent. However, since specimens seem not to have been sectioned, the extent of deficiency of brain was not determined. Encephalocele was usually located in the midparietal region. Metabolic studies cited by Chaube and Murphy (1966) indicated that in rats the greater part of injected hydroxyurea is excreted within 4 hours. The multiple treatments given thus indicated that certain of the effects of the drug on embryonic development were cumulative, varying directly with the total dose, regardless of how fractionated.

Various malformations of the axial skeleton and central nervous system were produced (Jackson *et al.* 1967) in Osborne-Mendel rats by single intra-peritoneal injections of 250 mg/kg hydroxyurea on the 9th day of pregnancy, including exencephaly, various degrees of encephalocele, and spina bifida (whether aperta was not indicated).

Exencephaly and spina bifida were produced in hamsters by single intra-venous injections of 50 mg hydroxyurea on the 8th day of pregnancy (Ferm 1965*b*, 1966*a*). This amount (5–10 mg/kg) was far less than the minimal teratogenic dose for rats, mentioned above.

Other substances tested by Chaube and Murphy (1966) were hydroxyure-than, acetohydroxamic acid, and hydroxylamine. No qualitative differences were found between the former 2 and hydroxyurea, all 3 producing the same types of malformations, including exencephaly and encephalocele. Hydro-xyurethan, however, appeared somewhat more active than the other 2. Hydroxylamine, on the other hand, caused a relatively high incidence of fetal resorption, but no abnormalities in near-term survivors.

Miscellaneous Substances

Congenital malformations of the central nervous system were occasionally obtained in studies using a wide variety of substances. The following is a brief summary of some reports.

Phenothiazine Derivatives

Roux (1959) administered prochlorpemazine (2-chloro-10[3-(1-methyl-4-

piperazinyl)propyl]phenothiazine) to rats and mice. Among the few malformed offspring seen was a rat with craniorachischisis (treated 10th day) and a mouse with exencephaly (treated 9th day). A double monster also occurred and was described (Roux 1962). Brock and Kreybig (1964) gave rats of 2 stocks 10 mg/kg chlorpromazine [2-chloro-10-(3-dimethylaminopropyl)-phenothiazine] intraperitoneally on the 4th day of pregnancy. Congenital malformations, including some of the central nervous system, were found in 13th-day embryos examined. In several other studies, such drugs were non-teratogenic (Chambon 1955; Murphree, Monroe, and Seager 1962; Ordy *et al.* 1963).

Serotonin

Serotonin [5-hydroxytryptamine; 3-(2-aminoethyl)-5-indolol] caused congenital malformations in mice (Poulson, Robson, and Sullivan 1963; Seller 1964) and rats (Reddy, Adams, and Baird 1963), but not rabbits (Robson, Poulson, and Sullivan 1965). Single subcutaneous injections on the 6th to 11th days of gestation in mice produced a total of 13.2 per cent (18/136) malformations with a 2.0 mg daily dose and 4.5 per cent (19/424) with 0.5 mg. The highest incidence occurred after injection on about the 9th day. Among the defects were "brain and skull deformities" and a case of cyclopia (Poulson, Robson, and Sullivan 1963). Treatment of pregnant rats with 1.5 mg daily, presumably throughout the gestation period, caused malformations in 4 offspring, including hydrocephalus and exencephaly (Reddy, Adams, and Baird 1963).

The lethal action of serotonin on fetuses may be due to its interference with placental function (Robson and Sullivan 1963a), and its mode of tera-togenic action may also be related to such interference, although this possibility was by no means clearly established. But the rise in fetal serotonin level after maternal injection indicated that a high local concentration may be responsible for abnormal prenatal development (Poulson, Robson, and Sullivan 1963). Support of the possibility that the embryotoxic and teratogenic effects of serotonin in mice were due to interferences with placental function was provided by a preliminary study (Honey *et al.* 1964), in which both its placental disturbances and embryopathic effects may have been partly prevented by administration of certain antagonists of serotonin.

Triparanol

Triparanol (MER-29; 1-[p-(β-diethylaminoethoxy)phenyl]-1-(p-tolyl)-2-(p-chlorophenyl)ethanol), an anticholesterolemic, produced severe congenital malformations of the central nervous system in Wistar rats (Roux and Dupuis 1961; Roux 1964). Single doses of 100 mg given orally on the 4th to 10th days of gestation produced 4 to 80 per cent external congenital malformations in survivors. The defects included craniorachischisis extending from the rhombencephalon to the inferior extremity of the spinal cord, exencephaly in the region of the diencephalon, and lumbosacral spina bifida. It was commonly observed in these malformations, resulting from failure of neural tube closure, that by the end of pregnancy almost complete destruction of exposed nervous tissue had occurred; so that in the spinal area the dorsal face of vertebrae had become superficial owing to disappearance of all traces of the cord, while in the head region a voluminous angiomatous mass had formed, producing a typical "anencephaly."

There also occurred a syndrome of malformation of the face and forebrain. The most significant facial defect was shortness of the upper jaw accompanied by proboscoid elongation of the nasal region. In severe cases the nostrils were approximated and sometimes fused, as evidenced by the presence of but one nostril. These features often occur in cyclopia; but the eye defects that give this condition its name—approximation or fusion of orbits and other optic structures—was seen but once, despite other eye defects—microphthalmia and anophthalmia—being the most frequent malformations induced.

Internally, the nasal fossae were small, deformed, and lacked communication with the pharynx. Nevertheless, the olfactory apparatus seemed well developed, and sent nerve fibers toward the brain.

Abnormalities of the brain in these specimens were mainly of the telencephalon and diencephalon, while the mesencephalon and rhombencephalon were apparently normal. The telencephalon was often maldivided, presumably univentricular, while abnormalities of the diencephalon consisted of ventricular expansion and associated anomalies.

The hydrocephalus, which involved dilatation of the lateral and 3rd ventricles and the foramina of Monro, may have been due to the abundant choroid plexuses found, and to reduction in size of the aqueduct of Sylvius. In this condition the general volume of the brain was reduced and the walls of the cerebrum were more or less thinned. In addition, the walls of the hemispheres contained porencephalic-like cavitations, which sometimes communicated with each other or with the cerebral ventricles.

In a number of animals with abnormalities of the brain, defects of the pituitary also occurred. In 3 cases the pituitary was small and sometimes presented a pharyngeal diverticulum, which may have been a remnant of a craniopharyngeal duct. In 8 other cases the pituitary was completely absent. Animals with craniorachischisis sometimes also had iniencephaly.

Another unusual property of triparanol was that it produced malformations when given during preimplantation stages of gestation, as early as the 4th day (Roux 1964). However, the highest incidence of craniorachischisis (32%) was produced by treatment on the 6th day of pregnancy, and of anterior brain defects (57%) by treatment on the 7th day.

Similar defects of the central nervous system were produced in rats by

Vichi *et al.* (1965*a*) following Roux's (1964) methodology. A somewhat different array (encephalocele, microcephaly, spina bifida) occurred in rats after oral treatment with 20 to 30 mg/kg daily beginning soon after fertilization (Yakovleva and Shakhnazarova 1965).

Vichi *et al.* (1965*a*) gave pregnant mice a dose (12 mg) comparable to that found teratogenic in rats, but produced no defects. Roux and Dupuis (1966) also found mice refractory, and were forced to use large doses (200 mg/kg/day from the 1st–14th days of gestation) to induce malformations (39/61 = 63.9%). The defects included craniorachischisis (1 case) and defects of the nose and eye such as were seen in triparanol-treated rats. Another inhibitor of cholesterol synthesis, AY 9944 [trans-1 bis(2 chlorobenzylami-noethyl) cyclohexane dihydrochloride] was also found to be teratogenic in rats (Roux and Aubry 1966) and to induce defects similar in part to those caused by triparanol.

Imipramine

Robson and Sullivan (1963*b*) gave imipramine [5-(2-dimethylaminopropyl)-10, 11-dihydro-5H-dibenz[b,f]azepine hydrochloride] to 12 rabbits of several strains from the 1st to the 13th, 17th, or 20th days of pregnancy. Daily doses averaging about 15 mg/kg (5–30 mg) given subcutaneously produced some defects, whose incidence was not stated. Abnormalities of the cranium were especially noted. Two offspring showed more gross central nervous system defects. The first had a large encephalocele that consisted of a protrusion, through a fault in the parietal cranium, of the region of the brain between the cerebral hemispheres and the cerebellum. The brain was covered by meninges, which were directly attached to the skin. The second animal had a large "cranial swelling" and, microscopically, spina bifida occulta. Other offspring had cranial swelling and a hemorrhagic area on the skull. Two malformed rabbits (absent kidney, short tail) were produced in a different study with imipramines (Larsen 1963).

Harper, Palmer, and Davies (1965) studied the effects of imipramine in rabbits, mice, and rats. New Zealand White rabbits were treated orally or subcutaneously with 5, 15, or 30 mg/kg daily from the 7th to 17th days of pregnancy and killed several days before term. Oral administration (5–15 mg) resulted in 1/46 abnormal fetuses (ectopic kidney). The lower doses given parenterally produced fetal loss but no defects in survivors; while the largest subcutaneous dose (30 mg), which was toxic to pregnant animals, induced anomalies in 4/29 viable survivors: 2 with hydrocephalus and brain tissue protruding through a cranial fault; one with craniorachischisis; and one with an absent kidney. Sprague–Dawley rats were given imipramine in the diet over a long period of time, beginning at least 60 days before breeding. This method of administration caused no observable abnormalities in offspring. Outbred mice treated orally and subcutaneously with 10 to 150 mg/kg daily from the 6th to 17th days of pregnancy had 2/953 malformed offspring. One of these was exencephalic but a case of this defect was also seen among the 605 control young. In distinction to the rabbits, large doses had no observable toxic effects on pregnant mice. While in this study imipramine was apparently without teratogenic effect in mice, Robson (1963) stated, without giving any details, that the drug produced malformations when used by him.

Steroid Substances

Several adrenal steroids were reported to cause congenital malformations of the central nervous system. Soludecadron (dexamethasone) produced low incidences of such defects after single or multiple injection of pregnant rabbits, resulting altogether in one case of anencephaly, 3 of exencephaly, and 4 of spina bifida (apparently occulta), in 112 offspring (Buck, Clavert, and Rumpler 1962). Cleft palate and cardiovascular and other defects were also obtained (Clavert *et al.* 1965); and a phase-specific response was noted (Clavert, Rumpler, and Ruch 1965). Hydrocortisone given to pregnant guinea pigs produced spinal abnormalities in a small number of young (Hoar 1962). It was claimed (Gordon, Peer, and Bernhard 1961) that cortisone caused a low incidence of spinal abnormalities and hydrocephalus in mice, and that concurrent injection of adenosine triphosphate (Gordon *et al.* 1962, 1963) reduced the incidence of these defects. It may merely be mentioned that in a large number of studies of the teratogenic action of cortisone in mice (Kalter and Warkany 1959*a*) no congenital malformations of the central nervous system attributable to the treatment were reported. The spina bifida in an offspring of a pregnant A/J mouse given desoxycorticosterone tri-methylacetate (Walker 1965) was probably not caused by the treatment.

A progestogen, chlormadinone acetate, was teratogenic in mice and rabbits (Takano *et al.* 1966). The most common defect in mice was cleft palate; no central nervous system anomaly was seen. In rabbits, however, of 257 late fetuses examined, cyclopia occurred in one and exencephaly in 4 cases. One offspring from a pregnant rabbit given a different progestogen, norethisterone, had spina bifida; but the same defect occurred in a control rabbit offspring. Masculinization of female mouse and rabbit fetuses was not produced by chlormadinone. In another study (Chambon, Depagne, and Le Veve 1966), a chlormadinone-treated rabbit had an acephalic offspring. A number of synthetic estrogens and estrogen antagonists induced a few malformations of the central nervous system in rabbits (Morris *et al.* 1967*b*).

Miscellaneous Therapeutic Agents

Quinine was given in various doses at different (unstated) times during gestation to guinea pigs (Mosher 1938). Hemorrhage was found in fetal cochleae. The same result was obtained by giving sodium salicylate and oxophenarsine hydrochloride, an arsenical. Belkina (1958) gave rabbits 130 mg/kg quinine daily for 4 to 8 days during the first half of pregnancy and found pronounced deformities of the brain (anencephaly, microcephaly, etc.) in 3.2 per cent of the young. Klosovskii (1963, pp. 190–94) gave several doses (90–150 mg/kg/day) of quinine dihydrochloride to pregnant chinchillas for one to 8 days during the 4th to 14th days of gestation. Some defective offspring resulted, and the anomalies included decreased size of cerebral hemispheres and cerebellum. Three offspring had gross brain defects, one with anencephaly, one with microcephaly, and one with widely dilated lateral ventricles. Neuweiler and Richter (1964) treated several stocks of rats with quinine hydrochloride by various routes. No sign of fetal damage was seen except for an offspring with multiple defects, including an odd-shaped head.

Barbiturates caused fetal death (Olivecrona 1964) and some defects (Setälä and Nyyssönen 1964) in mice, and a few abnormal rat offspring, among which was one with exencephaly (Persaud 1965). Skeletal defects, but no external anomalies, were seen in rats by McColl, Robinson, and Globus (1967).

Intramuscular *epinephrine* (0.5 to 1.0 mg/kg) on the 10th day of pregnancy may have been responsible for the 3 cases (in 250 offspring) of exencephaly seen in Sprague–Dawley rats (Goldman and Yakovac 1965).

Caffeine given to mice by Nishimura and Nakai (1960) produced skeletal defects; and by Knocke and König (1964), some skeletal defects, one exencephaly, and one encephalocele. In a study by Bertrand et al. (1966) BALB/c mice were quite resistant to any harmful prenatal effects of caffeine, while Wistar rats showed only ectrodactyly.

Various doses of *disulfiram* were given (Favre-Tissot and Delatour 1965) to rats from the 5th to 10th days of pregnancy, but only one malformed offspring was found, which had craniorachischisis.

The tuberculostatic drug *ethionamide* was found to be teratogenic in rats; malformation included a low incidence (2.7%) of exencephaly (Fujimori et al. 1965). In mice, it was without significant teratogenic effect, except when combined with isoniazid or hydroxymethylpyrimidine, a pyridoxine antagonist. When combined with the former only skeletal defects occurred, while with the latter, exencephaly also appeared (Takekoshi 1965a).

Other Substances

Large doses of *sulfonamides* given to pregnant animals caused fetal resorption (Kalter and Warkany 1959a). In recent studies (Paget and Thorpe 1964; Bertazzoli, Chieli, and Grandi 1965), a long-acting sulfonamide, sulfamoprine (sulfadimethoxy pyrimidine), led to skeletal and dental defects in rats, but another one, 2-sulfanilamide,3-methoxy-pyrazine, did not (Bertazzoli, Chieli, and Grandi 1965).

Thiadiazole (2-ethyl-1,3,4-thiadiazole) was given to rats on the 10th, 12th, or 13th day of pregnancy (Murphy, Dagg, and Karnofsky 1957). Encephalocele occurred after treatment on the 13th day with 100 or 200 mg/kg. Cleared abnormal specimens showed circular defects of the frontal, parietal, interparietal, and occipital bones. Nicotinamide did not prevent the defects (Murphy 1960), although for some systems thiadiazole is a nicotinamide antagonist.

Subjecting pregnant mice to *fuel gas* for one hour on the 8th day of gestation (Kato 1958) or to *phenylmercuric acetate* applied intravaginally on the 7th or subcutaneously on the 8th day (Murakami, Kameyama, and Kato 1956*a*) produced various abnormalities of the central nervous system.

A diet containing 5 to 10 g/kg *sugar* was fed to female rabbits (Sumi 1960). When the regime was started about 11 weeks before conception, hydrocephalus resulted in offspring. There was marked dilatation of the lateral and 3rd ventricles, but no abnormal proliferation of ependymal cells of the choroid plexus, usually held to be associated with oversecretion of cerebrospinal fluid. The cerebral aqueduct was narrower than in controls and the cisternas of the midbrain region were reduced in size, possibly owing to compression of the brain by surrounding bones. Whether there was absolute overgrowth of the brain was not mentioned.

The abnormalities produced in mice by *2,3-dimercaptopropanol* were all skeletal except for one case of exencephaly (Nishimura and Takagaki 1959*b*). A low incidence of exencephaly was produced in mice by *iodoacetate* (Runner and Dagg 1960).

Various common industrial solvents were noted to be teratogenic. *Monomethylformamide* given to pregnant mice (0.1 mg/kg daily, intraperitoneally, on the 11th and 12th days of gestation; or 0.01 mg/kg, percutaneously, on the 11th day) caused exencephaly, spina bifida, and other malformations in about 50 per cent of surviving offspring (Oettel and Frohberg 1964). The same substance administered percutaneously to pregnant Wistar rats on the 10th and 11th or 11th and 12th days of gestation caused various degrees of encephalocele and, more rarely, exencephaly (Tuchmann-Duplessis and Mercier-Parot 1965). *Formamide* also caused malformations, but not of the central nervous system; *dimethylformamide* was not teratogenic (Thiersch 1962*c*; Oettel and Frohberg 1964), nor were certain *acetamides* (Thiersch 1962*c*).

A compound related to the monoamine oxidase inhibitor, phenelzine, was found to be teratogenic. This substance, *WL 27* (o-chloro-beta-phenylethylhydrazine dihydrogen sulfate), did not cause maldevelopment in mice, but when given to rabbits a grossly abnormal offspring was found. The head was half the normal size, and the skin and cranial bones of the top of the head were missing, exposing the brain (Poulson and Robson 1964).

Triton WR-1339 (p-isooctylpolyoxyethylphenol polymer), a detergent with surface-tension-reducing properties, which causes hypercholesterolemia and hyperlipemia, was teratogenic in mice, rats, and rabbits (Tuchmann-Duplessis and Mercier-Parot 1964*d, e*). Daily intraperitoneal injections of

200 or 400 mg/kg, given to mice for 3 days beginning the 6th or 7th day of pregnancy, caused 20 and 6 to 9 per cent congenital malformations, respectively. The majority of abnormal offspring had exencephaly and encephalocele or eye defects (Tuchmann-Duplessis and Mercier-Parot 1964*d*). To produce malformations in rats, 600 and 800 mg/kg had to be used. In rabbits, doses of 100 mg/kg or greater caused almost complete fetal destruction. A low incidence of defects occurred with smaller doses, but no malformations of the central nervous system were reported (Tuchmann-Duplessis and Mercier-Parot 1964*e*).

Hydrocephalus was produced in Long–Evans rats by maternal ingestion of nontoxic amounts of metallic *tellurium* in ground laboratory chow during pregnancy (Garro and Pentschew 1964). With 2500 ppm the yield was 100 per cent; with 1500 ppm it varied between 60 and 90 per cent; however, in certain colonies even 500 ppm produced some defective offspring. The abnormality was congenital if the amount fed was greater than 2500 ppm or if the 2500-ppm diet was not suspended 3 to 5 days before delivery. If less than 2500 ppm were given or if, as was necessary to avoid abortion, a normal diet was instituted a few days before delivery, the condition usually first appeared soon after birth.

In latter cases, hydrocephalus was most prominent in the lateral ventricles but progressed with time and eventually was characterized by dilatation of the entire ventricular system, reaching its greatest dimension around 3 weeks after birth. Lethality was about 99 per cent, the longest survival period being about one month. No obstruction of the ventricular passages or of the cerebrospinal-fluid drainage system was found. In early stages (at 1–2 days of age), no tissue damage could be seen, but porencephalic changes occurred later as well as almost complete destruction of the telencephalon, including the septum pellucidum and corpus callosum.

The carcinogen *methylnitrosourea* (20 mg/kg) given (Kreybig 1965*b, d*) intravenously on the 13th or 14th day of pregnancy to 2 stocks of rats, produced high incidences of malformations, mainly of the extremities and brain. Treatment (Druckrey, Ivanković, and Preussmann 1966) of inbred rats on the 15th day of pregnancy with 80 mg/kg *ethylnitrosourea* caused paw defects in newborn offspring. Several that survived to about 165 days of age showed nervous symptoms and were discovered at autopsy to have malignant neurinomata at various sites.

Sublethal doses of 7 different mineral salts were fed to pregnant sheep (James, Lazar, and Binns 1966). One given *bismuth tartrate* had a malformed offspring, but the defects were apparently not of the central nervous system.

Dimethyl sulfoxide (*DMSO*), a relatively simple organic compound, was teratogenic in golden hamsters (Ferm 1966*b, c*). Females were given single intraperitoneal or intravenous injections of 50 to 8250 mg/kg on the 8th day of pregnancy and killed mostly on the 11th day. The most frequent defect produced was exencephaly, but its incidence was not stated. As early as 24 hours after treatment, i.e., on the 9th day, embryos were noted with nonclosure of the anterior neural tube, which normally by this time in hamster development has already closed. In studies with rats and rabbits (Schumacher and Gillette 1966), DMSO enhanced the teratogenic effects of thalidomide, but had little if any prenatal effect itself. Doses of DMSO given were not stated. Caujolle *et al.* (1965) found that single or repeated administration of various doses of DMSO to pregnant mice, rats, and rabbits produced no malformations; but when higher doses and a slightly different technique were used (Caujolle *et al.* 1967), low frequencies of anomalies occurred, among which were some of the central nervous system.

Spatz, Dougherty, and Smith (1967) gave golden hamster females, on the 8th day of pregnancy, single intravenous injections of *methylazoxymethanol*, the aglycone of cycasin (methylazoxymethanol-β-D-glucoside), which occurs naturally in the seeds of the tropical plants *Cycas circinalis* and *C. revoluta.* Twelfth-day fetuses were examined grossly for defects. None occurred in young of females given 12 mg/kg, but all 165 from those given about 25 mg/kg, were abnormal, and the malformations included exencephaly, spina bifida, and craniorachischisis. Thin-layer chromatography established the presence of methylazoxymethanol in embryos after intragastric administration of cycasin to mothers. Cycasin was also discovered to be carcinogenic when administered transplacentally, but evidence (see Spatz, Dougherty, and Smith 1967, for references) suggested that this substance is deglucosylated to methylazoxymethanol, which is the proximate carcinogen.

A large, and ever growing, number of chemical, pharmacological, and biological substances have been tested teratologically (Baker 1960; Cahen 1964; Fave 1964; Salzgeber and Wolff 1964; Karnofsky 1965; Vichi *et al.* 1966). Many were teratogenic but did not produce malformations of the central nervous system, at least under the conditions used. Hence these numerous agents will not be mentioned here.

7

Other Teratogenic Procedures

Maternal Immunization

Only studies in which congenital malformations of the central nervous system resulted from maternal immunization, and certain related investigations, will be discussed here. Other aspects of this topic can be found in recent reviews (Brent 1965, 1966b).

The earliest experiment of this sort in which central nervous system defects were induced was that of Gluecksohn-Waelsch (1957). Two series of studies were made. In the first, BALB/c strain female mice were injected prior to conception with an antigenic emulsion prepared from brains of Swiss Webster mice. Twenty of 305 (6.6%) living embryos examined on the 11th day of gestation had abnormalities of the central nervous system. But these results were inconclusive (since the induced frequency was not very different from the spontaneous one, 11/272 = 4.0%); and, hence, a second study was made using mice of the DBA/1 strain, which had no spontaneous brain defects.

DBA/1 females were injected with brain or heart emulsion at different periods before conception. Embryos of females treated with brain tissue showed brain abnormalities (20/228 = 8.8%), whereas those from females treated with heart tissue were all free of such defects (0/191), but one had a heart anomaly. Thus not only was it apparently shown that maternal immunization produces malformation but that there appears to be a specific embryonic organ response to immunization with different tissues. The central nervous system abnormalities—as seen in 11th-day embryos—consisted of suppression of nervous tissue differentiation in the region of the brain and anterior spinal cord, microcephaly, and abnormalities of closure of neural folds.

What we are uneasy about in this work is not that maternal immunization was teratogenic, but that a claim was made that specific maternal antibodies were directed against specific embryonic organs. Thus the study requires scrutiny. As Brent (1965) pointed out, embryos only were examined at a young age, when dying ones are likely to have distortions and retardations of the central nervous system. Furthermore, some supposedly abnormal embryos came from mothers whose sera had no antibrain antibodies. Following Gluecksohn-Waelsch's (1957) technique, Barber, Willis, and Afeman (1961) produced eye defects but no abnormalities of the brain. Finally, in studies in which treatment was made during pregnancy, tissue-specific antisera did not produce specific malformations.

Brent, Averich, and Drapiewski (1961) injected female rats intravenously with rabbit anti-rat-kidney antisera on the 9th day of pregnancy and produced numerous types of congenital malformations, including anencephaly, exencephaly, and hydrocephalus. Subsequently the immunization technique was applied to rat embryos of various ages (Brent 1964*b*), with the result that somewhat different arrays of malformations were produced by treating on any one of several different days of pregnancy, although a great deal of overlapping occurred. Thus, so far as congenital malformations of the central nervous system are concerned, anencephaly occurred in 2.4 and 3.3 per cent of offspring treated on the 9th or 10th day, respectively; meningocele in 1.2 per cent treated on the 9th day; exencephaly in 3.9, 15.5, and 3.3 per cent treated on the 8th, 9th, or 10th day, respectively; and hydrocephalus in 49.0, 75.0, 47.5, and 78.7 per cent treated on the 8th, 9th, 10th, or 11th day, respectively. As seen in a photograph, the hydrocephalus involved the lateral and 3rd ventricles, but the condition was not described. Placental antiserum was also teratogenic, and the defects resembled those induced by kidney antiserum (Brent 1964*b*); but rabbit antisera to rat red blood cells, muscle, brain, serum, and fetal skin and liver were not teratogenic (Brent, Averich, and Drapiewski 1961).

David, Mercier-Parot, and Tuchmann-Duplessis (1963), following the same general procedure, gave single intravenous injections of rabbit anti-rat-kidney antiserum to female rats on the 8th, 9th, 10th, or 11th day of pregnancy. To some extent, different malformations were caused by treating on different days. Apparently, the only congenital malformation of the central nervous system found was exencephaly, several grades of which occurred after treatment on the 9th day and a case of which was found after treatment on the 10th day. Facial anomalies included otocephaly-like signs (David *et al.* 1966), i.e., low-set external ears and apparent absence of the lower jaw.

The work was repeated with mice (Mercier-Parot, David, and Tuchmann-Duplessis 1963). Single intravenous injections of rabbit anti-mouse-kidney antiserum were given on the 6th to 11th days of pregnancy. The effective period was narrower than in rats, with malformations resulting only after treatment on the 8th or 9th day. The sole congenital malformation of the central nervous system was exencephaly, and it was produced only by treatment on the 9th day. Rabbit anti-rat-kidney antiserum was also given to pregnant mice (Mercier-Parot, David, and Tuchmann-Duplessis 1963), but no congenital malformations resulted, suggesting that some type of specific response is involved.

It was determined by fluorescent techniques that teratogenic rat kidney and placental antisera became localized in maternal glomerular basement membrane and certain other maternal sites and parietal yolk-sac membrane, but not in young embryos, trophoblast, or amnion (Slotnick and Brent 1966). This and other evidence, e.g., that the teratogenic factors of active antisera lie in γ globulins (Brent 1966a), appear to indicate that the teratogenic mechanism may be an immunologically caused disturbance of yolk-sac function.

Other clues to mechanism came from a study (Brent 1966a) of several variables, including route of administration, which revealed the following. Teratogenic antiserum was ineffective when administered orally (indicating that the active component is a protein), but produced defects when given intravenously, intraperitoneally, subcutaneously, or directly into the uterine lumen. The intravenous route was most sensitive, however. Malformations also resulted from treatment before implantation (4th gestation day). But this result was probably due to persistence of the teratogenic milieu for a few days, as indicated by (1) the failure of 30 minutes of uterine vascular clamping to protect against antiserum teratogenesis, and (2) the fairly uniform qualitative teratogenic response obtained after treatment on any one of several days.

Infection

Several studies have been made in which pregnant animals were inoculated with various infectious agents. The outcome of these procedures was often fetal destruction but only rarely fetal maldevelopment, and only in some of the latter instances were abnormalities of the central nervous system noted. In addition, anomalous and malformed animals have sometimes been born to females suffering from natural infections during pregnancy.

Pregnant rats were injected intracardially with rubella virus on different days of gestation (Cohlan and Stone 1955). Histological sections of offspring revealed brain abnormalities consisting of hydrocephalus, marked narrowing of the cerebral aqueduct and parts of the 3rd ventricle, and meningeal adhesions to the base of the brain. The defects were most frequent after treatment on the 5th or 6th day of pregnancy but did not occur after treatment on the 8th day. These results remain unconfirmed.

No congenital malformations occurred in the offspring of 5 rhesus monkeys inoculated intravenously with rubella virus between the 25th and 28th days of gestation (Sever *et al.* 1966). In a sketchy account (Delahunt 1966) of another study with rhesus monkeys, cataracts and other, unspecified, effects, "similar to those reported in human embryos damaged by rubella," were noted in 2 offspring from females injected with rubella virus material on the 20th and later days of gestation.

Mice were bred immediately after intranasal injection with influenza virus (Adams *et al.* 1956). Among the dead offspring were 2 with abnormalities of cephalic areas, which were not described. The offspring of mice infected with lymphocytic choriomeningitis (Kreshover and Hancock 1956) occasionally showed dental abnormalities. Intranasal (Ohba 1958) or intravenous (Ohba 1959*a*) administration of HVJ (hemagglutinating virus of Japan) to mice early in pregnancy resulted in occasional abnormalities of the central nervous system, such as exencephaly, hydrocephalus, hydromyelia, and other defects of brain and spinal cord. Similar anomalies occurred after injection of the endotoxin of pathogenic coli bacillus (Ohba 1959*b*).

Golden hamsters injected intravenously with the H-1 strain of rat virus (RV) during the middle third of pregnancy had malformed offspring, including some with exencephaly, microcephaly, and spina bifida (Ferm and Kilham 1964, 1965). Dilution of the viral inoculum decreased the incidence of fetal death and maldevelopment. Virus was recovered from fetal tissues, showing that it had crossed the placenta. This finding and the fact that there was widespread distribution of intranuclear inclusion bodies in fetal tissues led to the conclusion that the H-1 virus has a direct teratogenic effect on hamster embryos (Ferm and Kilham 1965). Several other viruses produced no defects in hamsters or rats, nor was there indication that they crossed the placenta (Ferm and Kilham 1963*a*, *b*, 1965; Kilham and Ferm 1964; Ferm and Low 1965).

A high incidence of stillbirth and encephalomalacia or internal hydrocephalus in offspring of pregnant sows inapparently infected with Japanese encephalitis virus (Burns 1950) suggested a relation between these phenomena, which was tested experimentally by Shimizu *et al.* (1954). A number of mature Yorkshire hybrid female pigs, free of neutralizing antibody to the virus, were intravenously injected with a dilution of Japanese encephalitis virus on several days of gestation (36th–97th days) and then killed at various intervals or permitted to deliver. One female injected on the 46th day of pregnancy and killed 62 days later had 4 resorbed and 3 hydrocephalic offspring. No other malformed young were seen. The cranial cavity and ventricles of the defective young were filled with clear fluid and the cerebral cortex consisted of a thin membrane. Virus was recovered from a number of normal fetuses, but not from the hydrocephalics, possibly owing to the many days they were permitted to develop before being examined. It was also noted in natural cases of the disease that virus was difficult to isolate from hydrocephalic fetuses. It thus appeared that a long period of time was necessary for hydrocephalus to develop following fetal infection.

Hydrocephalus in newborn calves was found in Japan, following and possibly caused by epidemics of Japanese encephalitis (Tajima, Yamagiwa, and Iwamori 1951; Tabuchi *et al.* 1953). The abnormalities are described elsewhere (see p. 297).

Pregnant pigs were injected intramuscularly with modified live hog cholera virus 10 to 16 days after breeding (Young *et al.* 1955). Various malformations occurred in the young, but the central nervous system apparently escaped damage. In earlier reports (Sautter *et al.* 1953; Kitchell, Sautter, and Young 1953), however, cephalic asymmetry (narrow head) was mentioned. More recently, definite malformation of the central nervous system was seen in several offspring of Duroc sows given standard doses of commercial tissue-culture-modified hog cholera virus during pregnancy (Emerson and Delez 1965). In addition to clinical signs, such as muscular tremors, the following defects were noted: hydrocephalus (not described) in one pig; small cerebral gyri in one; and rudimentary or small cerebellum in 10.

A pregnant pig was inoculated (Harding and Done 1956) with an attenuated strain of swine fever virus on the 21st day after service. Various malformations occurred in her litter of 11, including cyclopia.

Gitter and Bowen (1962) noted several young pigs with various degrees of muscular tremors and other nervous symptoms. Two 2-day-old Landrace–Large White hybrids were examined and found to have marked cerebellar hypoplasia. The vermis was almost absent and only the nodules were discernable. The cerebellar hemispheres were represented by 2 small portions joined by a flat bridge of tissue in place of the vermis. The brainstem and cerebral hemispheres were normal. There was no evidence of involvement of hereditary factors. On the contrary, the history of the herd indicated that the condition was possibly associated with a mild infection of swine fever to which sows were exposed during pregnancy.

Evidence of the possible infectious basis for congenital tremors and cerebellar hypoplasia in pigs was gathered by Harding, Done, and Darbyshire (1966). Investigations were made on a large number of herds in which sows were not vaccinated against swine fever and gave birth to early-dying, congenitally-trembling pigs. The study was made in parts of England, Scotland, and Wales from March, 1963 to June, 1965, during which interval the incidence of swine fever was relatively high (average monthly outbreaks, 15). The brains of 1,115 pigs with congenital tremors were examined, and 138 (12.4%) found to have cerebellar hypoplasia. The criterion used for diagnosing the condition was a ratio of cerebellum weight to whole-brain weight of less than 0.08. The incidence was far greater in pigs 3 or less days old than in those over 3 days of age, indicating that deformed piglets tended not to live longer than 3 days. Of 33 herds producing young with cerebellar hypoplasia, and which could be investigated completely, in 32 one or more sows gave evidence of immunity to swine fever. The authors thus concluded that the circumstantial evidence indicated an association between the malformation and the agent that immunized the sows against swine fever. After June, 1965, the average monthly number of outbreaks of the disease dropped to 3, and in 167 brains examined between that date and February, 1966, no cerebellar hypoplasia was found.

Congenital neuropathies were found in newborn progeny of sheep vaccinated with live bluetongue virus early in pregnancy (Shultz and DeLay 1955). Hydranencephaly was recognized grossly in more severely affected lambs. In less extreme forms of the abnormality the principal feature was cystic cavities in subcortical tissues of the neopallium and cerebellum accompanied by dilatation of the lateral ventricles (Cordy and Shultz 1961). In a study dealing with experimental reproduction of the disease, bluetongue virus was given subcutaneously to pregnant sheep on the 40th day of gestation (Young and Cordy 1964). Brain lesions were produced in a number of offspring; the abnormalities were considered, however, not the outcome of teratological processes, but the result of viral action on the fetal vascular system. No abnormalities were produced by maternal infection on the 19th to 29th days of pregnancy. Malformations similar to those observed in lambs from ewes inoculated with bluetongue virus were found in lambs from a flock that had probably been infected with the virus (Griner *et al.* 1964).

Mechanical Procedures

Hypoxia

Subjecting pregnant mammals to reduced atmospheric pressures caused various congenital malformations, especially of the skeleton. The teratogenesis of this procedure has generally been interpreted as due to hypoxia. The work done between 1950—when prenatal damage in mammals by reduced atmospheric pressure was first reported (Werthemann and Reiniger 1950)—and 1958, was summarized by Kalter and Warkany (1959*a*).

Hypoxia produced only a very small incidence of central nervous system malformations, in some studies. Ingalls, Curley, and Prindle (1950, 1952) subjected pregnant "white mice" to atmospheric pressures of 260 or 280 mm Hg for 5 hours between the 2nd and 18th days of pregnancy and noted a variety of developmental defects. Among the surviving offspring of females exposed on the 9th day were 3 (5.7%) with exencephaly. Hydrocephalus was also said to have been produced, but no details were given (Ingalls, Curley, and Prindle 1952). In addition, there were 2 cases of spina bifida occulta (vertebral defects only), but which occurred in young from mothers treated on the 4th day of pregnancy, i.e., before implantation and long before the time of organogenesis.

Further evidence that hypoxia only rarely disturbs development of the central nervous system was obtained in a study in which 5 inbred strains of mice were used (Ingalls *et al.* 1953). Only 10/545 young had exencephaly; 4 of these occurred in the BALB/c strain in which there also were 2 exencephalic control young, and another was from a female treated on the 15th day of gestation, long after the mouse neural tube is closed. It is therefore not likely that these defects were due to the treatment. No other central nervous system defects were mentioned (Ingalls *et al.* 1953), and in a subsequent extensive study (Ingalls and Curley 1957*b*), no defects of the central nervous system appeared at all.

Likewise, very few or no instances of exencephaly were found in other hypoxia experiments with mice (Murakami, Kameyama, and Kato 1956*b*; Freye and Freye 1959; Runner and Dagg 1960; Baird and Cook 1960, 1962, 1966; Murakami, Kameyama, and Nogami 1962; Vierck and Meier 1963). Certain apparent brain and cord abnormalities were noted (Murakami and Kameyama 1954; Murakami, Kameyama and Kato 1954) in 13th-day fetuses, but some of these may have been postmortem changes. Craniofacial dysplasias, with which brain disorders were correlated, were found in some strains of mice only rarely, and only after exposure to extreme oxygen deficiency (Degenhardt, Badtke, and Lund 1961; Lund 1966).

Rabbits are also susceptible to the teratogenic effects of hypoxia. Again, however, very few instances of defects of the central nervous system were found. Among 96/281 abnormal young, only 2 had exencephaly (Degenhardt 1954; Degenhardt and Kladetzky 1955). Subsequently (Badtke, Degenhardt, and Lund 1959; Degenhardt 1960*a*), a cyclopic offspring with a median proboscis was found. The animal was microcephalic and also had an encephalocele in the frontonasal region. Only axial skeletal defects were produced in rabbits by Grote (1965).

Pregnant cats were placed in a hermetically sealed chamber for 30 to 60 minutes during the middle of pregnancy. This treatment led to postnatal abnormalities of behavior and decreased weight and size of the brain (Klosovskii 1963, pp. 127–31).

Rats are apparently less susceptible than mice and rabbits to the teratogenic effects of hypoxia. In the earliest report dealing with this subject in mammals (Werthemann and Reiniger 1950), it was claimed that lowered atmospheric pressures produced defects of the rat eye. Critical evaluation (Kalter and Warkany 1959*a*) indicated that the results are untrustworthy. Since then, few reports have appeared of clear-cut congenital malformations produced by hypoxia in rats (Vidovic 1952; Fernandez-Cano 1959; Robertson 1959; Via, Elwood, and Bebin 1959). When studied at the age of 2 months, rats subjected to prenatal hypoxia had disturbances in brain development and vasculature (Klosovskii 1963; pp. 127–31). Some studies have suggested that hypoxia may produce certain cardiovascular defects in rats (Haring 1965; Clemmer and Telford 1966), and that heart abnormalities may also result from exposure to increased concentrations of CO_2 in the presence of normal or decreased oxygen (Haring and Polli 1957; Haring 1960, 1966). Moderate hydrocephalus was noted in 25/530 (4.7%) newborn offspring of Sprague–Dawley female rats exposed to 6 per cent CO_2 and 20% oxygen during pregnancy (Haring 1960). The method of fixation, the manner of examination, and the defect itself were not described.

Hamsters also seemed (Ferm 1964) resistant to the teratogenic effects of hypoxia (reduced atmospheric pressure equivalent to 18,000 ft elevation for 12 hours).

Hyperoxia

Golden hamster females were subjected (Ferm 1964) for 2 or 3 hours on the 6th, 7th, or 8th day of gestation to 30 or 40 lb per square inch of oxygen (i.e., 3.0, 3.6, and 4.0 atmospheres, respectively). Only the 2 larger amounts were teratogenic. Gross congenital malformations, including exencephaly and spina bifida, were noted in a small number of fetuses recovered 2 or 3 days before term.

Uterine Clamping

Fetal death and resorption, growth retardation, and congenital malformations were induced in rat embryos by temporarily shutting off the maternal circulation to a pregnant uterine horn (Brent and Franklin 1960). Isolation of the horn was accomplished by clamping it and the uterine blood vessels at the cervical and ovarian ends. Uterine hemostasis was confirmed by failure of detection of trypan blue, fluorescent dyes, or radioiodinated serum albumin in the isolated horn after intravenous injection of pregnant females with these substances.

The horn was clamped once for $\frac{1}{2}$ to 3 hours on the 4th to 15th days of gestation (Brent and Franklin 1960; Franklin and Brent 1960, 1964). The unclamped horn provided the control offspring, 2.6 per cent (26/1005) of which were found to be malformed. In offspring clamped on the 7th or earlier days and on the 12th or later days the rate of malformations was similar to that found in controls. Increased frequencies occurred in offspring clamped on the 8th to 11th days, the total being 12.3 per cent (55/448). The highest frequency was induced by treatment on the 9th day (37/141 = 26.2%) and the largest percentage (10/17 = 58.8%) by $2\frac{1}{2}$ hours of clamping (Franklin and Brent 1964).

There appeared to be little difference in the type of malformations produced by clamping on different days. So far as abnormalities of the central nervous system are concerned, hydrocephalus, considered to be any degree of ventricular dilatation, but not further described, occurred after treatment on the 8th, 9th, or 10th day of gestation; anencephaly on the 9th or 10th day; meningocele on the 9th day; and small cerebral hemisphere on the 11th day. The commonest defect was hydrocephalus; 36 cases occurred, 32 after clamping on the 9th day. In 14 cases hydrocephalus was an isolated defect and in 22 cases it was combined with other defects. When combined with other defects, the degree of dilatation was greater than when it occurred alone. In general the incidence, severity, and multiplicity of the malformations, numerous other types of which were also found, increased with increasing duration of clamping (Brent and Franklin 1960; Franklin and Brent 1960, 1964).

The same technique was used by Feild, Kreshover, and Lieberman (1960) for periods up to one hour on the 8th to 18th days of pregnancy. One instance of a central nervous system abnormality, exencephaly, occurred after treatment on the 13th day; later treatment produced cleft palate and limb defects only. All vessels supplying blood to the uterus of pregnant cats were temporarily clamped (Kiseleva 1955, cited by Klosovskii 1963, pp. 127–31). When done for 8 minutes during the 13th and 14th days of gestation, death and resorption of embryos occurred. Lesser durations caused decreased brain size and postnatal behavioral changes.

Uterine clamping was combined with other procedures to assess the role of embryonic accessibility of teratogens. Early data (Brent, Averich, and Drapiewski 1961) indicated that injection of kidney antisera produced a higher incidence of congenital malformations in offspring in unclamped uterine horns than in those from unclamped horns, but a later study (Brent 1966a) failed to confirm this result. Clamping afforded marked protection against the terato-genic effects of X rays and 5-fluorouracil and slight protection against the toxic effects of aminopterin, but on the other hand the incidence of congenital malformations was higher on the clamped side after maternal treatment with nitrogen mustard and trypan blue (Brent et al. 1962). Little or no difference in rate of defects between clamped and unclamped horns was found after injection of progestational compounds (Franklin et al. 1963).

The embryocidal, growth-retarding, and teratogenic effects of $2\frac{1}{2}$ hours of clamping on the 9th day of gestation were decreased by lowering the uterine temperature (George, Franklin, and Brent 1957). At 4°C the incidence of malformations was restored to the control level.

Hyperthermia

Exposure of pregnant animals of various species to increased ambient tem-perature was associated with suppressed ovulation, embryonic mortality, and fetal growth retardation, but only rarely with malformation (Hsu 1948; Shah 1956; MacFarlane, Pennycuik, and Thrift 1957; Yeates 1958; Chang and Fernandez-Cano 1959; Fernandez-Cano 1959; Dutt 1960, 1963; Aldred, Stob, and Andrews 1961; Pennycuik 1964, 1965; Shelton 1964; Vincent and Ulberg 1965; and others). Eye defects noted in 2 rats may well have been spontaneous occurrences (Hsu 1948). Histological abnormalities of dental structures were reported in rats (Kreshover and Clough 1953). Gross con-genital malformations, but not of the central nervous system, were noted in mice by Pennycuik (1965) and Lecyk (1966). A pyrogen administered early in pregnancy to rabbits elevated the embryonic death rate (Chang 1957).

Offspring of female guinea pigs exposed (Edwards 1967) to high ambient temperature (which increased rectal temperature to about 110°F) for an hour a day on 8 consecutive days beginning the 18th, 25th, etc. day of pregnancy bore some offspring with ataxia, uncoordinated movements, and other abnormal behavior. Dissection revealed the young to have brains smaller than those of controls, even though their birth weights may not have been affected. In general, the frequency of micrencephaly decreased with later treatment during pregnancy. The cerebral hemispheres and cerebellum were smaller in all dimensions, the former especially posteromedially, allowing the colliculi to be seen. In a preliminary study 4 cases of hydranencephaly occurred.

Other techniques for raising the temperature of pregnant animals or for directly exposing embryos to heat were more damaging to prenatal development. By injecting cooked milk into female rabbits on the 7th and 8th days of pregnancy the maternal body temperature was increased on the days treated (Brinsmade and Rübsaamen 1957). Three grossly defective offspring, with microcephaly or microcephaly and encephalocele, and various histological changes in the central nervous system, were found.

Relatively high incidences of frank congenital malformations were produced (Škreb and Frank 1963) by immersing a uterine horn of pregnant rats into hot water (40–41°C) for 40 to 60 minutes on the 9th to 16th days of pregnancy. Malformations were not found in embryos exposed on the 8th day even for 90 minutes. Exposure on the 9th and later days for 40 minutes was sufficient to induce abnormalities, which were, according to the authors, specific for each phase of development. Malformations of the central nervous system included abnormal prosencephalon, anencephaly, meningocele, and histological defects (rosettes) of the telencephalon. Treatment at later times produced brain changes similar to those found after X irradiation, such as rosettes in areas of the cerebral hemispheres, thin corpus callosum, and slight overall reduction in brain size. In a later study (Škreb 1965) the critical temperature was found to be 42°C, and the yield of malformations ranged from 5.6 to 8.8 per cent. The immediate histological effect of the temperature shock on embryos was irregularly distributed pycnotic cells.

Malformations were induced in offspring of female rats subjected to various intensities and durations of abdominal shortwave diathermy from the 5th to 14th days of gestation (Hofmann and Dietzel 1966). A few young with exencephaly were seen after treatments with intensities of 70 to 100 watts for 10 minutes usually on the 9th or 10th day of pregnancy. To a large extent specific effects resulted from treatment at different stages of pregnancy. Rectal temperatures rose during treatment.

Hypothermia

Subjecting pregnant animals to low temperatures was usually nonteratogenic. Such procedures caused reduced litter size (Barnett and Manly 1954), embryonic degeneration regardless of time of treatment (Fernandez-Cano 1959), interruption of pregnancy when applied at certain times during gestation

(Courrier and Marois 1953), but not at others (Courrier and Marois 1954), and in one case no apparent effect on litter size or fetal development (Vidovic 1952).

In a Wistar stock of rats with 2 per cent spontaneous cardiovascular anomalies, cold increased the rate of heart maldevelopment (Sobin 1955) in survivors ($32/240 = 13.3\%$), according to the author, by probably facilitating "some already present process or tendency to abnormality."

Pregnant female hamsters were frozen for 30 to 45 minutes and then thawed and reanimated (Smith 1957). Treatment for 30 minutes on the 1st to 9th days or on the 13th day of gestation did not harm the embryos; when done on the 10th or 11th day most embryos were killed. Treatment for 45 minutes on the 10th to 12th days usually caused embryonic death, but 5 females exposed on the 3rd, 7th, 8th, or 9th day had 34 offspring, 32 of which were grossly malformed. The abnormalities included hydrocephalus, anencephaly, exencephaly, spina bifida, and defects of various other parts. Malformations of the axial skeleton were found in offspring of pregnant mice subjected to lowered temperature (Lecyk 1965).

Noise

Intermittent, daily auditory stimulation for several months did not cause reproductive dysfunction in mice (Anthony 1955). Exposure to periods of loud noise on 4 successive days of pregnancy did no fetal damage in mice (Warkany and Kalter 1962). Audiovisual stimulation applied to rats throughout pregnancy caused abortion in 25 per cent of the females, but surviving litters were normal in number, average weight, and morphology (Soiva, Grönroos, and Aho 1959). No malformations were produced in rats and mice by audiovisual stimulation or noise during pregnancy, nor were the teratogenic effects of hypervitaminosis A modified by such factors (Härtel and Härtel 1960; Takekoshi 1961).

Intermittent, audiovisual stimulation for 3 weeks before conception and throughout pregnancy caused 11.6 per cent (24/207) malformations in newborn rats, but no central nervous system defects were mentioned (Árvay, Nagy, and Bazsó 1961). A low incidence of such defects ($14/3052 = 0.46\%$ interparietal meningocele; $17/3052 = 0.56\%$ thoracic or lumbar spina bifida) was noted (Geber 1966) in offspring of pregnant Sprague–Dawley rats exposed to intermittent audiovisual stimuli throughout pregnancy. Spina bifida also occurred in controls ($3/4880 = 0.06\%$). The explanation offered is that "the experimental procedure merely produced an upset in the physiological balance of the [maternal] nervous, vascular and endocrine systems . . ."

A Japanese strain of mice was exposed to different levels of noise for 6 hours a day on the 11th to 14th days of pregnancy (Ishii and Yokobori 1960). The highest level produced abnormalities in 7/130 living offspring, including 4 with exencephaly and one with anencephaly. The rate of abnormality may have been increased by additional treatment with trypan blue. While noise produced no congenital malformations in rats (Shidara 1963; Okuda 1964), noise plus trypan blue caused a higher rate of abnormality than did trypan blue alone; and the teratogenic effect of this combined treatment was significantly lowered by bilaterally adrenalectomizing pregnant rats (Shidara 1963).

Surgical and Other Procedures

Among the offspring of female rabbits ovariectomized on the 12th day of gestation, about 30 hours after being administered estradiol, were 2 with defects of the central nervous system, one with exencephaly and the other with spina bifida (Courrier and Jost 1939).

Female guinea pigs were adrenalectomized in 2 stages, the right adrenal being removed a week or so before mating and the left within 10 hours after insemination (Hoar and Salem 1962). Malformations, among which were spinal abnormalities, were found in survivors examined near the end of gestation. Surprisingly, similar malformations also occurred in offspring of pregnant guinea pigs injected with hydrocortisone (Hoar 1962). Female rats bilaterally adrenalectomized on the 12th day of pregnancy had young without congenital malformations (Angervall 1962). Developmental abnormalities did not occur after hypophysectomy of pregnant rats (Knobil and Caton 1953; Angervall and Lundin 1962).

Hypothalamic lesions at certain locations produced (Averill and Purves 1963) in young nonpregnant female rats were associated with reproductive difficulties, but congenital malformations were apparently not seen. Similar effects occurred after such lesions were made in pregnant rats (Gall 1959). Various hypothalamic areas of pregnant rabbits were stimulated or destroyed on the 10th to 14th days of gestation (Takakusu *et al.* 1962). A number of malformed offspring were found, including some with flexed spinal cord, slight hydromyelia, microcephaly, malclosure in the rhombencephalic area, and exencephaly. Amniotic-sac puncture induced cleft palate in mouse (Trasler, Walker, and Fraser 1956; Walker 1959) and rat (Jost 1956) fetuses, but no other abnormalities were seen.

Delayed fertilization in guinea pigs resulted in an increased number of pregnancies ending in embryonic death and abortion, but no defective offspring were noted (Blandau and Young 1939). In similar studies with rats, 2 grossly abnormal young were found, but neither had defects of the central nervous system (Blandau and Jordan 1941). Such studies with rabbits, however, yielded 6 per cent abnormal 24-day-old fetuses, including some with exposure of the brain and spinal cord (Chang 1952).

A number of malformed 29-day-old rabbit fetuses, among whose defects exencephaly was one of the most common, were produced by females that were superovulated. The abnormalities were attributed to intrauterine overcrowding (Hafez 1964).

Gates (1965*a*) superovulated BALB/c mice, cultured the ova in vitro for

3 days, and then transplanted them to suitable pseudopregnant female mice. Among the live offspring, examined near term, were 2 with malformations, one exencephalic, and another that was duplicated posteriorly, with 2 umbilical cords and a fused placenta. The latter specimen was not further described, but a front-view photograph showed it to have a thick upper body, wide head, 2 tails, 8 limbs, and a large omphalocele. Gates (1965a, p. 259, in the discussion following his article) mentioned that no other abnormal offspring occurred in about 500 young derived from transplanted eggs. He also stated that the fused placenta of the duplicated animal was similar to that observed by McLaren and Michie (*J. Exp. Zool.* 141: 47, 1959), where it was certain that 2 implantation sites were involved. A further point of interest is that both defective offspring occurred in an experiment in which 5 eggs were transplanted: of which, one resorbed, one was normal, and—as stated—one was exencephalic and one duplicated. The fifth egg was therefore unaccounted for—except if the duplicated offspring was in reality 2 originally separate organisms fused. As Gates (1965a, p. 259) said, "The possibility exists that two blastocysts fused, fell into one uterine crypt, and then proceeded to form two placentas. I have observed many fused placentas in immature superovulated mice."

Part Two

Spontaneous Malformations

8

Introduction

Part Two of this book deals with spontaneous malformations of the central nervous system in laboratory, agricultural, domestic, and other mammals. Spontaneous malformations, for our purposes, are all those not brought about by known extrinsic teratologic means.

A negative definition such as this is of course unsatisfactory, since it immediately raises the question, what *does* cause such congenital malformations? And the answer, it is almost needless to say, is that there is no one answer.

In the chapter on congenital malformations in their *Comparative Neuropathology*, Innes and Saunders (1962, pp. 267–68) divided such defects, essentially, into those usually occurring as individual, isolated cases, and therefore rarely amenable to etiological inquiry; and those for which a hereditary basis is well, or not so well, established. The inadequacy of this classification is due partly to its being based on the existing scarcity of useful information and partly to the limited view of the authors.

It may be profitable to mention briefly the similar problem of classification that faces investigators of congenital malformations in human beings and note that defects in our species have been broadly divided into those with clear environmental causation, those with clear genetic or chromosomal causation, and those, perhaps the vast bulk, that are the outcome of no one specific cause, but probably due to combined and interacting environmental and hereditary factors (Fraser 1961; Warkany and Kalter 1961). It is likely that a similar scheme is valid for the congenital defects of all species of mammals, whether the details differ or not.

Having discussed in Part One malformations that are environmentally caused—experimentally or otherwise—we turn in following chapters to defects that are hereditary, or suspected of being so, and to those that appear sporadically and thus for which a cause is not usually assignable.

Except for mice, which have been favored with special attention, very few methodical investigations of congenital malformations have been made in animals—whether morphological, embryological, genetical, epidemiological, and so on. Consequently, although numerous cases of defective animals have been recorded in the world scientific and other literature, understanding of various problems entailed in such conditions is still in but a primitive state of advancement. So elementary a question, e.g., as the frequency of congenital malformations in, let us say, cattle, in many respects the best-studied, large, nonhuman mammal, is almost totally unanswered.

Why this should be so is not difficult to understand. As Innes and Saunders (1962, p. 268) stated, breeders the world over are reluctant to admit the presence of inherited, or supposedly inherited, disease in their prize stocks and breeds, and not a fraction of newborn animals with conditions incompatible with life are called to the attention of the veterinary pathologist, most just being quietly buried.

Some information on frequency of malformations in cattle was supplied by a survey made in Ohio (Herschler, Fechheimer, and Gilmore 1962) of the number of abnormal calves born in a $3\frac{1}{2}$-year period, in which, of 4,980 reported calves, 312 (6.3%) were considered abnormal. No significant association of total frequency of abnormality was found with breed (Guernsey, Holstein, and Jersey), all having approximately the same proportion of anomalous calves. But when the abnormalities were broken down into 5 categories—general (i.e., affecting the animal as a whole); muscle, bone, joint, or cartilage; nerve (eye); epithelium; and stillbirth—definite associations were found of certain types of abnormality with specific breeds. Unfortunately, the abnormalities could not be more explicitly classified, and hence the data did not reveal the frequency of particular congenital malformations, such as those of the central nervous system.

Other information was furnished by a sampling of 1,008 bovine fetuses (including 31 pairs of twins) gathered in an abbattoir during a 9-month period (Mammerickx and Leunen 1964). Fetal age ranged from 4 to $8\frac{1}{2}$ months. Among them were 2 monsters, 19 with defects of the urogenital system, and 9 with various other anomalies, for a total of 30/1008, or 2.98 per cent defective. It may well be that other internal abnormalities were overlooked; but the low incidence of external malformations is surprising. Only 3 fetuses with malformations of the central nervous system were noted: a duplication monster with spina bifida, a hydrocephalic, and one with a small meningocele.

Brief reference to the incidence of congenital malformations in cattle was made by Frauchiger and Fankhauser (1957, p. 39), who found it to be 3.3 per cent in their collection. In a 1-year study of 243 calves (mostly Holstein) born in Michigan, 53 (21.8%) showed congenital heart, organic, and skeletal defects (Rothenbacher 1962). Weber (1949) mentioned that in his experience of 30 years, 16 per cent of malformed calves had defects of the brain.

Another pertinent study (Mead, Gregory, and Regan 1946*a*) revealed the prevalence of harmful genes, a situation that may exist in many herds of cattle. In breeding experiments with 6 unrelated bulls, chosen at random, it was found that, among them, these individuals were heterozygous for 8 different autosomal recessive genes, one animal even being heterozygous for 3 of them. Two of the genes were lethals (epitheliogenesis imperfecta and a recessive chondrodystrophy) and the 6 others nonlethals. Weber (1946*a*) estimated that the gene frequency for congenital malformations in cattle, based on a 30-year study in the Bern Canton, was between 1.2 and 1.6 per cent. Stegenga (1964) noted in Friesian cattle that the frequency of congenital malformations depended partly on factors such as season of birth and maternal age.

Also relevant to our discussion are genes causing prenatal death, since in some cases such genes may work by producing anatomical deviations. Indirect estimates of the average number of lethal gene equivalents per individual have been made in animals, using Morton, Crow and Muller's (1956) method, which utilizes observed increases in mortality and other detrimental effects occurring in the offspring of consanguineous, compared with nonconsanguineous, matings. A lethal equivalent corresponds to a lethal gene with 100 per cent probability of causing death, to 2 genes each with a 50 per cent average probability of causing death, etc.

When these and other methods were applied to prenatal and neonatal losses in cattle and swine, only low estimates of attributability to lethal genes were forthcoming. Pisani and Kerr (1961), using data collected by Regan, Mead, and Gregory (1947), calculated that Jersey and Holstein cattle possess very low average lethal equivalents affecting prenatal life, with the value for the latter not differing statistically from zero. In fact, the only significant value found was for genes affecting early postnatal mortality in Jersey calves, a phenomenon that may be of little concern to us here.

Based on embryonic and fetal deaths following 1,404 artificial inseminations in an experimental Holstein-Friesian herd, Conneally *et al.* (1963) also estimated that the average number of lethal equivalents was low; and concluded that most of the prenatal deaths were due not to recurrent gene mutation, but to nongenetic factors (trauma, infection, etc.) and to such genetic factors as chromosomal aberrations, interactions between maternal and fetal genotypes, etc.

On the other hand, significant values were estimated for 2 other mammals. Data for the wisent or European bison (*Bison bonasus*, L.) enabled Slatis (1960) to conclude that the average individual in some herds possessed about 2.5 fully penetrant recessive genes or their equivalents responsible for perinatal death. Using Hodgson's (1935) data for Poland-China pigs, Pisani and Kerr

(1961) calculated that an average of approximately 2 lethal equivalents per animal affected prenatal and neonatal life.

So far as can be determined, even fewer data of these types are available for other domesticated species, such as horses, sheep, goats, dogs, and cats. It was estimated (O'Hara and Shortridge 1966) that in New Zealand swine 2.3 per cent of preweaning deaths are attributable to congenital abnormalities.

The fact that such statistics, despite their inadequacy, are available for cattle and seem not to have been gathered for many other species may be due to congenital malformations being more frequent in cattle, as the records presented by Weber (1946a) and Frauchiger and Fankhauser (1957, p. 38) indicated. Even Saint-Hilaire (1832–37, vol. 3, p. 357), almost a century and a half ago, to some extent noted the same phenomenon. While these may well be spurious observations, there can be little doubt, as the following chapters will document, that some types of congenital malformations of the central nervous system are more common in certain species than in others.

9

Mouse

Introduction

In many ways, the mammal whose genetics has been most fully explored is the common house mouse *Mus musculus*, and the discovery of new genes in mice ever quickens (fig. 16). In the July, 1966 issue, number 35, of the Mouse News Letter, 351 established mutant genes were listed—not including the large number of recessive alleles recognized at the *t* locus—as well as 46 new and provisional ones. Multiple alleles have been discovered at many loci, and 19 of the mouse's 20 theoretical linkage groups are known.

The virtues of the mouse for the investigation of the multitudinous facets of heredity are well recognized and need not be dilated here (Green 1966). It should only be remarked that the embryology of many hereditary characteristics in mice have been intensively studied and debated (Grüneberg 1952*b*, 1963). In the following pages the known inherited congenital malformations of the central nervous system in this species are described and discussed. The headings of the following sections refer, of course, to the effects of the genes on the central nervous system.

Genes Causing Hydrocephalus

Hydrocephalus-1

Hydrocephalus determined by a simple autosomal recessive gene (symbol *hy-1*), now extinct, was discovered by Clark (1932) in mice derived from Hunt's flexed-tail stock. The gene was probably already present in this line, since Hunt informed Clark he had previously noted hydrocephalus.

The time of onset of the condition was variable (Clark 1932, 1934). It was occasionally expressed as a slight swelling of the head at birth but was not usually detectable until 12 to 15 days after birth. Affected mice had uncoordinated movements and in advanced stages showed nervous derangements and irritability. The condition was always eventually lethal; most animals died between 40 and 60 days of age (probably from emaciation owing to inability to find food and water). Some reached sexual maturity (60–90 days), but died soon afterward; these were of normal size and fertile.

Affected offspring had a domeshaped head due to pressure of accumulated clear fluid in the lateral cerebral ventricles that distended the skull outward. In more extreme cases the head was transilluminable. Anatomical studies (Clark 1934) in both adult and newborn mice showed that the hydrocephalus was of the internal obstructive type, with occlusion of the aqueduct of Sylvius and enormous dilatation of the lateral and 3rd ventricles and the foramina of Monro. The 4th ventricle, on the other hand, appeared normal though the cerebellum was flattened in extreme cases and deformed in shape in less severe ones. Some secondary effects were stretched and thinned cerebral cortex, great reduction, or, in extreme cases, obliteration of the corpus callosum, presumably due to pressure atrophy, and occasional rupture of cerebral hemispheres causing subarachnoid spaces to become filled with bloody fluid, giving the appearance of external hydrocephalus.

Several years later, by the time Bonnevie (1943) had taken over the stock, the condition had become milder (possibly, Grüneberg 1952b, p. 168, believed, by the accumulation of modifying genes), in all but one subline. In the large majority of homozygotes it was not recognizable during their lifetime, which was of normal duration, and classification had to be based on postmortem examination. In the few mice in which external signs—a faint convexity above the eyes—were present, they were poorly correlated with the degree of internal abnormality (Bonnevie 1943).

Examination of brains of young affected mice revealed (Bonnevie 1943) a pattern of malformations similar in some respects to that reported by Clark (1934) and different in others. The lateral ventricles were expanded and their walls and roof were thin. The 3rd ventricle was enlarged only ventrally. The aqueduct was constricted rostrally, but posteriorly rapidly opened into the widely expanded 4th ventricle. However, the most characteristic feature of the hydrocephalic brain, and already recognizable at birth, was partial or seemingly complete absence of the cerebellar vermis, leaving a gap between the cerebellar hemispheres that was covered by a thin membrane. The amount of medial cerebellar tissue missing varied greatly, and it was learned that this variability was nongenetic in origin.

In embryological studies Bonnevie (1943) traced the earliest morphological appearance of the hydrocephalus to 12th-day embryos. The first sign was ventricular enlargement, including that of the 4th ventricle, accompanied by a stretched and bulging state of the epithelial roof of the latter. Because of this stretching, the anterior membranous region of the roof—called the area membranacea superior ventriculi quarti by Weed (1917), and the foramen anterius by Bonnevie (1934)—which would normally have already disappeared by incorporation into the rostral fold of the choroid plexus, was still present.

As a consequence of this abnormality and possibly also because of excessive intraventricular pressure, median parts of the cerebellar plate were dislocated and characteristic cerebellar defects resulted, i.e., absence or under-development of the vermis (Brodal, Bonnevie, and Harkmark 1946). Brodal (1946) described these and other changes in detail.

As for occlusion of the Sylvian aqueduct, observed by Clark (1934), Bonnevie (1943) believed it to be a secondary phenomenon, appearing during the last days of pregnancy and due to compression resulting indirectly from rapid growth of the cerebral hemispheres; as a result of which the hydrocephalus was augmented near term and postnatally.

Bonnevie's (1945) attempt to trace the development of the condition further back in embryogenesis than the 12th day led her to believe that the very earliest manifestation of the gene occurred on the 4th day of gestation, just before and during implantation, and that it consisted of irregularities in the formation and rupturing of the trophoblast. This abnormality, she assumed, was followed by maternal fluids entering embryonic tissues, then being transferred to the ventricular channels, and there producing hydrocephalus. Grüneberg (1952b, pp. 171–72) was not convinced by these deductions and criticized Bonnevie's study from several points of view; the most telling of which was that Bonnevie may not have been sure of the genotypes of the embryos she was dealing with, since some of the matings from which they came were of types that yielded normal as well as affected offspring.

As mentioned above, there were several discrepancies between Clark's (1934) description of the condition and Bonnevie's (1943). In a number of ways Clark's animals were apparently much more severely affected than those of all but one subline of Bonnevie's. In Clark's mice the condition was expressed and diagnosable before death, which occurred relatively early, while in Bonnevie's the diagnosis usually had to await postmortem examination, after a normal lifespan. Other differences concerned the anatomy of the abnormality. In Clark's mice the aqueduct was occluded and the anterior ventricles were dilated, but the 4th ventricle and cerebellum were essentially normal. In Bonnevie's material, however, the entire ventricular system was enlarged, including the 4th ventricle, and the cerebellum was malformed. This last feature, in fact, was so consistent, though variable in extent, that the diagnosis of hydrocephalus could be made on the basis of it alone. Furthermore, this total dilatation occurred with the presence, in newborn and young mice, of a somewhat constricted but occluded aqueduct, thus signifying that occlusion was a secondary phenomenon.

These differences are so great that it is difficult to believe they could have come about through the workings of modifying genetic factors alone; one is left wondering whether these authors may not have been working with different alleles or even genes at different loci.

The morphology and embryology of hydrocephalus-1, as described by

Bonnevie (1943), were very similar to those of the hydrocephalus produced (Kalter and Warkany 1957; Kalter 1963*b*) in mice by galactoflavin-induced riboflavin deficiency (see p. 22). In both conditions the external appearance of the head was an unreliable index of the state of the brain; the entire ventricular system, but especially the 4th ventricle, was dilated; and the cerebellum, especially in medial areas, was aplastic. The cerebellar defect, furthermore, was the most characteristic and consistent feature of both conditions. In both conditions the first embryonic expression occurred early in gestation. (Bonnevie 1943 did not state how she timed the pregnancies of her animals, and therefore the apparent slight disagreement in time of earliest appearance of the abnormality between her mice and mine must remain unreconciled.) Finally, the most conspicuous embryonic abnormality in both consisted of dilatation of the 4th ventricle and persistence of the area membranacea superior. It is the most improbable of suggestions, and entirely untestable— until the gene recurs—but in the light of the very similar condition produced by acute maternal riboflavin deficiency, might not the *hy-1* gene have worked, through one means or another, by inducing a degree of riboflavin deficiency.

Hydrocephalus-2

Hydrocephalus-2 (symbol *hy-2*) was discovered by Zimmermann (1933) in the offspring of wild mice caught in the cellar of the Genetics Department of the Institute of Brain Research in Berlin-Buch. Whether the subjects were seeking genetic counseling or psychiatric advice was never ascertained. Like *hy-1*, this gene was a regular autosomal recessive and is now extinct. It was invariably associated with sterility in both sexes, and so to determine whether the *hy* mutations were identical it was necessary to mate heterogyzotes ($+/hy-1 \times +/hy-2$). Since no affected offspring resulted the genes were proved nonallelic (Clark 1935).

The external signs of hydrocephalus-2 were very much like those of hydrocephalus-1, but perhaps even more severe. The skull was domeshaped and the cranial bones were thin and the sutures often open owing to increased intracranial pressure. Brain abnormalities were always present, even at 4 days, the earliest age investigated. In all cases internal hydrocephalus was found, but no other description of the condition and no information concerning its possible anatomical basis were given (Zimmermann 1935).

Hydrocephalus-3

Hydrocephalus-3 (symbol *hy-3*) was discovered by Grüneberg (1943*a*) upon inbreeding a heterogeneous stock of mice. The condition is due to a single autosomal recessive gene with variable manifestation, producing visible hydrocephalus in about 70 per cent of homozygotes and changes such as growth retardation and mild internal hydrocephalus in the remaining ones.

In certain respects the abnormality resembled the picture presented by hydrocephalus-1 and hydrocephalus-2. The head was sometimes domeshaped, but often its shape was not appreciably abnormal. When skinned the skull showed a slight bulging not recognizable in the living animal, but even in the absence of such bulging dissection revealed mild internal hydrocephalus. In typical cases the lateral ventricles were dilated (cranial capacities of as much as 0.75–0.88 ml were found; normal capacity was 0.40–0.44 ml). There was extreme thinning of the pallium but relatively mild changes in the basal ganglia. In far-progressed cases hemorrhages into the pia-arachnoid spaces were common.

Hydrocephalus-3 was manifested relatively late. The earliest successful diagnosis was made at 5 days of age, but usually the abnormality developed during the second week and occasionally even later (21–36 days). Berry (1961), however, was able to identify most hydrocephalic offspring from their external appearance by 3 to 5 days of age, and in some instances, even at one day after birth. The possible reasons for the earlier recognizability in this study were not discussed. Hydrocephalic offspring were always retarded in growth, never reached normal size, and usually died by 4 to 6 weeks of age in the earlier study (Grüneberg 1943a) and by the time of weaning in the later (Berry 1961), possibly owing to emaciation. Near the end of life they developed spasticity of the hindlimbs. Maternal parity had no effect on penetrance of the gene.

The condition was extensively described by Berry (1961), whose study of its pathogenesis is discussed below. Animals aged one to 4 days, and some older, were sectioned. There was gross enlargement of the lateral ventricles, which increased progressively with age. In presumably hydrocephalic newborn animals these spaces were only slightly dilated. Further enlargement occurred through expansion of the posterior horns of the lateral ventricles and by the formation of diverticula from them that ruptured the ependyma. The foramina of Monro were greatly widened and the 3rd ventricle was dilated. The aqueduct of Sylvius was not much affected. Only in severe cases was the 4th ventricle somewhat expanded. Most hydrocephalics had some increase in size of the ventral subarachnoid cistern, i.e., a degree of external hydrocephalus.

Injection of colloidal carbon and Prussian blue into the ventricles and the subarachnoid system indicated no block in the ventricular pathway or the basal cisternal system. The injected material was never found in the subcalvarial arachnoid spaces, however, and it was therefore concluded that a defect of these spaces was the cause of the hydrocephalus.

Histological examination of the meninges revealed "cloudy" degenerative appearances, probably in all layers, which were believed to have caused blockage of cerebrospinal-fluid circulation. These pathological changes were not found in fetuses one day before term but were noted in newborn offspring. In the latter the changes were limited to the regions adjoining the foramina of Luschka and over the otic capsules, but in older animals they were somewhat more widespread.

All newborn to 5-day-old offspring classified as hydrocephalic on the basis of ventricular dilatation showed striking degrees of "cloudiness" in certain areas. In addition, many nonhydrocephalic young showed similar but less pronounced changes. Such animals were considered to be heterozygous for the gene on the basis of the proportion of them present (17 normal, 31 "intermediate," and 15 hydrocephalic, which conformed with the 1 : 2 : 1 ratio of genotypes expected from crosses of heterozygotes). Naturally, whole litters were examined.

It was postulated that the meningeal abnormalities were somehow related to ossification. This idea was based, first, on the finding that the pathological changes were associated with areas of active ossification in the calvaria and, second, that the effects of the gene appeared to be systemic, since the hydrocephalics were runts. But abnormalities of ossification were not found (Barnicot 1947; Berry 1961). *hy-3* has not been tested for allelism with *hy-1* or *hy-2*.

Congenital Hydrocephalus

Congenital hydrocephalus (symbol *ch*) is caused by a single autosomal recessive gene, which arose in laboratory mice by spontaneous mutation (Grüneberg 1943*b*). The forehead of affected newborn animals rose steeply from a shortened snout and consisted of bilateral bulging regions corresponding to greatly enlarged cerebral hemispheres. The bulges were covered by normal skin but had no bony protection. These and other signs were very uniform in all abnormal offspring observed, with no apparent variation and no milder degrees of the anomaly.

A study (Grüneberg 1943*b*) of the anatomy and development of the condition revealed that the hydrocephalus had as its ontogenic basis an anomaly of cartilage, which was first expressed on the 13th day of gestation. The anomaly consisted of shortening of the cartilaginous basicranium and nasal septum owing to delay in chondrification, which was preceded by reduction in size of mesenchymal condensation (Grüneberg 1953). The retardation was apparently transitory, but the eventual appearance of cartilage normal in histology and growth did not restore the situation to normal. Thus, through continued retardation, by the 14th day of pregnancy there developed a considerable shortening of the base of the skull, which forced the normally growing telencephalon to bulge dorsally. The brain could be distorted in this way without hindrance, since at this stage the cranial bones are not yet developed.

Sections of 13th-day affected embryos showed that the lateral ventricles were already somewhat dilated but that the pallium was not very different in thickness from that of controls. By the 17th day the lateral ventricles were enormously expanded and were in wide communication with each other except most anteriorly and posteriorly; the choroid plexus was poorly developed and hung down from the dorsal midline area of the joined ventricles; and the pallium was considerably thinned. Dilatation was confined to the lateral ventricles. The 3rd and 4th ventricles and the aqueduct, on the contrary, were somewhat compressed; but the continuity of the entire ventricular system was nowhere obstructed.

It seemed likely that the compression of the middle and hind cerebral channels resulted from telescoping of the lower parts of the brain through counterpressure of the elastic skin against the bulging hemispheres; and that the circulation of cerebrospinal fluid was thereby interfered with in the region of the foramen of Magendie (but see p. 204), which in turn produced expansion of the lateral ventricles by hydrostatic pressure. A further ramification of these processes was the thinning of the osteogenic membrane over the bulging hemispheres, preventing formation of bone in this area. In addition, strain on the blood sinuses led to extensive intracerebral hemorrhages during the last days of pregnancy, which together with brain damage was responsible for death of neonates.

A pedigree of causal events was thus established; and the principle enunciated that gene action is cell- or tissue-specific and that all apparently unrelated parts of a hereditary syndrome can be traced to the gene's primary action (Grüneberg 1953).

Dreher

Dreher (symbol *dr*) is one of a large number (Sidman, Green, and Appel 1965) of hereditary disorders of the labyrinth in mice producing "circler" or "waltzer" behavior. The gene arose in the wild, presumably by spontaneous mutation, and was found to be a simple autosomal recessive (Falconer and Sierts-Roth 1951). The abnormalities of equilibrium were found to be due to malformations of the inner ear (Hertwig 1951; Fischer 1956); the embryology of these defects was investigated by Fischer (1958), and their basis discovered by Deol (1964*a*) invariably to be localized abnormalities of the rhombencephalon, which were recognizable one day before those of the inner ear. Deol (1964*a*) believed it improbable that the early changes in the neural tube disappear without leaving a permanent mark on the myelencephalon, and that their later effects may account for the behavior of dreher mice. It is also possible that these changes are responsible for, or involved in, the development of the hydrocephalus to be discussed. Parenthetically, Deol (1966*a*) recently found that the neural tube abnormalities produced by homozygosis for the Splotch and Loop-tail genes were related to abnormal differentiation of the inner ear.

It was noted (Falconer and Sierts-Roth 1951) that 5 per cent (4/80) of homozygous drehers had hydrocephalus, as was also reported several years later (Fischer 1956). In his study, Bierwolf (1956) noted 11 per cent of all new-born offspring to be hydrocephalic, and, furthermore, only animals with a severe degree of hydrocephalus were considered abnormal. This increased frequency was believed to have resulted from continued inbreeding of the stock and their different genetic background.

Most of the severely hydrocephalic offspring died within a few days of birth (Bierwolf 1956). Surviving hydrocephalics continued to exhibit the characteristic excessive curvature of the head. In a 4-week-old extremely abnormal animal the cerebellum was completely absent, except for small rests, and the forebrain consisted only of a thin sheet of brain substance covering the ventricles.

The age of 4 weeks apparently presented a second period of crisis, after which, if successfully traversed, the mice developed into normal-appearing adults. After a time the curvature of the head disappeared and the condition was no longer recognizable externally. Upon dissection, however, the brain of such adults showed a wide range of degrees of malformation with numerous intermediate grades. In milder cases almost no anomaly was found except for a slight indentation or fissure in the vermis of the cerebellum as well as a more or less distinct flattening of the sulci. In progressively greater abnormality the fissure became broader and deeper and finally turned into a hole covered only by pia mater. In some cerebellums a small bridge remained between the 2 hemispheres; in severely affected cases the bridge disappeared and the hemispheres were completely separated by a wide gap. In addition, the hemispheres were reduced in size, but not to the same extent as was the vermis. The region of the mesencephalon was affected by reduction of the colliculi. In all cases the cerebral hemispheres were enlarged owing to dilatation of the lateral ventricles.

There was also a graded series of brain abnormalities in newborn animals. While more severe hydrocephalus was recognized by the appearance of the head, less severe states were only detected by gross inspection of the brain. Macroscopic examination of newborn hydrocephalics revealed the following brain defects. The 4th ventricle was considerably dilated—with relatively thin, sometimes transparent, overlying brain substance—and pouched into the mesencephalon, inflating it. At birth the normal cerebellum lies as a compact bulge behind the mesencephalon. In defective brains this bulge was hollow and its wall was greatly thinned. In milder cases, only a thin roof of brain substance and pia mater was present in the region of the vermis; in severely defective animals the entire vermis was replaced by a hole, which was covered by pia.

The aqueduct of Sylvius was not occluded. A slight constriction was sometimes found in adult hydrocephalics, which probably resulted from pressure of the growing cerebral hemispheres. Newborn animals, on the contrary, always had a slight dilatation of the aqueduct.

A study of the embryology of the condition revealed a remarkable sequence of events (Bierwolf 1958). On the 11th day of gestation the caudal region of the roof of the 4th ventricle, corresponding to the area membranacea inferior, became thickened, which, according to the author, prevented the later development of the "foramen of Magendie." (For a short discussion of the existence of the foramina of the roof of the 4th ventricle in small animals see p. 204). This thickening ostensibly sealed the 4th ventricle, and mounting internal pressure of cerebrospinal fluid ensued. The apparent result, as seen in 15th-day fetuses, was the occurrence of an expansion or cystlike bulging of different sizes between the cerebellum and choroid plexus, causing these parts to be far separated from each other. This secondary dilatation continued to exist for the remainder of fetal life and may have been present at birth. The thickened inferior membrane, however, remained attached to the choroid plexus. In addition, in severe cases, the lateral apertures of the 4th ventricle (foramina of Luschka) may have remained closed.

The abnormalities of the cerebellum were thus apparently brought about by inhibition of brain tissue development in the neighborhood of the dilated 4th ventricle, especially near the midline, i.e., in the region of the vermis.

The spectrum of abnormalities caused by the *dr* gene in newborn hydrocephalics—mainly, dilatation of the 4th ventricle and cerebellar malformations—greatly resembled that produced by *hy-1*. In origin, however, it was quite different, since hydrocephalus-1 resulted from anomalous development of the area membranacea superior (Bonnevie and Brodal 1946), while in *dr/dr* homozygotes the hydrocephalus was caused by anomalous development of the area membranacea inferior (Bierwolf 1958).

Leukencephalosis

Fischer (1959*a, b*) described a dilatation of the entire cerebral ventricular system produced by a completely penetrant autosomal recessive gene (no symbol assigned). Externally, affected mice had a very accentuated angle between the nasal and frontal bones and marked arching in the parietal region. In serial sections the lateral ventricles were seen to be greatly expanded and often combined into a single large space. The foramina of Monro were dilated and the aqueduct of Sylvius was widened throughout its entire length. In some cases the 3rd and 4th ventricles were moderately enlarged.

The hydrocephalus was interpreted as being the secondary *ex vacuo* result of widespread tissue destruction. Necrosis began in the white matter (leukodystrophy) of the occipital cortex and spread rostrally and medially to involve various regions. The entire posterior portion of the corpus callosum and posterior limbs of the anterior commissure were destroyed, causing enlargement and coalescence of the lateral ventricles. The cortex was less affected laterally and anteriorly and the lateral ventricles were correspondingly less expanded in these areas. The olfactory bulbs were reduced in size, either because of poor development or degeneration. The colliculi were reduced in volume. The cerebellum was of fairly normal size and shape.

Fischer (1959*a, b*) failed to indicate to what extent, if any, the condition was congenital, and this and other questions will remain unanswered—unless the mutation recurs—since the leukodystrophic stock was lost during an epidemic (Sidman, Green, and Appel 1965, pp. 34–35).

Double-Toe

A recently discovered (Green 1964–65) radiation-induced mutation ("double-toe") produced preaxial polydactyly often accompanied by slight to severe hydrocephalus. The latter condition was not described.

Cerebral Degeneration

Cerebral degeneration (symbol *cb*), a condition produced by a recently discovered autosomal recessive gene (Deol and Truslove 1965), has as yet been only briefly described. "The degeneration causes an *ex vacuo* hydrocephalus which is clearly visible in the living animal. The time of onset of the anomalies varies, but classification is usually possible at birth. The most susceptible parts of the brain are the cerebral hemispheres and the olfactory lobes. In later stages the epithelium of the nose and the trachea also degenerates. The involvement of the skull is believed to be secondary. The homozygotes generally die before reaching maturity, but if they live on they are always sterile."

Droopy-Ear

Droopy-ear (symbol *de*), a fully penetrant autosomal recessive gene (Curry 1959), caused widespread skeletal changes some of which resembled those found in certain chondrodystrophies. A transient hydrocephalus, not further described, was found to be clearly present at the age of 6 weeks, but was not discernable in those 3 to 7 months old.

Visceral Inversion

Visceral inversion was caused by an incompletely penetrant autosomal recessive gene (symbol *vi*), probably now extinct, which possibly produced some prenatal mortality in homozygotes (Tihen, Charles, and Sipple 1948). The visceral inversion was chiefly associated with probable hydrocephalus. The latter was not described, aside from brief mention of swollen cranium, thin, distended skullcap, and a foramen between the parietal and interparietal bones. The homozygotes were small and weak at birth and died within a few weeks.

Similar visceral abnormalities (Hummel and Chapman 1959) were produced by a different recessive gene (symbol *iv*, for situs inversus viscerum). But this condition was not accompanied by abnormalities of the central nervous system and *iv/iv* homozygotes were fairly viable and fertile.

Hydrocephalic-Polydactyl

Offspring with hydrocephalus and double hallux appeared in a partially inbred stock derived from an X-rayed male (Hollander 1966). Each of the 2 malformations sometimes occurred alone. Both conditions were variable in degree, but even moderate hydrocephalus was associated with poor growth and early death. Those with polydactyly only usually matured well, but the males were consistently sterile. The internal anatomy of the brain defect was not mentioned. The syndrome was probably due to a single recessive gene (symbol *hyp*). Apparent incomplete penetrance noted may disappear when anatomical studies are made.

Other Simply-Inherited Hydrocephaluses

A hydrocephalus similar to that produced by *hy-3* arose in a stock of mice with defects of the pinna (Kobozieff and Pomriaskinsky-Kobozieff 1947). It was due to a single autosomal recessive gene with variable manifestation. The hydrocephalics were rarely recognizable at birth, except for their abnormally low weight. The condition was expressed, beginning at the age of 7 days, by increase of different amounts in size of the head, ranging from slight convexity to very distinct enlargement. In extreme cases the facial skeleton was overshadowed by the enormous size of the cranium, and since the snout was slender the head was pearshaped. The parietal bones were thin and widely separated and the fontanelles were therefore large and covered only by skin. The brain itself was not described. Most affected mice died before reaching 3 weeks of age.

About 50 per cent of hydrocephalic animals also had abnormalities of the ear, eye, or both. It was not made clear whether these anomalies were caused by the gene for hydrocephalus, but it was found that ear abnormalities occurred much more frequently in offspring with hydrocephalus than in those without it (Kobozieff, Pomriaskinsky-Kobozieff, and Migne 1955).

Hydrocephalic mice with "characteristic domed-shaped head" were found in animals of 4 strains (Eaton 1952). The condition was not further described. In most cases the growth rate of abnormal offspring was slower than that of normal littermates, and their mortality was high (about 75% of them being dead by 4 months of age). The condition was apparently not recognizable before 15 days of age, and in some cases not until 60 days. Those dying before 15 days were, it seems, not autopsied, and in any case not classified. About 13 per cent of those alive at 15 days were hydrocephalic. If all those born dead or dying before 15 days are considered also hydrocephalic the departure from a 3 : 1 ratio is not significant. The author thus considered the abnormality as due to a recessive gene. The evidence for this assumption is tenuous. In addition to the skepticism aroused by "the" condition arising in 4 different strains, it is sustained by the fact that no controlled crosses between mice of known genotypes were apparently made.

Snaker

A constant and clearly distinguishable variant phenotype arose in descendants of mice treated with a chemical mutagen (Cattanach 1965). Variant animals were recognized at birth by their small size and domed heads. The condition was apparently semilethal, since only about half the young survived beyond 3 weeks of age. The reduced body size and domed head persisted into adulthood, but the most obvious characteristic in older animals was a weaving behavior, which gave the trait its name, Snaker. While the unusual head shape may have been due to congenital hydrocephalus, its anatomical basis was apparently not investigated.

Breeding tests were interpreted as indicating that 2 genetic factors were involved in the inheritance of the character; one, a dominant, producing the mutant phenotype, and the other, having no phenotype of its own, but suppressing the action of the first when both were present together. Although cytological studies were negative, it was postulated that the 2 factors were chromosomal rearrangements.

Multifactorial Hydrocephalus

Several congenital malformations in mice are probably due to the cumulative action of relatively small numbers of genes. Such abnormalities do not appear in the well-known mendelian ratios but range in frequency from less than one per cent to perhaps 10 to 15 per cent, depending on the number of genetic factors and the subsidiary environmental variables involved.

The hydrocephalus that occurs spontaneously in animals of the C57BL/6 and C57BL/10 inbred strains of mice is probably in this category of defect. In the stocks of these strains maintained by The Jackson Laboratory, Bar Harbor, Maine, hydrocephalus occurred with a frequency of about 1 per cent in the former and was less common in the latter (Inbred Strains of Mice No. 5, p. 28, 1967).

In the C57BL (substrain not indicated) colony of Baylor University College of Medicine, the frequency of spontaneous hydrocephalus was 4.3 per cent (Carton et al. 1956). Attempts to increase it by selective breeding were, not surprisingly, unsuccessful. Irradiating pregnant females at various stages of gestation also failed to increase the frequency of hydrocephalus, although several other congenital malformations were produced.

In gross appearance (Carton et al. 1956) hydrocephalic mice were usually recognizable at birth or shortly afterwards because of their small size, but the head at birth was apparently not enlarged or distorted in shape. With advancing age, the usually sloping forehead was replaced by a slight bump in the occipital area, eventually producing a high-domed head accompanied by a foreshortened skull base. Early in the course of the disease hydrocephalics were quite active and seemed somewhat hyperirritable. As the condition progressed and the head enlarged further they became lethargic, sat in a hunched-up position, and had poor eating habits. The fur lost its sleek appearance and became ruffled.

In advanced stages dissection revealed an almost paper-thin dorsal cranium with occasional hemorrhagic areas in the subdural region visible through the skull. The cerebral cortex was often extremely thin, especially in the occipital region, and holes or diverticula were common. The lateral ventricles were markedly enlarged, but the foramina of Monro and the 3rd ventricle appeared normal. The aqueduct and 4th ventricle were not enlarged but were frequently patent. By aspiration, the ventricular system yielded 0.1 to 0.15 ml of cerebrospinal fluid in early stages of hydrocephalus (Perry 1961) and 0.2 to 0.35 in later stages (Carton *et al.* 1956), compared with 0.03 to 0.05 in controls.

India ink or trypan blue injected into the lateral ventricles was usually concentrated in the lateral and 3rd ventricles; little or none was found in the aqueduct, 4th ventricle, or subarachnoid spaces. Ventriculograms made with air or with air and an opaque contrast material showed no air beyond the 3rd ventricle. Yet serial sections of early hydrocephalus showed no evidence of atresia or deformity of the aqueduct (Carton *et al.* 1956; Perry 1961).

Efforts were made to prolong the life of hydrocephalic mice by several procedures. Repeated ventricular taps plus the ventriculograms mentioned above were performed. In addition, ventriculoperitoneostomy with small polyethylene tubes worked successfully for short periods of time.

Brain Hernia

See below.

Genes Causing Encephalocele

Shaker-Short

Shaker-short (symbol *st*), a now extinct, recessive gene, produced shortened tail, severe disturbance in equilibration and behavior, and sterility (Dunn 1934). In addition, many abnormal newborn offspring had a marked lesion near the median point of the occipitoparietal (lambdoidal) suture of the skull. This lesion, when sectioned, was found (Bonnevie 1935) to consist of skin-covered cerebral herniations (encephalocele), which dried to small scabs, sometimes even by the time of birth, and were apparently not incompatible with life.

The prenatal development of the brain and ear anomalies was studied by Bonnevie (1936*a, b*). In 8th-day embryos, i.e., before closure of the neural tube, there was abnormal compression of neural structures, especially in the "neck" region, followed at the closure stage by coalescence between the young epidermis and the dorsal median line of the myelencephalon, which was associated with reduction in dimensions of the roof of the 4th ventricle and other defects of the developing brain. As a direct consequence of these occurrences the choroid plexus of the 4th ventricle remained rudimentary, and no "foramen of Magendie" formed.

(An extended aside is called for. To my knowledge, rodents have never been conclusively shown to have a true foramen of Magendie. In fact, although the long controversy over whether there is such an aperture in human beings was settled in favor of its existence (see, e.g., Barr 1948), the question whether this structure is present in many of the lower mammalia is still quite unresolved (Millen and Woollam 1962, p. 56). In an extensive study, Blake (1900) discovered that the foramen of Magendie appeared to be formed in human fetuses by means of absorption of a saccular evagination of the posterior region of the roof of the 4th ventricle; but, he concluded, "in the lower mammalia the caudal protrusion as a rule remains closed." In a recent study, Coben (1967) examined sections of brains of 2 rabbits, 3 cats, 3 dogs, and 2 goats—all adults—and could not find the foramen of Magendie in any of them.

Although in Bonnevie's numerous publications concerning mice a foramen of Magendie was mentioned as present, it appears that something different from a true aperture was meant, since in the discussion in part 4 of the series of papers devoted to hydrocephalus-1 the following statement appeared (Bonnevie and Brodal 1946, pp. 50–51): "In fact the 'foramina' Magendii and Luschkae have in the mouse at all stages appeared as continuous though very tiny membranes." As for the foramina of Luschka, Strong and Alban (1932) found that they were closed in rats until some hours before birth. But Coupin (1920) found no foramina, either of Magendie or Luschka, in mice, rats, cats, rabbits, and guinea pigs.)

Continuing with Bonnevie's findings, it was noted that in the region of adherence between the epidermis and medullary tube there was a serious hampering of development of the meninges. In 16th-day fetuses, the lumina of all brain ventricles were extremely narrow while the walls, especially their ependymal parts, were abnormally thickened and richly supplied with tiny blood capillaries, perhaps, as Bonnevie suggested, in compensation for disturbed drainage of cerebrospinal fluid. During the last days of development all these abnormalities combined to lead to "brain-catastrophy," producing complete rupture (on the 17th day) of the roof of the mesencephalon and cerebellum, which together with blood and cerebrospinal fluid erupted into one or two big hernias.

Brain Hernia

Brain hernia (symbol *bh*) is a simple autosomal recessive gene with complete penetrance, somewhat variable expressivity, and normal viability in newborn homozygotes (Bennett 1959). A few homozygotes proved fertile, and matings between them gave 17 affected, and one apparently normal, offspring, the latter probably being a rare normal overlap.

External defects of the brain present at birth consisted of variable-sized herniation (encephalocele) ranging from a barely noticeable blister to a bloody sac several millimeters in diameter in the midfrontoparietal region. The defect was always covered by skin. Defects of the bony cranium were seen in cleared specimens. In the most extreme cases there was wide median separation of the paired frontal and parietal bones; in less severe ones only the frontals were separated, sometimes only partially.

Numerous newborn homozygotes showed no frank encephalocele, but did have various degrees of hydrocephalus. This abnormality was not further described, but a photograph of an older affected mouse showed a rotundity of the head above the eyes. In extreme cases of encephalocele, hydrocephalus was absent, and vice versa. In other instances both defects were present simultaneously.

In 65 homozygotes scored at birth or soon after, 11 (16.9%) had encephalocele alone; 38 (58.5%), hydrocephalus alone; 14 (21.5%), both conditions; and 2 (3.1%), neither. In addition to these defects, anophthalmia and microphthalmia occurred in about 75 per cent of *bh*/*bh* newborn offspring.

Hydrocephalus-Like

This condition arose in a noninbred stock being developed in to the CFWS strain (Mauer 1963, 1964*b*). Genetic analysis indicated it to be due to a simple recessive gene. The malformations were apparently similar to some of those produced by the brain hernia gene, ranging in expression from minor brain contusion to encephalocele. Affected offspring died within a few days of birth. It is not clear why the condition was named "hydrocephalus-like."

Grizzled

Grizzled (symbol *gr*), a recessive gene with pigmentary effects, was associated with reduced viability (Bloom and Falconer 1966). Homozygotes died at all stages from the 10th day of gestation to some time after birth. Some living embryos had external malformations, most frequently shortening of the snout and swellings in the optic and occipital regions. These defects were not dissected.

Genes Causing Only or Primarily Exencephaly

Blebs

In 1923 Little and Bagg reported an experiment in which some mice were X rayed for the purpose of inducing mutations. Among the third and fourth generation descendants of 2 of 13 irradiated animals some mice were found with hereditary malformations that were shown to be due to the same mutant gene. Since it seems unlikely that the same mutation would have been induced twice in the relatively small number irradiated, it is possible that the gene changes were not caused by the X-ray treatment (Grüneberg 1952*b*, p. 147).

The gene was recessive and caused a large variety of congenital defects including those of eyes, feet, and urogenital and central nervous systems. Jaw anomalies also occurred, but these were probably independent of the other defects. The jaw abnormalities are discussed below (see p. 232).

Based on Bonnevie's (1934) embryological studies, which traced the abnormalities to an apparent oversecretion of cerebrospinal fluid from the foramen anterius or area membranacea superior of the roof of the 4th ventricle during early embryogenesis, the gene was given the symbol *my* for myelencephalic blebs. Although the symbol has stuck, reinvestigation of the problem (Carter 1959) threw doubt on Bonnevie's theory that all the abnormalities were due to blebs filled with fluid derived from central nervous system leakage. In fact, it may be that the blebs were merely another of the numerous effects of the gene. (See p. 230, dealing with the tail kinks gene, for further discussion of the question of leakage of cerebrospinal fluid.)

Few discussions of the central nervous system defects are found in the earlier reports, despite an enormous number of studies of the *my* gene. (By 1951, when Grüneberg's 1952*b*, pp. 147–62 and 560–62, review of the literature ended, 37 publications had appeared.) Plagens (1933), in fact, who also disagreed with Bonnevie's conclusions, did not mention abnormalities of the central nervous system at all, although he described the appearance and development of various other defects quite well. The explanation may be that genetic differences among various stocks carrying the mutation arose quite early in the history of the line.

Little and Bagg (1923) noted "acraniate" or "acephalic" specimens and obtained evidence that they were born exencephalic, not anencephalic. The hereditary condition pseudencephaly (see below), studied by Bonnevie (1936*c*), arose in the *my* stock of mice; but she considered it to be genetically independent of the *my* gene. Carter (1959) did not believe her evidence satisfactorily proved this contention.

The genetics and embryology of the Little and Bagg X-rayed mouse stock were comprehensively reinvestigated by Carter (1956, 1959). He concluded that the various malformations commonly or rarely found in *my/my* homozygotes were all parts of one and the same syndrome, which was produced by the main gene *my*, and that different parts of the syndrome were probably each influenced by different sets of modifying genes.

Three families of mice, A, B, and C, were derived from a group obtained from G. D. Snell (Carter 1956). These families were inbred and selected for increased frequency of different facets of the syndrome. In families A and C, which were selected for abnormalities other than those of the central nervous system, the rate of exencephaly changed little during several generations of inbreeding and averaged during this period 2.0 and 0.3 per cent, respectively. In family B, which was selected for defects of the central nervous system, exencephaly occurred in 8.7 per cent of generation 3 and rose rapidly to 22.0

per cent in generation 4 and 36.6 per cent in generation 5. Further increases did not occur during another 2 generations. It would thus appear that relatively few modifying genes were involved in the expression of this abnormality.

In the embryological study (Carter 1959), 116 9th- to 19th-day embryos and fetuses, 40 of which were exencephalic, were examined from crosses of mice of family B. Exencephalic offspring were recognizable from the 10th day, at which time there was failure of the neural ridges to close in the area of the mesencephalon. With further growth the neural ridges became flattened and the whole dorsal surface of the head consisted of exposed neural tissue. Simultaneously, the closed parts of the anterior neural tube, i.e., forebrain and hindbrain, failed to become distended—as normally happens when the tube fills with cerebrospinal fluid—giving the neural tube a crumpled appearance; the latter feature was more obvious in 12th-day than in younger embryos. The full development of exencephaly in later stages was considered to be a mechanical consequence of the open mesencephalon and crumpled myelencephalon. No evidence was found to support Bonnevie's (1936c) belief that some exencephaly was due to secondary reopening of the closed neural tube. On the contrary, the observations suggested that the condition arose only through failure of primary closure of the neural tube.

Exencephalic offspring were found at all prenatal stages studied, and their incidence did not decrease later in pregnancy, which indicated that their prenatal viability was not impaired. From the 17th day their amniotic fluid contained blood. At dissection the encephalic defect found was always exencephaly, never anencephaly.

Pseudencephaly

Embryos with pseudencephaly (i.e., exencephaly) were found (Bonnevie 1936c) in a stock that also carried the gene for myelencephalic blebs. Bonnevie believed that pseudencephaly was genetically independent of the bleb condition, but, according to Carter (1956, 1959), this belief was unsatisfactorily documented. The malformation may have been due to a recessive gene, but the customary 3 : 1 ratio of unaffected to affected offspring obtained from crossing heterozygotes to each other was only poorly approached, possibly because a large proportion of homozygotes died early in pregnancy and were resorbed, or perhaps because the condition was not a simply-inherited one.

In malformed animals the brain was fully exposed to the surface, protruding through an extensive fault in the roof of the cranium. It thus formed a large, thick, naked, icebag-like cap on top of the head, which extended in all directions and partly covered the snout, eyes, and back of the neck.

Although all parts of the brain underwent almost normal histological differentiation, their topographical relations were greatly upset. In other words the abnormality was not one of a normal brain that was merely exposed to the surface. Essentially the brain was partly turned inside out so that deeper structures were brought to the surface, while less deep ones were everted laterally. Thus the thalamus formed the top of the icebag and the pallium was situated ventrally and laterally on each side of it, with the choroid plexuses of the lateral ventricles being carried on each side to a position near the eyes. This description is very reminiscent of those of exencephalies that have frequently resulted from teratogenic procedures, e.g., excess vitamin A (see p. 49).

In a detailed study of the mechanism responsible for the brain ectopia, and of its development, Bonnevie (1936c) found that the condition was purely a mechanical consequence of increased tension owing to abnormal curvatures of the neural tube in the cervical region—curvatures that were already present in embryos 6 mm long. In young embryos it was found, contrary to the usual belief concerning the genesis of exencephaly, that there was no primary inability of the neural tube to close. Instead, it was held that the posterior part of the roof of the mesencephalon was weak because of the curvatures that were present, and thereby offered an area where dorsal closure, whether complete or incomplete, gave way to tension. Thus the weakness of the mesencephalic roof was a consequence of irregularity of the neural tube, while abnormalities in its closure were a further result of these curvatures. Studying the condition at earlier stages of gestation indicated that the curvatures were the outcome of enlargement of the neural tube as a whole in relation to its mesodermal surroundings; flexures thus represented accommodation of the tube to the available space. This disproportion seemed to be due to retarded separation of the primary embryonic germ layers, which in severe cases led to death soon afterwards, while less marked deviations, permitting further development, but causing growth disturbances, were assumed to be responsible for the brain abnormality.

Summing up, Bonnevie (1936c) believed that pseudencephaly was caused by a mechanical situation originating outside the brain and that the brain's intrinsic state was not at all involved; that the ability of the anterior end of the neural tube to close was not impaired; and that in some cases, in fact, the neural folds had already met dorsally but were reopened secondarily. This is the crucial point and one on which insufficient evidence was presented. It must therefore remain questionable, in this condition, whether the ability of the neural tube to close was actually unimpaired.

Since the gene studied by Bonnevie is apparently extinct, the problem so far as this particular hereditary defect is concerned must rest where is it now; it is of course quite possible that its mechanism was unique. It is also possible, however, that some, or even most, of its pathogenetic routes can be mimicked by teratologic methods. What is now known of the embryology of exencephaly suggests, contrary to Bonnevie's theories, that this defect can be traced back to a neural tube that fails to close.

Carter's (1959) study of the development of exencephaly induced by the *my* gene, which may in fact be identical to the gene for pseudencephaly, also suggested that Bonnevie's interpretations are quite erroneous.

Crooked-Tail

Crooked-tail (symbol *Cd*), an autosomal semidominant gene with partial lethality in homozygotes, arose by spontaneous mutation in the inbred A strain (Morgan 1953). The gene produced crooked-tail and other axial skeletal abnormalities, in heterozygotes and homozygotes, perhaps of somewhat greater severity in the latter than in the former.

Homozygotes were also affected in numerous other ways. Examination of 12th- to 19th-day fetuses from crosses of heterozygotes revealed the following. Of the 25 per cent of *Cd/Cd* homozygotes expected, approximately half (11.9 %) died before term; and 4.0 per cent were alive at examination but had exencephaly (exencephalics on the 18th and 19th days had bloody amniotic fluid). The remainder were apparently normal, except for frequent tail defects. The latter class was born and remained alive but exhibited various abnormalities, some of which developed postnatally, including absent and small lower incisors, eye defects, nervous head movements, and (2 %) hydrocephalus. One curiosity is that none of the offspring dying between implantation and parturition had exencephaly.

Three anencephalics were found in newborn litters; but Morgan (1953) recorded the interesting observation that a live exencephalic whose birth he watched was dead and anencephalic the next morning. Apparently the mother relished the tidbit.

Disorganization

Disorganization (symbol *Ds*), a semidominant autosomal gene that arose spontaneously in an inbred strain (Hummel 1958), was incompletely penetrant and variably expressive in heterozygotes and usually lethal in homozygotes. The time of death of *Ds/Ds* embryos was not precisely determined, and little was discovered about the cause of their death and the type of abnormalities they had. Penetrance in heterozygotes (but not expressivity) was greatly influenced by the genetic background, and some evidence was found as well for maternal (i.e., physiological) influence.

The gene caused a great variety of malformations of the skeleton and viscera, which occurred in a wide range of severity. The abnormalities affected the face, mouth, eyes, ears, neck, ventral body wall, digestive tract, central nervous and urogenital systems, limbs, axial skeleton, and integument. Malformations of the central nervous system included encephalocele, exencephaly, spina bifida aperta, craniorachischisis, and hydrocephalus. Different degrees of cerebral herniation occurred in 53 per cent of a sample of 500 offspring, and thoracolumbar spina bifida in 4 per cent; the other central nervous system defects were less frequent.

Cerebral herniation varied in extent from that involving small holes to complete absence of all cranial bones. In exencephaly the protruding brain was sometimes covered by membranes but more commonly was naked and showed erosion, the effect of extensive bleeding into the amniotic cavity. Small fissures with encephalocele occurred most frequently in the parietal and inter-parietal bones. Smaller hernias were also found at sutures. Defects such as unilateral atresia of cerebral hemispheres, overgrowth of cerebral regions, and hydrocephalus were also noted but not studied in detail.

Rib Fusions

Rib fusions, a semidominant autosomal gene (symbol *Rf*), caused relatively mild axial skeletal defects in heterozygotes and marked abnormalities and prenatal death in homozygotes (Mackensen and Stevens 1960). In hetero-zygotes the ribs were the most consistently affected part of the skeleton, 85 per cent of such offspring having unilateral or bilateral rib fusions. Five extremely abnormal newborn offspring, with very extensive and bizarre fusions of ribs and vertebrae, were considered to be homozygotes. Two of these animals were exencephalic, and one had spina bifida. A third exencephalic offspring was otherwise only slightly abnormal and may have been a heterozygote.

Homozygous embryos were first recognizable (Theiler and Stevens 1960) early on the 9th day of pregnancy, through their invariably malformed somites. Another uniform manifestation was irregularly-shaped neural plate and tube, with a sharp constriction at the boundary of the open and closed portions of the neural folds, which probably represented an early stage of exencephaly. In 10th-day normal embryos the head folds are completely closed, and there-fore the exencephalic ones were easily spotted. Approximately two-thirds of early homozygous embryos had exencephaly. In 2 specimens the entire neural plate was open. Most neural tissue of homozygotes was histologically normal, but there were some areas of degeneration. The notochord was normal.

Extra Toes and Brachyphalangy

In heterozygotes the autosomal dominant gene Extra toes (symbol *Xt*) produced slight preaxial polydactyly, and in homozygotes acted as a lethal and resulted in extreme polydactyly of all limbs, often accompanied by exen-cephaly (Lyon, Phillips, and Searle 1964). Another semidominant gene causing digital changes and frequently exencephaly as well was called brachy-phalangy and symbolized *Bph* (Searle 1965), until it was discovered (Johnson 1967) to be allelic with Extra toes; its symbol is now thus Xt^{bph}.

Bent-Tail

Bent-tail (symbol *Bn*) is a dominant sex-linked gene discovered by Garber (1952). The anatomy of the tail defects it produces was thoroughly examined by Grüneberg (1955*a*). Both authors noted a deficiency of affected newborn males and reasoned that it was caused by their prenatal death and elimination. The basis of this lethality was recently uncovered. Butler and Lyon (1967) dissected pregnant females on the 14th day of gestation and later and found some offspring with exencephaly or spina bifida. At the earlier stages, in addition to young with similar defects, others had completely open neural tube.

Genes Causing Only or Primarily Spina Bifida

Pigtail

The condition pigtail, now extinct, was a recessively inherited characteristic, variable in expressivity and penetrance (Crew and Auerbach 1941). The most frequent abnormality consisted of various degrees of curling of the tail, which occurred in about 24 per cent of offspring of parents manifesting tail defects. In addition, spina bifida, which was not described, occurred in 3.4 per cent (20/596) of newborn offspring.

Several lines of evidence indicated that the malformations were influenced by nongenetic factors. First, the incidence of pigtail decreased with litter size; and second, although the penetrance of the tail defect was only 22.3 per cent in all genetically pigtail litters, it was 56.6 per cent in litters containing young with spina bifida. No radiological evidence of spina bifida occulta was found in older animals with pigtail or in phenotypically normal, genotypically pigtail, individuals. Spina bifida does not seem to have been produced by an apparent recurrence of the mutation causing pigtail (Chase 1943). This gene is also now extinct.

Curly-Tail

Curly-tail (symbol *ct*), an autosomal recessive gene whose manifestation was strongly influenced by the genetic background (Grüneberg 1954), may also have been a recurrence of the pigtail gene(s) of Crew and Auerbach (1941) and Chase (1943). It, however, caused more severe congenital defects. The expression of the tail anomaly was variable, consisting of curling or spiraling, usually combined with shortening. In addition to this type of defect, lumbo-sacrocaudal spina bifida aperta (myeloschisis) was very common.

The gene was incompletely penetrant: 36.8 per cent of newborn offspring of crosses between abnormal mice were malformed, while in offspring examined before birth the frequency was 50.6 per cent. In newborn mice spina bifida (with or without tail defects) occurred in 18.6 per cent of all young and in 50.5 per cent of otherwise defective ones, while in prenatal mice spina bifida occurred in 40.7 per cent of the total and in 80.5 per cent of abnormals. Spina bifida occulta was not found in normal overlaps but was common in abnormals. A high correlation was found between the occurrence of spina bifida and tail defects. Of 417 abnormal mice, 4 had spina bifida alone, 262 had both types of malformations, and 151 had tail defects alone.

In addition to these abnormalities, 8 prenatal mice had exencephaly (out of a total of 194 abnormals, of which 128 had spina bifida). Six of the exencephalics also had spina bifida; in the remaining 2 only the brain defect occurred. The degree of exencephaly varied. In extreme forms the entire brain from the telencephalon to the myelencephalon was open dorsally and turned inside out; in mild types only the roof of the hindbrain was open.

The spina bifida was variable in length, ranging over numerous intermediate degrees from an extensive lesion to confinement to the base of the tail. Offspring with larger defects were stillborn or died soon after birth; those with a smaller defect often survived and even bred. In latter cases the malformation usually healed completely during the first few days after birth (it was improbable that prenatal healing occurred), with the skin closing over the small sacrally-located defect, thus preventing its external recognition. In 4 such animals examined as adults, open neural arches extended from S2 or S3 to Ca5, the last vertebra with a neural arch in mice.

Study of the development of these abnormalities revealed the following (Grüneberg 1954). In late fetuses with spina bifida the tail abnormality was always situated closely behind the spinal defect and flexed back toward the neural plate. The close spatial relation between the 2 anomalies pointed to their causal dependence. It was clear that the growth of the spinal cord next to the spina bifida was reduced while that of ventral structures of the tail continued normally. As a result of this growth disparity the tail curled up and subsequently turned into a spiral. The picture was not much different in younger specimens, except that the spina bifida bulged more above the level of the surrounding skin than in older fetuses or neonates.

In 12th-day and older conceptuses the spina bifida did not extend further caudally than the root of the tail. But in younger ones it extended throughout the whole length of the tail and thus included a region no longer affected later on. Apparently, therefore, the most distal parts of the neural plate could still undergo closure even when more proximal parts were unable to do so. In any case, the caudal part of the neural tube normally degenerates in later fetal life. In some young embryos an open neural plate (posterior neuropore) was found only in the distal region of the tail, in which case it was associated with a twist in this part of the tail. Had such embryos continued their development, the open plate would have closed, but the tail twist would have remained as evidence of its transitory presence. There was little doubt that these events were the cause of tail twist in otherwise normal offspring.

The tail defects, therefore, were caused mechanically by a spina bifida that persisted or by delayed closure of the posterior neuropore. Hence the defect of the central nervous system was primary and that of the skeleton secondary, just the reverse of the situation in congenital hydrocephalus in the mouse (see p. 196).

Splotch

Splotch (symbol *Sp*), an autosomal dominant gene discovered in C57BL mice

(Russell 1947), caused spotting in heterozygotes and prenatal death in homozygotes. *Sp/Sp* animals died on about the 14th day of gestation and were characterized by kinky tail and spina bifida aperta. The fact that such malformed fetuses were Splotch homozygotes was demonstrated (Russell and Gower 1950) by a delicate experiment in which ovaries of defective fetuses were transplanted to normal (+/+) hosts, which were then mated to +/+ males and had only *Sp/+* offspring.

The embryology of the malformations was studied by Auerbach (1954). Homozygous embryos could first be recognized on the 10th day of pregnancy, since it is at this time that closure of the neural folds normally occurs, whereas in Splotch homozygotes the neural folds remained open in the region of the hind legs. This phenomenon (spina bifida aperta, myeloschisis, or rachischisis) was accompanied by lateral overgrowth of the unclosed neural plate. Excess neural tissue was not found in embryos at stages before neural fold closure normally occurs, and hence it appeared concurrently with the nonclosure. The extent of the area of nonclosure was highly variable even at the earliest recognizable time and continued to be so in older embryos. Most frequently the defect was confined to a discrete part of the lumbosacral region, but in some cases it extended from this area to the tip of the tail.

The degree of neural overgrowth flanking the bifidous area was also variable; but while the bifida increased in size only proportionate to the growth of the embryo, the neural overgrowth became more pronounced with time until by the 12th day it was sometimes manifested externally by large flaps of tissue projecting laterally from the embryo; more usually, however, it merely formed a bulging mass. In histological sections the ventral area of the neural "tube" appeared normal, and the excess tissue seemed to be derived by proliferation from its dorsal regions.

In the lumbosacral region, apparently in association with the spina bifida, spinal ganglia were absent except for occasional vestiges. Other abnormalities of the neural tube consisted of erratic curvatures and narrowing, obliteration, and dilatation of the spinal canal. Abnormalities of dorsal root and sympathetic ganglia were also found.

Abnormalities of the brain occurred frequently in prenatal specimens. Open neural folds of the head region (exencephaly) were found in 56 per cent of Splotch homozygotes old enough for this condition to be recognizable (10 days and older). Exencephaly was limited to the hindbrain region and was invariably associated with overgrowth of neural tissue, which also became increasingly more pronounced with advancing embryonic development. Histological sections revealed other abnormalities of the brain in all Splotch homozygotes 10 days or older, consisting of partial collapse or obliteration of the entire ventricular system because of abnormal overgrowth of neural tissue.

In the light of this pervasive overgrowth of neural tissue, it is of interest that a higher mitotic rate was found in neural epithelium of Splotch homozygotes than in that of normal embryos but that overgrowth did not appear to be the cause of the spina bifida, since the entire neuraxis was retarded during early formative stages (Hsu and Van Dyke 1948).

An allele of Splotch (symbol Sp^d) was recently discovered (Dickie 1964). It is a semidominant lethal and consistently produced spina bifida aperta, but never exencephaly, in all homozygotes. Furthermore, all abnormal offspring of pregnant females killed at different times during pregnancy were alive when examined; thus the superscript d in the gene's symbol indicates delayed death of Sp^d homozygotes in comparison with Sp homozygotes. Crosses between $Sp^d/+ \times Sp/+$ produced approximately 25 per cent abnormal (Sp^d/Sp) offspring similar in appearance to Sp^d homozygotes. The Splotch locus appears to be prone to mutate, since several recurrences of the mutation have been found (Dickie and Belden 1964–65).

Tail-Short

Tail-short (symbol Ts) was discovered by Morgan (1950) in the BALB/c inbred strain. It acted as an autosomal dominant, causing short, flexed tail in heterozygotes, and complete prenatal lethality in homozygotes. It also apparently caused some embryonic death in heterozygotes of certain genotypes and death of all heterozygotes on another genetic background. Crosses of $Ts/+$ BALB/c mice to $+/+$ C3H mice produced tailless F_1 heterozygotes some of which had exencephaly and some spina bifida. No incidence figure or description was given.

It may thus be that a more severe, or similar but more frequent, expression of the gene in heterozygous condition on some genetic backgrounds or in homozygous condition was responsible for prenatal death. This question remains problematical, since the development of Ts/Ts embryos has not yet been worked out. A study of the embryology of $Ts/+$ BALB/c mice (Deol 1961) revealed some irregularities in morphology of the spinal cord and changes in shape of the brain. The latter were probably secondary to changes in shape of the skull.

Posterior Duplication

This condition may have been due to a recessive gene with low penetrance, but other possible modes of inheritance were not excluded. Danforth (1925) was able, by selection, to increase the frequency of abnormal offspring to about 12 per cent in one stock and to about 20 per cent in another.

The condition consisted (Danforth 1930) of various degrees of duplication of posterior parts of the body, ranging from pronounced to scarcely deviating from normal. The most usual type was of intermediate severity and manifested one or more supernumerary hindlimbs, polydactyly, duplicated phallus, etc. The central nervous system of such animals was normal. Abnormalities of the central nervous system occurred in the most deviant specimens, in which numerous structures, skeletal and visceral, were doubled. These defects consisted of doubling of the spinal cord up to the lumbar or thoracic region, with various intergradations in severity. A not infrequent condition was failure of posterior neural tube closure (i.e., lumbosacral spina bifida aperta), in which the neural tissue hypertrophied and spread out in a cauliflower-like mass. Some duplicated mice died before birth, and the viability of the others was low, but a few reached maturity and were occasionally fertile.

Danforth and Center (1967), in a recent abstract, speculated that the condition is in effect a recessive but with a multifactorial basis, and that possibly 3 genes are involved. As to its embryological basis, they contend that the effects are due to an accessory growth center.

Fused

Fused (symbol *Fu*) is a semidominant autosomal gene whose penetrance greatly depended on the genetic background. In Reed's (1937) study its most frequent expressions were different types of asymmetrical fusions of vertebrae, absence of part or all of the tail, and rib fusions. In later studies (Dunn and Glucksohn-Waelsch 1954), the gene was also found to cause waltzing behavior and deafness and, in occasional newborn animals, imperforate anus, urogenital abnormalities, sirenoid malformations, exencephaly, and spina bifida. In newborn animals, Theiler and Glucksohn-Waelsch (1956) found different types and degrees of spina bifida aperta and occulta in the lumbar, sacral, and caudal regions of homozygotes and heterozygotes.

Reed (1937) noted that the first observable embryological abnormalities were "poor alignment of the notochord and distinct curves and angles of the neural crests." Gross examination of homozygous embryos (Theiler and Glucksohn-Waelsch 1956) revealed abnormalities of the head, neural folds, and tail. That of the head region consisted of failure of normal brain-fold closure leading to exencephaly (in 7/88 cases) and one microcephaly. Failure of normal neural-fold closure also occurred in the trunk region, leading (in 21/88 cases) to spina bifida. With the exception of one craniorachischisis, all instances of failure of neural-fold closure were restricted to the head or lumbosacral region.

Sectioned material yielded other abnormalities. No defects occurred in 8th-day embryos, but in 9th-day ones neural tube irregularities were seen, and in later development abnormalities of the central nervous system were the most constant features. These defects were expressed, in addition to early waviness, as ventral budding and posterior duplications of the neural tube and were in general believed to be due to overgrowth of neural tissue. The effect on the notochord was less striking than that on the neural tube.

Kinky

Kinky (symbol Fu^{ki}), first described by Caspari and David (1940), is a semi-dominant allele of Fused (Dunn and Caspari 1945; Dunn and Gluecksohn-Waelsch 1954) whose effects in heterozygous condition were very much like those in Fused heterozygotes; but unlike Fused, Kinky homozygotes regularly died on the 8th to 10th days of gestation.

The development of homozygotes was studied by Gluecksohn-Schoen-heimer (1949). They were easily recognized on the 7th day of pregnancy by the presence of multiple embryonic axes, which probably resulted from hyperplasia of embryonic tissues. In later stages of development these peculiarities led to various grades of embryonic twinning and duplication of organs. Living 9th-day embryos had severe abnormalities of the neural head folds; those surviving to the 10th day occasionally had microcephaly, a strange double vesicle in the region of the myelencephalon, and some doubling of the neural tube in the posterior trunk region.

A recent attempt (Deol 1966*b*) to correlate anomalies of behavior and malformation of the inner ear in $Fu^{ki}/+$ heterozygotes of various ages indicated that they are related collaterally rather than lineally, and it was suggested that both originate in some early abnormality of the central nervous system.

Brachyury and Anury

The short-tail or Brachyury gene (symbol T), discovered by Dobrovolskaïa-Zavadskaïa (1927), is semidominant and lethal in homozygous condition. In heterozygotes it produced variable shortening of the tail, which gave the condition its name. The prenatal lethality of T/T homozygotes was inferred (Dobrovolskaïa-Zavadskaïa and Kobozieff 1927) from 3 facts. (1) Heterozygotes ($T/+$) mated to each other produced litters of less than normal size; (2) in such matings short-tailed and normal-tailed offspring were produced in a ratio of 2 : 1 instead of the expected ratio of 3 : 1; and (3) short-tailed animals were always heterozygotes. Furthermore, prenatal examination of $T/+$ females mated to $T/+$ males revealed about 25 per cent dead conceptuses (Chesley 1935; Ephrussi 1935).

The anatomy of $T/+$ heterozygotes was studied by Dobrovolskaïa-Zavadskaïa, Kobozieff, and Veretennikoff (1934) and Kobozieff (1935), and that of a recent recurrence of the gene ($T^{hg}/+$) by Kuminek (1959). Characteristic skeletal abnormalities were found, including different types and degrees of nonclosure of vertebral arches, with or without involvement of the spinal cord.

The prenatal development of heterozygotes and homozygotes for this gene was studied in great detail by Chesley (1935). Heterozygotes were grossly distinguishable from normals beginning the 11th day of gestation. At this time the distal part of the tail lacked a neural tube and notochord, while later this part of the tail regressed and disappeared. In sectioned material notochordal abnormalities first appeared at about $8\frac{3}{4}$ days of gestation. Irregularities of the neural tube were always accompanied by abnormalities of the notochord in the tail, but in the lumbosacral region notochordal abnormalities were common without those of the neural tube. It appeared, therefore, that the notochord was the structure on which the Brachyury gene primarily had its effects.

Chesley (1932) recognized that T/T homozygotes occurred as a characteristic type in matings of $T/+ \times T/+$, forming as they did a homogeneous group that died shortly before the 11th day of gestation. In 9th-day T/T embryos the posterior end of the neural tube had marked lateral deviations from the midline, contrasted with the straight neural tube in controls. These irregularities did not usually occur before neural-tube closure and later became more pronounced, sometimes extending anteriorly to the region of the liver.

Somewhat later the neural tube sent out branches with secondary lumina, which often became larger than the primary neural tube. On the 10th day of gestation and later the nervous tissue in the posterior region little resembled the normal neural tube. In some cases the neural tube ruptured and was continuous with the amniotic cavity. At the extreme posterior end the nervous tissue was represented by an amorphous mass. No regular segmental dorsal ganglia were formed, as in normal 10th-day embryos, but ganglionic tissue was found. In one embryo, one of the 2 dorsal aortae was completely obliterated by a neural tube diverticulum.

By the 10th day, when normal mouse embryos have 25 to 30 somites, anterior limb buds well started, and posterior limb buds just beginning, the posterior part of the body of T/T embryos was greatly reduced and no posterior limb buds were present. Gluecksohn-Schoenheimer (1944) discovered that as a consequence of shortening of the body, the allantois of T/T mice, in contrast to that of normal embryos, did not increase in length and appeared shrunken, with the result that umbilical vessels did not develop and the embryonic and maternal circulations remained separated. Thus, she wrote, the "embryo dies at the time when maternal circulation becomes all-important for the nutrition of the embryo."

From the stock of short-tailed mice 3 lines were obtained that differed from the original animals (Dobrovolskaïa-Zavadskaïa and Kobozieff 1932). The derived mice were tailless and bred true for taillessness, i.e., no brachyuric or normal-tailed young were produced. The genetics of this situation, which is of great interest from various aspects, was analyzed in great detail by Dunn and his associates, beginning with the work of Chesley and Dunn (1936). It was found that tailless mice bred true because of a system of "balanced lethals." By breeding tests it was learned that the tailless mice of 2 of the lines (A and 29) were heterozygotes of the types T/t^0 and T/t^1, respectively, where t^0 and t^1 may be alleles of T. When animals of these lines were bred *inter se*, young of 3 genotypes were produced from each type of cross:

	Line A	Line 29
P	$T/t^0 \times T/t^0$	$T/t^1 \times T/t^1$
F_1	$T/T, T/t^0, t^0/t^0$	$T/T, T/t^1, t^1/t^1$

However, the homozygotes (T/T, t^0/t^0, t^1/t^1) died and only the heterozygotes (T/t^0 and T/t^1), which were tailless, lived.

The anatomy and embryology of these viable mice were studied by Gluecksohn-Schoenheimer (1938a) and found to be apparently identical in both stocks. T/t^0 or T/t^1 adults were tailless or, more usually, had a short caudal filament consisting of skin and connective tissue only. Spinal malformations were present in the form of fusions of lumbar vertebrae with each other or with the sacrum, as well as of fusions of other combinations of elements. There was much variability in the manner of termination of the spine, which occurred between S1 and Ca4. Newborn tailless mice often had sacral lesions consisting of subepidermal blebs or hematomata, which represented cysts of spinal cord tissue. The spine terminated anterior to the lesion, and the last part of the cord, not finding any protective vertebrae, formed a cyst. In adults, however, no trace of the lesion was found externally. In a few extreme cases, paralysis of hindlimbs, probably due to absence of nerves or great shortening of the cord, was observed at birth. In one dissection no ventral roots were found in the last part of the cord.

Gross examinations of embryos indicated that the tail of future tailless mice developed normally up to the 11th day of gestation, after which constriction occurred at its base and regression set in, resulting by the 14th day in almost total loss of the tail. The constricted tail contained somites, neural tube, and hindgut, but no notochord after the 10th or 11th day of gestation. After the 12th day there was no neural tube or hindgut in the tail filament; next, somites disappeared, and finally only mesenchyme was left.

The notochord was reduced in the posterior trunk region and sent off ventral branches. The neural tube was also reduced at times and had diverticula in this region. Malformations of the neural tube, however, were never found without simultaneous notochordal abnormalities, whereas in younger stages abnormalities of the notochord were present without associated abnormalities of the neural tube. The evidence therefore again pointed to the malformations of the neural tube being secondary to those of the notochord. On the 12th day of gestation, termination of the neural tube occurred in the most distal part of the trunk, but no filamentum terminale was present and the neural tube ended rather abruptly and was often not straight but curled. In the neighborhood of the termination of the neural tube small fragments of neural tissue were found in the surrounding mesenchyme.

In all essentials, therefore, the picture was very much like that described by Chesley (1935) for $T/+$ embryos, except that the constriction of the $T/+$ tail occurred almost anywhere, whereas in T/t^0 and T/t^1 mice it always occurred at or near the base of the tail. Problems concerning the effects of these genes on notochordal development were reinvestigated by Grüneberg (1958*a*).

t^0/t^0 homozygotes died very early in embryogenesis (Gluecksohn-Schoenheimer 1940), their development ceasing $5\frac{1}{4}$ days after fertilization, and though they continued to live for some hours afterwards, there were no signs of further growth and organization or of mesoderm formation. t^1/t^1 embryos apparently died before implantation, since no group of dying embryos ascribable to this genotype was found in $+/t^1$ females bred to $+/t^1$ males (Gluecksohn-Schoenheimer 1938*b*). Contradictory results on this point were recently reported (Pai and Gluecksohn-Waelsch 1961).

Crosses between lines A and 29 (Dunn and Gluecksohn-Schoenheimer 1943) produced the following offspring.

	Line A			Line 29	
P	T/t^0		×	T/t^1	
F_1	T/T	T/t^0		T/t^1	t^0/t^1
	died	tailless		tailless	normal tail

The new type (t^0/t^1) had a normal tail but was otherwise often far from normal. Such mice had an increased prenatal mortality, and many showed congenital malformations such as microphthalmia, microcephaly, and exencephaly. The same was true of t^0/t^1 mice from the cross $+/t^0 \times +/t^1$. A study of t^0/t^1 embryos (Pai and Gluecksohn-Waelsch 1961) revealed atypical development of head and neural structures as well as several with herniated hearts.

A mating between 2 T/t^1 individuals produced an exceptional animal, which, contrary to expectation, had a normal tail. It was analyzed and found to be carrying a new t factor, which was called t^3, and to have the genetic constitution t^1/t^3 (Dunn and Gluecksohn-Waelsch 1951). By similar breeding techniques a large number of new t factors have been discovered in laboratory stocks of mice and in wild mice. Many of these new factors are lethal or have other prenatal effects in homozygous condition, which have been analyzed embryologically.

The lethals of independent laboratory origin proved different by complementarity tests and by their known prenatal effects in homozygotes, in addition to T, t^0, and t^1, are t^4, t^9, t^{12}, t^{14}, and t^{20}. Homozygotes for t^4 died at 7 to 8 days of gestation at the egg-cylinder stage, with abnormal development of the archenteron region, from which the notochord-mesoderm arises. In t^9/t^9 embryos, which died at 9 days or later, there occurred duplications of the embryonic axis and neural folds (Gluecksohn-Waelsch 1954; Dunn 1956). t^{12}/t^{12} embryos never progressed beyond the morula stage and died at 3 to $4\frac{1}{2}$ days, with clear indications of ribonucleic-acid deficiency and failure of blastocyst formation. This lethal has the earliest detectable effects of any such mammalian gene (Smith 1956). Compound heterozygotes of the constitution t^1/t^{12} usually died 12 to 19 days after mating, but the cause of death was not indicated (Smith 1956). t^{14} and t^{20} were also mentioned as being lethals (Dunn 1957; Dunn, Bennett, and Beasley 1962). The development of t^{12}/t^{12} morulae was studied in vitro (Silagi 1963; Mintz 1964).

A large number of t alleles (t^{wx}), many of which are lethal, have been found in wild mice collected from various parts of the U.S.A. and Canada (Dunn and Morgan 1953; Dunn and Suckling 1956; Dunn 1957; Bennett and Dunn 1958; Bennett, Dunn, and Badenhausen 1959; Dunn and Bennett 1960; Dunn, Bennett, and Beasley 1962; Anderson 1964). The lethal alleles were separable into several groups, those in each group being indistinguishable embryologically or genetically.

Alleles in group II (t^{w1}, t^{w3}, t^{w12}, t^{w20}, and t^{w21}) had an extended lethal period, ranging from 8 or 9 days after fertilization to birth (Bennett, Baden-hausen, and Dunn 1959; Dunn, Bennett, and Beasley 1962). Abnormal off-spring recovered alive had a typically uniform external appearance, regardless of genotype. All were considerably reduced in size and had normal tails. Variable microcephaly was present, complicated by hydrocephalus, which caused bulging of the skin-covered cerebral hemispheres through an abnormal opening in the bony cranial vault. Cleft palate and various other skeletal and neural abnormalities also occurred and were described in detail (Bennett, Badenhausen, and Dunn 1959).

The t^{wx} alleles in group III (t^{w5}, t^{w6}, t^{w10}, t^{w11}, t^{w13}, t^{w14}, t^{w15}, t^{w16}, and t^{w17}) produced lethal homozygotes and lethal compound heterozygotes in-distinguishable from one another (Bennett and Dunn 1958; Dunn and Bennett 1960; Dunn, Bennett, and Beasley 1962). The embryology of 5 of these alleles was studied in detail (Bennett and Dunn 1958). Homozygotes were recognized as abnormal at $6\frac{1}{2}$ to 7 days after fertilization, the major abnor-mality consisting of lack of differentiation of endoderm and embryonic ecto-derm. Mesoderm and notochord formation were apparently not affected.

Two additional alleles, t^{w18} and t^{w32}, did not fall into any other group (Dunn, Bennett, and Beasley 1962). A detailed embryological study of t^{w18}/t^{w18} homozygotes showed (Bennett and Dunn 1960) that the lethal period was 8 to 11 days after fertilization. The first morphologically recognizable defect was overgrowth of the primitive streak, seen when this feature forms at 7 days, which became especially prominent with further growth on the next day. The usual result was mechanically produced, partial or complete, duplication of the neural tube. No other structures, including the notochord, became doubled. These defects were quite similar to those produced by 3 other mutations on the same chromosome, t^9, at the same locus, and Fu and Fu^{ki}, a short distance away. t^{w30} homozygotes and t^{w18}/t^{w30} heterozygotes showed exactly comparable growth disturbances to those produced by homo-zygosity for t^{w18}, and the embryological effects of t^{w32} were indistinguishable from those of t^{12} (Bennett and Dunn 1964).

The development of embryos homozygous for the semilethal t^{w8} was recently reported (Bruch 1966, 1967). Such mice died throughout gestation, but in those dying after the 12th day several malformations were recognizable, viz., various degrees of malclosure of the anterior neural tube ranging from encephalocele to exencephaly, different grades of otocephaly, and internal hydrocephalus. Homozygotes for the semilethal t^{w49} usually died before the 12th day, with defects similar to those occurring in t^{w8}/t^{w8} offspring (Bennett 1966). Of a group examined on the 15th day only 6 were still alive, and 4 of these were extreme otocephalics.

Selection for increased tail length in T/t^{w18} heterozygotes produced a hindrance of about a day in the lethal effects of homozygosity for either of these alleles (Bennett 1964*a*). But no gross change in specific abnormalities resulted.

A study of the prenatal development of t^0/t^{12} heterozygotes (Silagi 1962) showed that on the 7th day of gestation such embryos were always retarded and that their most consistent defect was overgrowth of the primitive streak, much as in t^{w18} homozygotes (Bennett and Dunn 1960). By the 9th day several degrees of abnormality were exhibited, ranging from degeneration and extreme retardation to smallness, with reduced or completely absent telencephalon in some cases. On the 11th day extremely small and abnormal embryos were beginning to die, though many remained alive for another day. A large number of them showed asymmetrical brain and eye development. Less abnormal ones continued to develop and near term were all found to have normal tails but to be smaller than normal. Some showed congenital malformations, such as eye defects, maxillary and mandibular abnormalities, and occasional microcephaly and otocephaly (Bennett and Dunn 1960). Some animals of the compound genotypes T/t^0, T/t^{12}, T/t^{w1}, T/t^{w5}, and T/t^{w18} had spina bifida (Bennett 1964*b*).

In addition to the original T gene (Dobrovolskaïa-Zavadskaïa 1927), 3 other dominants have been found at this locus. Hertwig's allele, T^{hg}, appeared to be a recurrence of T (Kuminek 1959, 1960). Homozygotes for the Harwell allele, T^h (Lyon 1959), were already abnormal and dead on the 8th day of pregnancy, at an earlier stage of gestation than that at which the T allele produced its lethal effects. The third allele, T^c (for curtailed), a fully penetrant dominant, was recently discovered (Searle 1966). Typical heterozygotes had an abnormal tail consisting of a short, boneless, caudal filament. Rarely, newborn curtailed mice had other defects as well, including small hematomata just dorsal to the caudal filament associated with low-grade spina bifida, and paralysis of the hindlimbs, possibly owing to spina bifida occulta.

Intercrosses of $T^c/+$ mice produced abnormal-tailed offspring in a ratio of about 2 : 1, indicating that homozygotes for the dominant died prenatally. This presumption was supported by observation of abnormalities in embryos from females of such crosses killed on the 9th to 11th days of pregnancy.

The abnormalities resembled those found in T/T embryos but were more severe, consisting of great posterior reduction of the body, failure of closure of the neural tube in the trunk region, and irregularities of the spinal cord on each side of the open neural folds. In crosses between a curtailed heterozygote and a t^{h7}/t^{h3} mouse, the presumed T^c/t^{h3} offspring were more severely affected than $T^c/+$ mice, since many died before 2 weeks of age, and quite a few had congenital dorsal hematomata as well as paralyzed hindlimbs. It thus seemed probable that there was a high incidence of spina bifida occulta.

Shaker-3

This gene (symbol *Sh-3*), a semidominant, arose in a stock of mixed origin (Gates 1965*b*). Heterozygotes behave in very much the same way as do homozygotes for the shaker-1 and shaker-2 genes. Homozygous Shaker-3 offspring, however, were malformed and died immediately after birth. Among their defects were spina bifida and exencephaly. A fuller description of the effects of the mutation has not yet been published.

Quinky

Quinky (symbol *Q*) is a semidominant gene with variable effects on skeleton, pigment, and behavior. Most homozygotes died soon after implantation, but 3 presumed homozygotes survived to about the 13th day of gestation. One lacked development posterior to the forelimb buds, and the other 2 showed irregular closure of the neural tube. These effects have not yet been more fully described (Schaible 1961).

Danforth's Short-Tail

The gene for Danforth's short-tail (symbol *Sd*), an autosomal semidominant, killed homozygotes soon after birth (Dunn and Glueksohn-Schoenheimer 1938). The expression of the gene was highly influenced by the genetic background (Grüneberg 1952*b*, pp. 379–86). Two organ systems were especially affected, the axial skeleton and the urogenital system. In addition, newborn homozygotes frequently had a subcutaneous hematoma in the lumbar region, which was found to be a symptom of spina bifida occulta (Dunn, Glueksohn-Schoenheimer, and Bryson 1940).

Dissection (Glueksohn-Schoenheimer 1943) revealed the spina bifida to be located in the lumbosacral region. The spinal cord was partly unprotected by the vertebral column, which was due to absence of all caudal and sacral vertebrae or to ventral clefts in the few lumbar vertebrae present. The cord itself was of normal length, and therefore acquired an abnormal shape and often ended in a cyst, which occurred anywhere in the sacral region, sometimes directly beneath the dorsal epithelium. In embryological studies (Glueksohn-Schoenheimer 1945) *Sd/Sd* homozygous embryos were easily recognized by the 11th day by the presence of a large, transparent, epidermal bleb in the sacral region. It could be seen through the bleb that this region was characterized by failure of the neural folds to close.

The striking influence of the genetic background on the expression of the *Sd* gene was illustrated by the complete absence of spina bifida in Grüneberg's (1958*b*) study of the effects of this¹ mutation.

Short-Ear

The autosomal recessive gene, short-ear (symbol *se*), in addition to its effects on the pinna, caused widespread skeletal abnormalities and deviations and some visceral anomalies (Grüneberg 1952*b*, pp. 279–85). There were several differences in the manifestation of spina bifida occulta between 2 inbred strains of mice carrying the *se* gene (McNutt 1957). In the SEC-*dse* strain the condition affected the cervical and thoracic spine and involved only one bifid vertebra per affected mouse, whereas in the SEA-*se* strain the defect was located in the thoracolumbar region and involved up to 5 bifid vertebrae per affected animal. The incidence of spina bifida in the SEC-*dse* mice was 5.5 per cent (11/200); it was apparently much greater in the SEA-*se* mice, but the absolute frequency was not stated. In the SEC-*dse* strain, short-ear mice (i.e., *se/se* homozygotes) were not spina bifidous more often than normal-eared mice (i.e., +/*se* heterozygotes); in the SEA-*se* strain the incidence of spina bifida was greater in short-ear than in normal-eared mice.

Although, so far as its effects on the ear are concerned, *se* is a recessive gene, in other regards it is an irregular dominant (Grüneberg 1952*b*, p. 280). Furthermore, many of its pleiotropic effects were greatly influenced by the genetic background. It is conceivable, therefore, that spina bifida occulta was another of the irregular dominant effects of the gene, present more commonly in homozygotes than heterozygotes, the penetrance and expressivity of which were modified by the hereditary milieu in the 2 strains discussed above.

Gene Combinations

The recessive gene urogenital (symbol *ur*) caused a lethal syndrome, of gut, tail, and urogenital abnormalities in homozygotes (Dunn and Gluecksohn-Schoenheimer 1947). When combined with genes at the *T* locus, the *ur/ur* genotype produced a urorectocaudal syndrome (Grüneberg 1952*b*, pp. 386–89), including imperforate anus and a genuine cloaca without external opening. In addition, among offspring with this combination of genes, there were several with spina bifida aperta (Dunn and Gluecksohn-Schoenheimer 1947).

T alleles combined with the Fused and Kinky genes also produced spina bifida (Dunn and Gluecksohn-Schoenheimer 1944; Dunn and Caspari 1945). A severe form of the malformation occurred quite often (34/84 = 40.5%) in offspring of the cross $Fu^{ki}T/++ \times t^0/t^1$ (Dunn and Caspari 1945), probably in those of the genotype $Fu^{ki}T/+t^0$ or $Fu^{ki}T/+t^1$. The defect was less frequent and apparently milder in $Fu^{ki}T/++$ animals.

In crosses of heterozygotes for the genes Crooked-tail and Tail-short $(Cd/+ \times Ts/+)$ the F_1 litter size was small, suggesting prenatal lethality (Morgan 1954). In late fetuses from such crosses a "high incidence" of exencephaly and/or omphalocele was found. Exencephaly occurred in Cd/Cd homozygotes, but not in $Cd/+$ heterozygotes; and the Ts gene produced low frequencies of this defect on certain genetic backgrounds only. Thus in double heterozygotes $(Cd/+, Ts/+)$ there was interaction of gene effects, which produced increased rates of abnormality.

A low frequency of sirenomelia occurred (Gluecksohn-Schoenheimer 1945; Dunn and Gluecksohn-Schoenheimer 1947) in offspring from crosses involving combinations of Fu or ur with alleles at the T locus. All such abnormal young had severe spinal defects ranging from spina bifida occulta to spina bifida aperta as well as abnormalities of the cord associated with the sirenoid condition.

Genes Causing Only or Primarily Craniorachischisis

Loop-Tail

Loop-tail arose in the A strain and was first described by Strong and Hollander (1949). The gene (symbol Lp) is semidominant and lethal in homozygotes, with variable expressivity and incomplete penetrance in heterozygotes. In the latter, the contortion of the tail, which gives the condition its name, varied from extreme pretzel twists to minor angular crooks and curves; but in some cases the tail was straight. X rays of randomly chosen adult heterozygotes with defective tails showed no spinal abnormalities anterior to the tail region. Associated anomalies were variable nervous rocking or wobbling of the head, without deafness, tending to mild choreic activity in a few cases, which also occurred at times in normal-tailed heterozygotes; and imperforate vagina in about one-third of females with tail or behavioral abnormalities.

In matings of heterozygotes $(Lp/+ \times Lp/+)$, the litter size was markedly reduced. Prenatal mortality being suspected, pregnant females were killed. From 24 such crosses there were obtained 67 normal-tailed offspring, 40 loop-tails, 11 resorbing and unclassifiable, and 44 young with craniorachischisis. The last were about 25 per cent of the total, and thus were probably the homozygote class (Lp/Lp). Fetuses with this malformation were generally alive in the last 2 days of pregnancy but never survived birth, apparently always being eaten by the mother.

These monsters showed surprisingly little variability in the form of the defect and were readily recognized macroscopically after about the 10th day of pregnancy. The neural tissue failed to form a neural tube and thus developed as a herniated cranial mass with 2 broad tracts down the back with a narrow groove between them. In the last 2 or 3 days of pregnancy the neural tracts usually degenerated in the lumbar region with considerable hemorrhage into the amniotic fluid (Strong and Hollander 1949).

Additional descriptions of the gross defects in such fetuses were given by Stein and Rudin (1953) and Smith and Stein (1962). Skin was absent over all portions of the central nervous system. The neural tissue, from the posterior border of the metencephalon to the extremely shortened tail, consisted of a flat plate with a deep median groove. Abnormal space relations existed in the forebrain and the portion of the midbrain that was closed. The lateral ventricles were collapsed, but the choroid plexuses were present and normally differentiated. Flaps of mesencephalic tissue frequently protruded forward, making a median dorsal extension that overlay the diencephalon and the cerebral hemispheres and sometimes overhung the face.

Associated anomalies occurred in homozygotes. Strong and Hollander (1949) found a small umbilical hernia in a fair proportion and 2 cases of eventration of heart, lungs, liver, and intestines. Smith and Stein (1962) reported that such defects had disappeared from all their lines but one, in which herniation of liver and intestines affected all Lp/Lp homozygotes. They also discovered that older abnormal fetuses had umbilical cords roughly half the normal length, but did not record the state of the umbilical vessels. Finally, animals with craniorachischisis were markedly smaller than their normal siblings, and the decrease was not proportional for all parts of the body, the trunk seeming relatively short for the size of the head and the nervous system looking too large for the body.

Strong and Hollander (1949) found one specimen with exencephaly alone, which they classified as a homozygote. Stein and Mackensen (1957) disagreed with this interpretation, since in 14 different matings of loop-tailed by straight-tailed mice they found 21 exencephalics and thus considered these defectives as heterozygotes. No data were given in this paper to support this belief further; but more recently Smith and Stein (1962) reported 9 exencephalics in litters from 6 crosses of loop-tailed by straight-tailed parents, in which there were no craniorachischitic offspring. Certain puzzling features, however, appeared in their Tables 1 and 2 (*ibid.*, pp. 74–75). For example, 3/9 exencephalics from these crosses were straight-tailed mice. Further only one exencephaly occurred in 10 crosses of $Lp/+ \times Lp/+$, and that in a straight-tailed animal. Last, crosses of heterozygotes of certain lines yielded fewer Lp/Lp fetuses than the expected 25 per cent; in line 71, e.g., only 10 per cent Lp/Lp's were found.

The prenatal development of Lp/Lp homozygotes was studied in mice of various strains by Stein and Rudin (1953), who were not able to identify homozygotes before closure of the neural tube, which occurs on about the 9th day of gestation. Histological differentiation of nervous tissue appeared normal, and gray and white matter were formed in approximately similar proportions. Aside from the gross morphological malformation, which resulted from failure of the neural tube to fuse, rather than from a secondary breakdown of the roof of the neural tube, the only deviant feature was an increased number of mitoses. Because of an apparent excess of neural tissue, especially in the open regions of the mid- and hindbrain, counts were made between the optic stalk and auditory vesicle and in the lower level of the cord. There was no evidence of proliferation in the latter location, but more mitotic figures may have existed in the brain region of the abnormal animals than in normal littermates. The results were interpreted as indicating a localized effect of the gene on this region of the developing nervous system. It was believed that there were no such differences in the cord area because the region of the first closure of the neural tube was within the localized region affected by the brain, and if this area failed to close, the entire neural plate remained open.

Total cell counts in 10th-day embryos (Stein, Lievre, and Smoller 1960) confirmed the presence of increased numbers of dividing cells, and though cell counts in the hindbrain region were not consistently higher, those in the cervical cord region were always increased. In addition, 10th- to 13th-day abnormals exhibited a unique histological picture of sparse, loosely arranged cells in some parts of the hindbrain or spinal cord, lateral portions of the open plate usually being affected rather than median ones, and anterior levels rather than posterior. This observation was confirmed (Smith and Stein 1962), and it was noted that despite areas of decreased cell density, tract formation in *Lp/Lp* embryos was essentially normal.

The only other gross abnormalities were sequelae of the open central nervous system, i.e., skeletal defects such as anomalies of vertebral arches (Stein and Rudin 1953) and of the thoracic skeleton (Stein and Mackensen 1957). Cranial and spinal ganglia and nerves were normal, as were the pituitary, thyroid, adrenals, gonads, and kidneys. The various elements of the auditory anlage—utriculus, sacculus, semicircular canals, cochlea, and endolymphatic ducts—were present and superficially normal. A detailed histological study of these parts was not made, but morphologically the entire anlage, in wax reconstruction, seemed flattened, perhaps because of lack of mechanical stimuli that usually occur in the presence of a closing or closed hindbrain (Stein and Rudin 1953). The appearance, development, and transformations of the notochord were normal, as was the development of mesoderm; and it therefore seemed that the abnormalities of the nervous system were not secondary to effects of the gene on organizer tissue (Stein and Rudin 1953).

The primitive streak of 9- to 9½-day *Lp/Lp* embryos (Smith and Stein 1961, 1962) was longer than in normal littermates, and although its length decreased during this period in both classes of embryos, the decrease occurred less rapidly in the abnormals. In addition, the gut and neural tissue were considerably shorter and the posterior portion of the notochord was thicker in *Lp/Lp* embryos, with relatively smaller increase in length of the gut and notochord than of neural tissue. Thus the effect of the mutation was delay in shortening, and perhaps in regression of, the primitive streak during and following the period of closure of the neural tube and, possibly as a direct consequence, reduced axial elongation of the notochord and its associated somites and neural tissue. However that may be, the failure of the neural plate to close appeared to result from its failure to elongate.

The *Lp* gene apparently interacted with the *T* (Brachyury) and *Fu* (Fused) genes, double heterozygotes often having spina bifida aperta, a defect not found in *Lp/+* individuals (Strong and Hollander 1949).

Coiled

Coiled (symbol *co*), a recessive, arose in the A strain (Morgan 1952). Many dead coiled offspring had "rachischisis totalis" (craniorachischisis?), and were phenotypically indistinguishable from Loop-tail offspring. The mutation is probably now extinct.

Genes Causing Other Brain or Spinal Cord Defects

Absent Corpus Callosum

In anatomical studies of the brains of mice with hereditary absence of the rod cells of the retina, the corpus callosum was noted to be missing in several cases (King and Keeler 1932). The brain abnormality was unrelated to the retinal defect. By laborious efforts it was established that absent corpus callosum was due to a recessive gene (symbol *ac*), which has long been extinct but, happily, has now been refound (Wimer 1965). In subsequent studies (Keeler 1933; King 1936), some exceptions to recessive inheritance were noted, i.e., a few apparently normal offspring were produced by malformed parents.

Histological examination (King and Keeler 1932) of affected mice revealed that the longitudinal fissure extended all the way to the hippocampal commissure, owing to absence of the corpus callosum, and thus that there was no dorsal connection between the hemispheres. Posterior to the hippocampal commissure, the longitudinal fissure extended without interruption to the roof of the 3rd ventricle. Dorsal to the hippocampal commissure, an aberrant bundle of fibers was sometimes seen. This bundle has no homologue in the normal brain and thus may have represented the abortive anlage of the corpus callosum. No other gross abnormality was associated with the condition, and other tracts were normal or nearly so. Mice lacking the corpus callosum were indistinguishable from normal ones on casual inspection.

In the preliminary study (King and Keeler 1932) no quantitative variations were mentioned, but in a more detailed report (King 1936) several intermediate degrees of the abnormality were described. Three distinct types of abnormality, each with slight variations, were found, corresponding roughly to similar categories in man. (1) Complete absence of the corpus callosum, in which the aberrant longitudinal callosal bundle, mentioned above, gave rise to no commissural fibers. This bundle (called Balkenlängsbündel in the German literature, see p. 295) consisted of a group of fibers running predominantly sagitally in the dorsomedial part of the hemisphere; it was believed to be composed of fibers from cells of origin of the corpus callosum, fibers hindered early from crossing to the opposite hemisphere, which thus turned sagitally and ran in the ipsilateral hemisphere. (2) Partial presence of an atypical corpus callosum, found in the anterior part of the brain, but not at the genu. (3) Partial presence posteriorly, in which commissural fibers arose from the posterior half to form a well-defined splenium, similar in many respects to the normal.

In all 3 types, fibers from the anterior part of the bundle proceeded to the midline but appeared to end blindly. In the second type additional fibers from the bundle met across the midline to form a variable-sized corpus callosum over the psalterium. In the third type, a partial corpus callosum, also derived from the bundle, formed a splenium in the posterior part of the brain. In all types the cytoarchitecture of the cortex was normal and, further, no defects of the brain, other than those secondary to the callosal malformation, were found. The incidence of each of the types was not stated.

These variations of the abnormality may have represented variable expressivity of the gene, possibly owing to modifying genetic factors. This interpretation is supported by the fact that the type of defect in offspring sometimes differed from that in their parents. The possible genetic basis of these variations was not investigated.

To the joy of numerous neuropathologists and mammalian geneticists, Wimer (1965) recently announced the discovery that a condition not discernably different from that produced by the *ac* gene exists in the BALB/cJ and 129/J inbred mouse strains. Sidman, Green and Appel (1965, p. 10) stated that the abnormality in the BALB/cJ mice is apparently identical with the one described by King (1936), but that in the 129/J mice the callosal defects are somewhat different.

Strong's Luxoid

Numerous hereditary hemimelias have been discovered and intensively studied in mice (Grüneberg 1963, pp. 193–211), but only one of these conditions, that produced by the luxoid gene of Strong (symbol *lst*), was possibly associated with abnormalities of the central nervous system (Strong and Hardy 1956). The gene, a semidominant, produced preaxial polydactyly of the hindfoot in many heterozygotes, and the hemimelic syndrome in homozygotes.

Strong and Hardy (1956) noted hydrocephalus, signalled by domeshaped skull, and, rarely, cranioschisis in their stock. The effects of the *lst* gene were studied further by Forsthoefel (1962). He found various changes in the skull of homozygotes, including shortening of all elements of the cranial base and relative expansion of dorsal parts, which resulted in a short head with abruptly elevated cranium (i.e., bulldog profile)—an appearance commonly seen in cases of hydrocephalus. But true hydrocephalus was not found at birth or in adults. However, dissections revealed other morphological deviations of the brain, consisting mainly of changes in the proportion of parts. Posteromedial areas of the cerebral hemispheres were indented, completely exposing the colliculi. Cerebellar changes included compression and absence of parts. Examination of the brain in sections showed no enlargement of ventricles or thinning of walls. In some cases the ventral part of the corpus callosum was degenerated.

Study of the prenatal development of *lst/lst* homozygotes (Forsthoefel 1963) showed that the skull anomalies were all related to deficient growth of the anterior part of the head, including facial processes, which was first observed on the 12th day of pregnancy. This retardation shortened the anterior growth of the chondrocranium and restricted the forward expansion of the rapidly growing brain. Other anomalies of the brain were apparently all consequences of these primary events.

Flexed-Tail

Flexed-tail (symbol *f*) is a recessive gene whose well-known effects are transitory siderocytic anemia, belly spots, and anomalies of the axial skeleton (Grüneberg 1952*b*, pp. 239–48). In addition, Kamenoff (1935), in a study of the embryonic development of the effects of the gene, found abnormalities of the neural tube and notochord in 20/100 sectioned embryos. The defects of the spinal cord included irregularities in the shape of its lumen and localized duplications of the cord with discontinuous spinal canal.

Vestigial-Tail

Vestigial-tail (symbol *vt*) is a recessive gene producing variable shortening of the tail (Heston 1951). In an embryological study of its effects, Grüneberg (1957*a*) observed that obvious abnormalities regularly developed on the ventral aspect of the neural tube in 10th-day *vt/vt* embryos. Unlike normal embryos, there was no progressive diminution of the neural tube in the tail, but instead a segment of the tube split off, increased in size in the caudal direction, and acquired secondary lumina; so that in sectioned material several extra neural tubes were present in the tail. Similar splittings-off, with or without formation of lumina, sometimes occurred more cranially and came to lie in the sacral region. These anomalies developed later than those in the tail and never proceeded very far. The remainder of the neural tube was normal. In 12th-day fetuses constrictions appeared in the tail, separating it from its base, and a day later a condition was reached very much like that present at birth, with no tail at all, a thin filament, or a short stump.

The gross deformities of the neural tube in vestigial-tail embryos were considered (Grüneberg 1957*b*) to be secondary to reduction in size or absence of a transitory embryonic structure, discovered by Grüneberg (1956*b*), called the ventral ectodermal ridge of the tail, which in normal animals may play an important part in the growth of that organ.

Truncate

Truncate (symbol *tr*) is a simple recessive gene with slightly reduced penetrance, which caused variable shortening of the tail, lumbosacral agenesis, and absence of the median ventral fissure of the spinal cord (Theiler 1959). In adults the interruption of the spine sometimes led to compression of the cord and paralysis of the hind legs. Investigation of the embryonic development of the condition revealed that the abnormalities were due to disturbance of formation of the notochord and sclerotomes in early embryonic life, which led to malstructure of the ventral neural tube in the region of absence of the notochord.

Lumbarless

Only a brief description of the lumbarless condition has been published (Gluecksohn-Waelsch 1963). It is caused by a recessive gene that produced death of some homozygotes in early adulthood as the result of paralysis of the posterior part of the trunk and the posterior extremities. The paralysis was due to abnormalities of the spinal cord and vertebral column in the lumbar region, consisting of various degrees of defectiveness or absence of lumbar vertebrae, accompanied by constriction and thinness of the cord.

Tail-Kinks

This condition is due to a simple recessive gene (symbol *tk*) whose major effects are confined to the axial skeleton (Grüneberg 1955*b*). While the vertebral column was most severely affected at both ends, a few instances of defects of vertebrae at the lumbosacral border were seen. These abnormalities consisted of spina bifida occulta, a condition that is apparently quite rare in mice, though commonly produced by the curly-tail gene (see p. 211). The spinal cord itself, however, was seemingly normal in *tk/tk* mice.

An apparently transient effect of the *tk* gene on structures connected with the central nervous system was noted in 13th-day embryos (Grüneberg 1955*b*). In 2 sectioned specimens there was a striking and uniform widening of the pia-arachnoid spaces in the cervical and upper thoracic regions. Dorsally, the distance between the medulla and the overlying dura mater was twice as wide as normal, and laterally the spinal ganglia occupied more ventral positions than normal. The impression gotten was that the whole dural sac was blown up by excess cerebrospinal fluid and that the ganglia were dislocated by the same pressure. Evidence pointed to the excess of cerebrospinal fluid being a secondary phenomenon, caused by weakening of the mechanical support the dura mater normally receives from the vertebrae, owing to vertebral abnormalities in this part of the axial skeleton of *tk/tk* embryos.

These observations prompted Grüneberg (1955*b*) to recall Bonnevie's (1934) theory of the leakage of cerebrospinal fluid from the roof of the 4th ventricle in the bleb syndrome (see p. 205). Grüneberg's (1955*b*) finding that the pia-arachnoid spaces were expanded by excess cerebrospinal fluid indicated that the fluid, at this stage of embryonic life, as in the adult, is confined to the meninges and does not escape from the 4th ventricle, contrary to Bonnevie's contention.

Patch

Patch (symbol *Ph*), a dominant, arose as a spontaneous mutation in a C57BL mouse. Its effects were studied in CBA mice (Grüneberg and Truslove 1960). It caused spotting with sharply defined pigmented and white areas in heterozygotes, and prenatal death in homozygotes. The earliest visible effects in homozygotes were seen in 9th-day embryos, in which there occurred localized accumulations of clear liquid at various specific sites in the body. More extremely affected *Ph/Ph* embryos died on about the 10th day; others survived to later stages of pregnancy. The latter had a large bleb of liquid in the middle of the face that mechanically interfered with formation of the nose and palate and produced a "cleft" condition. Abnormalities of the central nervous system were few and were probably consequences of the hydropic condition of the embryos. The ventricular system of the brain was dilated, and the brain walls were attenuated. The neural tube was wavy, and a small hole was sometimes found in the roof of the myelencephalon.

Dorsal Excrescences

This condition consisted of a group of manifestations characterized by nodular tissue or accessory tufts of hair occurring on the head or at various places along the mid-dorsal line (Center 1960). Morphologically, some excrescences appeared to be masses of neural tissue or surrounding meninges that were forced outside the usual limits of the neural tube. Excrescences were recognized at birth as fluid-filled sacs or spurlike processes of tissue. In the head region, the nodules were usually directly over or adjacent to a cranial suture; or were sometimes connected to the underlying meninges by a stalk that passed through a foramen. The excrescences sometimes possessed a high degree of organization: a lumbosacral appendage, e.g., consisted of an accessory spinal cord with the accompanying ganglia. Available evidence indicated that there was an underlying genetic mechanism responsible for the condition, but that the mode of inheritance was complex.

Steel

Steel (symbol *Sl*) is a dominant gene causing pigmentary and hematological effects in heterozygotes and prenatal lethality in homozygotes (Sarvella and Russell 1956). In 413 morphologically observable embryos and fetuses from crosses between $Sl/+$ heterozygotes, 9 were found with malformations of the central nervous system: one, exencephaly and spina bifida; 2, exencephaly; 3, spina bifida; 2, collapsed brain; and one with other defects. No such anomalies occurred in 166 offspring from crosses of $Sl/+ \times +/+$. However, since the abnormalities occurred in nonanemic as well as anemic offspring and, further, since these malformations were apparently not found in another developmental study (Bennett 1956) of the effects of Sl, it is unlikely that this gene was responsible for them.

Neurological Mutants

A large number of genes have been discovered in mice that affect equilibrium, hearing, and neuromuscular function (Sidman, Green, and Appel 1965). Many have histopathological effects, but few produce gross morphological alterations in the brain. Some have already been discussed in previous pages.

Shaker-1 (symbol *sh-1*), a recessive, was briefly mentioned (Zimmermann 1935) as causing atrophy of the striatum accompanied by a slight secondary internal hydrocephalus of the lateral ventricles. Whether these changes were congenital was not stated.

In leaner (symbol *la*) and weaver (symbol *wv*), both recessives, the cerebellum was reduced in size, but its condition in neonates has not yet been reported (Sidman, Green, and Appel 1965). Staggerer (symbol *sg*), a recessive, reduced the cerebellum to less than one-third normal size. The abnormality was recognized at 4 days after birth but was not detected at birth (Sidman, Lane, and Dickie 1962). The cerebellum was also grossly reduced in size in weanlings homozygous for the recessive reeler (symbol *rl*) (Meier and Hoag 1962), but in this case certain gross cerebellar abnormalities were already present at birth (Hamburgh 1963). The recessive fidget (symbol *fi*) was associated with a congenital abnormality of the shape of the paraflocular lobe of the cerebellum caused by absence of the subarcuate fossa of the auditory capsule, into which the lobe ordinarily fits (Truslove 1956).

The recessive kreisler (symbol *kr*) was subjected to a detailed embryological study by Hertwig (1944). She noted that large, cystlike evaginations from the embryonic inner ear encroached on areas of the cerebellum and interfered with its development. Deol (1964*b*) confirmed the presence of cysts and also found changes in the structure of the neural tube, as early as the 9th day of gestation, which consisted of faulty segmentation in the region of the rhombencephalon and degeneration in the 4th rhombomere. It was undetermined whether these changes left any permanent imprint on the brain.

Otocephaly

Little and Bagg (1924) reported a number of congenital abnormalities in the descendants of some irradiated mice, in an experiment that also led to the discovery of the gene for myelencephalic blebs, discussed earlier. One of the abnormalities was a heritable jaw defect, which seemed to be due to a single recessive gene (symbol *j*), now apparently extinct.

The jaw anomaly was lethal in the great majority of cases, over 90 per cent of affected offspring being stillborn or failing to reach weaning age. The head was round or square in appearance, and the lower jaw was variably reduced (micrognathia) or sometimes completely absent (agnathia). In micrognathia the opening of the mouth was decreased in size (microstomia), depending on the degree of reduction of the lower jaw, and in agnathia was sometimes apparently absent (astomia). The eyes were sometimes fused together, and the snout sometimes extended like a proboscis, with the fused eyes ventral or dorsal to it. In other words, it seemed that the defect fell into the category of otocephaly.

A number of affected offspring were described in some detail by Johnson (1926), but he failed to mention whether brain abnormalities were present, as they were in extreme otocephaly in, e.g., guinea pigs (Wright and Wagner 1934). Photographs of histological sections of some affected mice showed no gross defect of the brain. Thus, while this abnormality of mice may not be of direct importance to us, it is of great interest for other reasons, and a bit more space will be devoted to it.

The jaw anomaly appeared in 3 different lines of mice descended from the irradiated individuals and in these lines behaved as though due to a recessive gene. However, because the defect also occurred in some animals of the unirradiated control stock, it did not seem that the gene had been induced by the X rays.

But several bits of evidence make it doubtful that the condition in the control mice was the same as the one in the experimental animals. (1) The abnormality occurred (Little and Bagg 1924) "in its most aggravated form" in the controls. (2) Its relative infrequency in the controls may indicate that in them it was not produced by a simple genetic situation, as it was in the experimental groups, and this possibility is reinforced by the subsequent history of the control line. This line originated with a cross between a heterogeneous sib pair, female 57 black and male 52, also black, both obtained from the Lathrop Mouse Farm. This mating gave rise to the inbred strain known as C57BL, which was split before 1937 into the C57BL/6 and C57BL/10 sublines (Staats 1964).

In my laboratory, the C57BL/6 substrain has been noted, even today, 40 years and hundreds of generations later, still to throw an occasional "otocephalic" offspring (fig. 17). In 354 litters born between June, 1958 and October, 1965, 12/2466 (0.49 %) offspring were found with the "jaw anomaly." This consisted of various degrees of micrognathia and microstomia, agnathia and astomia, low-set ears, small or absent tongue, and, where examination was possible, cleft palate. Eye defects were present in some cases, but they were the types occurring rather frequently in this strain (microphthalmia, anophthalmia, coloboma iridis, etc.) and were not defects of the cyclopean variety. No proboscises were found. However, the fact that the ears were low set, especially in more severe cases of reduction of the lower jaw, probably indicates that the condition represents low-grade stages of otocephaly. The heads of 4 of these animals were serially sectioned. The abnormalities seen, often bizarre, were predominantly orofacial, optic, otic, and pharyngeal. No gross brain defects were present.

Higher grade otocephalics, such as occurred in guinea pigs (Wright and Wagner 1934), were not seen by Little and Bagg (1924) or by me. The mouse and guinea pig abnormality differed in sex ratio of affected animals, since in the 12 cases in mice mentioned above no great sex difference in incidence occurred, while in guinea pigs the condition was about twice as frequent in females as in males (Wright 1960).

The facts discussed in the last 2 paragraphs thus make it possible that the jaw anomaly that occurred in the experimental lines of Little and Bagg (1924) was radiation induced, after all.

10

Rat

Spontaneous or sporadic congenital malformations of the central nervous system have seldom been reported in rats. The reason for the apparent lack of such defects in laboratory stocks of this species can only be speculated on. Parts of the answer may be: (1) Rats are mostly randombred, or at least not inbred, and hence deleterious recessive genes are largely prevented from acting, and developmental homeostasis is maintained. (2) Abnormal animals and their parents are usually routinely destroyed by commercial breeders, and thus any contributory genetic factors are selectively reduced or eliminated. (3) Disinterest or casual observation results in their being overlooked.

The paucity of such malformations or, indeed, of malformations in general, in this species, can be gauged by the little space devoted to the subject in Robinson's (1965) recent book on rat genetics: malformations of the central nervous system accounted for less than one (p. 221) of the 730 pages of text.

Isolated and Sporadic Hydrocephalus and Other Defects

Symptoms possibly due to hydrocephalus occurred in 4 Wistar rats (3 males, 1 female) from 2 litters (Colton 1929). The frontal region of the cranium was quite bulbous, so that the profile of the face was concave and not slightly convex as it normally is. Skulls of 2 of the animals were domeshaped and wider than normal. The brain was apparently not examined. Two of the males died at 21 and 44 days, respectively; the female—unable to face life—drowned in a bowl of milk at 28 days of age. The surviving male (who lived 508 days) was mated to 2 normal sisters, but the condition did not recur in their offspring, grandchildren, or great-grandchildren. Nor had it been seen in 611 rats observed in the preceding $3\frac{1}{2}$-year period.

Definite hydrocephalus was seen in one animal of a litter of "albino" rats (Houck 1930). Enlargement of the head was noticed on the 5th day after birth. The animal was sluggish, its movements and locomotion were uncertain, and it tended to walk in circles. The symptoms progressively worsened until death occurred at 25 days of age.

At that time the head was enlarged in the frontal and parietal regions, producing a domed shape. When dissected, the cranial cavity was found to contain a mass of fluid. The cerebral tissue was so flattened by intracranial pressure that it was paper thin and closely adherent to the membranous cranium. Ganglia and other structures of the brainstem stood out in bold relief. The corpus callosum, corona radiata, septum pellucidum, and most of the fornix were lacking. The only parts of the cerebrum in good condition were the basal areas of the corpora striata. The brainstem appeared almost completely intact. The cerebellum was displaced posteriorly and was somewhat herniated into the foramen magnum. The lesion underlying the condition could not be determined.

Fifteen cases of hydrocephalus, which were not described, appeared (Hain 1937) in a stock also showing eye and urogenital defects. All 3 types of anomalies were regarded as belonging to the same syndrome, but no evidence for this possibility was presented.

In a study of the teratogenic effects of uterine clamping in rats (see p. 179), there were a small number ($26/1005 = 2.6\%$) of malformed term fetuses among those that had developed in the unclamped uterine horn (Franklin and Brent 1964). Single malformations occurred in 24, 2 malformations in one, and 3 in another. The most common defect ($11/1005 = 1.1\%$) was hydrocephalus, diagnosed as any degree of ventricular dilatation; other abnormalities affected heart, kidney, limb, palate, eye, etc. Low incidences of spontaneous hydrocephalus were also found in 2 other rat colonies; O'Dell, Whitley, and Hogan (1948) noted the defect in $3/1212$ (0.25%) weaned young, and Gillman et al. (1951) in $5/5886$ (0.08%) newborn offspring.

Observations of control rats over a $6\frac{1}{2}$-year period provided the following data (Takacs, personal communication). From May, 1958, to December, 1964, 4328 newborn offspring and 2662 fetuses (12th–22nd days of gestation) of Long–Evans and Wistar-derived stocks were carefully examined for gross malformations. Twenty-eight young had observable defects of the central nervous system. Only one neonate had such a condition—hydrocephalus; it survived to 30 days of age—whereas 27 fetuses (1.01%) were affected, 6 with exencephaly, 21 with irregularly-shaped brain. Since the latter abnormalities were not found in newborn offspring, the defects were transitory, or young with such defects died before birth or were eaten at birth before they could be examined.

Bertrand et al. (1966) noted one rat with a small frontal protruberance, corresponding, according to the authors, to a "microexencephaly," in 512 late fetuses from Wistar females.

A Genetic Syndrome Including Brain Abnormalities

A polydactylous female rat was born in 1958 in the colony of Wistar-derived animals of the Teratology Division of the Children's Hospital Research Foundation, Cincinnati, Ohio. She was bred to a male littermate, and, from the results found in their progeny and immediate descendants, it soon became apparent that the polydactyly was probably due to an autosomal recessive gene (symbol *po*).

The following data were accumulated in the next several years. (1) Eighteen crosses between polydactylous (*po/po*) females and heterozygous (*+/po*) males (abnormal males were sterile) produced 96 offspring, of which 40 (41.7%) were affected. (2) Sixty-six crosses between heterozygotes gave 105/550 (19.1%) affected. (3) Fifteen crosses between heterozygotes and animals homozygous for the normal allele produced 0/117 affected. Somewhat fewer abnormal offspring were thus obtained in crosses 1 and 2 than expected on the basis of recessive inheritance (41.7% vs. 50%, $\chi^2 = 1.0$, P = 0.3; and 19.1% vs. 25%, $\chi^2 = 5.2$, P = 0.02, respectively).

Judging from cross 1, the deficiency of affected offspring may have been due to increased prenatal mortality, since the mean litter size was lower (5.3) than in cross 3 (7.8). But this explanation does not hold for the deficiency of abnormal young in cross 2, since its mean litter size (8.3) was not less than usual for the colony. It may thus be that the gene lacked full penetrance. If so, the penetrance in cross 1 was 83 per cent and in cross 2, 76 per cent.

Usually one, rarely 2 or 3, extra preaxial digits were present on each paw. Most affected animals died soon after birth. The few surviving males, although given ample opportunity, sired no litters; surviving females bred poorly and, as indicated above, had relatively small litters.

Sixteen polydactylous newborn offspring were serially sectioned. Aside from polydactyly, defects were noted only in the head and primarily involved the forebrain, pituitary, and eye. One or, more usually, both olfactory bulbs were partly or completely absent in 12 cases and irregular in 2 others. The place of absent bulbs was taken by large, disorganized masses of olfactory nerve, which ended without joining the brain (fig. 18).

The posterior lobe of the pituitary was entirely missing in 3 and was either small or abnormal and small in 3 others (fig. 19). In one of the latter there was no infundibular communication with the 3rd ventricle. The anterior lobe of the pituitary was completely missing in one animal (that also lacked the posterior lobe). In 2 it was abnormal in shape, lacked a lumen, and was far rostral to its normal location; and in 4 others it was small or asymmetrical. In one case both lobes, though aberrant, were present but were far separated from each other, a condition known as dystopic pituitary in human pathology. Five animals had a craniopharyngeal duct, which originated from the naso-pharynx, traversed the presphenoid, and entered or coalesced with the parenchyma of the anterior pituitary. In another, the duct did not reach the pituitary.

Other neural defects also occurred. In 2 a pearshaped projection, with its apex superior, rose from the floor of the 3rd ventricle in the area of the infundibulum; in one it was large and was associated with great widening of the ventricle in its neighborhood. One had a narrow corpus callosum. Various complex histological disarrangements of the basal ganglia and other cerebral areas were found. The posterior horns of the lateral ventricles were enlarged in one case.

It is quite possible that the pleiotropy, variable expressivity, and reduced penetrance exhibited by the *po* gene were at least partly due to the heterogeneity of the genetic background upon which it acted in these randombred animals. Unfortunately, the gene is now extinct.

Other Abnormalities

Chidester (1914) found 2 abnormal rats in a litter of 6 offspring. One, not further described, had "anterior hydrencephalocele." The second had "anophthalmia cyclopica." Gross examination of the brain showed 3 cerebral vesicles, one slightly anterior to paired lateral ones. The cerebellum was pushed back to a ventral position, and its hemispheres were slightly separated from the vermis. The cerebral peduncles were absent, as were the cranial nerves anterior to the 4th. The whole brain was reduced in size. Sections of the brain revealed apparent absence of the corpus callosum; slightly enlarged ventricles, but without marked hydrocephalus (no external indication of hydrocephalus was seen); and apparent absence of the pituitary. There was no external or internal indication of eyes. The animal had no proboscis.

Conrow (1917) discovered a rat in the colony of the Wistar Institute with posterior duplication that lived in good health for about 15 months. The vertebral column was single and normal as far back as the 5th lumbar vertebra, and deformed and duplicated from that point caudally. The condition of the cord, however, was not mentioned.

Veerappa and Bourne (1966) noted a double central canal in histological sections of the midthoracic spinal cord of a rat of unstated age. One central canal was in the normal position and the other was slightly ventral to it on the midline in the anterior white commissure. The ependymal lining of both canals was cytologically similar. Followed anteriorly, it was seen that the ventrally located, presumably supernumerary, canal was derived from, and directly continuous with, the central canal. The posterior cord was unexaminable. The cord was otherwise apparently normal in morphology. There were no apparent neurological signs of the condition.

11

Guinea Pig

Otocephaly

The only study of the inheritance of otocephaly and the most extensive study of its range of manifestations were made in guinea pigs by Wright and his colleagues (see below). Hence it is logical to consider otocephaly at length in this chapter and to refer to it only briefly elsewhere. Since the malformations present in this condition sometimes apparently overlap those presented by cyclopia, and because the classification and nomenclature of these states is confusingly intertwined, it will be useful to discuss these aberrations together.

Based on the reports of others', as well as on his own observations, Saint-Hilaire (1832–37, vol. 2, pp. 423–24) classified certain major forms of human and animal facial defects into 2 "families": cyclocephaly and otocephaly. The former is characterized by approach or variable union of the orbits and their contents, with the ears remaining normally situated; while the latter is characterized by approach or union of the external and middle ears on the midline, reduction or absence of the mandible, and sometimes approximation or fusion of the orbits and ocular structures as well.

Cyclocephaly consists of a graded series of defects culminating in severer forms commonly known as cyclopia (whose synonyms are cyclocephaly, cyclencephaly, synopsia, monopsia, synophthalmia, and monophthalmia). Saint-Hilaire (*ibid.*) recognized the following 2 divisions and 5 subdivisions, each succeeding grade containing features of the preceding one. I. Orbits approximated, but eyes separate. (1) Ethmocephaly (ethmos = sieve): nasal proboscis above orbits. (2) Cebocephaly (kebos = longtailed monkey): nose atrophic, usually with one median nostril, but normally situated. II. Single median orbit and united contents. (3) Rhinocephaly (rhinos = nose): nasal proboscis above orbits. (4) Cyclocephaly proper (kyklos = circle): no nasal proboscis. (5) Stomocephaly (stoma = mouth): small lower jaw and mouth, buccal swelling or "proboscis."

The 2 mildest grades, ethmocephaly and cebocephaly, which sometimes occur in conjunction with median or lateral cleft lip, were called arhinencephaly by Kundrat (1882), since their most characteristic feature is absence of at least the olfactory bulbs and tracts, although other defects more common in severer forms of cyclocephaly, such as more or less complete fusion of the cerebral hemispheres, may also be found. A description of several types of arhinencephaly was given by Ernst (1909, pp. 135–37), and his account translated into English by Currarino and Silverman (1960).

The brain defects typical of higher grades of cyclocephaly are usually confined to the fore- and midbrain. The central hemispheres are most often completely fused, and the falx, interhemispheric fissure, corpus callosum, and septum pellucidum are absent or incomplete. Internally, there is thus only a single, large, anterior cavity, comprising the confluent lateral and 3rd ventricles, which may be hydrocephalically distended. A thinwalled, dilated "dorsal sac" is frequently present between the forebrain and cerebellum, communicating freely with the large single ventricle. The olfactory bulbs and nerves are missing, and the optic nerves are defective, fused, or absent. Descriptions of these defects as well as those of the skeleton, nasal apparatus, eyes, and other structures, in human cyclopia, were given by Ballantyne (1904, pp. 395–400); Schwalbe and Josephy (1913, pp. 210–30); Potter (1961, pp. 492–98); and Duke-Elder (1963, pp. 429–45).

Of late, Kundrat's term, arhinencephaly, has been challenged as not being precise enough, since in some cases olfactory structures are present, while in others more than olfactory structures are involved. Based on neuro-tectonic studies of several cases, Yakovlev (1959) suggested the term "holo-telencephaly" to denote this syndrome of brain malformations. This expression did not satisfy DeMyer and Zeman (1963), because they felt it did not reflect certain features of the condition. Instead they proposed the generic term "holoprosencephaly," since to them the morphology of the brain in these states is determined by arrest of cleavage of the prosencephalon, upon which other aspects may or may not be superimposed. As with any respectable genus, this one subsumes various specific and subspecific divisions and subdivisions, e.g., lobar, semilobar, and alobar holoprosencephaly. The entire classification covers several pages (DeMyer and Zeman 1963, pp. 22–25). Thus a perfectly sound term, arhinencephaly, that designates, and is known by its users to designate, milder degrees of certain combinations of malformations of the brain, is to be replaced, because it is more precise, by the following: genus holoprosencephaly, species alobar, subspecies, B, C, and D (subspecies A includes not only cyclopia, but otocephaly as well!).

It is laudable that efforts should be made to devise classifications whose goal is the reduction of ambiguity. But will descriptive precision (whether possible of achievement we will not discuss) lead by itself to greater under-standing of efficient cause? Not if teratologic variations in kind and degree are—as they well may be—but adventitious reflections of subsidiary genetic and nongenetic factors.

Let us turn now to the second of Saint-Hilaire's families—otocephaly—whose essential characteristic he believed to be ventral approximation or union of the ears, and of which he at first recognized (*ibid.*) 3 divisions and 5 subdivisions. I. Eyes well separated. (1) Sphenocephaly (i.e., referring to the condition of the sphenoid): ears approximated or united ventrally under the head, but lower jaw, mouth, and nose normal. II. Eyes partly or wholly united in one median orbit; ears as in sphenocephaly. (2) Otocephaly proper (otos = ear): proboscoid nose, mouth present. (3) Edocephaly (aidoion = genital, referring to the fancied resemblance of the proboscis to a penis): fused eyes with united ears below them and nasal proboscis above; jaws atrophic, no mouth. (4) Opocephaly (ops = face): no, or small, proboscis, no mouth, atrophic jaws. III. Eyes absent. (5) Triocephaly (tri = 3, i.e., all 3—mouth, nose, eyes—absent): in addition to the features of opocephaly, eyes entirely absent; thus all that apparently remains of the head are the fused ears occupying the apex of the neck; hence, true otocephaly.

Saint-Hilaire's otocephaly thus comprised a series of defects at one end of the scale of which only ears and jaws were involved, while the other end included more extensive facial defects, including approximation and fusion of eyes. However, these eye abnormalities are not exactly the same as occur in cyclopia, since in the latter the migration of the eyes is toward the midline of the front of the face, whereas in otocephaly the movement is down the face toward the neck.

To Gurlt (1877), whose viewpoint was colored by the way the condition appeared in animals, the most important feature of otocephaly was not the state of the ears, as it was for Saint-Hilaire, but that of the lower jaw; and on the basis of degree of abnormality of this part he divided his cases into those with brachygnathia, micrognathia, and agnathia. The main difference between the first 2 was extent of jaw reduction, while in the last the lower jaw was entirely absent or seemed so.

Not content with these schemes, Taruffi (1884–91, vol. 6, pp. 391–92) suggested another system of classification. All conditions that include defective development of the lower part of the face he grouped together and called hypoprosopo-aplasia, which was subdivided into hypomicrognathia (small lower jaw) and hypoagnathia (absent lower jaw). A separate group, cyclops hypoagnathia, consisted of specimens with fused eye and absent lower jaw; and, finally, a last category, aprosopia (a term introduced by Dugès 1827), comprised those with no eyes, nose, and mouth. Hannover (1882–84, p. 160) gave the name synotia to such specimens. As Ballantyne (1904, p. 424) commented, Taruffi's and Saint-Hilaire's classifications correspond to some extent but are not entirely reconcilable.

A heroic *fin de siècle* effort was made by Blanc (1895) to bring harmony and logic to this nomenclatorial and conceptual chaos by the use of intermediate and combinational categories. Furthermore, he introduced additional criteria, such as degree and type of malformations of the middle and external ears and, especially, the brain. His classification follows.

I. Transitional (from normal). Small chin or no chin, without approximation of external ears, but with nasopharyngeal atresia in some cases. II. Otocephaly. A. Brain well formed. (1) Ageniocephaly (geneion = chin): micrognathia or agnathia, occlusion of isthmus faucium forming pharyngeal sac, approximation or fusion of middle ears, sometimes approximation of external ears, cranium and sense organs well formed, mouth present. (2) Sphenocephaly: as in (1), plus abnormalities of craniofacial skeleton, approximation or median fusion of external ears and tympanic cavities; includes 3 subvarieties, partly according to amount of descent of external ears and fusion of external auditory canals. (3) Agnathocephaly (gnathos = jaw): as above, except for shift of eyes to lower part of face, no mouth, other facial skeletal defects. (4) Strophocephaly (strophos = twisted): as above, except maxillae fused and atrophied, no zygomatic arch, eyes very close in one large orbit under anterior sphenoid.

B. Brain vesicular. (5) Edocephaly: much as in (4), viz., absent or rudimentary lower jaw, occlusion of isthmus faucium, pharyngeal sac, external ears approximated or fused, no mouth, maxillae fused and rudimentary, no zygomatic arch, nasal proboscis present, eyes close together or fused under anterior sphenoid, tympanic cavities approximated or fused, auditory ossicles deformed. New feature is vesicular brain, i.e., defects described above as characteristic of cyclopia. The medulla, cerebellum, and colliculi are well developed. A single median optic nerve is present. The single anterior cerebral cavity is full of liquid. The olfactory bulbs and nerves are rudimentary. (6) Opocephaly: as in (5), except no nasal proboscis, no facial bones, frontal very reduced. (7) Spherocephaly (sphaira = ball): as above, except usually no eye, no anterior sphenoid.

C. No brain anterior to medulla and pons. (8) Triocephaly: cranium reduced to the occipital petrosals (approximated or fused on midline), and a rudimentary parietal; no jaws, no mouth, no eye, no nasal proboscis, external ears very close together or fused; brain reduced to the medulla, which may be topped by a sort of impaired acoustic and other nerves.

III. Combinational, called cyclotia, composite of essential features of cyclopia and otocephaly; i.e., atrophy of mandible and approximation of ears associated with union of eyes above upper jaw, with or without nasal proboscis above orbit.

Ballantyne (1904, p. 426) considered Blanc's arrangement far too complicated for use in human teratology, especially as many of the types are not recorded in human fetuses. But it was indeed because cyclopia and otocephaly appear to be far more common in many animal species than they are in man that the construction of elaborate schemes of classification and interrelation was possible.

Blanc (1895) regarded the supermaxillary location of the approximated or fused eyes in cyclocephaly, and their location under the head in types of otocephaly, as indicating that they are quite different abnormalities. Wright and Wagner (1934), on the other hand, regarded the difference in location of the defects as superficial, since anatomically they are essentially identical.

Wright and Wagner (1934) thus ignored this distinction, and drew up a "2-dimensional" classificatory scheme for the cyclopia-otocephaly syndromes. In one dimension they placed the series of defects the mandible is heir to. (1) Brachygnathia: mandible short, but of normal width. (2) Micrognathia: mandible diminutive, ventral approach of ears. (3) Hypoagnathus: mandible absent, ear ossicles united. (4) Synzygo-agnathus: as in (3), with fusion of zygomatic arches. (5) Azygo-agnathus: as in (3), with absent or vestigial zygomatic arch.

The second dimension was occupied by a series of premaxillary and associated defects. (a) Brachyrhynchus: premaxilla reduced or absent, brain normal. (b) Arhinencephaly: as in (a), with defect of olfactory bulbs and variable union of cerebral hemispheres, usually one nostril (monorhinia). (c) Rhinocyclops: forebrain vesicular, eyes more or less fused, nasal proboscis above single orbit. (d) Cyclops arhinus: as in (c), except proboscis absent. (3) Anops: as in (d), except eye absent. (f) Aprosopus: cerebellum and fore- and midbrain absent. (g) Monoto-aprosopus: as in (f), with united ear vesicles.

It was supposed that any one of the types of the first and of the second series, by itself or combined with the other, corresponds to the array of anomalies presented by the majority of defective specimens. E.g., according to Wright and Wagner (1934), at the intersection of hypoagnathus and arhinencephaly are found specimens having the features in the sheep illustrated (and called sphenocephalus) by Josephy (1913, fig. 188, p. 258); or azygo-agnathus combined with anops results in the sphenocephaly of Saint-Hilaire. In practice, no doubt, there are as many cases that do not fit this scheme as do, and indeed Wright and Wagner (1934) themselves noted several exceptions.

Regardless of whether the ophthalmic defects in the severer varieties of otocephaly are similar to, or even identical anatomically with, those in cyclopia, the possibility is not excluded that they originate in different ways or develop in distinct manners or both. As we have seen in the chapters devoted to experimental teratogenesis, structural analogy of malformations does not prove their homology.

Blanc's (1895) case for the creation of his new defect category cyclotia, intermediate between cyclopia and otocephaly, rests on 3 specimens collected by other authors. They are not adequate to the task of supporting the foundation of a new disease entity; especially since in the 70 or so years that have passed, Blanc's belief that in cyclotia a series of defects would be discovered running parallel with the different varieties of cyclopia and otocephaly has not been vindicated.

Otocephaly in a guinea pig was apparently first reported in this century by Bujard (1919), who noted it in a 5 cm-long fetus. Defects were found only on the head, which was small and had a large median eye. Beneath the eye was a transverse groove uniting the pinnae and the orifices of the external auditory canals. Nose and mouth were absent. The cranium was very small, as was the cranial mass it contained. The brain was not further described. The specimen apparently corresponded to the type opocephaly.

As stated above, definitive studies of otocephaly in guinea pigs were made by Wright and his collaborators, beginning with the preliminary report by Wright and Eaton (1923), in which the condition was classified into a sequence of 12 grades of increasing defectiveness. These grades, later augmented (Wright and Wagner 1934) by several minor exceptional categories, were collectively referred to as otocephaly.

The lowest grades (1–5) were characterized by defects of the lower jaw—micrognathia and agnathia—combined with ventrally approximated or fused ears. In higher grades (6–9) agnathia was joined by eye and brain defects. The highest grades (10–12), lacking most of the face and head, were aprosopics.

Detailed descriptions of the various degrees and types of the condition exhibited by 316 abnormal specimens were given by Wright and Wagner (1934). Another 3 animals, called grade A, had abnormalities only of the upper jaw; they have not been included in what follows. The description of each grade includes or extends the defects of those preceding. Animals of grade 1 sometimes lived for a few days; all others were stillborn or died within a few minutes of birth.

Grade 1 (7.0% of 316): lower jaw short, usually with a median or no incisor. Grade 2 (13.6%): lower jaw reduced in length and width with adjacent parts of skull involved; external ears low set; oral cavity small and atretic; pharynx communicated anteriorly with middle ear cavities. Eyes normal despite aberrant position of zygomatic arches. Grade 3 (18.4%): ear openings separated only by bare skin of ears; mandible absent or reduced to minute proportions; zygomatic arches closely approximated posteriorly. Grade 4 (44.0%): single median ventral ear opening; pharynx in broad communication with single middle ear cavity; ear ossicles of both sides fused; nose and eyes normal; brain appeared normal.

Grade 5, including variants (5.1%): defective upper jaw; usually no mouth or oral cavity; single median or no zygomatic arch; hydrocephalus in one case. This grade showed much diversity in abnormalities of facial skeleton and certain other features. One variant differed superficially from grade 5 in having single median nostril; from higher grades, by complete separation of eyes, though they were variably approximated. Grade 6 (3.5%): single, median nostril; absent premaxilla. Most important difference from preceding grades was condition of brain. All specimens examined had a forebrain consisting of a thickwalled sac with no indication of separation into hemispheres. Outwardly its form was normal, except that it was considerably reduced in size relative to the normal-appearing cerebellum. Two optic nerves emerged from a single large foramen.

Grade 7 (1.3%): eyes partially united below nasal proboscis; no snout between eye and ear openings; forebrain sac further reduced; both optic nerves present in 2 cases examined. Grade 8 (1.3%): single median eye below proboscis; no nostril; middle ear cavity much reduced; fused ear ossicle small. The telencephalon was a small, thickwalled, unconvoluted sac, forming a cup over the diencephalon, but not extending as far as the colliculi; in size about as large as the normal-appearing cerebellum. Single optic nerve to fused eye. Grade 9 (1.6%): single median eye with no supraorbital nasal proboscis or suborbital upper jaw. Forebrain as in grade 8.

Grade 10 (3.2%): no eye; shallow median orbit; brain further reduced anteriorly; no optic nerve. Grade 11 (0.3%): no ear opening, and for first time ears much reduced in size; small skull composed entirely of a small occipital ring and 2 petrosals. Brain consisted solely of a short continuation of the spinal cord, undoubtedly representing part of the medulla. Grade 12 (0.3%): most extreme defect found. Head consisted merely of rounded prominence in front of shoulders, without any orifices, but with a small median external ear at its apex. Cranial cavity largely filled by bulky ear vesicles; no trace of inner ear. Cavity of pharynx communicated anteriorly with esophagus, but neither had an external opening.

Wright and Wagner (1934) noted that the lower jaw was the region most consistently affected, with all but 3 abnormal animals having defective mandible, while in over 80 per cent the defect was restricted to the lower jaw and related parts of the head (grades 1–4). By further analyzing the frequency of abnormality of the various structures involved in this complex of malformations, they concluded that it appeared that all the abnormalities could be traced to a small number of embryonic centers, which in their usual order of frequency were the ventral mandibular arch, frontonasal process, maxillary process, etc.; and that these may in turn be related to inhibition of the anterior medullary plate and associated ectodermal placodes, e.g., through interference with formation and migration of mesectodermal cells from the neural crest.

The genetics of the condition was exhaustively investigated by Wright (1934a, b). Records of 24 inbred strains kept since 1906 showed that otocephaly never occurred in many of them, and only rarely in most of the others, so that the overall incidence in 23 of the strains was less than 0.05 per cent. Most of the otocephalic young, which numbered over 500 several years ago (Wright 1960), appeared in one strain—family 13. In its early generations family 13 had a 1 per cent incidence of the condition but later gave rise to a branch giving 5 per cent in all but one of its sub-branches. The exceptional branch produced about 28 per cent defectives and was maintained at this level for 15 years by selection from high-producing matings (Wright 1960).

The high percentage in this line resulted from a dominant mutation in the 19th generation of inbreeding; but analysis of the voluminous data indicated that the general tendency to defectiveness depended on an interaction of both hereditary and environmental factors. Aside, however, from a slight increase in frequency in small litters and in the winter and early spring, no clue was forthcoming as to what nongenetic mechanisms were acting.

As in sporadic monstrosities of this sort in most other species, about twice as many of the abnormal young were females as were males. But while in man and lower animals sporadic cyclopia and otocephaly are frequently associated with various other congenital malformations, such as cleft lip, polydactyly, anencephaly, etc. (Ballantyne 1904, pp. 400, 427, 430), no such associations were noted in family 13 of guinea pigs. Finally, evidence indicated that certain differences in expression of the condition among various lines might have had genetic bases (Wright 1934a).

The only other instances of (probable) otocephaly in guinea pigs that I have found mention of are 2 cases reported in 1872 by L. B. Thomson (cited by Taruffi 1881–94, vol. 6, p. 428). The animals were aprosopic, with external ears fused at their base. The tympanic cavities were also fused. The presence of an atrophic eye indicated a severe grade of the defect. The brain does not seem to have been described.

The Polydactylous Monster

Wright (1934c, 1935) reported a semidominant gene (symbol *Px*, for pollex) in guinea pigs, causing polydactyly in heterozygotes and a lethal syndrome of congenital malformations in homozygotes. The anomalies were described by Scott (1938). Newborn homozygotes were exencephalic or had an enlarged skull with a soft spot in the parietal region. In the latter case, the lateral and 3rd ventricles were fused into a common, blood-filled cavity, which did not connect with the swollen aqueduct. The cerebral hemispheres were unjoined, the callosal commissure being absent. The olfactory bulbs were rotated sideways. The diencephalon was greatly enlarged and touched the roof of the skull where the brain tissue was thickened. The colliculi and optic nerves were absent. The cerebellum was asymmetrical and lacked the vermis. The medulla was enlarged. No brain defects occurred in heterozygotes.

An embryological study (Scott 1937) revealed nothing startling. The youngest recognizable homozygous *Px/Px* embryos were possibly found in a 19th-day litter, the only sign being an irregular waviness of the neural folds in the region of the cervical flexure.

From these observations Scott (1937) concluded that the *Px/Px* state was caused by accelerated growth of parts developing most rapidly at the time of the first action of the gene (about the 18th day of gestation), i.e., so far as neural parts are concerned, of the roof of the diencephalon and the region of the cervical flexure, and that all defects could be traced to these beginnings.

Other Abnormalities

A guinea pig duplication monstrosity was found by Regnault (cited by Saint-Hilaire 1832–37, vol. 3, p. 129), and another was recorded by Taruffi (1881–94, vol. 2, pp. 310–15). A syncephalus thoracopagus janiceps with one normal face and the other an otocephalic of grade 6, and a duplication monstrosity with single but partly doubled head, were mentioned by Wright (1934a). Previously, Wright (1922) noted that several other sporadic defects had been seen. In family 13, a nonotocephalic animal was found "with a hole in the skull through which the brain protruded," i.e., it was exencephalic. In other families 10 more of the same sort were noted. Three others had an abnormally large head, but were not further described. Hoeve (1938) reported a case of cyclopia in a guinea pig.

Hydrocephalus has apparently not occurred often in this species. In a study of irradiation effects, Strandskov (1932) found 2 hydrocephalic guinea pigs in controls as well as 2 in offspring of irradiated males. Wright and Wagner (1934) stated that from time to time it was seen in otherwise normal guinea pigs of strains not producing otocephaly. Finally, hydrocephalus was noted (Gatz and Allen 1961) in amelic guinea pigs. The cerebrum was thin-walled and without gyri and had enlarged ventricles. Cerebellar folia were absent. Urogenital malformations also occurred. The amelia seemed to have a hereditary basis, possibly recessive.

12

Rabbit

Hydrocephalus
Several patterns of occurrence of hydrocephalus have been noted in rabbits:
epidemic-like occurrence with no discernable cause; inherited types, either
isolated or associated with achondroplasia and other conditions; and sporadic
forms.

Hydrocephalus Epidemics
Hyde (1940) reported an epidemic-like wave of hydrocephalus in a mixture of
American and Dutch Blue rabbits, which began in the fall of 1932, reached
its apex in 1933, and all but disappeared by 1934. The condition occurred in
143/810 offspring of females given injections of various substances during
pregnancy and of females not treated at all. All defective offspring were born
in a laboratory, but none was seen in the colony, situated in an isolated
country district, from which the animals were transported to the laboratory
as needed. Furthermore, females that bore hydrocephalic young in the laboratory had only normal young when returned to the colony. Conditions under
which the rabbits were kept at the 2 places were similar except for the type of
cage used and the fact that the diet fed at the colony was occasionally supplemented with hay and kale.

Hydrocephalus was evident at birth in a few cases, but more often newborn
rabbits were normal with symptoms developing soon afterward. Signs of the
condition varied in degree, but in general the head was enlarged and domeshaped, the fontanelles were widened, and the ventricles were distended with
fluid. In more severe cases the frontal and parietal bones were incompletely
formed and the top of the skull was soft and membranous; such animals
exhibited loss of balance and disturbed motor function, which were temporarily relieved by removal of cerebrospinal fluid, as much as 6 ml being obtained.

The great majority of severe cases died before one week of age. Some of the milder ones survived and were bred but failed to transmit the condition. A few in which hydrocephalus was not suspected were found to have moderate ventricular enlargement at autopsy. In severe cases, ventricular dilatation was so great that the cerebral cortex was only about 1 mm thick. Injection of India ink into the lateral ventricles showed a closed aqueduct in some animals but not in others. In the latter, ink entered the 4th ventricle but not subarachnoid spaces, indicating a block in the basal foramina.

Taking into consideration all the evidence, the condition was not explicable on a hereditary, infectious, or nutritional basis, and was and remains a mystery.

A second outbreak of a possible epidemic of hydrocephalus was recently noted in stocks of rabbits maintained by the Phipps Institute of Philadelphia (Robertson, Samankova, and Ingalls 1966). In a 2-year period 148/1103 (13.4%) young were born with hydrocephalus, cleft palate, or both, the last group being the most common (45%). The defects did not appear to have a simple genetic etiology. The hydrocephalus was not described, except for the remark that in all cases it was internal.

Hereditary Hydrocephalus

Rosa (1946) described a hydrocephalus that behaved as though due to a simple autosomal semidominant gene with reduced penetrance. The breed in which it was found was not stated. The condition was often recognizable at birth by the presence of a cranial vault wider and more convex than normal. In severely affected offspring the vault was soft and easily depressed on palpation, while in others these phenomena were less marked, and positive identification was not always possible. The convexity increased after birth and reached its maximum at about one month of age. But from this time the hydrocephalus subsided, and abnormal animals that reached adulthood were of normal size and reproduced well. But they remained recognizably abnormal because of a wide cranium, irregularities in the sagittal suture, and the frequent presence of ocular defects, which were considered to be secondary to the hydrocephalus. While some of the eye defects (microphthalmia) could conceivably have been associated with the hydrocephalus, others (e.g., coloboma of iris and choroid) are less easily explained in this manner.

Upon dissection, the condition was diagnosed as internal hydrocephalus. The cerebral hemispheres were dilated, both lateral and 3rd ventricles being involved. It was felt that the condition was due to a disturbance in development of the aqueduct, but this aspect was not investigated.

The author supposed that severely affected animals were homozygous for the mutant gene and that those with less obvious defects were heterozygotes; and, furthermore, that some of the latter were not recognizably defective and thus constituted a class of normal overlaps. He also postulated the existence of genes modifying the expression of the character.

Genetic evidence supporting this scheme was fragmentary. The appearance of the abnormality in offspring of outcrosses of a mildly affected, presumably heterozygous, male to several unrelated females makes it difficult to doubt the working of a dominant factor. The crosses produced 25/76 hydrocephalic young, which is 68 per cent of the number expected on the basis of a dominant —a deficiency that the author explained as due to incomplete penetrance. Crosses between presumably heterozygous animals produced 14/24 hydrocephalic offspring, which represents a penetrance of 78 per cent. Far poorer results were obtained from crosses of presumably heterozygous males to their apparently normal sisters, since but 2/17 abnormal young resulted. The author explained this great deficiency by invoking the effects of dominant modifying genes. More valuable than such *ad hoc* reasoning would have been a more ambitious gathering of data.

Hydrocephalus in Dwarfism and Achondroplasia

The effects of a semidominant gene (symbol *Dw*) producing proportionate dwarfism in Polish rabbits were described by Greene, Hu, and Brown (1934), Rosahn and Greene (1935), and Greene (1940). At birth heterozygotes had a moderately reduced body size while homozygotes were more severely affected and usually died within 4 days. The head of homozygotes was round and bombose and the skull was enlarged. These signs persisted in 4 survivors. Frequently the symptoms were so marked they suggested hydrocephalus, but no increase in cerebrospinal fluid or gross abnormalities of the brain were apparently present (Greene 1940). A dwarf mutation discovered by Kröning (1939) in German Ermine rabbits was very similar to (according to Robinson 1958, possibly identical with) Greene's mutant.

Nachtsheim (1937a, 1939) briefly described a lethal condition in mixed white Viennese and Dutch rabbits due to homozygosity for an incompletely dominant gene (called nanus and symbolized *nan* by Nachtsheim, and called Dahlem and symbolized *da* by Robinson 1958). It consisted of proportionate dwarfism accompanied by hydrocephalus and also included short upper jaw, which led to defects of lower incisors. The lifespan of dwarfs could be extended by administration of an anterior pituitary preparation (Preloban), but only to little more than 21 days of age.

Nachtsheim did not clearly state whether the hydrocephalus was congenital, but it seems that once it was established, its severity quickly increased. Even in animals living to 3 weeks the body and skull remained small, and the cranium had extensive unossified areas with large holes. An anatomical study of the hydrocephalus apparently was not made. Schnecke (1941) found that heterozygosity for this gene ($+/da$) combined with the Rex condition (r_1/r_1)

produced phenotypic dwarfism, probably due, according to Robinson (1958), to enhancement of the mild lethal tendency of the Rex gene.

Another form of proportionate dwarfism, produced by a recessive gene (symbol *zw*, for Zwergwuchs), was studied by Degenhardt (1960*b*) in an inbred line of Hermelin rabbits. Associated with the condition were some brain abnormalities: defective gyration of the cerebrum and both internal and external hydrocephalus, i.e., dilatation of the ventricular system and expansion of subarachnoid spaces. Also found were wide open fontanelle in the area of the sagittal suture and ossification defects in the parietal bones. In other forms of proportionate dwarfism there were apparently no defects of the central nervous system (Sawin 1955).

Two achondroplasias are known in rabbits (Sawin and Crary 1964). The first was caused by a recessive gene (symbol *ac*), lethal in homozygotes, which almost certainly originated in a Havana stock (Brown and Pearce 1945). The head of newborn achondroplastics was broad and square with a pronounced calvaria that frequently protruded in the posterior portion. These signs suggested hydrocephalus, but excess cerebrospinal fluid was found in only 2 cases (Pearce and Brown 1945*a, b*). In the second form of achondroplasia, caused by an incompletely dominant gene (symbol *Da*, for Dachs) there was no indication at all of hydrocephalus (Crary and Sawin 1952; Sawin and Crary 1957).

Hydrocephalus in Osteopetrosis

Pearce and Brown (1948) and Pearce (1950) described an osteopetrosis, first observed in progeny of purebred Dutch rabbits, which was inherited as a simple autosomal recessive trait. Internal hydrocephalus occurred in a few affected animals. In some it was present at birth, but in most it developed during the first week of life. In the most unmistakable cases, progressive domelike expansion of the calvaria occurred over a period of a few days. The hydrocephalus sometimes gradually regressed and only minor degrees of it were found at autopsy. Hydrocephalus was also found in a few animals that were not suspected of having it during life. Even in definite cases, i.e., those in which the diagnosis was made during life and confirmed at autopsy, variable degrees of hydrocephalus were found. The brain and meninges were normal, except for the ventricular dilatation. Seemingly associated symptoms, e.g., exophthalmos and uncoordinated and athetoid movements, were apparently unrelated to the hydrocephalus.

Other Hydrocephalus

Variations in cranial shape resulting from craniosynostosis were studied by Greene (1933). Hydrocephalus in any form was not associated with oxycephaly or trigonocephaly. But internal hydrocephalus was occasionally found in plagiocephaly, in which case the otherwise normal side was bombose and showed numerous areas of deficient calcification, while the fused side showed nothing but its characteristic deformity. Although not common in scapho-cephaly, hydrocephalus was unusually frequent in the noncraniosynostotic littermates of one line. The brain of hydrocephalic individuals was not described. The brain in all these variations of the skull, although apparently not changed in size, was modified in shape to conform to that of the altered cranial cavity.

Sawin (1955) illustrated a litter of newborn rabbits with various degrees of muscle contracture; some of the offspring also had hydrocephalus, which may or may not have been another effect of the gene causing the muscular abnormality.

Spina Bifida

Hammond (personal communication), in unpublished observations (also cited by Grüneberg 1947, p. 35, and by Nachtsheim 1958, p. 332), noted spina bifida in a line of inbred rabbits. The condition, a simple recessive character, ranged from complete opening of the spine from head to tail to small pustules on the head or rump. Severely abnormal young were usually born alive but died soon afterward. Those with minor manifestations were raised to adult-hood but had tremors and could not be gotten to mate. Photographs of 3 of Hammond's newborn rabbits with different grades of the severe defect were reproduced by Nachtsheim (*ibid.*).

External and histological features of myeloschisis in a term fetus were described by Patten (1953). Exposed neural tissue was almost completely disintegrated.

Sawin and Crary (1955) observed scoliosis in 41 rabbits of several un-related races over a number of generations. The condition varied in severity and in the location and magnitude of the area affected, and included absence of neural arches (i.e., spina bifida occulta). At first the scoliosis appeared to be sporadic but later seemed to be due to homozygosity for 2 recessive genes. More recently this hypothesis was found to be untenable (Sawin and Crary 1964).

Crary, Fox, and Sawin (1966) discovered a form of spina bifida in rabbits of the Dutch belted AC stock, which carried the *ac* (achondroplasia) gene. The defect appeared to be transmitted as a simple autosomal recessive trait, governed by a gene symbolized *sb*. The abnormality affected the entire spine, sometimes extending from the posterior part of the skull into the tail. All affected young were stillborn. The characteristics of the lesion were as follows. In most cases the neural tube was closed and dorsally was in direct contact with a thin, transparent layer of skin. The condition of the meninges was not mentioned. In cleared specimens, it was seen that vertebral spines were absent and vertebral arches flared out laterally. Hence the defect can be classified as an extensive spina bifida occulta. Occasionally open areas were seen in the neural tube, but these appeared to result from secondary degeneration. Numerous other malformations occurred in spina bifidous animals, viz., cleft lip; cleft palate; skeletal, cardiovascular, respiratory, and urogenital anomalies; 3 cases of acephaly; and 3 of exencephaly. Exencephaly was also seen in 5 *ac/ac* homozygotes, and encephalocele in 1/159 otherwise normal young.

Sporadic Malformations of Various Types

Sporadic congenital malformations of the central nervous system are apparently not uncommon in some stocks of rabbits while in others they are far rarer. Defective rabbits and hares have been observed throughout the ages, and Saint-Hilaire early in the last century cited the experiences of several writers as well as his own with animals of these species with cyclopia, otocephaly, and various types of duplication abnormalities (1832–37, vol. 2, pp. 386, 399, 404, 426; vol. 3, pp. 128–29, 148–49, 357). At one point he remarked (*ibid.*, vol. 2, p. 404) that he had seen 2 cyclopic rabbits in the same litter. Other older writers who found or cited cases of rabbits or hares with these anomalies are Vrolik (1854, pl. 58, figs. 1–5); Rayer (1863); Gurlt (1877, p. 56); Panum (1878); Taruffi (1881–94, vol. 2, pp. 310–15; vol. 8, p. 393); and Hannover (1882–84, pp. 123, 160). An aprosopic hare was found by Thomson (cited by Taruffi 1881–94, vol. 6, p. 428). An anomalous canal in a fetal rabbit brain was observed by Breglia (1894–95).

These and other malformations have been recorded with some frequency in our century. Aplasia of the fore- and midbrain associated with bilateral anophthalmia was noted in a 12th-day rabbit embryo (Kubik 1923). Pickard (1933) remarked that otocephaly was more prevalent in certain stocks of fancy English rabbits than in others, which suggested that it was a heritable defect. Robinson (1958), citing unpublished findings of Pickard, stated that the latter found 3 cases of otocephaly in 16 years. Three cases of otocephaly were seen in a line of chinchilla rabbits (Menschow 1934). Only the external appearance of the condition was described and that very briefly. Ancel (1950, p. 240) mentioned a newborn rabbit with triocephaly (a severe grade of otocephaly), in which the pituitary was lacking. A cyclopic hare with a large, single, median eye and a large, supraoptic proboscis was figured by Stupka (1933). The forebrain was severely malformed. Rosa (1946) noted one case of exencephaly. During a 35-year period, Nachtsheim (1958, pp. 330–32) examined about 40,000 rabbits, but found very few with sporadic defects. One individual with a proboscoid structure had arhinencephaly. A case of meningoencephalocele was seen by Frauchigher (1959). Duplication monsters in rabbits were recorded by Engel (1931) and Cock (1950), and in a hare, by Fischer (1929).

Sawin (1955) noted hydrocephalus in various races, but in no case did it appear with a clear-cut hereditary pattern. There also occurred, during an

18-year period, 58 cases of spina bifida in several stocks, more than half of which occurred during the last $3\frac{1}{2}$ years of this interval. Furthermore, the proportion of affected individuals in certain breeds seemed to increase considerably, although there was no conscious effort to achieve this result. Sawin (1955) stated, somewhat ambiguously, that of the later-discovered cases, a substantial number consisted of those that would be classified as cranium bifidum.

Chai and Degenhardt (1962) collected data from 2 partially inbred stocks, BRY and CA, and found hydrocephalus in 6/167 and 0/185, and exencephaly in 3/167 and 2/185, respectively. The hydrocephalus was not described. In exencephaly there was complete absence of parietal bones and reduced size of frontal and occipital bones. A case of complete absence of the head above the mandibles (called cephalodysplasia) was also found. Since other defects were also more common in BRY than in CA animals, the results suggested that the stocks were genetically different. The authors discussed the possible bases of this difference: differential loss of developmental homeostasis accompanying inbreeding; new single mutations; and a multigenic interpretation.

Baird *et al.* (1964) saw 52 malformations in an unstated breed of rabbits. The number of abnormal young and the total number examined were not mentioned. The malformations, none of which was described, included anencephaly, cephalocele, hydrocephalus, and hydranencephaly. Epidemiological studies of the possible genetic, viral, nutritional, toxic, hormonal, seasonal, and other factors were unsuccessful in establishing the etiology of the malformations.

In several studies only few defective offspring were uncovered. Loosli (1964) examined about 7000 rabbits of the Füllinsdorf breed from 1961 to 1963 and noted 3 malformed young: one posterior duplication, one anencephaly, and one microcephaly with a scalp defect. Tuchmann-Duplessis and Mercier-Parot (1964*f*), in an unstated breed, recorded an acephalic offspring and a microcephalic one with gross deficiency of the top of the head. Yeary (1964) found 3 hydrocephalic offspring in a litter of 4 from a Dutch Belted female. K. H. Harper (personal communication) examined 3951 late fetal rabbits (of unspecified breed); defects of the central nervous system noted were one case each of anencephaly, hydrocephalus, cyclopia, and craniorachischisis.

In distinction to these observations, which were made on newborn or near-term animals, Sawin and Crary (1964) reported the incidence of malformations discovered in 12th- to 30th-day rabbit fetuses of a number of races. Out of 2640 examined, there were 18 with hydrocephalus, 6 with exencephaly, 3 with acephaly, and one with microcephaly. Certain racial differences were noted. Cozens (1965) examined 3935 fetuses of the New Zealand white breed on the 29th day of gestation and found 34 (0.9%) with abnormalities of the skeleton or external form. Among the defective young were 2 anencephalics, one acephalic, and one cyclopic.

Syringomyelia

This condition was discovered in descendants of a Rex rabbit imported from France to Germany. Clinically it consisted of asymmetrical spastic paralysis usually affecting only one leg, more often hindlimbs than forelimbs. Paralysis most often appeared between 4 and 6 months of age, sometimes much earlier or much later. Its course varied considerably, and remissions sometimes occurred. Early onset was often accompanied by greater severity.

The disease was first observed in 1927 but was not reported for several years (Nachtsheim 1931). Further descriptions and results followed (Nachtsheim 1937*b*). Genetic studies indicated the condition to be due, essentially, to a main gene, in general recessive, which interacted with a group of modifiers to produce variable expressivity. Later, Nachtsheim (1958, p. 344) stated that exogenous as well as endogenous modifying factors were involved and that the interaction between them made it hopeless to demonstrate a Mendelian mode of inheritance, especially since clinically symptomless animals were occasionally found to have anatomical defects, and those without the latter were sometimes clinically affected.

The anatomical basis of the disease was established by Ostertag (1930*a, b*, 1934). Three grades of severity were noted, but in general the abnormalities consisted of extensive cavitations in the substance of the entire hind spinal cord, hydromyelia, imperfect closure of the dorsal raphe of the cord, as well as progressive gliosis.

13

Cat

Congenital malformations of, or involving, the central nervous system have been recorded with an appreciable frequency in cats. But the gross malformations that have been the main concern of most other chapters of this book—such as hydrocephalus, exencephaly, and spina bifida—apparently seldom occur in cats or, at any rate, have not often been reported.

Hydrocephalus

Hydrocephalus in the apparent absence of other defects of the brain has rarely been noted in cats. Milks (1918), in an 11-line report, mentioned a litter of 6 kittens, 4 of which displayed loss of coordination. Autopsied at about 8 weeks of age, 2 of them were found to have hydrocephalus, which was not described. The condition of the cerebellum was not mentioned.

Fankhauser (1959) noted a 10-day-old kitten with clinically-established hydrocephalus. It had a balloon-like distention of the cranium with corresponding reduction of the face. The cranium was paper-thin, and the cerebral hemispheres consisted of fluid-filled, dilated sacs. Sections showed that the aqueduct was divided into several narrow channels, i.e., was forked.

In a series of necropsies (Blahser and Labie 1964), hydrocephalus was encountered in certain families of Persian cats; but the frequency was not stated. The animals usually died at birth because of injury to the thin bones of the enlarged head. In all cases the lateral ventricles were greatly dilated and full of clear fluid, but the 3rd and 4th ventricles were normal.

Hydrocephalus of one or both lateral cerebral ventricles was found in several cats with cerebellar defects (Cornwall 1927; Verhaart 1948; Carpenter and Harter 1954; Gillilan and Lockard 1956; Frauchiger and Fankhauser 1957, pp. 38, 40; Kilham and Margolis 1966).

Exencephaly

Exencephaly has similarly seldom been recorded. Daubenton (cited by Taruffi 1881–94, vol. 6, p. 142) described a cat with "hemicephaly." Two newborn cats with encephalocele were mentioned by Otto. One (Otto 1824, p. 159) had a small hole in the left frontal area, from which protruded a liquid-filled extension of the left ventricle. The second (Otto, cited by Taruffi 1881–94, vol. 8, p. 246) had a small cranium with bilateral frontal hernias, formed by saclike lobes of the corresponding hemispheres. This animal also had cleft lip and palate. Dareste (1852) described a posteriorly duplicated newborn cat with a deformed head, which was single except for a small, parasitic, supernumerary lower jaw. The vault of the cranium was replaced by a large opening through which the base of the skull was visible; the animal was thus apparently anencephalic. Continuous with this defect was a large opening in the cervical area, representing a cleft condition of the spinal elements of the nape. An acephalic cat was seen by Gurlt (1877, p. 2). Weber (1946a) included a cat with "absent brain" in a table of abnormal animals discovered in the Canton of Bern.

Malformations of The Cerebellum

Judging from the number of observations recorded in the veterinary and medical literature, cerebellar defects are probably the commonest type of malformation of the central nervous system in cats. The greatest interest in these abnormalities has centered about their morphology, histopathology, the behavior they are associated with, and the relations among these phenomena. However, since this book is limited to considering gross aspects of anomalies of the brain and spinal cord, it is the macroscopic morphology of the conditions that will primarily be discussed. In addition, the possible etiology and congenital nature of the defects will be considered.

Rumpf's (1885) is the earliest article on the subject of cerebellar defects in cats that I am aware of. He examined an 8-week-old cat with a diagnosis of "Kleinhirnerkrankung," which showed the same behavior patterns from the first day of independent movement. At autopsy, symmetrical overall reduction in size of the cerebellum was found.

Herringham and Andrewes (1888) described a litter of 4 young whose mother was a half bred Persian cat. All showed similar signs of nervous disease, 2 when they started to walk, and the other 2 when a few weeks old. The first 2 were killed when young but not examined. The latter 2, which were probably less severely affected, were killed and examined, one at 4 months of age and the other at 8 months. In both, the cerebellum was very small, especially the vermis, which hardly projected at all beyond the hemispheres and did not reach the calamus scriptorius. The smallness of the cerebellum left a gap between it and the cerebrum through which the colliculi were seen. The cerebrum and cord were normal.

Krohn's (1892) cat, one of a litter of 2, suddenly showed ataxic signs at 3 months of age, which persisted until 11 months, when it was killed. Examination of the central nervous system revealed only that the cerebellum was slightly smaller than normal and seemed shrunken.

Russell (1895*a*) did not state how old his subject was when its nervous symptoms first appeared, nor its age when he examined it. The whole cerebellum was smaller than normal, but in addition the right hemisphere was further reduced in all dimensions, being about one-third the size of the left one. This right-sided atrophy extended to other parts of the brain as well. Thus the right half of the pons and medulla were somewhat reduced in size; the right colliculi were about one-third the size of the left; the right cerebral hemisphere appeared generally a little smaller than the left, but without special defect; and the right cranial nerves were smaller than the left ones.

Langelaan (1907) painstakingly described the behavior of an ataxic cat. It exhibited abnormal behavior soon after birth and was recognized as ataxic when it began to walk. At autopsy the cerebral gyri were flat and the sulci narrow and shallow. The cerebellum was very small and embryonic in its general features. Histopathological study showed that only the cerebellar cortex was affected.

Jelgersma (1917) described cerebellar atrophy in 3 cats, 2 of which were from the same litter. The latter 2 were killed at 3 months of age, the third at about one year. In the younger animals the cerebellum was markedly reduced in size, making the hind poles of the cerebral hemispheres visible. The macroscopic state of the third animal's brain was not explicitly mentioned.

Poenaru and Vechiu (1922) reported an affected cat from a litter of 5, 2 of which were stillborn or died soon after birth; the mother had previously had a litter that were all stillborn. The principal symptom of the defective animal was congenital cerebellar ataxia. It was killed when 3 months old, but anatomical findings, if any, were not described.

Cornwall (1927, 1929) examined a 2-month-old kitten, one of a litter of 4, that showed pronounced nervous symptoms from birth. The cerebellum was reduced in all dimensions, but more so anteroposteriorly than transversely. The cerebrum was also defective, in the right frontal and parietal areas. The right ventricle was dilated and lacked, or was deficient in, ependymal lining cells. In many other regions the ependymal cells were grouped in clusters forming irregular nodular masses. The left ventricle was not dilated but also contained some cellular changes. Another member of the litter was stillborn and greatly retarded in development, and a third died soon after birth.

Cobb's (1928) kitten, one of a litter of 3, had a peculiar gait that appeared when it first began to walk. It died at 13 months. The cerebellum was distinctly aplastic and symmetrically small in all dimensions and had a simplified lobular arrangement. Its general appearance indicated aplasia of the vermis, an impression that was strengthened by the fact that the pons was extremely small. Chaillous, Robin, and Mollaret (1931) reported a 3-month-old cat with nervous signs and cataract from birth. Apparently no dissection was made.

Brouwer (1934) saw 2 siblings with a striking cerebellar functional disorder syndrome, which apparently was manifested soon after birth. One, killed at about a month of age, had isolated olivopontocerebellar hypoplasia. The second died at 22 months of age and was found (Finley 1935) to have a smaller cerebellum than normal, most marked in the hemispheres. The rest of the central nervous system was entirely normal. The type and degree of hypoplasia in the 2 animals were remarkably similar. Sholl, Sales, and Langham (1939) described a 2-week-old kitten that had never been able to walk. The cerebellum was greatly reduced in size, leaving a considerable space through which the colliculi were visible. A 2½-month-old cat examined by Panu, Mihailesco, and Adamşteanu (1939) presented a very much reduced cerebellum. The cerebral gyri were few and thick, and the lateral ventricles were slightly dilated.

Spuhler (1944) reported 2 ataxic siblings; the third cat in the litter was stillborn and was discarded. Both had symmetrically reduced cerebellum with absence of the posterior vermis, but the defects were somewhat more severe in one than in the other. The cerebral hemispheres were slightly small and contained fewer, smaller, and flatter convolutions than normal.

Blood (1946) saw 2 abnormal kittens, each the only affected animal in its litter. No breeding history was available. Peculiarities of gait and posture were noted as soon as they began to walk. At autopsy, the only macroscopic abnormality was obvious smallness of the cerebellum. Schut (1946) described defects found in an adult cat. The brain had normal dimensions except for bilateral symmetrical reduction in size of the cerebellum. Since all cerebellar lobes were identified, the reduction did not appear due to agenesis but possibly to atrophy. Verlinde and Ojemann (1946) observed 6 young cats with cerebellar hypoplasia, 3 of which occurred in the same litter. These authors also cited a similar finding by E. Gyarmati, who described cerebellar defects in 2 cats from the same litter.

Verhaart (1948) examined the brain of an 8-year-old cat that had exhibited ataxic symptoms from the age of at least one month. The cerebellum showed a general atrophy. The cerebrum was grossly normal, except that the right hemisphere was somewhat small. In transverse section, the right lateral ventricle was seen to be much distended, and the white matter over the right pyramid within the pons and the medulla was absent. Frauchiger and Fankhauser (1949, p. 140) briefly mentioned a 3-month-old, congenitally ataxic Angora kitten with severe cerebellar hypoplasia.

Verlinde (1949) advanced the possibility that congenital cerebellar ataxia and marked histological cerebellar alterations in 2 cats were caused by latent infection of the pregnant females with the virus of infectious feline enteritis. Fankhauser (1955), however, stated that he had no evidence for such events occurring in his cases of nonpurulent inflammatory processes leading to cerebellar changes in cats.

Carpenter and Penny (1952) reported the sudden onset and persistence of truncal ataxia in a cat about 5 years old. The cerebellum was greatly reduced in size; the anterior lobe seemed normal, but the pyramis, uvula, and hemispheres were greatly reduced. There was no apparent clue to the condition's etiology and pathogenesis. Scheidy (1953) noted a cerebellar behavioral syndrome that appeared shortly after birth in 3 littermates. Grossly identical findings were seen in all 3 when autopsied at about one year of age. There was marked symmetrical cerebellar hypoplasia, the organ being about one-quarter to one-third normal size. The only divisions macroscopically visible were the vermis and hemispheres.

Collet *et al.* (1954) found cerebellar defects in 3 cats. The first 2 were siblings from a litter of 3, the third of which was found dead at or near term. They both showed nervous symptoms at 6 to 8 weeks of age. They were killed by a ferocious dog when 4 years, 3 months old. The first had a volumetric reduction of the cerebellum, which was more or less restricted to the hemispheres. The second had a similar condition, but the vermis was more involved and the hemispheres were more atrophied. The third cat was 4 months old when seen, but also probably had a congenital disorder. The cerebellum was atrophied, but in this case the vermis and hemispheres were equally affected.

Kobozieff and Gruner (1954) studied several litters in which there were defective animals. Two litters were produced by a small female bred to her father. The first consisted of 4 kittens that were killed when they became weak, but which were apparently not examined further. The second litter also contained 4 animals. Two, which manifested nervous signs early, were discarded. The others, as in Herringham and Andrewes' (1888) experience, developed symptoms somewhat later. One was killed at 5 months, but again was apparently not dissected. The fourth, killed at 22 months, was autopsied. A third litter, produced by a different female, also a dwarf, contained 3 kittens. One was stillborn; the second manifested a cerebellar syndrome, but was not kept; the third showed later-appearing signs, and was autopsied at 2 months of age. In both autopsied specimens identical abnormalities were found: intense cerebellar atrophy. Compared to controls, the cerebellum was volumetrically reduced to scarcely one-tenth of normal, with vermis and hemispheres both affected. In the 2, the cerebrum was rather small, although well proportioned.

Gillilan and Lockard (1954) and Lockard and Gillilan (1956) described 5 defective cats. The first, one of a litter of 3, apparently began acting abnormally when about one to two weeks old, and died at one year of age. The cerebellum was greatly reduced in size in all dimensions exposing the posterior medullary velum and the inferior colliculi. The cerebrum was slightly small and had somewhat maldeveloped convolutions. The lateral ventricles were greatly enlarged at the expense of white matter. The 3rd ventricle was irregularly shaped, but the aqueduct and 4th ventricle were fairly normal. The corpus callosum was very small. The second and third animals, killed at about 4 years of age, were littermates that had been abnormal since birth. In both, the entire brain was smaller than normal, being foreshortened; but in addition, parts of the cerebellum were further decreased in size. The pons was very small in width and bulk.

The last 2 animals, a male and a female, were bred and had 2 litters. The sole survivor of their first litter, a male, was the fourth of the authors' cases. The second litter, probably containing 2 offspring, was immediately eaten by the mother and her idiot firstborn. The authors thus assumed this litter was abnormal. Of course, the mother may just have been driven to distraction by her young, unbalanced son. He, too, had a small brain but had not, by 14 months of age, grown to adult size. The brain was also foreshortened, and the cerebellum and pons were small but without gross defects.

The fifth cat, unrelated to any of the others, showed early, marked lack of balance. Autopsied at one year of age, it had a small cerebellum, the hemispheres being especially affected. The cerebrum was normal.

Koch, Fischer, and Stubbe (1955) studied several abnormal cats. The work of these authors will be discussed below, since it is the only attempt, however inadequate, that has been made to study the genetics of cerebellar disease in cats. Fankhauser (1955) noted 6 cats with cerebellar atrophy.

Carpenter and Harter (1956) added to the record 5 defective kittens from 3 litters, all of which displayed unequivocal evidence of cerebellar deficits from or soon after birth. In the first, one of a litter of 4, there was marked reduction in cerebellar size, which permitted the colliculi and posterior part of the rhomboid fossa to be seen without retraction. The cerebellum, in fact, merely consisted of a small cystic piece of tissue, lacking division into vermis and hemispheres, lying on the dorsal surface of the brainstem. Folial pattern was completely lacking. Although the cerebral hemispheres were normal in size and configuration, there was bilateral symmetrical dilatation of the lateral ventricles.

Another 3 were littermates whose fourth sibling was normal. One had a markedly small cerebellum with the hemispheres most affected. Viewed from above, the inferior colliculi and lower part of the rhomboid fossa were seen simultaneously. The second had a brain grossly like that of the first, but with a somewhat larger cerebellum. The vermis was less affected than the hemispheres. The third was more severely ataxic than its littermates. The cerebellum, especially the hemispheres, was greatly reduced in size. The posterior lobe was very small, and thus the caudal part of the rhomboid fossa was easily seen.

The last kitten, also from a litter of 4, had a grossly normal brain except for a slight reduction in the transverse diameter of the cerebellum, which was due to underdevelopment of the hemispheres. The brain of a nonataxic littermate said to have had an aberrant gait appeared normal but displayed some histological peculiarities.

Frauchiger and Fankhauser (1957) listed 8 cats with cerebellar atrophy in their collection of defective animals (pp. 38, 232–33), and included photographs of a 1-month-old cat brain that was megalencephalic, pachygyric, and hydrocephalic, and whose cerebellum was hypoplastic (p. 40), and of another of the same age with lissencephaly and hypoplasia of the cerebellum (p. 41). Kilham and Margolis (1966) found a grossly hypoplastic cerebellum in a 5- to 6-week-old markedly ataxic kitten. The other 3 in the litter showed similar neurological symptoms. In a brief report, Escobar and Dow (1966) described a kitten with hypoplasia of the entire cerebellum.

Despite cerebellar abnormalities in cats thus being rather common and having been recognized and investigated for over 80 years, the etiology of the condition (or, as is more likely, the etiologies of the conditions) remains all but unknown.

Among the cases described, many have been familial, i.e., involved more than one affected animal per litter (Herringham and Andrewes 1888; Jelgersma 1917; Cornwall 1927—possibly; Brouwer 1934; Spuhler 1944; Scheidy 1953; Collet *et al.* 1954; Kobozieff and Gruner 1954; Koch, Fischer, and Stubbe 1955; Carpenter and Harter 1956; Lockard and Gillilan 1956). While this fact alone is hardly conclusive proof that the condition may sometimes be gene mediated, it suggests such an interpretation.

This possibility is reinforced by several bits of evidence. Kobozieff and Gruner (1954) obtained 2 litters from a dwarf female crossed to her father. The first litter consisted of 4 kittens that were "weak"; but they seem not to have been autopsied and thus cannot be considered abnormal with certainty. In the second litter, all 4 had symptoms indicating cerebellar disease. For some reason, though, only one was dissected; its cerebellum was very small.

Abnormal animals were bred by several investigators, with the production of both affected and normal offspring. Cobb (1928) mated an abnormal male to 4 different normal females; the 12 offspring all behaved normally and had normal brains. Verhaart (1948) stated that of all the progeny of his ataxic cat, only one grandchild manifested the same disturbances. Collet *et al.* (1954) bred 2 abnormal siblings, apparently to unrelated cats; they each had several litters, but all offspring were normal. Lockard and Gillilan (1956) obtained 2 litters from crosses of an abnormal female to her abnormal littermate brother. The sole survivor of the first litter had abnormalities of the cerebellum, but they were not as severe as those of his parents. The second litter was eaten as soon as delivered and may thus also have contained affected offspring.

Koch, Fischer, and Stubbe (1955) investigated a litter of 4 cats, 3 (1 male, 2 females) of which showed severe signs of congenital cerebellar ataxia, but whose anatomical basis does not appear to have been ascertained. The ataxic male was crossed to (1) an affected sister, (2) a phenotypically normal daughter from the first mating, and (3) a normal, unrelated female; seemingly a single litter from each mating was considered sufficient.

Many of the young in the litters of the first 2 crosses were stillborn or died soon after birth (the total born was not stated). The survivors (their number also not given) showed no ataxic symptoms. Various abnormalities of brain, eyes, skeleton, and viscera were found in the kittens that were dead at birth or died soon afterwards, but whether any defects occurred in the survivors was apparently not determined. The brain defects consisted of overall reduction in size, absence of cerebral and cerebellar convolutions, symmetrical but underdeveloped cerebellum, and in one animal, absence of the vermis.

The third cross (ataxic male to unrelated normal female) resulted in 6 offspring. One died at 5 days of age but was free of symptoms indicating ataxia. The other 5 showed extreme ataxic signs, beginning in one case at 3 days of age. An especially small and severely affected male, which died at 7 days of age, had a slightly asymmetrical cerebrum, but apparently the cerebellum was macroscopically normal. The 4 survivors continued being ataxic until 10 to 12 weeks of age, when the signs slowly disappeared; but they remained somewhat dwarfed. It was not stated whether the brains of these 4 were examined.

On the basis of these scanty, ambiguous, and incomplete findings the authors attempted to erect a theory—that ataxia may be due to a dominant gene with variable expressivity and reduced penetrance. Hence, the possibly hereditary nature of the disease is still unproven.

Recently, Kilham and Margolis (1966), on the basis of an experimental study, suggested that feline ataxia may be of viral origin. An agent was isolated from the cerebellum of a spontaneously ataxic kitten, which, when administered to other kittens or ferrets, induced marked degrees of cerebellar hypoplasia and ataxia after a 4- to 5-week period. Especially severe cerebellar damage was found in a newborn kitten following in utero inoculation 3 weeks previously. The transmitting agent was filterable and heat resistant and was neutralized by sera from kittens convalescent from the spontaneous disease. Especially pertinent was the finding that the agent spread spontaneously from infected to control kittens. In a later report (Johnson, Margolis, and Kilham 1967), the agent was identified with feline panleucopenia virus.

Spina Bifida

Vertebral defects and occasional spina bifida are apparently not uncommon in cats with short or absent tail (see Robinson 1959, p. 313, for references to earlier observations). In a recent study, Kerruish (1964), upon examining a large number of Manx cats, found that quite a high proportion of the tailless ones had symptoms indicating lack of control over hindleg movement, and urination or defecation, or both. Animals with a "stumpy" tail did not show these involvements, while usually only tailless animals with a distinct hollow at the base of the spine had uncoordinated hindleg movement. The spinal cord of tailless kittens ended at the tip of the sacrum, and the cauda equina could not be seen because the nerve roots all passed directly sideways. Among the Manx cats examined (number unstated), 3 had conditions resembling spina bifida: one with defects of dorsal elements of the sacrum (spina bifida occulta), one with swelling of the dura (meningocele) in some areas, and one with a similarly placed cyst. Todd (1964) also reported much the same situation, and found at least 2 cases of spina bifida in Manx animals.

It may be of interest to discuss what is known of the inheritance of taillessness in cats. A summary (Robinson 1959, pp. 313–14) of the few earlier studies of the genetics of anury and brachyury in cats disclosed that the evidence regarding its mode or modes of transmission was contradictory and that the problem was far from resolved by the 1950's.

Some recent studies with Manx cats may have partly clarified this topic. Howell and Siegel (1963) showed that different tail lengths in Manx cats are apparently due to incomplete penetrance (*sic*; the authors seem to have meant variable expressivity) of a gene, which Todd's (1961) work indicated to be an autosomal dominant.

Todd (1961) remarked that despite years of selection aimed at producing a "pure" (i.e., consistently tailless) strain of Manx cats, almost all Manxes tested behaved as if heterozygous for taillessness. Crosses of tailless males and females led to litters of reduced size (others reported the same thing; see references in Todd 1961, and Howell and Siegel 1963); and of the offspring of known heterozygotes, 55 were tailless and 27 tailed, an almost perfect 2 : 1 ratio (although by a miscalculation Todd failed to perceive this proportion). These facts (reduced litter size and 2 : 1 ratio) appear to indicate the working of an autosomal gene producing taillessness in heterozygotes and prenatal death in homozygotes.

It would certainly be of great interest to learn the cause of intrauterine death of the presumed homozygotes. It may turn out, in the light of the fact that among viable tailless Manxes some degree of spinal dysraphism occurs (Kerruish 1964; Todd 1964), that homozygotes are similarly but more severely affected and that this accounts for their prenatal elimination.

A different spinal defect was reported by Frye and McFarland (1965). A 1-day-old crossbred Siamese kitten had an open mid-dorsal lesion extending from the midthorax to the sacrum. The tail was apparently of normal length for the animal's size (about 25% smaller than its normal littermates). The lesion was moist and glistening, was bright red, and had smooth edges where the skin and fur ended. The kitten was active, but its hindquarters were immobile and were dragged along as it crawled.

It was killed when 3 days old and further examined. There was no evidence of spinal-cord tissue within the area of the lesion. But it was possible to pass a thin probe into the anterior end of the spinal canal. No further description of the defect was given, and hence the composition of the external surface of the lesion is not known. It may be guessed, however, that it consisted of an epithelialized meningeal sac and therefore corresponded to myelomeningocele as seen in children (Warkany, Wilson, and Geiger 1958).

Cyclopia

A fair number of cyclopic cats have been discovered. Two cases, of different degrees of severity, were seen by Saint-Hilaire (1832–37, vol. 2, pp. 387, 404); in addition he cited a case found by Regnault (*ibid.*, pp. 402–3) and stated that a total of 4 instances of this defect were known in cats (*ibid.*, p. 399). In another place (*ibid.*, vol. 3, p. 357), however, he included 7 cyclopic cats in a table listing abnormal animals.

Taruffi, in 2 places (1881–94, vol. 6, pp. 378–79, 433) mentioned that this defect was recorded 7 times in the literature, but elsewhere (*ibid.*, vol. 8, pp. 392–93) listed only 6 references to cyclopia, dated between 1671 and 1872. Two cyclopic cats with mandibular defect were also listed (*ibid.*, vol. 6, p. 433). Hannover (1882–84, pp. 123, 160) managed to collect 11 or 12 cases from the literature known to him, 2 of which were duplication monstrosities; 12 others had cyclopic and otocephalic features combined.

Atkinson (1833) figured a newborn cat, which he called monoculus, and described it as having a single eye in the middle of the forehead, with total obliteration of the nose. The illustration showed well-developed jaws and normally positioned pinnae. Keil (1912) recorded a newborn cat with a fused median eye and 4 fused eyelids. Both external auditory canals were atretic, but the pinnae were normal in size and location. The brain, which was but briefly described, had poorly developed convolutions and was bilaterally hydrocephalic. Lamb (1936) presented a full-term, newborn cyclopic kitten that lived for several hours. It had a partly ossified cranial vault of apparently normal expanse and shape but which, when opened, was noted to be almost empty. The cerebral hemispheres were absent; only the posterior part of the brainstem and the cerebellum were present.

In several instances cyclopia was found in duplicated individuals (Panum 1878; Taruffi 1881–94, vol. 2, pp. 310–15; Hannover 1882–84, p. 160).

Otocephaly

Saint-Hilaire (1832–37, vol. 2, pp. 426, 429, 431–32) mentioned a few otocephalic cats found by various observers. Taruffi (1881–94, vol. 6, pp. 425–28, 433) noted 11 instances of aprosopus, i.e., severe otocephaly, recorded in earlier writings; in Thomson's cases, e.g. (*ibid.*, p. 428), one animal had fused tympanic cavities with but a single external auditory canal, which communicated with the pharynx; and in the second cat the external ears were fused at their base. Aside from the cats mentioned above, with both cyclopic and otocephalic features, Hannover (1882–84, p. 160) noted one with otocephaly only.

Radasch (1912) observed malformations of the head in a posteriorly duplicated cat. The head was astomic and agnathic, the ears were low-set and a transverse slit beneath the head extended from pinna to pinna and led into the pharynx. The brain was not described.

Duplication Monstrosity

Such phenomena have been noted on numerous occasions in cats, in both the earlier and the more recent literature (Ville 1755; Saint-Hilaire 1832–37, vol. 3, pp. 123, 128, 144, 196–97, 202–3, 357; Vrolik 1854, pl. 99, fig. 8; Vulpian 1855; Joly 1857; Macalister 1867; McIntosh 1868; Gurlt 1877, pp. 36–37; Panum 1878; Taruffi 1881–94, vol. 2, pp. 310–15; Hannover 1882–84, p. 160; Kerville 1885; Lesbre and Guinard 1891; Ozawa 1899; Pellegrin 1901; Neveu-Lemaire 1902; Rabaud 1905; Lesbre and Jarricot 1908; Wilder 1908; Guerrini 1909a; Reese 1911; Radasch 1912; Lima 1918a; Weber 1946a; Ellinger, Wotton, and Hall 1950; Voute and Dussen 1951).

Where described, the central nervous system, if involved, was sometimes partly duplicated and occasionally otherwise abnormal as well.

Other Defects

Absence of the corpus callosum was reported in 2 cats (Wilder 1883; Kisselewa 1934), and partial absence of this commissure in one cat (Frauchiger and Fankhauser 1957, p. 48). Microgyria was seen in 3 cats (Verlinde and Ojemann 1946).

"True" unilateral porencephaly was described by Ball and Auger (1926) in a 2-year-old dwarfed cat. The right cerebral hemisphere was atrophied and clearly smaller than the left one, and its convolutions were smaller than those on the left. In addition, the right cerebellar hemisphere was slightly atrophied. The porencephalic opening was present at the lateral border of the right hemisphere and led into the right lateral ventricle, which was enlarged. In the area of the opening the pia mater was slightly thickened and opalescent. The opening contained normal-appearing cerebrospinal fluid. Porencephaly was also found in some cats with cerebellar atrophy (Fankhauser 1955), but in these cases it appeared to be secondary to inflammatory processes.

14

Dog

Hydrocephalus

Miessner (1899) observed a young setter from about a month to one year of age, near the end of which it developed nervous symptoms and was discovered to be blind. Dissection revealed various brain abnormalities. Endosteal and meningeal irregularities and poorly developed cerebral convolutions were apparent. The lateral ventricles were dilated and full of fluid, and a hole between them permitted complete communication. The corpus callosum, hippocampus, and choroid plexuses of the lateral ventricles were absent; and lack of grooves between the colliculi caused the latter to appear as a single structure.

A 1-year-old rabid dog with hydrocephalus was briefly noted by Forgeot and Nicolas (1906). At autopsy, despite the presence of normal cerebral convolutions, the brain was completely hollow and filled with clear, serous liquid. The cerebral walls were extremely thin, in places not being more than a millimeter wide. Thinning affected white matter especially. The lateral ventricles were considerably dilated and communicated with each other, owing to absence of the septum pellucidum. In addition, the corpus callosum was missing, which indicated that the condition was congenital.

Oules (1909) described a 3-month-old Great Dane with an enormously enlarged skull and a short, underdeveloped face. When placed on the ground, the animal circled, always to the right. Only the cranium and brain were abnormal. The former was globular, thin, and exaggerated in its vertical dimensions. An open fontanelle was palpable in the right frontoparietal region. The brain had the appearance of a tremulous, distended sac. It contained about half a liter of clear liquid. The normal convolutional pattern was effaced. The cerebral hemispheres were united by a thin, transparent band on which were seen 2 whitish, longitudinal tracts, representing remains of the corpus callosum. All other commissural connections between the hemispheres were absent. There was no septum pellucidum, and consequently the lateral ventricles formed a single, enormously dilated vesicle, which communicated with the apparently normal 3rd ventricle through the foramina of Monro. The basal ganglia of the left hemisphere were well developed, but those of the right one were atrophic. The rest of the brain was fairly normal.

Dandy and Blackfan (1914) briefly described a dog with spontaneous internal hydrocephalus found by Dr. A. P. Jones. The lateral ventricles formed a single markedly expanded cavity, owing to absence of the septum pellucidum. The aqueduct was completely occluded, but beyond it the 4th ventricle was normal. Jakob (1916) noted internal hydrocephalus of the lateral ventricles in a 2-year-old dwarf terrier.

Dexler (1923) proposed that several miniature and dwarf breeds of dogs that normally have large heads, short legs, narrow pelves, and crooked tails, are afflicted with hereditary constitutional hydrocephalus. His observations were made on 30 dogs of a wide range of ages, in most of which there was variable widening of the lateral ventricles; in some of them additional defects were also found, such as dilatation of other ventricles, especially the 3rd, abnormalities of the septum pellucidum, partial absence of the corpus callosum, and anomalies of the cranium. Frauchiger and Fankhauser (1957, p. 46) were somewhat critical of some of Dexler's concepts; they believed that constitutional hydrocephalus is restricted to brachycephalic breeds.

Schroeder (1924) saw a 3-month-old fox terrier with a disproportionately large head and open fontanelles. The cranium was paper thin, the cerebral convolutions greatly flattened, the lateral ventricles markedly expanded and liquid-filled, and the cerebral cortex severely reduced in thickness.

Gunn (1924) described 3 dogs, which he diagnosed as having chronic internal hydrocephalus of acquired form, but none of the facts of the cases opposes the possibility that the conditions were congenital. The first dog, an Australian terrier of the age of about 8 months, had enlarged cerebral hemispheres, tremendously dilated lateral ventricles, and greatly thinned cerebral cortex. The second dog, a 4-year-old black pug, had an enlarged right lateral ventricle, but the cortex appeared normal. No obstruction was observed. The last animal, a 1-year-old black retriever, had a considerably enlarged left ventricle, which may have been caused by obstruction of the left foramen of Monro, since the rest of the ventricular system appeared normal, but the state of preservation of the brain prevented its close examination. Appended to these descriptions was a note in which it was solemnly recorded that the unusual behavior of the dogs included circling, and that this movement took place towards the side on which lateral ventricular dilatation existed, left or right in the 2 with unilateral enlargement, and in both directions (at different times) in the dog with symmetrical enlargement. He cautiously refrained from commenting on this phenomenon beyond remarking that "it may be significant."

Hutyra and Marek (1926, p. 358) stated that Fröhner saw hydrocephalus in 20/70,000 dogs, but whether these cases were congenital or not was not indicated. Filimonoff (1929) noted 2 cases of hydrocephalus at autopsies of 100 dogs; one of a moderate degree, the other of considerable extent. Only the second case was described. Both cerebral hemispheres were enormously dilated, and the corpus callosum was greatly thinned. The age of this animal was not stated, nor was it made clear whether the condition was regarded as congenital or not.

Engel (1931) found severe hydrocephalus in a posteriorly duplicated newborn dog. The cranium was very thin and soft and a large fontanelle was present. Although the head was outwardly single, there were 2 medullae oblongatae in the foramen magnum, and the spinal column and cord were duplicated.

Morrill (1932) examined several purebred and hybrid dogs. Four of 5 British bulldogs had marked internal hydrocephalus, while the fifth had practically none. Purebred Great Danes and St. Bernards did not commonly show internal hydrocephalus, but among hybrids various degrees of the condition were most often seen in Great Dane–St. Bernard crossbred offspring. Occasional instances were also found in other (unspecified) hybrid animals.

Serrano (1933) inspected a 2-month-old Pomeranian puppy with a bulging forehead. The lateral ventricles and foramina of Monro were enormously enlarged, and a great excess of cerebrospinal fluid was present. The cerebral cortex was very thin, and the optic nerves had undergone pressure atrophy. Enlargement of the head was said, by the owner, to have been progressive from the moment a nasal hemorrhage was first noted.

Schlotthauer (1934) described 2 dogs with hydrocephalus, an 18-month-old fox terrier, which at necropsy showed a rather marked dilatation of the lateral ventricles with enlargement of the cranium and, microscopically, flattening of the fornix and dilatation of the cavity of the septum pellucidum; and a wirehaired fox terrier of about 6 years of age with marked dilatation of the lateral ventricles and thinning of the walls of the cerebrum. The latter animal also had definite hydromyelia. In the younger one no apparent cause of the condition was discovered; in the older there was a diffuse, chronic encephalitis, which probably explained it.

Schlotthauer (1936) reported 5 further cases of internal hydrocephalus, all confirmed at autopsy. Four were congenital. The first was an 8-week-old bulldog that manifested progessive symptoms of nervous disease beginning 2 weeks previously. The owner mentioned that he had observed similar nervous signs in 4 other bulldogs, 3 of which (males) had all died quite young, while the fourth (a female) was then still alive and, in fact, pregnant at the age of more than a year. Further, all 4 were offspring of the same sire. At the death of the subject, which occurred suddenly at the age of 2 months, necropsy revealed no gross deformity of the skull and vertebral column, but bilateral internal hydrocephalus and definite hydromyelia were present. In addition, patency of the central spinal canal (i.e., spina bifida occulta) was found in the lumbar region.

Dilatation of the left lateral ventricle was found in case 2, a 3-month-old fox terrier. No other lesion was present, and the cause of the (presumed) obstruction of the ventricle was not discovered. In the third dog, a collie 4 or more years old, there was a moderate but well-marked dilatation of the lateral ventricles, also of undetermined origin. Case 4, a 4-year-old mongrel white bull terrier, had marked internal hydrocephalus, with dilation of the entire ventricular system, including the aqueduct, and the central spinal canal. The condition appeared grossly to be due to obstruction of the foramina of Luschka of the 4th ventricle or narrowing of the subarachnoid space at the level of the tentorium. The last case was a 10-year old British terrier that had had many convulsions, beginning at 2 years of age. At autopsy there was marked dilatation of the left lateral ventricle, but obstruction was found to be due to an old inflammatory adhesive lesion in the floor of the ventricle, and hence the condition was undoubtedly acquired postnatally.

Barber (1936) autopsied a 7½-month-old German shepherd that had shown nervous symptoms and found hydrocephalus on the left side. A thin cortical shell, filled with clear fluid, was practically all that was left of the brain on that side. The right lateral ventricle was slightly enlarged and seemed to communicate directly with the cystic left side. It was suspected that originally the lateral ventricles were not joined, but that an opening was made accidentally during examination. The cerebellum was apparently normal, as were the olfactory bulbs. The author believed that the condition was not congenital. Papez and Rundles (1938) studied the pathology of this German shepherd, and found that the cortical shell was composed of non-nervous material. A "congenital accident," it was believed, prevented the development of the thalamus.

Panu and Adamsteanu (1937) examined a 2½-month-old Maltese hybrid whose head was enlarged in the frontal and parietal regions. The cranial bones were very thin and soft. The brain was greatly enlarged, fluctuant, and poorly convoluted, but the cerebellum and pons appeared normal. Internally, the lateral ventricles, 3rd ventricle, and foramina of Monro were all greatly expanded, forming in effect one large, liquid-filled cavity. The corpus callosum and choroid plexuses were greatly diminished in size. The aqueduct of Sylvius was slightly dilated rostrally, and posteriorly enlarged greatly to enter the 4th ventricle, which may also have been somewhat dilated; the authors were not clear on this last point. Thus no ventricular constriction was found. The state of the roof of the 4th ventricle was not mentioned.

Klatt (1943) observed hydrocephalus in 4/15 French bulldogs, aged 7 months to about 6 years. Frauchiger and Fankhauser (1949, p. 94) mentioned a dog with hydrocephalus and cerebellar hypoplasia; and briefly described a 10-week-old poodle whose cranium was greatly expanded. After removing the thin cranial bones, a thin-walled cerebral sac was seen whose surface was almost devoid of convolutions.

Webb (1944) examined a 7-week-old French poodle. The frontal and parietal areas were enlarged, as were the fontanelles, and the cranial bones were thin and soft. The cerebral hemispheres were greatly enlarged and almost devoid of convolutions. The lateral ventricles were much dilated and filled with fluid, and the surrounding cortex was very thin, being 2 mm wide at its thickest. The corpus callosum, fornix, and septum pellucidum were absent, and the lateral ventricles thus freely communicated with each other. It would seem that lack of these parts, in conjunction with other factors, led to absence of the roof of the 3rd ventricle and to abnormal position of its tela choroidea. These conditions, together possibly with enlarged foramina of Monro—whose state the author did not mention—caused the 3rd ventricle to be largely joined to the lateral ones. On the floor of each lateral ventricle the caudate nucleus and the ectopic thalamus stood out boldly and seemed in no way atrophied. The pituitary was represented by a thin-walled sac, although there was a well-marked infundibular recess. The sphenoid bone was flat, with no sign of a sella turcica. The aqueduct was reduced to a vertical slit but was not atretic, and its ependymal lining was normal. The 4th ventricle and the foramina of Luschka were normal. The author explained the unusual features described above as resulting from arrest of embryonic development of certain features, which stemmed from disturbance of cerebrospinal dynamics beginning at a particular stage. While expansion of the anterior ventricles in the presence of a normal 4th ventricle is consonant with the constricted cerebral aqueduct found, the apparent stenosis was not felt to be the cause of the hydrocephalus.

Banks and Monlux (1952) described a young Chihuahua with marked hydrocephalus of the lateral ventricles. McGrath (1956, p. 71) showed a photograph of a hydrocephalic purebred beagle puppy, discovered to have extreme dilatation of the lateral ventricles. Innes and Saunders (1962, p. 281) showed an illustration of a Pekinese puppy with congenital hydrocephalus, supplied by Dr. P. Olafson. Green (1957) mentioned a syndrome of congenital malformations in families of inbred beagles, which included nervous seizures and hydrocephalus and other (unnamed) brain abnormalities. The defects did not have a simple genetic etiology but were definitely dependent to a large degree upon genetic factors. Frauchiger and Fankhauser (1957) recorded 5 dogs with congenital hydrocephalus in a collection of abnormal animals (p. 38) and showed a photograph of a 6-month-old poodle with an extreme grade of congenital internal hydrocephalus (p. 45). The poodle was later described (Fankhauser 1959). It had an expanded skullcap and flattened skullbase, and an aqueduct whose entire lumen was reduced to the diameter of a thread.

In an EEG study of nervous diseases in dogs (Croft 1962), a 4-month-old animal that had behaved strangely from birth and was subject to fits was found at autopsy to have internal hydrocephalus. All 3 puppies of a litter of Doberman pinschers were observed to have hydrocephalus, probably congenital (Murkibhavi *et al.* 1964). The head was enormously enlarged and the brain atrophied. No further description of the abnormalities was given, and one therefore cannot comment on the authors' diagnosis of the condition as external hydrocephalus.

Fankhauser (1965) described congenital internal hydrocephalus in a 7-week-old Appenzeller-Sennenhund hybrid. The cranial vault was considerably enlarged and thinned, but the fontanelles were closed. The cerebral hemispheres were very thin-walled and distended with fluid. The aqueduct was patent and widened, as was the 4th ventricle. The cerebellum was partially reduced in size. The marked ventricular dilatation was apparently caused by absence of the foramina of Luschka, the apertures normally present at the lateral recesses of the 4th ventricle. Since dogs and other lower mammalia probably lack a foramen of Magendie (see p. 204), it would seem that lack of communication between the ventricular system and the subarachnoid spaces was the cause of this animal's hydrocephalus.

McGrath (1965) examined a 3-month-old toy poodle with slight cranial enlargement and various clinical signs of hydrocephalus. Autopsy revealed severe hydrocephalus of the entire ventricular system and cerebellar herniation through the foramen magnum, and study of the spinal cord disclosed extensive syringomyelia throughout its length. The author also saw 4 cases of hydrocephalus, which were not described, in a large number of dogs of the Weimeraner breed with spinal cord abnormalities (see p. 279).

Yashon, Small, and Jane (1965) observed a 4-month-old Chihuahua with a disproportionately large head. A roentgenogram showed a large calvaria, open fontanelles, and a wide coronal suture. Dissection showed a markedly thin cerebral cortex, dilatation of the lateral and 3rd ventricles, and absence of the septum pellucidum. The basal ganglia were intact. The rostral portion of the aqueduct was expanded, but this widened area was followed by an abrupt stenosis, which ended in a blind diverticulum. However, a narrow channel, devoid of an ependymal lining, connected the aqueduct to the normal 4th ventricle, i.e., the aqueduct was forked.

DeLahunta and Cummings (1965) described the clinical, pathological, and electroencephalographic features of 3 hydrocephalic dogs. The first was a 3-month-old bulldog with slight enlargement of the cranium, which had been noticed by its owner. The fontanelles were not palpably open, and the cerebrospinal-fluid pressure was normal. The lateral ventricles were widely dilated and communicated with each other freely because of absence of the septum pellucidum. The cerebral cortex overlying the dilated areas was reduced in thickness. The foramina of Monro were widened, and the rest of the ventricular system, including the 3rd ventricle (and its infundibulum), aqueduct, and 4th ventricle, were also all enlarged. Otherwise, the general arrangement and size of the mesencephalon and rhombencephalon were not grossly affected, except for slight lateral flattening of the cerebellar hemispheres due to their partial herniation through the foramen magnum, the result, according to the authors, of increased pressure.

On the basis of (1) absence of anatomic block in the ventricular system, (2) lack of increased cerebrospinal-fluid pressure (measured at the cerebello-medullary cistern, and thus indicating a noncommunicating hydrocephalus), and (3) dilatation of the 4th ventricle, it was assumed that the block to the flow of cerebrospinal fluid occurred at the foramina of Luschka. However, no structural evidence of such a block was presented.

The other 2 dogs had lesser degrees of hydrocephalus. One was a 7-month-old Boston terrier whose cerebrospinal-fluid pressure, recorded at the cere-bellomedullary cistern, was normal, and a ventriculogram of which indicated a block at the foramina of Luschka. Necropsy revealed the following. The frontoparietal fontanelle was open. Although the gyri were only slightly flattened, the lateral ventricles were obviously dilated and the 3rd ventricle somewhat dilated; the aqueduct and 4th ventricle were normal. The body of the corpus callosum was reduced in thickness. The vermis was distinctly decreased, probably owing to compression of the cerebellum by the occipital lobes. Although, as mentioned above, the ventriculogram indicated lack of patency of the apertures of the 4th ventricle, no such feature was noted at autopsy.

The last dog was a 9-week-old beagle with a noticeably large head and a bilaterally palpable frontoparietal fontanelle. A ventriculogram demonstrated enlarged lateral ventricles and also showed the hydrocephalus to be communicating, i.e., no block was indicated between the ventricular system and subarachnoid spaces. At necropsy the gyri were only slightly compressed; the lateral ventricles were greatly enlarged and the 3rd ventricle moderately so; and the 4th ventricle, the cerebellum, and presumably the aqueduct, were normal. The electroencephalographic investigations showed that the hydro-cephaluses were associated with synchronized patterns of extremely high-voltage slow waves.

Of 62 dogs with noninfectious brain disorders examined in 2 years, Few (1966) diagnosed 22 as having internal hydrocephalus. Most of the diagnoses were confirmed at autopsy. The dogs consisted of 15 Chihuahuas ranging in age from 3 months to $4\frac{1}{2}$ years, and one each of 7 other breeds (dachshund, beagle, Pomeranian, German shepherd, miniature poodle, boxer, and toy fox terrier) ranging from 4 months to 5 years. The brain abnormalities were not described.

Fox (1963a) reported a 12-week-old dachshund with severe micrognathia (which the author called agnathia) and hydrocephalus. The skull was markedly domed, and palpation revealed a large patent fontanelle. The hydrocephalus (not described) was confirmed at postmortem. The author concluded that the hydrocephalus was a secondary developmental abnormality, but did not explain what was meant by this term, nor how this presumed secondary phenomenon came about. His premise was that the mandibular defect was a symptom of low-grade otocephaly, since types of the former are found in the otocephalic syndrome. Further—he seems to have reasoned—since cranial structures are also abnormal in otocephaly, the hydrocephalus in this case was thus a consequence of damage of this sort.

Fox's (1963a) assertion that the mandibular defect was equivalent to low-grade otocephaly cannot be accepted, since no other sign of this state, such as low-set ears or a buccopharyngeal membrane, was apparently present; especially since micrognathia has frequently been found as an isolated malformation in dogs (Georgi 1936; Grüneberg and Lea 1940; Phillips 1945), and skull defects, such as patent fontanelle, have been reported without brain abnormalities or mandibular malformation (Pullig 1952). In addition, in undoubted otocephaly, e.g., in guinea pigs (Wright and Wagner 1934), hydrocephalus appeared only in abnormal specimens with higher grades of the condition (see p. 244). Fox, of course, is not alone in believing that isolated mandibular defects are mild expressions of the otocephalic syndrome. Blanc (1895), e.g., cited several cases of such conditions in different species and referred to them as transitional forms.

In several other reports, Fox (1963b, 1964a, b) described malformations occurring in a stock of beagles. Skeletal abnormalities included delayed or incomplete closure of fontanelles, and micrognathia (not obvious at birth, but becoming apparent postnatally). Also seen was hydrocephalus (enlargement of lateral ventricles with abnormal gyrus formation and deficiency of cortical tissue). Again the author considered these malformations as constituting a syndrome of low-grade otocephaly and partially supported this contention by the occurrence of a deformed pup with unquestionable high-grade otocephalic defects, which included agnathia, astomia, and medioventral anastomosis of pinnae. The latter animal, however, was not a purebred beagle, but the product of a beagle-chow cross, and its defects, hence, may have been a fortuitous occurrence, unrelated to those in the purebred animals.

If, as the author intimated (Fox 1964b), the defects found in the beagle stock were multigenic in origin, it is highly unlikely that among the genes contributed by an unrelated dog (the chow) there would exist a complement, coinciding with those occurring in the beagles, that predisposed to the defects found in that stock. Therefore, it is improbable that the abnormalities in the crossbred dog were of the same origin as those in the purebred ones; and unjustified to draw analogies from the one set of defects to pertain to the other.

Other points that contradict the argument that the defects in the purebred beagles were low-grade otocephaly are the following. (1) As mentioned above, in true low-grade otocephaly, abnormalities of the pinna occur, such as ventral approximation. The ear abnormalities in the beagles were not of this class at all. (2) Rather than microglossia, which commonly accompanies reduction of the mandible in otocephaly, in defective beagles a relative macroglossia was found.

Exencephaly

Taruffi (1881–94, vol. 6, pp. 142–44) mentioned a dog with anterior "acrania," the remainder of whose skull was very elevated, probably by hydrocephalus. Weber (1948) described a newborn Sennenhund with "partial anencephaly," exophthalmia, and short upper jaw. A knob of brain material was present externally, adjacent to an extensive fault in the top of the cranium, and this part was almost all that remained of the brain. The cerebellum, medulla oblongata, and upper part of the spinal cord were entirely missing as well. No nervous connection existed between the brain rudiments and the remaining part of the cord.

Little (1948) reported an instance of a cocker spaniel with the "skull not grown together." McGrath (1956, p. 76) mentioned "anencephaly" and failure of cranial cap development in a stillborn puppy (breed unstated); the bulging brain substance was apparently poorly preserved. Frauchiger and Fankhauser (1957, p. 38) listed 2 anencephalic dogs in their collection of abnormal animals. Fox (1963b) found "cranioschisis" in a newborn beagle, accompanied by absence of much of the calvaria.

Soon after starting a program of inbreeding with standard beagles, Fuller (1956) found very atypical animals, with overshot jaws and twisted ears. The young were born dead and had incomplete closure of the skull. Whether abnormalities of the brain accompanied the skull defects was not stated. Analysis of the inheritance of the syndrome indicated that it was probably the result of a recessive gene.

Another lethal hereditary condition involving open fontanelle was studied by Pullig (1952) in cocker spaniels. No abnormality of the central nervous system apparently existed in these animals, despite Fox's (1965, p. 172) referring somewhat puzzlingly to the condition as "cranial defect (cranioschisis)." In one paper Fox (1963b) applied the term cranioschisis to frank exencephaly; in another (Fox 1965), to a skeletal defect. Confusion abounds as it is, in teratology. It seems needless to increase it by careless use of words.

Contrary to the situation commonly encountered in some species, especially cattle, hydrocephalus has not been found in canine chondrodystrophy (Millar and Tucker 1952; Tucker and Millar 1954; Mather 1956; D. L. Gardner 1959).

Malformations of the Cerebellum

Russell (1895b) reported a litter of puppies (breed unstated) all with signs of congenital ataxia. The brain of one of them was examined; the cerebellum was reduced to about three-quarters normal size but was symmetrical and had a normal shape. Stefani (1897) found a similar condition in a water spaniel. The animal's movements became irregular soon after weaning, and during the 6 months it was observed these and other signs became intensified. The brain was normal except for overall reduction of the cerebellum. The microscopic anatomy was described by Deganello and Spangaro (1899).

Finzi (1919) saw a 45-day-old white poodle whose peculiarities of gait and other behavior indicated the presence of a lesion of the central nervous system. At autopsy it was found that the cerebellum was divided into 2 distinct parts owing to complete absence of the vermis. Apparently no other superficial abnormalities of the brain were noted; but its internal condition seems not to have been explored.

Bertrand, Medynski, and Salles (1936) described in great detail a case of complete agenesis of the vermis and reduction in size of the cerebellar hemispheres in a 3-month-old French bulldog. The cerebral hemispheres, mesencephalon, colliculi, pons, and other parts appeared entirely normal, as apparently was the 4th ventricle, which was easily seen into because its roof, ordinarily covered by the vermis, was missing. The important point (see below) is that the brain was obviously not hydrocephalic. Baker and Graves (1936) noted brain defects in a Boston bull terrier–Manchester terrier hybrid. Retarded development was seen early, but the animal was kept under observation until 8 months old. The vermis was absent and the rest of the cerebellum markedly reduced in size. In addition, there was partial agenesis of the cerebral hemispheres, and the inferior olives appeared absent externally. There was no hydrocephalus.

Sholl, Sales, and Langham (1939) examined a 4-month-old wire-haired fox terrier that had difficulty standing from the age of 3 weeks, and found complete absence of the cerebellum and underdevelopment of the cerebral convolutions.

Dow (1940) studied 2 abnormal female Boston bull terriers from a litter of 4, which were recognized as defective soon after birth. Both dogs had identical cerebellar defects: complete absence of the middle lobe of the vermis and absence of most of the culmen. One of the animals, in addition, had a slight cerebral cortical asymmetry, a slight internal hydrocephalus, presumably of the lateral ventricles, and other small changes. One female was bred to a normal, related male, but their offspring showed no cerebellar abnormalities. Verlinde and Ojemann (1946) mentioned a 7-week-old Scotch terrier with partial cerebellar aplasia. Frauchiger and Fankhauser (1949) found 2 dogs with cerebellar hypoplasia; in one the condition was accompanied by hydrocephalus.

Cordy and Snelbaker (1952) investigated a family of Airedales with cerebellar hypoplasia. At least 6 puppies in as many litters showed ataxic symptoms, which usually became evident at about 12 weeks of age. Two animals were dissected and found to have very similar lesions consisting of small flattened cerebellum with a specific histological picture. The familial incidence suggested a hereditary etiology, but the incomplete breeding history of the family prevented genetic analysis.

Some writers (e.g., Brodal and Hauglie-Hanssen 1959) have equated cases of absence of the cerebellar vermis in dogs and other animals with the Dandy-Walker syndrome that occurs in man (see p. 22). In the latter condition, however, a *sine qua non* is cystlike dilatation of the 4th ventricle, a feature that was absent in the cases of partial agenesis of the cerebellum in the dogs described in the above paragraphs.

Spina Bifida

Boulard (1852*a, b*) was sent a stillborn, anomalous dog from a litter of 6, of which 5 were normal. In the occipital region there was a small tumor, apparently an encephalocele, formed of the cerebellum and a large part of the left cerebral hemisphere, which was herniated through the cranium, and which was covered by meninges but not by skin. The dog also had an extensive fault of the vertebral column and spinal cord. From the 10th dorsal vertebra to the caudal region the vertebral arches were completely missing, and the vertebral canal was represented solely by an osteofibrous gutter. Further, at the lumbar level the cord emerged through a long orifice, not covered by skin, and formed a button of tissue, thus leaving the spinal canal empty.

Tagand and Barone (1942) described abnormalities in a young puppy of the Berger Allemand breed. When first seen, at 10 days of age, the dog had a small fistulous wound in the lumbosacral region, said to have been present from birth, from which drained a small amount of serous fluid. At the second examination, 15 days later, the wound was completely cicatrized, but the hindlegs were inert and the animal painfully dragged itself along. It also had urinary incontinence. Palpation revealed a spina bifida occulta extending from the 4th or 5th lumbar vertebra to the middle of the sacrum. Death occurred several days later, but the cadaver was destroyed before it could be further explored.

Tagand and Barone (1943) also discovered spina bifida in a 3-year-old mongrel with abnormal external genitalia (viz., pseudohermaphroditism) and severe, persistent urinary incontinence. Examination disclosed a pronounced atrophy in the coccygeal region and a very short bent tail. At the anterior end of the sacral area there was a small, fleshy growth with a small tuft of hair at its end. Roentgenograms showed severe vertebral deviations in the sacrococcygeal region indicative of spina bifida occulta. The urinary incontinence was thus imputed, not to the imperfect state of the genital apparatus, but to nervous lesions associated with the spina bifida.

Spina bifida aperta was briefly recorded in one dog each by Winsser (1945) and Verlinde and Ojemann (1946). In both cases cerebral ventricles were enlarged and in the latter hydromyelia was present as well. Klatt (1939) found cleft vertebrae in several descendants of a cross between a French bulldog and an English whippet.

McGrath (1956, p. 136) reported spina bifida occulta associated with posterior paralysis in a 5-week-old Dalmatian. Externally there was dimpling of the skin in the region of T9. Necropsy disclosed other myelodysplasias characterized by cavitations (syringomyelia) in the lower thoracic and lumbar areas of the cord. Schlotthauer (1959) saw a case externally resembling spina bifida occulta in a 6-week-old puppy (breed unstated), and at autopsy it was found that the neural canal was not completely closed in the posterior midline of the distal lumbar region, and also that the spinal canal was incompletely closed, producing a small meningocele. Five other dogs of the same stock had similar clinical symptoms but were not further examined. A whippet puppy with spina bifida occulta was briefly described by Akker (1962). Other defects were large, polygyric cerebral hemispheres, displacement of the occipital lobes into the posterior fossa, and a very small cerebellum.

Curtis, English, and Kim (1964) investigated a short-tailed ("stub") condition in a stock of beagles, which appeared to be inherited as an autosomal dominant factor with reduced penetrance and variable expressivity. Selective breeding for shorter tail resulted in a smaller mean number of caudal vertebrae in succeeding generations, and the appearance in one dog of a bifid centrum at S1 and in 2 others, of spina bifida "manifesta" starting at L1 and L2.

Dogs with presumably hereditary, characteristic deformities of the spine, occurring sporadically in Japan, were first described by Suu (1956) and given the name short-spine dogs. Further studies (Ueshima 1961; Suu 1962) showed that the unusual outward appearance of the animals was due to extreme shortening of the entire vertebral column, while the skeleton of the head and extremities was normal. In addition, various types of vertebral bifidity were present. The spinal cord was apparently not investigated, nor was the possible genetic basis of the condition clarified. The same or a similar condition has occurred in several parts of the world (Burns and Fraser 1966, pp. 101–2).

Syringomyelia

So far as can be learned, prior to McGrath's (1965) study, syringomyelia had been seen in only 3 dogs. Besides a brief reference to the condition by Harbitz (1942) in an article on tumors in animals, and McGrath's (1956, p. 136) previous case, which was not described in any detail, only Liénaux (1897) found a dog with this condition. Liénaux's description is excellent. The subject was a 2-year-old Newfoundland affected with slight paralysis of the hindquarters. At autopsy the brain was externally normal, but the ventricular fluid was notably excessive. The spinal cord was also externally normal, but was flabby to the touch. On sectioning the cord, cavities were found in its substance, from which flowed a small amount of colorless liquid.

After fixation, these and other features became better distinguishable. It was then seen that the central canal was dilated throughout its entire length, but in a very unequal fashion, being much more enlarged in some areas than in others. In addition, the canal was quite irregularly shaped in places and a number of times communicated with the syringomyelic cavities. The original paper should be consulted for descriptions of the cellular changes noted.

McGrath (1965) made extensive clinical, neurological, and histopathological studies on a large number of purebred Weimeraner dogs. Clinical observations were made of 22 puppies and adults, all of which demonstrated various signs of nervous disorder. These signs first appeared at 4 to 6 weeks of age and always included a symmetrical, hopping hindlimb gait and a peculiar stance. Less constant signs also occurred, such as scoliosis of the spine in the lower thoracic to anterior lumbar region. These 22, and 56 other dogs obtained from a breeding program, were autopsied and studied anatomically, at ages from birth to 40 months. Structural abnormalities of the spinal cord existed in many animals; these comprised anomalies of the central canal, anomalies of the ventral median fissure, and syringomyelia.

Abnormalities of the central canal included hydromyelia with or without syringomyelia, duplication of the central canal, absence of the central canal, eccentric central canal, and unusually-shaped central canal. Abnormalities of the ventral median fissure consisted of variations in its size and culminated in its complete absence. Fissure defects, which were called dysraphic lesions, were found in obvious forms in all 22 clinically examined dogs, and in 17 of the other 56; less severe lesions occurred in 20 cases; in 14 no dysraphic lesion was seen; and the 5 remaining dogs were not examined.

The syringomyelia consisted of microscopic to gross cavitations of the spinal cord; gross defects were most frequently located in the thoracic region. This anomaly was found in 17 dogs older than 6 weeks of age but was not seen in animals younger than this age. The syndrome, nevertheless, had congenital aspects, since some lesions, e.g., hydromyelia, were found in newborn and young animals.

McGrath (1965) attempted a genetic investigation of the syndrome by making a number of matings, which produced 17 litters. He hesitated to interpret the results of these crosses, but judging from some of the pedigrees presented, the condition may have been determined by a dominant gene with reduced penetrance.

Syringomyelia, hydromyelia, and defects of the spinal cord were recently observed (Geib and Bistner 1967) in a 1½-year-old mongrel with signs of torticollis and scoliosis of the cervical spine.

Cyclopia

Numerous cyclopic dogs have been observed. Saint-Hilaire (1832–37, vol. 2, pp. 384, 386, 390, 396–97, 399, 402–4) cited 14 observations of his own and other writers of various grades of the deformity. Vrolik's specimen (1854, pl. 57, figs. 10–13) had a proboscis and a forebrain not divided into 2 hemispheres. Of the 123 cases of cyclopia that Taruffi (1881–94, vol. 6, pp. 378–79) garnered from the literature, 11 were in dogs (*ibid.*, vol. 8, pp. 384–85). He also cited 8 instances of cebocephaly and 7 of cyclopia with mandibular defects in dogs (*ibid.*, vol. 6, p. 433). Hannover (1882–84, p. 123) discovered 22 cases of canine cyclopia in the literature at his disposal. Seefelder (1910) mentioned cyclopia in a dog of a large breed.

Magendie (1821) dissected a cyclopic dog that died about 10 minutes after birth. It had a large, single, median, lidless eye; no nose, no mouth, and only rudiments of the tongue and lower jaw. The pinnae were normal, but the auditory canals were atretic. The cranium was largely filled with limpid, colorless, slightly viscous fluid, located between the dura mater, which was closely adherent to the skull, and the very small brain. The latter was free of convolutions and seemed to consist of a simple tubercle situated in the posterior part of the cranial cavity. The cerebral hemispheres consisted of a single mass formed only of grey matter with no corpus callosum, corpora striata, etc. The first 5 pairs of cranial nerves were absent. The hindbrain appeared to be well formed but was also composed entirely of grey matter. Numerous facial and skull bones were missing.

A case was briefly but well described by Gluge and Deroubaix (1840). Only the head was malformed. A single median eye and single optic nerve were present. The cerebral hemispheres were fused and formed one mass. Two cases of cyclopia in puppies were seen by Symington and Woodhead (1886).

One of the most detailed descriptions of cyclopia in a dog was made by Phisalix (1889). The eyes were incompletely united. Brain changes existed only in the prosencephalon. The cerebral hemispheres were represented by a single median lobe, which did not extend back as far as the colliculi. The lateral ventricles communicated freely with each other with hardly an indication of a separation between them. Entirely missing were the choroid plexuses of the lateral ventricles (a large, vascular mass in the cavity of the median lobe was considered to be the misplaced choroid plexus of the 3rd ventricle), hippocampus, anterior commissure, and corpus callosum. The 3rd ventricle was reduced to a cleft, but its surrounding structures were easily identifiable. Anteriorly it joined the cavity of the cerebral vesicle through a median cleft, representing a foramen of Monro.

Banchi (1905) reported a newborn cyclopic dog all of whose littermates were normal. It had a single, median orbit and eye above which was a large proboscis with a single apical aperture. The ears were normally situated. Grossly, the brain presented undivided hemispheres, nearly total absence of convolutions, no olfactory bulbs, and a single median optic nerve. In transverse section, owing to the absence of the septum pellucidum and the largeness of the single foramen of Monro, there was only one large ventricle in the frontal and parietal areas; but more posteriorly, in the region of the occipital lobe, the hemispheres were divided and lateral ventricles were present, though enlarged. The corpus callosum, too, was present posteriorly, but not anteriorly. A pituitary was present.

A prematurely born mongrel dog with cyclopia was recorded by Guerrini (1909*b*). Only the head was malformed. Beneath the single eye was a proboscoid projection. The mouth was large and the lower jaw fairly well formed. The brain terminated in a small globiform mass, with all parts rostral to the pyriform lobe almost completely absent, including the olfactory bulbs and the roots of the olfactory nerves. The optic nerves did not form a true chiasm. The rhombencephalon was normal.

Otocephaly

Otocephaly is apparently less common in dogs than is cyclopia. Cases were described by Otto (1814, cited by Ballantyne 1904, p. 428). Dugès (1827) noted an aprosopic, otocephalic, stillborn, term puppy, with fusion of the auricular conchae. The brain was not mentioned. Saint-Hilaire (1832–37, vol. 2, pp. 426, 429, 431–32; vol. 3, p. 357) reported a number of cases with various grades of otocephaly seen by himself and others. Panum (1860, p. 126) mentioned 9 dogs with facial defects, some of which were possibly otocephalic. Taruffi (1881–94, vol. 6, pp. 424–29) collected 18 dogs with what he called aprosopus, which were probably usually equivalent to severe grades of otocephaly. In Mégnin's case (see below), e.g., it is certain that the animal did have otocephaly. On the other hand, another aprosopic dog cited by Taruffi (*ibid.*) was probably not otocephalic, but had a partly duplicated, triophthalmic head (Gurlt 1877, p. 5). Hannover (1882–84, p. 160) mentioned 4 dogs with synotia and agnathia, which were almost certainly instances of otocephaly; as well as 27 dogs with conditions that combined cyclopic and otocephalic features.

Kerville (1891) briefly mentioned a young dog with triocephaly, the severest grade of the condition, according to Saint-Hilaire's (*ibid.*, p. 431, see p. 241 in this work) classification, in which no eyes, nose, mouth, or mandible are present, and the ears are approximated or fused medioventrally under the face. Kerville failed to describe the brain, but Blanc (1895) noted that in this degree of the defect the brain consists of little more than a bulblike extension of the spinal cord.

In Mégnin's (1878) case, the head was reduced to a rounded, skin-covered hillock below which the ears, normally developed but fused on the midline, were located. No eyes, mouth, or nares were present. The entire face, in fact, was absent. The cranium was reduced to a small tubercle, which must have enclosed a rudimentary brain. The animal was not dissected however. It was from a litter of 9 (the others were all normal) delivered prematurely by a primiparous griffon. A similar case in a stillborn dog was described by Brauer (1898).

Lesbre and Pécherot's (1913a) specimen, a stillborn dog, had opocephaly, a form of the condition somewhat less extreme than triocephaly. There was no trace of the lower jaw, mouth, or nose. The external ears were apparently fairly normal in size and location; but despite the separation of the auricular conchae, otocephaly was demonstrated by the middle ears' being situated side by side under the base of the cranium, and by their opening directly into the pharynx. The brain was not examined. In cases of opocephaly in other species, the brain consists anteriorly of a single vesicular lobe, while posteriorly it is practically normal (Blanc 1895).

What appears to be a type of triocephaly was described in some detail by Chidester (1924). It occurred in a newborn Scotch collie whose 7 littermates were all normal and viable. The nose and mouth were absent, the lower jaw was greatly reduced in size, there was no external indication of eyes, and the ears were fused medioventrally. Dissection showed the auditory capsules to be located almost exactly in the center of the cranial cavity, leaving practically no cranial fossa. The dura mater was rather thin and lacked a falx cerebri. All parts of the brain anterior to the thalamus were absent, as were the pineal and pituitary glands. The colliculi were small and abnormal. Bilateral symmetry was retained posterior to the thalamus. The cerebellum was small but well formed. There was no hydrocephalus.

Duplication Monsters

Duplication monstrosities apparently do not occur frequently in dogs. Saint-Hilaire (1832–37, vol. 3, pp. 128, 144–45, 357), Gurlt (1877, p. 5), and Taruffi (1881–94, vol. 2, pp. 310–15) mentioned a few cases. More recent reports were made by Pilcher (1880), Seefelder (1910), Guérin (1911), Horsley (1920), Raschke (1922), Mainland (1929), and Weber (1946a). Of these, only Mainland's (1929), concerning a newborn French bulldog with 4 hindlegs, specifically mentioned a defect of the central nervous system. The arch of the 3rd sacral vertebra was thin and membranous, distal to which there occurred a small meningocele, located dorsal to and left of the first 2 coccygeal vertebrae.

Other Abnormalities

Partial dorsoventral diplomyelia in a 6-month-old Weimaraner was described in detail by Kersten (1954). Porencephaly occurred in a one-year-old fox terrier (Schlotthauer 1959). Large areas that were degenerated or had failed to develop were located in the right hemisphere, and the right lateral ventricle communicated directly with the subarachnoid space. Frauchiger and Fankhauser (1949) reported a 21-month-old dachshund with porencephaly and microgyria of the right cerebral hemisphere.

Lethal deformities that "chiefly involved head structures," but were not further described, occurred in Brussels griffon-dachshund hybrids (Stockard 1941, p. 339). Partial absence of the corpus callosum occurred in a 2-month-old dog of the dwarf King Charles breed (Dexler 1923), and complete absence in a hydrocephalic setter (Miessner 1899).

A 5-month-old, severely dwarfed dog had a cystic malformation of the craniopharyngeal duct and absent or atrophic pituitary (Alexander 1962). In a routine postmortem, a 6-month-old corgi was discovered with complete duplication of the pituitary (Cozens and Mawdesley-Thomas 1966). Sections of the bifurcated infundibular area showed localized dilatation of the 3rd ventricle.

15

Swine

Hydrocephalus

It is remarkable that the first report of uncomplicated congenital hydrocephalus in swine did not appear until about 30 years age (Blunn and Hughes 1938). The condition occurred in a purebred herd of the Duroc Jersey breed and consisted of the external variety, with fluid accumulated outside of the brain in the subarachnoid spaces. Affected animals also had absent or very short tail and extremely light coat color. They were stillborn or died within 2 days of birth. The few born alive stood only with difficulty and were unable to coordinate their movements; their joints were stiff, and they quivered all over and squealed as if in pain.

Externally there was fullness of the posterior part of the skull. In the most markedly affected cases the skull was domeshaped, being wider, longer, and slightly higher in the crown than normal. Several degrees of unfused and wide-open frontal fontanelle were found. The pressure of fluid on the brain caused partial collapse and displacement of the cerebral hemispheres. A range of severity was noted, from animals with almost normal-appearing heads to those most abnormal in shape. But even where head shape seemed normal a short tail revealed a defective animal, and in these instances fluid was found in the cranium upon necropsy.

All abnormal pigs were descendants of one male, Elmer's Pride, and the condition first appeared in offspring he sired by his daughters. From these litters and others, produced by a son of Elmer's Pride and related females, 42/178 (23.6%) hydrocephalic piglets were obtained, closely approximating the incidence expected from the working of a simple autosomal recessive gene.

A similar, or possibly the same, condition was reported by Warwick, Chapman, and Ross (1943). It also occurred in Duroc Jersey animals, was accompanied by tail defects, was lethal, and may have been due to a recessive. The hydrocephalus was pronounced but was not further described.

Various types of congenital anomalies of the central nervous system in pigs were noted over a 9-year period by O'Hara and Shortridge (1966). Hydrocephalus occurred in 5 young in a litter of 17, and similar cases had occurred previously. At birth the head was domeshaped. The lateral ventricles were greatly enlarged and the cortex was quite thin. The 3rd ventricle was also distended, and the massa intermedia was absent. The aqueduct was widened, but the authors neglected to relate the condition of the 4th ventricle. The breeding history of the herd (breed unstated) suggested that the defect stemmed from 2 boars, a father and his son. Other reports of hydrocephalus in pigs were made by Blunn and Hughes (1938), Warwick, Chapman, and Ross (1943), Weber (1946a), Fankhauser and Wyler (1953), Kitchell and Stevens (1953), Holz (1956), Frauchiger (1959), and Thoonen and Hoorens (1960).

Meningocele and Related Brain Defects

Taruffi (1881–94, vol. 8, pp. 243–47) referred to the observations by different authors of several hydrencephalocelic pigs. Two neonates with frontal defects were seen by Otto (cited by Taruffi, *ibid.*). The first had a small cranium and hydropic ventricles, and the second a hernia consisting of prolongation of the anterior lobe of the left hemisphere that communicated with the left lateral ventricle. Three pigs with similar defects, i.e., partial cleft of the cranium and hydrencephalocele, were seen by Gurlt (1877, p. 16).

Bradley (1899) reported 2 malformed littermates delivered by a primiparous sow. One was stillborn, the other lived for a few minutes. On the forehead of the first there was a large, skin-covered protuberance divided in 2 parts by a shallow, anteroposterior, median groove. When the skin was removed, it could be seen that the large bags projected from separate holes in the frontal bones and consisted of herniated, fluid-containing cerebral tissue. The intracranial portion of the brain consisted of normal medulla, pons, cerebellum, and other parts as well as a small part of both cerebral hemispheres; while the extracranial portion consisted of the greater amount of the hemispheres. The corpus callosum was absent, as were the first 3 cranial nerves. The swelling on the forehead of the second animal was smaller, because the cerebral hemispheres were rudimentary. Otherwise the anomalies were similar in both piglets.

Williams (1909, p. 1069) discussed the occurrence of "hernia cerebri" in a family of pigs bred on a farm. From the description of how he believed the condition to develop and from an illustration of it (p. 296), it is apparent that the abnormality was meningoencephalocele. The female line of the family was maintained unbroken for generations, while the males used for breeding were regularly changed. Despite this practice, an ever increasing number of pigs were born with a protrusion in the frontal region. In some litters over half the offspring were affected. The defect was sometimes covered with skin and at other times only by an epithelial membrane. Some affected offspring died within a few days of birth with symptoms of epilepsy, while others slowly recovered as the condition receded and disappeared. The defects eventually became so frequent that it was necessary to discard the family (Williams 1936).

Hunter and Higgins (1923) reported a stillborn pig with posterior duplication of the body and part of the head and an unexamined, wartlike protruberance on top of the head.

Nordby (1929) reported defects in 5 purebred herds of pigs, chiefly of the Berkshire and Duroc Jersey breeds, involving the frontoparietal region. Various degrees of the abnormality were seen, ranging from epithelial imperfection, through typical meningocele involving protrusion of dura mater and arachnoid, to exencephaly, i.e., true rupture of brain tissue through a defect in the frontal part of the skull. In general the size of the hernia depended on the size of the opening in the skull.

Some abnormal fetuses died prenatally. This was indicated by the occurrence of partly resorbed (i.e., mummified) affected specimens, and also by the fact that in some cases litters of one-half to one-third normal size, containing all normal offspring, were produced by animals that had previously borne abnormal pigs.

Very few abnormal animals survived postnatally, and these few were susceptible to epileptoid convulsions. Postnatal survival was not related to the fissure's size, since some specimens with large herniation lived, while others with the slightest external and internal manifestations were stillborn. The condition was assumed to be hereditary, but the exact nature of its genetics was not determined.

Hughes and Hart (1934) found similar defects in a Poland China herd. Externally, a variable-sized protuberance, not covered by true outer epidermis but only by a thick membrane, was present in the center of the forehead. The skull defect involved the frontal and parietal bones. External manifestations were found in 4 animals, 2 of which exhibited abnormal equilibrium. The authors stated that the abnormality was probably recessively inherited, but their data failed to support this interpretation. Defective offspring resulted only from matings of male A-59995 to his daughters, or, in one case, from a mating of a son to a granddaughter of this male. In 20 such matings defects were noted in only 4/159 offspring, a frequency far short of that expected of a recessive trait. Hughes and Hart (1934) tried to explain the deficiency by assuming that abnormal young with minimal skull defects were not noticed.

Milne (1942) described a newborn pig with pronounced bulging of the frontal region and 2 outgrowths on the left side of the head anteriorly. The frontal bones were incomplete, and they and the parietals were abnormally thin and bulged anteriorly and laterally. The cerebral hemispheres were thin-walled and saclike, and were largely devoid of convolutions. The hemispheres were unconnected except ventrally. Olfactory bulbs were missing. One of the 2 outgrowths mentioned above was formed by a skin- and meninges-covered protrusion from the rhinencephalon; the other, which was only partially covered by skin, appeared to consist of dura mater and periosteum. It was suggested that the defects in this pig and in another, similar to it and seen about the same time, were caused by maternal vitamin A deficiency.

The malformations noted by Gilman (1956) ranged from small protrusion of fluid-filled dura, which did not involve cerebral tissue, to vast frontal herniation of fused skin and meninges that carried with it the cerebral hemispheres. When the sac of the latter type was opened one looked directly into the expanded 3rd ventricle and the cerebral aqueduct. In all cases there was an accumulation of cerebrospinal fluid in the subdural and subarachnoid spaces, which was slight in less extreme defects. In severe cases fluid accumulation also involved the lateral and 3rd ventricles.

The herd in which these defects occurred consisted of 12 sows of several breeds (Large English White, Canadian Yorkshire, and hybrid) and a Canadian Yorkshire male, F. All abnormal young, however, came from the English White and hybrid females. The incidence of abnormal offspring (8/45) was about that expected on the basis of recessive inheritance. But some doubt was cast on this form of inheritance by the fact that one of the sows, which bore 2 abnormal offspring when mated to F, never had defective young with another male thought to be responsible for transmitting the genetic factor to the hybrid sows.

The diet fed the sows was unusual, consisting of little else but yellow corn. To check this factor, further matings were made between F and 3 of the hybrid females, who were then fed an adequate diet throughout pregnancy. From these matings only 2/40 offspring occurred with meningocele, and the defect was minimal. It may therefore be that a dietary deficiency or imbalance contributed to the anomaly in this herd.

Meningocele was noted (Šterk and Sofrenović 1958) in 5/10 offspring (Resavka breed) of a half brother-sister mating. One defective piglet was stillborn and another died immediately after birth. A third died after the protruberance was operated upon at 12 days of age. The last 2 thrived, and when they were slaughtered at 57 days of age the defect had slightly increased in size in one but had disappeared in the other. A very inadequate description of the defects was given. The authors presumed that the condition was due to a recessive gene.

Cohrs *et al.* (1963) described hereditary meningocele and meningo-encephalocele in the Buntes breed of pigs, which occurred after a new boar was introduced. Animals were born with variable-sized prolapse, not covered by skin, of meninges alone or meninges and brain through a fissure between the frontal or parietal bones. More severely affected offspring were stillborn or died soon after birth. The various types of anomalies were described by

Trautwein and Meyer (1966). The defect was apparently due to an autosomal recessive gene; crosses of known carriers produced 15/75 malformed young, which approximated the proportion expected of this hereditary situation. One defective offspring also had other brain abnormalities, viz., micrencephaly, cerebellar hypoplasia, and defects of the brainstem.

In further breeding experiments (Meyer and Trautwein 1966), carriers (i.e., normal animals that had borne defective offspring) mated *inter se* had 28/122 (23.0%) malformed young, which again supported the possibility of the trait's being recessively inherited. However, when carriers were bred with surviving malformed pigs, instead of the expected 50 per cent abnormal young, only 23.6 per cent (13/55) were defective. Since the survival rate of newborn malformed offspring was less than 50 per cent, the deficiency in the number of affected piglets from the latter type of cross may have resulted from their prenatal elimination. But the litter size in these crosses was only slightly reduced. Thus, while the character was shown to be hereditary, its mode of inheritance was not fully explained.

Labík (1965) investigated an outbreak of brain herniations in a herd of Czech pigs. As in other occurrences the herniation was frontal, variable in extent, sometimes skin-covered, sometimes not, and appeared to be a simple autosomal recessive hereditary trait.

Brief reports of defects involving cranial herniations in pigs were also made by Butz and Böttger (1939); Weber (1946a); Fankhauser and Wyler (1953); Frauchiger (1959); Widmaier (1959; Thoonen and Hoorens (1960); Innes and Saunders (1962, photograph by Olafson, p. 277); and O'Hara and Shortridge (1966).

Cyclopia

Various types and grades of cyclopia occur quite often in pigs. An early summary of the brain defects commonly found in cyclopia was presented by Tiedemann (1826), who also recorded a case of the condition in a pig. The cerebral hemispheres are undivided, lack convolutions, and are small, the latter feature making the pineal gland and colliculi visible. The corpus callosum is lacking. The olfactory nerves are absent, and this feature is accompanied by variable reduction in size of the corpora striata and by absence or imperfect development of the fornix and cornua ammonis. Usually only a median optic nerve is present. Numerous other nerves ordinarily serving facial parts are absent. Malformations of the brain of a cyclopic pig fetus were noted by Meckel (1826).

Saint-Hilaire discussed this defect (1832–37, vol. 2, pp. 381–82, 384–86, 388, 395–96, 399, 402–4, 406, 411, 426, 432) and recorded a total of 50 cases in a table (*ibid.* vol. 3, p. 357). One of the 2 heads of a duplication monster described by Thiernesse (1850–51) was cyclopic. Vrolik (1854, pl. 53, fig. 4; pl. 54, fig. 7; pl. 55, figs. 1–7, 10; pl. 57, figs. 1–6; pl. 58, fig. 6) illustrated and described 7 cyclopic pigs. In one (*ibid.*, pl. 54, fig. 7) an undivided vesicle replaced the cerebral hemispheres, the optic nerve was single, and the corpus callosum, septum pellucidum, fornix, and choroid plexus were absent or vestigial. In a second pig (*ibid.*, pl. 55, fig. 2) olfactory bulbs and nerves were absent. Another (*ibid.*, pl. 58, fig. 6) was micrognathic, but had normal ears. In Wyman's (1858) case the cerebral hemispheres were also represented by a single hollow vesicle. Panum (1860, p. 125) noted that of 91 nonduplicated malformed pigs seen by various authors, 37 were cyclopic. Gurlt (1877, pp. 29–30) observed 26 cyclopic pigs and a duplicated cyclopic one (*ibid.*, pp. 54–55). Taruffi (1881–94, vol. 6, pp. 378–79) found mention of 47 cyclopic pigs in literature dating from 1619 to 1880. He listed these sources elsewhere (*ibid.*, vol. 8, pp. 393–95). These 47 included 25 of the 26 cases found by Gurlt and 22 by others. Ten cases of cebocephaly were listed (*ibid.*, vol. 6, p. 433; vol. 8, pp. 370–72) separately from cyclopia; as were 5 cases of cyclopia with otocephalic defects (*ibid.*, vol. 6, p. 433). In addition, 3 duplication monsters listed by him were cyclopic (*ibid.*, vol. 2, pp. 310–15). Hannover (1882–84, pp. 123, 160) collected 127 cyclopic pigs from the literature; 3 of these were double fetuses. Another 29, including 2 double fetuses, were specimens in which both cyclopic and otocephalic features were present. Cyclopic pigs described by Otto or found in a veterinary museum were mentioned by Gurlt (1878). Mégnin (1879) and Degoix (1879) each noted a stillborn cyclopic pig but did not describe the brain.

Symington and Woodhead (1886) examined 3 cyclopic pig fetuses. Each had a proboscis above its completely or incompletely single median eye. One was dissected and found to have a normal brain behind the origin of the 3rd nerves, "as is usual in these cases," while rostral structures were rudimentary, "thus there was no division into hemispheres, but only one smooth vesicle containing a single cavity." There was no trace of olfactory nerves.

Cyclopic pigs were also noted or described by Dehors (1894); Gabriélidès (1896); Moussu (1899); Lindsay (1900); Schmidt (1904); Gregory (1905); Wilder (1908); Schlegel (1909, 1914); Josephy (1911); Lannelongue and Ménard (cited by Schwalbe and Josephy 1913, p. 227); Schwalbe and Josephy (1913, pp. 207–8, 215, 217–18); and Smallwood (1914). Josephy's (1911) had a median eye and a large, backwardly-bent, supraoptic proboscis. The forebrain was greatly reduced, being only about half the size of the normal hindbrain, and consisted of a fluid-filled, dura-covered, single vesicle. There were no olfactory nerves and but a single optic nerve. This animal was also described and figured by Schwalbe and Josephy (1913, pp. 207–8). Seefelder (1910), in reviewing the literature of 1898 to 1910 concerning eye defects, listed 5 cases of cyclopia in pigs. An astomic, cyclopic pig described by Gravelotte was cited by Lesbre (1928a). Various grades of cyclopia were found in several sets of cephalothoracopagic specimens (Landois 1902; Glaser 1928).

Prior, Hunter, and Latham (1924) reported 2 stillborn cyclopic pigs, in 2 litters from a pedigreed Berkshire sow bred to different males of the same breed. One had a single, median eye and a proboscis, and the other a single, median orbit, but no well-defined eye, and no nostrils or nose. A roentgenogram of the first showed skull abnormalities and a small cranial capacity, but the brain was not described. The second animal was dissected. The skull bones were thick and the cranial cavity small. The cranial contents weighed nearly one gram and consisted of a tiny cerebellum and other, unidentified, nerve tissue. There was apparently no cerebrum. A pathology report indicated that associated with the cerebellar tissue was a bilateral sac composed of thin nervous tissue lined by typical ependyma, enclosing typical choroid plexus, and enveloped by meninges. The sac was believed to represent the vestiges of the lateral ventricles and cerebral hemispheres.

More recently several other cyclopic pigs were found. In Keller's (1941) case a proboscis was present superior to fused eyes. Ancel (1950, p. 240) noted 2 stillborn cyclopic pigs in which the pituitary was absent. Holz and Fortuin (1956) described a newborn pig with cyclopic features, in which there occurred external hydrocephalus, abnormalities of the telencephalon, and micrencephaly. Cyclopia with abnormalities of the rhinencephalon was mentioned by Frauchiger and Fankhauser (1957, pp. 50, 52). Cyclopia was noted in a newborn, multiply deformed pig, which also had a defective cranial suture and several open vertebrae (Dieckmann 1953), in a 100-day-old fetus (Hafez 1960), and in a neonate with a supraoptic proboscis (Thoonen and Hoorens 1960), but the brains were not described.

O'Hara and Shortridge's (1966) cyclopic animal had an incompletely fused median eye and no nostrils or nasal cavity. In the cranium, the meninges were closely applied to the skull and contained a large, fluid-filled space over the brain. The brain appeared normal from the thalamus back. The cerebrum consisted entirely of a small transverse band of solid nervous tissue with no indication of ventricles.

Otocephaly

Various grades of otocephaly have occurred fairly commonly in pigs (Vrolik 1854, pl. 58, figs. 7–10; Gurlt 1877, pp. 6–7; Taruffi 1881–94, vol. 2, pp. 310–15; vol. 6, pp. 424–29, 433; vol. 8, pp. 403–5; Hannover 1882–84, p. 160; Morot 1889; Marx 1911, p. 617; Josephy 1913, pp. 255–57; Wright and Wagner 1934).

Vrolik's case, which Blanc (1895) considered edocephalic, was agnathic and astomic, and had low-set, approximated ears, eye defects and a single cerebral vesicle. Similar defects in a newborn pig were seen by Otto (cited by Blanc 1895). The mouth was small, ended blindly, and had no tongue; the mandible was atrophic; and the ears were low-set. A pharyngeal sac was present and communicated by an orifice with the tympanic cavities. A single eye and long proboscis were prominent; the forebrain was vesicular, lacked olfactory nerves, and had only one optic nerve. This animal was one of the 3 that formed the basis of Blanc's (1895) transitional group, cyclotia (see p. 242). Another edocephalic newborn pig was described by Vitu and Houdinière (1934). A large, median eye was situated immediately below a proboscis. The mouth and lower jaw were vestigial. The external ears were low-set but not fused, and the auditory capsules were approximated. The brain was not described. Panum (1860, p. 26) mentioned 19 cases of facial defects in pigs, some of which were probably otocephalic. Morot's (1889) case was opocephalic.

Blanc (1895) summarized numerous reports of earlier and contemporary writers and described 3 otocephalic pigs he examined. One of these animals was edocephalic and had a forebrain consisting of a cerebral vesicle filled with liquid; only rudiments of the olfactory bulbs remained. Another had a duplicated head, one part of which was mildly otocephalic (sphenocephaly, in which brain defects are not found). The brain of the third pig was not described, but the condition was a grade (opocephaly) in which severe anomalies of the forebrain usually occur.

In the animal presented by Chidester (1914), the ears were fused medioventrally. The cerebrum was very thin; the 3rd and 4th ventricles were continuous, with no noticeable constriction to form an iter between them; and the cerebellum was ectopic, misshapen, and relatively large. A marked external hydrocephalus was present.

A pig with a severe grade of otocephaly (spherocephaly) was seen by Lima (1918*b*). The head lacked eyes, nose, and mouth; the pinnae, which were well developed, were turned ventrally toward the face and were closely approximated. The brain consisted only of a large cerebellum and other parts of the hindbrain, the entire fore- and midbrain apparently being absent. In the pig, a purebred Hampshire described by Kernkamp (1921), in addition to ear defects, there were approximation of the eyes, downwardly bent, elongated snout, agnathia, and astomia. The ears were low-set, so that the middle ear cavities almost joined each other on the ventral surface of the head, and the external auditory canals were very short and atretic. The brain was not examined.

Duplication Monsters

Numerous instances have been recorded of malformations of the head or central nervous system in pigs with incomplete duplications of different parts of the body. Saint-Hilaire (1832–37) discussed his own observations, and those of many others, of duplication monstrosities in pigs in volume 3 of his works (pp. 123, 129, 144, 203), and tabulated the various types (p. 357), which totalled 18 cases. Later in the century, Taruffi (1881–94, vol. 2, pp. 310–15) cited 30 cases. Other specimens were described by Thiernesse (1850–51);

Wyman (1861); Gurlt (1877, pp. 5, 41–43, 54–57); Otto (cited by Gurlt 1878); Dehors (1894); Lesbre (1894); Blanc (1895); Jacoby (1897); Alexander (1899); Landois (1902); Schwalbe (1907, pp. 207–8); Forsheim (1908); Wilder (1908); Marx (1911, pp. 621, 626); Schlegel (1912); Carey (1917); Williams and Rauch (1917); Crocker (1919a); Thuringer (1919); Bishop (1921); Hunter and Higgins (1923); Jordan, Davis, and Blackford (1923); Crampton (1926); Baumgartner (1928); Glaser (1928); Nordby and Taylor (1928); Engel (1931); Cohrs (1936); Weber (1946a); Frauchiger and Fankhauser (1957, p. 61); and Grass-nickel (1961).

The usual abnormalities of the central nervous system in the examined cases consisted of complete duplication of the brain and partial duplication of the spinal cord, in individuals with 2 complete heads, or various types and degrees of partial duplication where the head was not completely doubled.

An extremely early stage of a type of anterior duplication was described by George (1942). A serially sectioned, approximately 7 mm-long, pig embryo had a notochord bifurcated from the level of the cardiac end of the stomach, associated with which was a bifid neural canal and paired Rathke's pouches.

Other Defects

Jacoby (1897) described several malformed early pig embryos, one of which had a completely open neural plate; a second, partial absence of the brain, especially of rostral parts. Wilder (1908) painstakingly analyzed various specimens, among which was a newborn pig with partial duplication of the head (diprosopus triophthalmus) in which the single brain was everted (i.e., exencephalic) and the cranial cavity was very small. A 9-mm pig embryo with bilateral anophthalmia, encephalocele, and rachischisis was noted by Seefelder (cited by Kubik 1923), and an acephalic pig was recorded by Schmincke (1921).

A well-preserved, 8-mm exencephalic pig embryo was discovered by Baxter and Boyd (1938). Externally, the defect consisted of eversion and splaying out, on the surface of the head, of the neural tube, extending from the rostral limit of the metencephalon to the region of the upper border of the lamina terminalis. The condition could best be considered as a marked, upward buckling of the whole neural plate in the midbrain region. The roof of the hindbrain was essentially normal, as were the blood vessels of the head. Associated with the abnormality were absence of cranial nerves III, IV, and VI, and markedly retarded development of the optic primordia. The lesion was thus obviously due to nonclosure of the neural tube in the mesencephalic and diencephalic regions. Ordinarily, this abnormality could be regarded as the forerunner of "anencephaly," the defect seen in the newborn of species with a relatively long fetal lifespan, except for the presence of the optic anomalies.

A bizarre defect was noted by Duckworth (1908). The pig was aprosopic, its face being replaced by a smooth and spherical surface. The ears, though not normal, were widely separated, and hence the animal was probably not otocephalic. The skull was thick and dense and the braincase small. The brain was symmetrical but consisted only of the medulla, pons, and cerebellum, which were reduced in size. The author also mentioned several specimens of pigs with a similar "microcephalic" condition, in the teratological collection of the Hunterian Museum.

Schellenberg (1909) described a porencephalic pig. The condition was bilateral, there being a large hole between each lateral ventricle and the respective occipitoparietal subarachnoid space. The lateral ventricles, including the posterior horns, were enlarged, but no other ventricles were dilated. The corpus callosum was absent.

Gellatly (1957) mentioned 2 cases of absent corpus callosum, unassociated with any clinical signs, in 6- to 13-day-old Large White pigs; and one case of Arnold–Chiari malformation, associated with well-defined lumbar myelomeningocele and secondary hydrocephalus, in the same breed. A pig with the Arnold–Chiari malformation was also briefly described by Fankhauser (1959). An arhinencephalic specimen was listed by Frauchiger (1959).

Born (1962) observed a 3-day-old pig of the Vietnamese swaybacked breed with a massive, symmetrically dilated skull. The diagnosis was hydranencephaly, and it was regarded as an extreme form of porencephaly. The author's explanation of the origin of the defect—aseptic necrosis due to circulatory disturbance in the umbilical cord, possibly resulting from knotting or twisting of the latter—is most unlikely. A stillborn pig with arthrogryposis and brain defects called hydranencephaly was seen by O'Hara and Shortridge (1966). The brain was small, occupying but two-thirds of the normal-sized cranial cavity. The cerebral hemispheres were paper-thin and contained dilated, fluid-filled, lateral ventricles. Microscopically the hemispheres contained no recognizable neural tissue, but consisted of reticulate cells and primitive blood vessels. The ventricles were lined by flattened cells. The rest of the brain was small but seemed normal.

Symptomless partial aplasia of the cerebellar cortex was described by Cohrs and Schulz (1952). Holz (1954) found a case of congenital asymmetrical diplomyelia of the thoracic cord. O'Hara and Shortridge (1966) noted a 3-week-old pig with duplication of the spinal central canal. Done (1957) reported 3 cases of diastematomyelia of the lumbar cord, which appeared to cause the animals no inconvenience. Marked cerebellar hypoplasia noted (Gitter and Bowen 1962) in young pigs, was probably associated with mild infection of swine fever to which sows were exposed during pregnancy (see p. 176).

16

Cattle

Hydrocephalus

In this section, congenital hydrocephalus appearing as an isolated or relatively isolated phenomenon, or as part of no particular combination of defects, will be distinguished from hydrocephalus forming part of an established syndrome.

Isolated Hydrocephalus

Congenital hydrocephalus is a fairly common abnormality in cattle. It was apparently noted quite frequently in the last century (see, e.g., Lassartesse 1894) but not recorded in the literature to any great extent. Gurlt (1877, pp. 7, 31) saw 10 calves with this defect, one of which also had unilateral absence of the mandible. In the animal observed by Lassartesse (1894), the head was greatly enlarged and filled with fluid. The cerebral hemispheres and cerebellum were almost entirely destroyed, and in their place was a small, shapeless mass of nervous substance. Limb defects were also present. A hydrocephalic calf was mentioned by Regnault (1901); it had a large, bombose head with a greater transverse than anteroposterior diameter.

Troussier (1904) recorded a lethal hydrocephalus that occurred in both of opposite-sex twin calves of the Jurassic breed but did not describe the condition. He stated that hydrocephalus was not a rarity in veterinary obstetrics, but that its happening in both of a pair of twins was unusual and merited being reported. A multiply deformed calf was described in great detail by Lesbre and Forgeot (1905a). The lateral ventricles were greatly enlarged and filled with yellowish fluid. The septum pellucidum was vestigial and the lateral ventricles thus largely communicated. The olfactory bulbs were small, the corpus callosum was absent, the pineal was atrophied, and the anterior lobe of the pituitary was reduced. Owing to great enlargement of the 4th ventricle, the cerebellar vermis was practically reduced to a thin lamella, which appeared to consist of ependyma and pia mater. The state of the 3rd ventricle and aqueduct were not explicitly mentioned. Several authors (e.g., Brodal and Hauglie-Hanssen 1959) have called attention to the fact that the condition of the cerebellum and 4th ventricle in this cow resembled the state of these parts in a human malformation, the Dandy–Walker syndrome (see p. 22).

Another hydrocephalic calf noted by Lesbre and Forgeot (1905*b*) was stillborn. The head was enormously enlarged, and the face was small and short. The distended cranium was extremely thin and covered above by a fibrous membrane in which was an isolated bony plate. The cerebral hemispheres consisted of enormous fluctuant pockets whose walls, lacking all convolutions, were reduced to a thin, fragile, nervous lamina. In places this wall was so closely apposed to the meninges they appeared as one, while in other places they were separated by fluid-filled spaces. The olfactory bulbs were distinct, but the olfactory nerves were very slender. The corpus callosum and septum pellucidum were absent, and the greatly expanded lateral ventricles thus largely communicated with each other. The other ventricles were also dilated, and the colliculi and cerebellum were atrophied. The latter consisted in the midline merely of a thin fragile ependymal membrane. The central canal of the spinal cord was expanded and hydropic. Bifid tongue, cleft palate, and ectrodactyly and ankylosis of all limbs were also present.

Schellenberg (1909) noted twin, 4-week-old calves of the Simmental breed that both had unilateral enlargement of the cranium. The condition was pronounced in one of them, which upon dissection was discovered to have severe, right-sided hydrocephalus. Other defects were absence of the hippocampal commissure and of the commissure of the corpus callosum in its entire extent. In place of the latter, however, there was present a corresponding anlage in the form of a huge, longitudinal, callosal bundle (Balkenlängsbündel), apparently very similar to the structure found (King 1936) in some mice with hereditary absence of the corpus callosum (see p. 228).

Photographs of calves with enormously enlarged heads are found in Williams (1909, pp. 293, 736, 738). A calf with greatly enlarged cranium and congenital hydrocephalus was briefly mentioned by Crocker (1919*a*). The brain was thin-walled and the ventricles were distended by fluid. Gardner (1923), Götze (1923), and Gavrilescu (1924) each noted a hydrocephalic calf. Lesbre (1928*b*), citing observations of his own and others, described several malformed calves among which was one with hydrocephalus limited to the left cerebral hemisphere.

Houck (1930) described hydrocephalus in a grade Durham calf whose head was noticeably large at birth and bulged in the frontal and temporal regions. The calvaria was expanded and domeshaped with the ears and horns wide apart. When the head was opened a thin bag of water, as it was termed, was visible. The cerebral gyri and sulci were completely obliterated, and the dura was firmly adherent to the sutures of the skull. The cerebral cortex was thin, and the interior of the hemispheres appeared as a large chamber with the basal ganglia standing out in bold relief. The lateral ventricles were tremendously dilated, with loss of the septum pellucidum and the greater part of the corpus callosum. The choroid plexuses of the lateral ventricles were prominent. The ventricles of the rhinencephalon were also enlarged.

The foramina of Monro consisted of extremely narrow slits, and the 3rd ventricle was obliterated except for a narrow channel and appeared obstructed by a growth between the thalami (probably the massa intermedia, which is large in cows, Millen and Woollam 1962, p. 8). The ependymal lining of the 3rd ventricle was almost completely eroded. No pineal body was found, only the stalk remaining. The colliculi and 4th ventricle were fairly normal. The state of the aqueduct of Sylvius was not mentioned. The condition of the foramina of Magendie and Luschka could not be determined. The cerebellum was normal except for being pushed firmly down against the medulla oblongata and being close to the colliculi. The pons and the rest of the brainstem were noticeably flattened. The father of the calf, a Durham bull, was said to have had a noticeably large head and horns that were far apart, suggesting a low-grade hydrocephalus.

Sholl (1931) noted a 7-month-old Holstein calf that apparently was was normal at birth, but in which disturbances of equilibrium gradually developed. At autopsy the left side of the skull was seen to be somewhat larger than the right, and a marked unilateral hydrocephalus was noted, which had destroyed the major part of the left hemisphere. The ventricle, which was filled with clear, watery liquid, definitely communicated with the right one, but the latter was normal.

Williams (1931) described 15 malformed calves, all of dairy breeds, 2 of which had hydrocephalus. In one of the latter there was an unmistakable bulging of the cranium, and the condition may have involved the aqueduct of Sylvius. In the second the cranium was also clearly hydrocephalic, and the cerebral convolutions were gross and indistinct. Williams and Frost (1938) found "subdural" hydrocephalus in a young Holstein–Friesian calf. A large fluid-filled sac was present that was continuous with the intracranial dura mater and protruded through an enormously enlarged, persistent "anterior neuropore," to use the authors' term. The brain itself was compressed and reduced in size. The animal also had a cleft palate.

Ely, Hull, and Morrison (1939), in a study of agnathia in 4 Jersey calves noted possible hydrocephalus in a term specimen, as indicated by the shape of the head and the condition of the brain. In other agnathic calves (Annett 1939; Lalonde 1940), hydrocephalus was not reported. A photograph of an 8-month-old calf fetus with internal hydrocephalus was presented by Frauchiger and Hofmann (1941, p. 166). The condition was not described. These authors (*ibid.*, p. 174) also cited a study by Landtwing of a dicephalic calf one of whose heads had internal hydrocephalus.

Cole and Moore (1942) discovered lethal hydrocephalus in a herd of grade and purebred Holstein–Friesian cattle. Several affected calves were obtained in a breeding study that will be described below. The condition was of the internal variety and was accompanied by marked papilledema. The lateral ventricles were greatly distended and covered by a thin layer of cerebral cortex, but dissection revealed no apparent blockage of any sort. The position and angle of the foramen magnum were markedly altered. The authors believed that these and other bony changes may have been the primary abnormalities, with the hydrocephalus a secondary effect caused by occlusion of the foramina of Magendie and Luschka.

Weber (1946*a*) listed 13 cases of bovine hydrocephalus in the 30-year collection of malformed animals in the Canton of Bern. Faix (1950) noted a greatly expanded fluid-filled head in a stillborn calf of no special breed. Dissection revealed that only the dura mater was left, the brain being all but gone, probably owing, he believed, to pressure atrophy. Ankyloses of the joints of the hindlegs and lateral deviation of the upper jaw were also present.

In the spring of 1949, many cases of a type of hydrocephalus were observed in newborn calves in several neighboring districts around Lake Towada in Japan (Tabuchi *et al.* 1953). The condition was not related to breed, since it occurred in various stocks kept in the districts. It was seen predominantly in cattle pastured from May to October, and hardly at all in those kept in barns all year around. Neurological symptoms of affected calves varied from slight to serious, and in 28 autopsied cases the severity of the brain changes was proportional to that of the clinical symptoms. The lateral ventricles were dilated and contained excessive amounts of clear, cerebrospinal fluid. The cerebral cortex was thin, and in more severe cases the tissue areas between the ventricles were absent. In some cases the brainstem was also atrophied.

Infection with the virus of Japanese equine encephalitis, outbreaks of which occurred throughout Japan during July to October, 1948, was suspected (see p. 175) as the cause of the hydrocephalus. Isolation of a causative virus, however, was unsuccessful.

Tajima, Yamagiwa, and Iwamori (1951) found 5 cases of hydrocephalus (which they called hydromicrencephaly). The abnormalities consisted of great enlargement of the lateral ventricles, which contained 80 to 220 ml of clear, cerebrospinal fluid, severe thinning of the cerebral cortex, absent corpus callosum, and atrophy of the brain stem. The authors considered that the condition was partly secondary (i.e., compensatory). They also speculated that it might have been caused by an epidemic of encephalitis (see above), but they had little evidence for this possibility. Hydrocephalic calves with similar symptoms were also collected in Japan during these same years by Sugawa, Mochizuki, and Tsubahara (1951). They, too, were unable to find any evidence connecting the congenital condition to a virological or bacteriological agent. Innes and Saunders (1962, p. 288) believed that the condition that occurred in these Japanese cattle was hydranencephaly, not hydrocephalus (see p. 308).

Hughes (1952) found an extreme hydrocephalus and hydromyelia in a calf of an Ayrshire mother. In both the cranium and vertebral canal, nervous tissue had almost entirely disappeared, possibly owing to pressure atrophy, leaving only a very thin layer of nervous tissue supported by meninges enclosing fluid. The author suggested that the cause of the hydromyelia was failure of cerebrospinal fluid to reach the subarachnoid spaces because of occlusion of foramina of the 4th ventricle. Giannotti (1952) recorded 20 hydrocephalic calves of the Marche breed of Italy, in all of which the condition was internal. The amount of liquid in the lateral ventricles varied from few to many liters; in some cases, especially the severe ones, the brain tissue was thin. Nine of the animals also had ankyloses of the limbs and other limb deformities.

Bone (1953) reported congenital hydrocephalus in 2 purebred Jersey calves of an experimental herd. Both were born prematurely, had apparent doming of the skull at birth, and were sacrificed about a week after birth when their general condition declined. At autopsy internal hydrocephalus was found, principally of the left lateral ventricle and foramen of Monro in one, and of the lateral and 3rd ventricles and foramina of Monro in the other. In neither case was there evidence of inflammation or obstruction of ventricles, aqueduct, or foramina. The principle factor common to both cases was that the dams were second-generation members of a group carried experimentally on rations low in carotene and had received this regime for their entire lives. The possibility that the hydrocephalus in their offspring was nutritional in origin thus cannot be ignored.

Gilman (1956) described 6 cases of internal hydrocephalus that occurred in a period of about 8 months in a purebred Holstein–Friesian herd. All the animals died within a few days of birth. Only one had an abnormally large cranium. Different degrees of dilatation of the lateral ventricles existed, from slight to moderately severe, but even in the latter situation, in which the cerebral hemispheres were reduced to a thin shell, there was no visible distortion of the cranium. The lateral ventricles communicated in the area of the septum pellucidum. In no case was the 3rd ventricle apparently enlarged.

Whittem (1957) mentioned that he occasionally saw hydrocephalus with enlargement of the head and thinning of the calvaria. Frauchiger and Fankhauser (1957, p. 38) listed 5 cases of congenital hydrocephalus in their collection of malformed calves. A hydrocephalic calf of the Romagnolo breed was noted by Silvestri and Lughi (1959).

Fankhauser (1959) described hydrocephalus accompanied by cerebellar hypoplasia in a young calf of the Simmental breed. The middle and caudal parts of the lateral ventricles were widely dilated. Atrophy of the cerebral cortex was most marked in the occipital lobe. The corpus callosum was thin and the septum pellucidum shrunken. The midbrain was apparently normal, and the aqueduct was patent. The cerebellum was absent except for minute remnants. The author was of the opinion that the dilatation of the lateral ventricles represented a compensatory (i.e., *ex vacuo*) hydrocephalus.

Blackwell, Knox, and Cobb (1959) reported a lethal hydrocephalic condition in grade and purebred Hereford cattle. Affected calves were stillborn or died shortly after birth; while alive they were unable to stand or make direct motor movements. All had small bodies and bulging foreheads. The only abnormalities discovered at autopsy were those associated with marked internal hydrocephalus and domeshaped, and otherwise defective, skull. In more extreme cases skull ossification was incomplete. In all affected animals the supraorbital foramen was partly occluded and the supraorbital groove flattened, probably because of excessive cerebrospinal-fluid pressure. The supraorbital foramen has not been found to be affected in all bovine hydrocephaluses, thus possibly indicating that the nature of the condition differs in some way where it is affected from cases where it is not. The cranial cavity was increased in size, but the volume of brain tissue was probably within normal limits. The cerebellum was smaller than normal. Hydramnios occurred in some cases.

Blood *et al.* (1957) briefly recorded 2 Jersey calves from prolonged gestations. Both had pronounced hydrocephalus consisting of markedly dilated fluid-filled, lateral ventricles domed by thin-walled cerebral cortexes, as well as apparent total or partial absence of the pituitary. The authors believed the defects to be similar in both animals and that, since they came from consanguineous matings, a hereditary etiology was suggested. The defects, in fact, were far from similar. The first calf had hydrocephalus, skull defects, pituitary anomalies, and cleft lip and palate. The second was also hydrocephalic and had absent pituitary but also presented rather definite signs of cyclopia, such as median orbital cavity, partly fused eyes, single median optic nerve, a supraoptic proboscis, absence of many facial bones, and no olfactory bulbs. Since the cerebral hemispheres were apparently not fused, the condition was clearly a low grade of cyclopia, perhaps rhinocephaly (see p. 239).

Baker, Payne, and Baker (1961) studied the inheritance of hydrocephalus in cattle; this aspect will be discussed below. The abnormality will be described here. The breed investigated was not mentioned, but it was probably Hereford (see p. 301). Thirty affected calves, including 8 living ones, were examined. Hydrocephalics were usually born alive but were small, weak, made little effort to stand, and usually died soon after. The forehead was frequently bulging and the skull domeshaped. Hydramnios was common.

Gross inspection revealed direct relations among amount of cranial enlargement, ventricular size, volume of cerebrospinal fluid, and locomotor incoordination. Cerebrospinal-fluid pressure was not markedly elevated. Closure of cranial sutures was normal. The cerebral ventricles were greatly enlarged (a photograph of a gross section showed greatly dilated lateral ventricles; whether other ventricles were also expanded was not specified); and choroid plexus was greatly increased in size (again it was not clearly indicated whether only choroid plexuses of the lateral ventricles were enlarged or others also). Although not mentioned in the text, the corpus callosum was lacking in a photograph of a sectioned affected brain. Various means of examination revealed free flow of injected material from the lateral ventricles into the cerebral and spinal arachnoid spaces. There was no evidence of dwarfism in the animals.

A brief report of congenital hydrocephalus in Ayrshire cattle was made by Huston, Eldridge, and Oberst (1961). Some affected animals were premature and stillborn, while others were term stillbirths or died shortly after birth. Prematures were more severely hydrocephalic than term animals. Also noted were abnormalities of the cerebral hemispheres, colliculi, and cerebellum. These defects and the hydrocephalus were not further described. Belling and Holland (1952) examined the heads of 42 stillborn Hereford calves from herds with a high neonatal mortality rate. Three, although not enlarged, were extremely hydrocephalic, but the condition was poorly described. Several others (number unstated) had lesser degrees and, apparently different types of hydrocephalus. In addition, there were several (again, number not stated) with hypoplastic cerebellum as well as herniation of the cerebellar nodulus.

Barlow and Donald (1963) reported 15 hydrocephalic calves that were born in an Ayrshire herd in a 2-year period. All but one were liveborn but were unable to stand and died within 48 hours. Externally, the frontal region of the head was domed and the eyes protruded. Ten were dissected and found to have gross lesions in the head only. The cranium was enlarged and dome-shaped. In the more severe cases the fontanelles were open. The gyri were usually narrow and shrunken and the sulci shallow. The meninges appeared normal. The cerebral hemispheres were dilated and fluctuant and the distention was accompanied by thinning of the brain substance, especially at the occipital poles. The posterior extremities of the occipital lobes tended to overlay the cerebellum to a greater extent than normal. In 2 animals the optic nerves were narrowed, and in one of them the infundibulum was not apparent.

Sections showed massive dilatation of the lateral ventricles with cerebral brain substance reduced to a thin rind. The cortex was narrowed, and the septum pellucidum was fenestrated or represented by vestigial fragments hanging from the roof of the cavity. The hippocampus was thin in all affected animals examined, and in the 2 most severe cases the fornix was entirely membranous. The halves of the diencephalon were widely separated and usually showed some compression, probably because of intraventricular pressure. The 3rd ventricle was also dilated. There was pronounced lateral narrowing of the mesencephalon and overlaying of the posterior colliculi by the anterior ones. The aqueduct of Sylvius was reduced to a vertical slit that was extremely narrow at the isthmus; nevertheless, it was mechanically patent. The cerebellum was structurally normal in all cases but was reduced in size in one animal. There was no Arnold–Chiari malformation. The choroid plexuses, medulla, and cord were normal. The foramina of Luschka appeared patent. The most salient finding, according to the authors, was a severe peripheral vascular gliosis in the region of the narrowed mesencephalon, which occurred in all affected calves, and may thus have played a primary role in the development of the hydrocephalus.

Schutte (1963) noted a calf with peculiar behavior. It was killed at about 5 months of age and discovered to have enlarged lateral ventricles in the posterior region and a very small cerebellum. The author reasoned, unconvincingly that since no cranial malformation was present the hydrocephalus developed postnatally. A 7-month-old aborted fetus had (Herzog 1963) a skin defect in the frontal region and a noticeably large head, which was diagnosed as internal hydrocephalus. It also had a tumorous leukosis with particular localization in the skin.

Urman and Grace (1964) found hydrocephalus in 12 neonatal Hereford calves from the same area and in some of the same herds that the cases of Baker, Payne, and Baker (1961) came from. Affected animals were unable to stand. Enlargement of the forehead was a constant feature but was not always extensive. Principally, the calvaria was enlarged, but the sutures were closed. Upon dissection the gyri were seen to be narrow and the sulci deep. The lateral and 3rd ventricles, especially the former, were extremely dilated and filled with clear cerebrospinal fluid. There was no excess fluid in the subarachnoid spaces. The structure of the dorsal cortex did not indicate excessive pressure, but the basilar cerebral cortex was greatly reduced in thickness and its convolutions were diminished in size.

The midbrain was elongated and narrow, and the medulla oblongata was somewhat S-shaped. The fissure between the anterior and posterior colliculi was absent, and the colliculi themselves were misshapen. The aqueduct of Sylvius was narrowed at the isthmus and formed a vertical slit, possibly owing to mechanical displacement of the mesencephalon as indicated by its conspicuous, domeshaped curvature. In several cases diverticuli of the aqueduct were found. The cerebral occipital lobes appeared to extend more posteriorly than normal and almost entirely covered the small cerebellum. Many animals were microphthalmic, and all were congenitally blind. The optic nerves and tracts were narrowed, the retina was detached in all 12, and the lens was sometimes small. The degree of cranial enlargement varied in severity but was never great enough to be a positive means of diagnosing hydrocephalus. In doubtful cases, microphthalmia and other ocular signs and muscular weakness were helpful.

Microscopically, areas of depletion or absence of myelin were seen in the cerebellum, upper cervical cord and, to a lesser degree, the midbrain and cerebral cortex; and an apparent increase of vascularity was noted in the region of the mesencephalon. In addition, there was a generalized, progressive type of muscular dystrophy. Similar muscular changes in a hydrocephalic calf were seen by Hadlow (1962, p. 164).

Rhodes *et al.* (1962) measured the levels of several serum enzymes in hydrocephalic calves described by Urman and Grace (1964). The elevations found for some enzymes were believed to be associated with the muscular abnormalities of the animals.

A survey of a large number of fetuses revealed a near-term hydrocephalic calf (Mammerickx and Leunen 1964). The cranium was deformed and the brain contained a liquid-filled ventricular cavity the size of a "large egg."

While a hereditary etiology was presumed or conjectured for many of the hydrocephaluses mentioned above, in only few instances was evidence offered to support this belief: in 3 studies retrospective analysis was resorted to, and in 2 studies controlled matings were made between animals of known or suspected genotypes.

The 20 hydrocephalic calves reported by Giannotti (1952) were all descendants of a single bull, which was presumed to have carried a single recessive mutant gene responsible for the condition. All 6 hydrocephalic calves reported by Gilman (1956) were sired by the same bull, Don. The mothers of 5 of the calves were half-sisters, the offspring of another bull, Louis. The mother of the sixth calf was related to both Don and Louis. Herd records showed that 20 of Louis' daughters had been mated to Don, producing 27 normal and 5 hydrocephalic calves. The data were thus compatible with recessive inheritance. The same conclusion was drawn by Blackwell, Knox, and Cobb (1959), whose 19 abnormal calves all came from matings of animals that were descendants of a certain bull. The herd records showed that these 19 came from 154 matings between sires of abnormal calves and daughters of such sires.

Planned matings were made in 2 studies. Cole and Moore (1942) saw 2 hydrocephalic calves that were the products of cows mated to their sires. Since this coincidence suggested a hereditary situation, additional sire–daughter matings were made. From these crosses 27 calves were produced, 6 of which had hydrocephalus, which again permitted the conclusion that the the condition was probably due to a simple recessive gene.

As well as gathering retrospective data from several sources, which supported the hypothesis of a recessive mode of inheritance of the hydrocephalus they described, Baker, Payne, and Baker (1961) carried out a prospective study. Each year, for 2 years, they mated 40 cows known to have produced abnormal offspring to 2 bulls, one a known sire of abnormal calves, and the other a bull from an inbred line with no history of hydrocephalus. From the latter, the "noncarrier" bull, 37 normal and no hydrocephalic calves were obtained; from the "carrier" bull 28 normal and 6 hydrocephalic offspring were obtained. These figures, once more, suggested that the abnormality was a recessive trait. In Huston, Eldridge, and Oberst's (1961) study, also, though not conclusive, the available evidence pointed to recessive inheritance.

It was noted in an abstract (Nuss 1966) that a syndrome including hydrocephalus occurring in an experimental herd of Ayrshire cattle appeared in a ratio of abnormal to normal animals twice as great as would be expected if the syndrome were due to a single gene. Genetic studies, not further described, indicated the condition was due to "multiple-gene mutations." Studies of thymus DNA of normal and abnormal animals, which indicated a variation in base sequence somewhere along the DNA helix, supported, it was contended this conclusion!

Of course, it is impossible to say whether or not the putative recessive genes in these cases, or any others that may cause hydrocephalus in cattle, are identical or allelic until crosses between heterozygotes for different ones are performed. Descriptions of the malformations revealed various points of similarity and dissimilarity among them. But it would be a mistake to believe that morphological comparisons can settle the question of allelism, partly because the different genetic backgrounds and the different environmental conditions the genes were exposed to can be counted on to have also influenced the end results.

Hydrocephalus in Achondroplasia and Other Forms of Dwarfism

Symptoms of hydrocephalus have often been found in cattle afflicted with different types of dwarfism. Some of these states will be discussed.

Bulldog calves. Several achondroplasias have been recognized in cattle (Shrode and Lush 1947; Gilmore 1949; Stormont 1958). Two of these are apparently inherited as *dominant* traits. One type was first found in the Dexter breed (Stock 1902; Begg 1903; McLaren 1903; Seligmann 1904; Wilson 1909), but has since been reported in others as well (Nickerson 1917; Adametz 1925; Downs 1928; Williams 1936; Karnes 1941; Mead, Gregory, and Regan 1946b; Berger and Innes 1948; Weber 1949; Brüggemann 1951; Dollahon and Koger 1960).

The genetics of this condition is not yet entirely agreed upon. The salient point is that achondroplastic animals, of the type known as Dexter, when bred together, produce 3 types of offspring: (1) normal, i.e., longlegged, sometimes called Kerry; (2) shortlegged like themselves; and (3) gross malformed, nonviable ones, called "bulldog" calves, because of their markedly misshapen heads.

Crew (1923, 1924) postulated that shortleggedness was due to homozygosity for a main factor, S, the expression of which was modified by 2 additional factors, L_1, and L_2; and that when SS was combined with both modifying factors the lethal type resulted. On the other hand, Wilson (1909) concluded from his own and Seligmann's (1904) material that the production of bulldog calves was dependent upon one genetic factor only. According to this interpretation, which Mohr (1926) adopted, achondroplastic Dexters were heterozygous for a semidominant gene, which when homozygous produced the bulldog type. This hypothesis was fairly well supported by Young's (1951) study, in which from matings of Dexters he obtained 21 longlegged, 28 shortlegged, and 12 monster calves.

This mode of inheritance was recently challenged by Gregory, Tyler, and Julian (1960), who obtained characteristically bulldog calves by crossing a Dexter bull to dwarf cattle of non-Dexter varieties. The full report of these studies appeared recently (Gregory, Tyler and Julian, 1966). From crosses among different types of achondroplastic and dwarf cattle several animals were produced that resembled the Dexter type. Some of these Dexters were bred *inter se* and to registered Dexters and produced bulldog calves that according to various gross morphological criteria were very similar to bulldogs the authors produced by mating registered Dexters to each other. The proportion of all the offspring of these matings the bulldogs constituted was not stated.

On the basis of this evidence, i.e., that Dexter animals were apparently "reconstituted" from other dwarf varieties, and from the results of certain other crosses, it was postulated that all achondroplastic mutants in cattle are interrelated components of the same genetic complex; and that the assumed dominance of the genetic factors for some of the achondroplasias probably results from an interaction between a major recessive gene and alleles at 2 other loci, on the order of the scheme proposed by Crew (1924).

Bulldog calves, which were usually aborted several months prematurely, presented numerous defects, including stumped legs, massive umbilical hernia, opisthotonus, bulging cranium, cleft palate, and other characteristic abnormalities. Seligmann (1904) noted that while the appearance of the vault of the cranium in bulldog specimens suggested hydrocephalus, there was no excess cerebrospinal fluid in the ventricles. Lesbre and Forgeot (1904) described 2 bulldog-like, achondroplastic calves in great detail, one of which, a $6\frac{1}{2}$-month fetus, had hydrocephalus. Of 27 bulldog calves examined by Crew (1923), only one was hydrocephalic; in this case the condition was pronounced, with virtually no brain present. The distortion of the head in bulldogs, he found, was mainly due to great thickening and coalescence of the bones of the vault, and to a short basicranium. Marked hydrocephalus in bulldog calves was also noted by others (Karnes 1941; Berger and Innes 1948; Brüggemann 1951) but sometimes was insignificant or mild, with very little fluid in the ventricles (Williams 1936; Mead, Gregory, and Regan 1946*b*). In a case examined by Innes and Saunders (1962, p. 286) the cerebellum, midbrain, and medulla appeared normal, but the hemispheres, including the rhinencephalon, were reduced to an eggshell layer of substance. In Downs' (1928) case dissection revealed a remarkably thick skull and micrencephaly. Gregory, Tyler, and Julian (1966) saw 16 bulldogs, 6 from matings *inter se* of registered Dexters, of which 3 were hydrocephalic, and 10 from crosses of "reconstituted" Dexters with each other or with registered Dexters, of which 2 of 9 examined bulldogs had hydrocephalus.

The bulldog calves described by Dareste (1887) were apparently not identical in type with those just discussed; since, first, they were born alive and lived for a short time afterward; second, they were not mentioned as having short limbs (but did have joint deformities); and, last, in some cases they had other malformations not found in bulldog monsters, such as spina bifida, imperforate anus, and rectovesical fistula.

Dominant achondroplasia 2. Another achondroplasia, also probably the result of heterozygosity for a dominant gene, arose in Swedish Red and White cattle (Johansson 1953). Affected offspring occurred in 2 separate herds but were all sired by the same bull, a completely normal animal in whom the gene probably arose through mutation in pregerminal tissues. The total progeny of the bull were 25 malformed and 28 normal calves.

Abnormal animals showed typical signs of achondroplasia, including short, broad head and moderately bulging forehead. Bull calves consistently showed more pronounced symptoms of achondroplasia than heifers. The calves were born after a gestation of normal length. In many cases hydramnios was noted. The vigor of the animals improved after birth, but all except 6 were killed before 3 weeks of age.

One malformed bull and 4 malformed heifers were raised in the hope of breeding them. Unfortunately the bull proved to be sterile and the heifers showed greatly reduced fertility. The abnormal animals were apparently not dissected, and hence whether they were hydrocephalic was not ascertained.

Telemark achondroplasia. Several probably different *recessive* forms of achondroplasia have been found in cattle. The first of these types was reported by Wriedt (1925) in Telemark Norwegian cattle but has since been noted in other breeds as well (Weinkopff 1927; Carmichael 1933; Brandt 1941; Surrarrer 1943; Winters 1948, p. 140).

As described by Wriedt (1925), the appearance of the limbs and head resembled that of bulldog calves. The condition was more compatible with life, however, since the calves were born alive at term, although they usually died within a few days—of respiratory obstruction, it was believed. In none of the works cited above was the state of the brain mentioned, so it cannot be said with assurance that true hydrocephalus was present, despite photographs of such animals presented by Mohr (1926) and Wriedt (1930, pp. 70–71) that showed them to have greatly bulging heads.

A description of this achondroplasia was also given by Punnett (1936), reporting the studies of Riches. Heterozygotes were not visibly different from homozygous normal specimens. Homozygous recessive animals were born alive at term but died within a few days. Although the achondroplastic condition of the skull, limbs, and general body formation was evident, these signs were not so marked as in bulldog monsters.

Punnett (1936) also reported the results Riches obtained from crossing a heterozygous Telemark bull with 8 Dexter cows. From these crosses 24 calves and a mummy were produced. At least 11 of the F_1 hybrids were typical Dexters, i.e., shortlegged achondroplastics, clearly indicating that the responsible gene was a dominant; but none was a bulldog monster, which demonstrated with a high degree of probability that the 2 lethal genes are genetically independent, i.e., nonallelic. This conclusion was confirmed by segregation of the genes in F_2 progeny, which included a lethal of the Telemark variety and 3 of the bulldog variety.

Recessive achondroplasia 2. A second autosomal recessive achondroplasia was discovered in calves of a Jersey herd (Gregory, Mead, and Regan 1942). Certain morphological features, especially length of legs, which was fairly normal in this condition, distinguished it from the Telemark variety. The condition was usually postnatally lethal. The signs of achondroplasia varied greatly in extent, but all of the 10 defective calves described had short, broad heads and prominent foreheads. Cleft palate was common, especially in more severe cases, but not invariable. Extremely abnormal animals had a large, unclosed fontanelle, but they were apparently not dissected, and the existence of hydrocephalus was therefore not clearly established.

Snorter dwarfism. A form of proportional dwarfism, which came to be known as "snorter" or short-headed dwarfism, was noted first in Hereford herds (Johnson, Harshfield, and McCone 1950) but was later discovered in Angus and perhaps other breeds as well (Chambers, Whatley, and Stephens 1954; Burris and Priode 1956; Gregory and Carroll 1956; Bovard and Priode 1965). The condition was congenital but became more pronounced with age. Slightly bulging foreheads were common, but not invariable, in animals examined by Johnson, Harshfield, and McCone (1950) and by Pahnish *et al.* (1955). Gregory *et al.* (1951), on the other hand, felt that this sign was the most constant and diagnostic characteristic of dwarfs of any age. Few dwarfs lived more than 2 years. One calf that never stood was autopsied at 10 days of age and found to have excessive cerebrospinal fluid in the lateral ventricles (Johnson, Harshfield, and McCone 1950). The heads of 4 dwarf and 4 non-dwarf calves not more than 5 days of age were grossly sectioned. Hydrocephalus (not further described) occurred in an unstated number of the dwarfs, but not in all of them; and a moderate degree of hydrocephalus was found in a nondwarf (Pahnish *et al.* 1955).

The frequency and distribution of the defect indicated it to be due to a single autosomal recessive gene (Johnson, Harshfield, and McCone 1950), which was confirmed by experimental matings (Pahnish, Stanley, and Safley 1955). But this interpretation was considered to be an oversimplification by Gregory, Julian and Tyler (1964), who postulated that alleles segregating at 2 or more loci are capable of producing the same type of dwarf, and, further, that several different mutant types are components of the achondroplastic complex.

Other dwarfism. Several other proportional and nonproportional types of dwarfism have occurred in cattle. They were sometimes associated with skull defects such as occur in hydrocephalus, and sometimes not. The proportional dwarfism, of the long-headed or dolicocephalic variety, seen by Mead, Gregory, and Regan (1942) in Jersey animals and by Baker, Blunn, and Plum (1952) in Aberdeen-Angus herds, probably a recessive, was nonlethal. Affected calves were not recognizable at birth. The proportional dwarfs seen in Hereford cattle by Hafez, O'Mary, and Ensminger (1958) were quite different, since defective young had a short, broad head and bulging forehead. The brain was not described, however. Other forms of dwarfism and achondroplasia were listed by Gilmore (1949) and Stormont (1958); the possible genetic interrelatedness of several dwarfisms was argued by Gregory, Tyler, and Julian (1966).

Hydrocephalus in the Amputated Syndrome (Acroteriasis Congenita)

Amputated is an autosomal recessive character, first found in Swedish Holstein–Friesian cattle and described by Wriedt and Mohr (1928). Abnormal calves were fullterm but were almost always stillborn or died immediately after birth. They presented a very uniform appearance, consisting of severe malformations of the head and face and absence of the forelimbs or of all extremities distal to the elbow and hock. A pronounced hydrocephalus was found with all ventricles expanded to such a degree that cerebral matter was reduced to a thin capsule with flattened gyri. Amputated with marked or slight hydrocephalus was recently reported again in Friesian breeds (Dyrendahl and Hallgren 1956; Schindler 1956; Fischer 1959*c*; Bishop and Cembrowicz 1964; Zayed and Ghanem 1964).

Several other occurrences of hereditary ectromelia accompanied by abnormalities of the face, including those of the lower jaw, were found in Swedish Friesian cattle or related breeds (Gotink, Groot, and Stegenga 1955; Lauvergne and Cuq 1963), but in these cases hydrocephalus was not mentioned. Lauvergne and Cuq (1963) believed that the facial malformations in their amputated specimens were representative of a form of otocephaly. However, the essential feature of otocephaly (Blanc 1895)—approach of the ears toward or their union on the ventral midline—was absent in amputated cattle. And while in otocephaly ectopia of the external ears is always associated with reduction of the lower jaw, micrognathia or agnathia in the absence of low-set ears cannot always be regarded as low-grade otocephaly. In cases of possibly hereditary congenital amputation in Brown Swiss cattle (Duzgunes and Tuncay 1962), there were no malformations of the head and face and no hydrocephalus.

It may be appropriate to include in this section the observations of Saint-Hilaire (1832–37, vol. 2, pp. 212–13) of 3 calves with "phocomelia" (i.e., excessive shortness of all 4 limbs) that also possessed large heads clearly affected with hydrocephalus; he also remarked (*ibid.*) that 2 other such cases were recorded by Jaeger. In a further report on the same subject, Saint-Hilaire (1850) presented another calf with the same combination of defects, bringing the total of such animals he was aware of to 7. Additional calves of probably the same variety were described by Weyenbergh (1875) and Barrier (1885).

Hydranencephaly

Hydranencephaly is defined as complete or almost complete absence of the cerebral hemispheres, with replacement of the space they normally occupy by cerebrospinal fluid surrounded by a membranous covering—the dura or meninges plus a thin rind of cerebral substance. The rest of the brainstem and cerebellum may be normal. Hydranencephaly is distinguished from hydrocephalus by absence of: visible enlargement of the skull, delay in union of the sutures, evidence of increased intracranial pressure, or demonstrable obstruction of cerebrospinal-fluid circulation (Whittem 1957). The abnormality is believed not to be due to primary agenesis of the cerebral hemispheres nor to be the extreme end result of hydrocephalus.

The condition has been reported in cattle. Five cases were observed by Blood (1956) in newborn dairy calves in New South Wales, and many others occurred in the district but were not seen by him. The abnormality appeared in a number of different breeds (Shorthorn, Ayrshire, Jersey, Friesian, Guernsey, and Hereford). The condition had existed in the area for at least 10 years, but with a low prevalence except during 2 nonconsecutive years. In these 2 years it had a seasonal fluctuation, most cases appearing in September. Cows of all the breeds in the area (named above) bore abnormal calves in approximate proportion to their representation in the district. The disease did not appear to have a genetic etiology and no environmental factor seemed strongly associated with it.

All affected calves were weak at birth, stood and walked only with difficulty and with considerable incoordination of hindlegs, and were characterized by blindness and "imbecility." In only 2 cases was the size of the cranium slightly increased. Affected calves had various degrees of brain abnormality, from virtual absence of the brain to a state in which the cerebral hemispheres were reduced to a fluid-filled sac. In latter instances the midbrain, cerebellum, and medulla were normal. Some hydranencephalic calves also had arthrogryposis, and many arthrogrypotic animals had brain changes similar to hydranencephaly. The author considered the brain and joint abnormalities to be parts of the same syndrome.

The pathology was studied by Whittem (1957). He reported on 29 calves, 6 with hydranencephaly alone, 13 with arthrogryposis alone, and 10 with both. One of those with arthrogryposis alone also had a well-developed sacral spina bifida. Considering the cerebral defect only, in 4/15 examined animals the brain was for all practical purposes entirely absent, with merely a few edematous fragments of brain tissue left that floated in the fluid-filled cranial fossae. Dissection of these cases was not possible. In the 11 others the cerebral hemispheres were represented by a thin-walled, fluid-filled sac, but the rest of the brain was normal. The fluid of the lateral ventricles moved freely through an opening in a position corresponding to the septum pellucidum. The corpus callosum and fornix were absent as such but were probably incorporated into the thickened margins of the interventricular orifice. Vestiges of the hemispheres were thickest above the midbrain region, where a number of gyri were present. Elsewhere the cortex was reduced to a very thin membranous sheet. In the floor of the vesicle there was a clear-cut hippocampus separated from the caudate nucleus by a well-defined choroid plexus. The normal-sized cranial cavity also contained hollow olfactory bulbs. The roof of the 3rd ventricle was somewhat enlarged. The foramina of Monro were open, and the rest of the 3rd ventricle and the aqueduct also showed no obstruction; in fact the rostral portion of the aqueduct appeared slightly enlarged. The 4th ventricle was normal, the foramina of Luschka were patent, and there was no accumulation of cerebrospinal fluid in any part of the subarachnoid space. The calvaria was normal.

Thus in typical hydranencephaly there was absence of the cerebrum, especially the cortex, while there was preservation of the rhinencephalon, basal ganglia, midbrain, and contents of the posterior fossa. The eyes and optic nerves were macroscopically and microscopically normal in all cases examined. There was no evidence of encephalitis or encephalomalacia.

Recently, 16 additional cases of hydranencephaly, arthrogryposis, or both, occurred in a district of Australia during a relatively short period of time (Bonner, Mylrea, and Doyle 1961). In 7 autopsied calves the cerebral hemispheres were partly or seemingly completely absent, the deficiencies being made up by fluid-filled membranes.

Huston and Gier (1958) noted a malformed grade Holstein–Friesian calf. Externally, the head was somewhat misshapen and had an elongated area from the forehead to the bridge of the nose from which the hair was missing and in the center of which there was a meningocele. Removal of skin from the top of the head revealed that the frontal, parietal, and nasal bones were widely separated. The dura mater was missing from this region and the rhinencephalon, cerebrum, thalamus, and cerebellum were completely absent. The authors interpreted this condition as being the result of hydrocephalus early in gestation. Their reasoning was unconvincing. Innes and Saunders (1962, p. 282) believed the condition to be hydranencephaly with meningocele.

Herniation of the Brain

Exencephaly and other types and degrees of herniation of the brain have been recorded rather infrequently in cattle. Taruffi (1881–94, vol. 6, p. 30) said that the first case of probable encephalocele in a domestic animal was noted by Nicola Tenone in 1671 in a calf with hydrocephalus and a "serious tumor" at the roof of the nose. He also stated (*ibid.*) that Gurlt in his *Lehrbuch der Pathologischen Anatomie* of 1832 collected 20 cases of meningocele or hydrencephalocele in cattle, including one in which the hernia was interorbital.

Saint-Hilaire (1832–37, vol. 2, p. 328) cited the observation of Waldschmidt in 1797 of a calf with probable "pseudencephaly." Otto (1824, pp. 158–59) described a newborn calf with a round, fluctuant tumor at the crown of the head. The mass was discovered to be a hydrencephalocele, which originated from a hole formed by absence of part of the anterior skull. A calf with pseudencephaly was described by Rayer (1852). The cranium was largely open and was surmounted by a "cellulo-vasculaire" tumor. Only vestiges of the brain remained in the cranial cavity. The animal also had agnathia, imperforate anus, and very short, splayed-out, fore- and hindlimbs. A calf with an unusual defect was reported by Monell (1846). It had a median cleftlike formation of the upper jaw, which continued to the region of the skull where a wedge-shaped defect was present, in which area the head appeared to be covered only by meninges.

Joly and Lavocat (1855) affirmed that theirs was the first authentic case of anencephaly found in animals. The calf was well preserved and clearly showed a cranium that was wide open anteriorly and posteriorly. The brain was "absent" and the spine was cleft throughout its entire length; thus, the animal had craniorachischisis. The authors did not wish to mislead; they explained that it was more exact to say, not that the brain was absent, but that is was represented simply by a remnant in the frontal area and by the membranes that ordinarily protect it. The calf also had a very short muzzle, protruding tongue, cleft palate, absent tail, and imperforate anus.

Walley (1875) described a small but possibly full-term calf with a defect of the frontoparietal region. A large sac, apparently composed of skin covered with hair, hung from this area. On removing the skin, the cranial bones collapsed. The frontals were large but unjoined at the longitudinal suture. The cranial cavity, which was devoid of brain matter, communicated with the sac through a large posterior fontanelle. Gurlt (1877, p. 11) mentioned and figured (pl. 6, legend on p. 89) a calf with absence of forelimbs and a hindlimb, which had a large hydrocephalic brain fully exposed through a cranial fault. He also listed (*ibid.*, p. 16) 8 calves with partial cleft of the cranium and hydrencephalocele, and one with missing skullcap.

Taruffi (1881–94, vol. 8, pp. 243–47), in addition to those he discussed elsewhere (see above), cited the observations by numerous authors of encephalocele in calves, including the following: a calf with a voluminous cerebral hernia that protruded through a frontal defect (Chouard); one with a large frontal tumor, comprising the major part of the brain (Taiche); 3 with hydrencephalocele, one of which had a hernial aperture (Otto); 2 with a voluminous tumor on the top of the head, in one of which the hernia occurred through a large aperture at the lambdoid suture and partly consisted of the hydropic posterior cerebral lobes (Otto); a calf with suboccipital hydrencephalocele and hydrocephalus of the 4th ventricle (Otto); a 40-day-old calf with a large, midfrontal aperture, through which a part of the anterior cerebral lobes protruded (Alessandrini); another, killed at 55 days of age, which had a large occipital pouch formed of skin containing fluid and the major part of the cerebellum (Alessandrini); a fetal calf with hydrencephalocele (Lombardini); and hydrencephalocele in 9 others (Siedamgrotzky, Gurlt) including Gurlt's 8 cases mentioned above. Taruffi (1881–94, vol. 6, pp. 142–44) also stated that he knew of 4 museum specimens with "acrania," by which, it seems certain, he was referring to forms of exencephaly. Two of these cases also had facial cleft, and a third had cervical spina bifida.

A midfrontal encephalocele was well described in a stillborn calf under the name proencephaly by Malet (1885). Externally the protrusion had the appearance of a soft tumor the size of a small chicken egg. It consisted of a herniation of part of the brain through a large opening in the anterior wall of the cranium and was covered by thin, hairless skin mingled with meninges. The cranium and cranial cavity were small and distorted in shape.

An unusual case was noted by Boizy and Blanc (1893). A calf that seemed normal at birth developed a frontal tumor during its second week of life. Killed when 20 days old, it was found to have a hydropic meningeal herniation through a large hole in the frontonasal region. In addition, the left cerebral hemisphere was apparently absent, leaving only its meningeal coverings, although the right one was normal except for being slightly small. The cranial cavity was reduced in size. Dubois and Lapoulot (1899) saw a calf with a large frontal encephalocele, which was connected by a stalk to a fairly normal brain.

A stillborn calf noted by Antoine (1906) had a peculiarly malformed skull and short face. On top of the very small head was a hairless, round area, consisting of vascular tissue, which was surrounded by bone. The bones of the head were defective, so that rostral to the occipital area the cranial cavity consisted only of sphenoid and small temporal bones. The spinal cord was normal except in the cervical area where there were but 4 pairs of spinal nerves. The medulla was not covered by the cerebellum, which was atrophied and consisted solely of the vermis, and thus the floor of the 4th ventricle was visible. Anterior to this region, little of the brain was left apart from rudimentary cerebral peduncles, which supported the pituitary.

Ballantyne (1904, p. 358) stated that "cephalocele" was rare in animals, including calves, and that when it occurred it was most often found at the frontal end of the cranium. Albrecht (1911) described a multiply deformed calf, which had a midfrontal hydrencephalocele and absent sacral and caudal vertebrae. Radasch (1912) examined a term calf with a partially duplicated face. At the vertex of the skull the skin was absent and the cranium not fully developed, and hence the dura was exposed. Furthermore, a small hole in the dura allowed the brain to be seen. Lesbre (1912, 1928b) mentioned calves with large median frontal encephalocele and others with frontal hydrencephalocele. Schlegel (1913) noted a near-term dwarf calf with a frontal hydrencephalocele, partly rudimentary cerebellum, and totally absent spinal cord and spinal canal. Gebhardt (1920, cited by Schlegel 1921) saw 3 calves with hydrencephalomeningocele and another with hemicephaly. Micucci (1926) briefly noted 2 newborn calves with large hydrencephalocele protruding through a large cranial fault. Keller and Niedoba (1937) found 2 calves with what was called anencephaly in a group of duplication monsters examined.

Shaw (1938) described skull defects in 2 Holstein–Friesian calves, a brother and his full sister; the former was stillborn, the latter died within a few hours of birth. The external defect consisted of a frontoparietal brain hernia that was not covered by meninges or, apparently, by skin. The defect was somewhat more severe in the female, in which the opening in the skull was larger and more brain tissue protruded.

Five exencephalic or anencephalic calves occurred (Weber 1946a) in the Canton of Bern in a 30-year period. Weber (1949) recorded a 6-week-old cow fetus with exencephaly in the occipital region. The diencephalon and mesencephalon were affected, and the 3rd ventricle was open to the surface. He also saw a newborn calf with a skin-covered brain defect. Schulz (1955) observed a stillborn calf with a small cranial defect in the frontal region through which a portion of the brain protruded. Various associated cerebral defects were present.

Frauchiger and Fankhauser (1957, p. 44) briefly described a newborn calf with frontoparietal meningoencephalocele, in which the cerebrum was replaced by an area cerebrovasculosa. The animal also had a deformed cerebellum and an open 4th ventricle. They (ibid., p. 51) also presented photographs of a newborn calf with a huge frontal meningoencephalocele and an absent left olfactory bulb. Other instances of meningoencephalocele were also listed (ibid., pp. 53–54).

Koch, Fischer, and Schumann (1957, p. 80) mentioned a calf with a large opening in the frontoparietal region, through which protruded a large, liquid-filled membranous sac. Also present were short upper jaw, cleft lip and palate, and microphthalmia. A calf with a similar set of abnormalities was recorded by Crocker (1919*b*). Hatziolos (1960) saw an 8-month fetal calf with incompletely fused cranial bones and an encephalocele. The animal also had a lymphoblastic lymphoma. Finally, Mammerickx and Leunen (1964) noted a fetus with a pigeon-egg-sized meningocele.

Defects of the Rhinencephalon

A lethal condition discovered by Ilančić (1940) involved the brain. A healthy bull sired 33 normal and 37 abnormal calves. The abnormal young had atresia of the nostrils and defective skulls and died at birth or soon after. In 3 that were autopsied the rhinencephalon was incompletely developed. The bull was not closely related to the cows he was bred to, although all were descended from animals of the Montafon breed imported from Austria. The genetic situation postulated to explain the defect was that the bull was heterozygous for a lethal dominant gene and a suppressing allele, and that abnormal calves were those inheriting the lethal from the bull without receiving a suppressing allele from the mother. Other possible explanations come to mind. For example, a dominant mutation arising during prenatal development of the bull may have produced gonadal mosaicism for the gene.

Arhinencephaly was described in a Simmental calf by Weber (1946*a*), and this condition was represented 4 times in Frauchiger and Fankhauser's (1957, p. 32) collection of malformed calves. The latter authors also discussed other occurrences of this defect. Malformations of the olfactory bulbs were described by Godglück (1952), who called the condition encephalocysto-meningocele. Frauchiger and Fankhauser (1957, p. 53) criticized the use of this term.

Weber's (1946*a*) case and 2 others were described in detail by Morsier (1962). The Simmental calf had malformed nasal structures, including absence of both nostrils and nasal cavities. There was complete agenesis of olfactory bulbs, defective cerebral convolutions, small cerebral hemispheres, and enlargement of lateral ventricles. The second animal had small, malformed olfactory bulbs and a small cerebellum as well as bilateral microphthalmia and a right cleft lip that reached the level of the eye. In the third animal the olfactory bulbs were almost completely absent, the cerebellum was small but well formed, and the 4th ventricle and cerebellum extended caudally, resembling a mild Chiari malformation. It also had bilateral microphthalmia.

Defects of the Cerebellum

Malformations of the cerebellum have been encountered a number of times in cattle. *Sporadic* cases of cerebellar aplasia or hypoplasia were reported on several occasions. Robin (1911) noted a calf with an extremely small cerebellum, as did Frauchiger (1940). Weber (1946*b*) saw 2 calves with absent cerebellum. Anderson and Davis (1950) briefly described a 3-month-old Holstein–Friesian animal with an extremely rudimentary cerebellum, which showed no division into vermis and hemispheres. A large amount of fluid was present in the space normally occupied by the cerebellum. The calf was unable to stand at birth; as it developed the ability to walk it did so with a staggering gait. Jennings and Sumner (1951) examined a 6-month-old Ayrshire calf that had exhibited nervous symptoms from birth. The cerebellum was smaller than normal and had a reduced amount of white matter in all lobes.

Cerebellar hypoplasia was found in grade Hereford cattle (Sippel 1951) and in purebred Herefords (Young, cited by Innes and Saunders 1962, p. 303). Cerebellar atrophy in calves was illustrated and discussed by Fankhauser (1955, 1957, 1959). Frauchiger and Fankhauser (1957, pp. 232–33) listed 7 cases seen personally; 2 with agenesis of the vermis; 2, total aplasia; and 3, atrophy, presumably due to inflammation. Other defects present were hydrocephalus in all cases, hypoplastic corpus callosum in 3, and occipital meningocele in 2. Tsiroyannis *et al.* (1957) noted congenital cerebellar ataxia in a Pie Noir breed calf with agenesis of the vermis and left cerebellar hemisphere and marked aplasia of the right cerebellar hemisphere. A calf of a Dutch breed with congenital cerebellar ataxia was found by Monti and Guarda (1961) to have severe overall reduction in cerebellar volume. As noted above, Morsier (1962) found cerebellar defects in 2 calves with abnormal or absent olfactory bulbs. In a study of 243 calves ranging in age from one day to 8 weeks, 2 were found with congenital cerebellar hypoplasia (Rothenbacher 1962). A very small cerebellum occurred in a 5-month-old calf that also had some dilation of the lateral ventricles (Schutte 1963).

Two Ayrshire calves, born in the same herd within a month of each other, but probably unrelated, exhibited nervous signs at birth (Howell and Ritchie 1966). Dissection revealed that both had gross abnormalities of the pons and reduction or absence of many parts of the cerebellum. The latter defects were thought to be the result of partial cerebellar agenesis complicated by subsequent degenerative changes. These are the only cases of cerebellar malformation that were seen in 10 years of constant observation of this herd.

Familial cerebellar defects in cattle have also been reported. A condition probably known to English cattlemen for many years was first investigated by Innes, Russell, and Wilsdon (1940). Affected calves all presented the same nervous symptoms. Tissue was examined from 5 purebred Hereford calves, 1 to 20 days of age, from 3 widely separated herds. Macroscopically the cerebellum was abnormally small and histologically showed degenerative changes. The brainstem and cerebrum were entirely normal. The disease was considered hereditary since defective calves were born only when Hereford bulls were bred to Hereford cows; in 2 instances replacement of a bull siring defective calves was followed by cessation of the condition. No genetic study was made, however. What may be the same condition was observed by Malm (cited by Innes and Saunders 1962, p. 301). Nine bulls were recorded as producing affected offspring. Also possibly the same defect was a familial cerebellar hypoplasia noted by Finnie and Leaver (1965) in 6 newborn Shorthorn calves.

Another type of cerebellar defect in cattle was described by Johnson *et al.* (1958). Eight calves with spastic symptoms occurred in 2 related herds of Holstein–Friesian cattle over a 2-year period. The symptoms—incoordination or ataxia—became apparent at about 6 weeks of age and were similar in all cases. Five affected calves were autopsied at 6 to 13 months of age and showed similar brain defects. The entire brain was small, cerebellar convolutions were small and closely packed together, the dura appeared to be thickened over the area of the cerebellum, and the tentorium was very small and poorly developed. Neuronal degeneration was found in the cerebrum, thalamus, and cerebellum. There appeared to be some distortion and reduction in size of the cranial cavity.

All affected calves had a common male ancestor, but none of their parents had nervous symptoms, which indicated that the condition, if hereditary, may have been recessive. A known "carrier" bull was bred to related females. One of the 3 resulting calves was affected. Ataxic calves stopped appearing after known carriers were removed from the herds.

The Arnold–Chiari Malformation

The Arnold–Chiari malformation, a well-known human condition (Feigin 1956; Cameron 1957), consists of congenital defects of the hindbrain: abnormalities of the pons, medulla, and cerebellum, with elongation and protrusion of parts of the last through the foramen magnum into the upper cervical spinal canal. It is often associated with spina bifida cystica and sometimes with hydrocephalus (see pp. 67–71).

So far as can be determined, the Arnold–Chiari malformation has been reported only twice in cattle. The first case, found only surprisingly recently, was noted by Frauchiger and Fankhauser (1952). The affected animal was a 2-day-old calf of the Brown Swiss breed. The brain defects were typical. The cerebellum was one-third normal size, and its median parts were stretched and herniated through the foramen magnum and reached the level of the 3rd cervical vertebra. There were also other hindbrain defects, and the lateral ventricles were moderately dilated.

A lesion indicative of spina bifida was located in the midline sacral area. It consisted of a lozenge-shaped, hairless region, the skin of which was reddish and wet like a mucous membrane. At one end of the defect was a small fistula, from which flowed a yellowish, opaque liquid, and through which a probe reached the spinal canal. By such probing the animal's hindlegs were made to twitch.

In sections, the hairless area was found to lack dorsal parts of the corresponding vertebrae. The termination of the spinal cord and its coverings were transformed into a gelatinous vesicle, which extended caudally beneath the area of the lesion. The defect was probably a myelomeningocele.

The second case of Arnold–Chiari malformation in cattle (of unstated breed), presented by Akker (1962), was briefly and inadequately described. Spinal defects were not visible, but the hindlegs were paralyzed, which may have been caused by spina bifida occulta. Abnormalities of the brain mentioned were elongation of the brainstem, enlargement of the cerebrum (without hydrocephalus), and protrusion of the occipital lobes into the posterior fossa.

Appended to a paper (Saunders *et al.* 1952) dealing with congenital ataxia in Jersey calves were photographs of the brain of a Guernsey animal with a caudally displaced cerebellar vermis, resembling this feature in the Arnold–Chiari malformation. The calf also had partial agenesis of the corpus callosum and defects of the anterior colliculi, but apparently no spinal defects.

Spina Bifida

Spina bifida has been found infrequently in cattle. The earliest record I have been able to find is Davaine's (1862), of a newborn calf with a spinal cord that was cleft in the lumbosacral region. Gurlt (1877, p. 23) saw a calf with spina bifida occulta involving dorsal cleft of the 7th to 13th vertebrae. Taruffi (1881–94, vol. 6, pp. 142–44) mentioned a specimen with exencephaly and cervical spina bifida but did not state whether the 2 defects coalesced. A 14-day-old calf with a relatively large cystic myelomeningocele and urinary incontinence and fecal retention was seen by Jackschath (1899). The cyst hung like a bag (from which half a liter of fluid was drained) and was formed by herniation of the spinal cord through a relatively narrow dorsal opening in the 6th thoracic vertebra. The animal also had an abundance of fluid in all cerebral ventricles. A 9-day-old calf with a lumbosacral defect was noted by Dobler (1903). He called the malformation rachischisis, but the text figure clearly indicates it to be a myelomeningocele. Ballantyne (1904, p. 301) mentioned that a few cases of spina bifida had been noted in calves but gave no details.

Gratia and Antoine (1913) described a stillborn calf with a lumbosacral defect. The skin was perforated but covered by a thin vascular membrane. The sacrococcygeal vertebrae were defective, and dorsal and lateral elements were absent. The spinal cord was normal caudally to about the 5th lumbar vertebra. At this point the meninges were dilated and formed a swelling, whose dorsal surface consisted of the exposed vascular-nervous membrane. Microscopic examination of the cord at the level of the 5th lumbar vertebra showed it to be deformed and flattened. The dorsal fissure was absent and the central canal was defective. A thoracic myelomeningocele occurred in a calf with a supernumerary parasitic extremity (Magnusson 1917, 1918). Adelmann (1920) saw an extreme spina bifida in a near-term fetus. The spinal column was dorsally and ventrally cleft almost throughout the entire lumbar region, and in addition in a part of this region the spinal cord was divided into 2 halves. Through this area of division of the cord and column passed a well-marked dorsal herniation of abdominal visceral parts, with the halves of the cord passing around this defect. The calf's head was not examined. Holmdahl (1926) discussed and presented illustrations (figs. 83 and 84, pp. 188–89) of a 7-mm calf embryo in which the posterior neural plate was still joined to the superficial ectoderm and speculated that this condition may have been an early stage of lumbosacral spina bifida.

Weber (1946*a*) recorded 2 cases of spina bifida in cattle. Whittem (1957) found a well-developed sacral spina bifida in a calf with arthrogryposis. Myelomeningocele in a calf was described by McFarland (1959). Externally the defect consisted of a sacrally-located, circular, hairless lesion. Radiographically it was seen that the neural arches of the last 2 lumbar and the sacral vertebrae were incompletely fused. The macerated skeleton showed failure of laminar fusion from the 5th lumbar to the 5th sacral vertebrae inclusive. Beneath the hairless area there was a cavity lined by dura mater and bordered by the incompletely fused laminae. Within the cavity, at the level of the 4th lumbar vertebra, the cord terminated in an atypical cauda equina, but sections of the terminal spinal cord showed no pathological alterations.

Nes (1959) noted spina bifida occulta or aperta in 9 calves of the Norwegian Red and White breed. The abnormality was always associated with muscle contracture of the hindlimbs and in several cases was accompanied by other malformations. The author regarded the different defects as parts of the same lethal or sublethal syndrome, which seemed to him to be inherited as a dominant trait with low penetrance and variable expressivity. But the pedigree presented does not appear to support this interpretation.

Spina bifida occulta with diastematomyelia (i.e., lumbosacral diplomyelia) in a 6-day-old calf was described by Hjärre (1926). In the spina bifida occulta seen by Goss and Hull (1933), the cord disappeared in the region of the 8th thoracic vertebra, and at that point the spinal canal was completely restricted. The vertebral arches of the 9th to 11th thoracic vertebrae were absent and no cord could be found from the 9th to 10th. The cord was therefore present at the 11th but was covered by soft tissues only. Below the 12th thoracic vertebra the spinal canal contained a cord, and the vertebrae were closed in a normal fashion. Obviously the bifida in this animal was part of a multiple anomalous situation that included interruption of the spinal cord, a much more serious defect. Goss and Hull (1933) also cited a communication to them from a Dr. Heizer who had seen a comparable situation in 3 calves sired by a bull mated to its paternal half sisters.

In a case described by Krölling (1922) of an 8-cm calf fetus with duplication of the head and neck and partial duplication of the spinal column and spinal cord, spina bifida aperta was present from the 11th thoracic to the 2nd caudal vertebra, in the region where the cord was single. In a study of a large number of duplication monsters in cows, Keller and Niedoba (1937) found 4 animals with spina bifida occulta of greater or lesser extent. A photograph of a 2-headed newborn calf with spina bifida aperta was presented by Frauchiger and Hofmann (1941, p. 215). Spina bifida aperta in the lumbar area was seen in a 2-headed fetus by Mammerickx and Leunen (1964). It was not further described. The skeletons of 2 calves, one of which was dicephalic, in the Teratology Museum of the Lyon Veterinary School, contained bifidous vertebrae (Tagand and Barone 1942).

Williams (1931) mentioned several cases of sacrococcygeal and lumbo-sacrococcygeal agenesis in cattle but did not state whether neural defects were also seen. In another calf the sacrum and tail were missing, and the spinal cord ended at the 3rd lumbar vertebra.

The "spina bifida" of zebu cattle, discussed by Epstein (1955), whose paper has been cited as dealing with a malformation, consists of the normal bifidity of the spinal process of certain vertebrae in this breed and is not a pathological trait at all. Obviously the term spina bifida was ill-chosen to describe this feature.

Cyclopia

Cyclopia has been noted relatively infrequently in cattle. Jaeger (1830) described one case, Saint-Hilaire mentioned 4 (1832–37, vol. 2, pp. 379–80, 399, 402–4; vol. 3, p. 357); Gurlt, 5 (1877, pp. 29–30); Hannover, 30 (1882–84, p. 123); and Taruffi, 10 (1881–94, vol. 6, pp. 378–79, 433; vol. 8, pp. 385–87), which included Gurlt's specimens. In an animal described by Gurlt (*ibid.*) there was a herniated hydrencephalic area found in place of the eyes. Taruffi (1881–94, vol. 6, p. 433) also listed cebocephaly in 2 calves, one of which may have been that noted by Meckel (*ibid.*, vol. 8, pp. 370–72), which had approximated eyes and a midline protuberance above the orbit. One member of a sternopygic pair had a cyclopic head, with an imperfect median eye that opened perpendicularly (B. 1862). Cyclopia in a duplication monster was also listed by Taruffi (1881–94, vol. 2, pp. 310–15).

A stillborn cyclopic calf was noted by Molinier (1879). He did not mention the brain, but found that the spinal cord and nerves were absent beyond the 6th thoracic vertebra. A 6-month fetal calf with cyclopia was described by Storch (1884). It had a single eye, a proboscis, and a large mouth. The cerebrum consisted of a serum-filled single vesicle covered by a thin layer of poorly convoluted gray matter. The cerebellum was normal. Weber (1885) described a cyclopic calf fetus but did not mention the brain. A very young cyclopic fetus, possibly of a calf, was noted by Symington and Woodhead (1886). Jefimoff (1898) and Gallier (1898) each recorded a cyclopic calf.

Brady (1904) found a full-term liveborn cyclopic calf with marked aplasia of the brain and apparent absence of the cerebral hemispheres. The hindbrain occupied about one-third of the cranial cavity, and the rest of it was filled with a hydrocephalic dural sac.

Lesbre (1928*b*) described unusual malformations in a calf, small for its age, born dead at 8 months of gestation. The mouth was extremely large, which was due to the cheeks' being totally cleft right to the (normally situated) ears; the clefts, in fact, continued even further back and divided each pinna into an upper and lower part. So extensive was the cleft state that the entire face was divided into 2 parts, the upper of which contained an enormous median eye and a rearwardly-directed proboscis, which overlay the back of the neck. Some cranial bones were absent, and others were atrophied; those of the cranial vault were prematurely fused, but still presented perforations at several places. The forebrain consisted solely of a hydropic sac, but most of the rest of the brain, including the colliculi, cerebellum, and medulla oblongata, was fairly normal. The cyclopic Jersey calf seen by Blood *et al.* (1957) was discussed previously (see p. 299). A cyclopic calf was seen by Silvestri and Lughi (1959), and a syndrome of malformations including cyclopia was reported in a calf by King (1965), but in neither case was the brain described.

Otocephaly

Panum (1860, p. 126) noted 18 cases of facial defects in cows described in earlier monographs, some of which were undoubtedly instances of otocephaly. An otocephalic calf was described by Barrier (1876). Only the head was deformed. The ears were approximated ventromedially and were fused together by a transverse cleft, located at the fold between the head and neck. The eyes and nose were apparently normal, but the mouth and lower jaw were defective. The skeletal features were recorded in great detail, but abnormalities of the brain were not mentioned. Gurlt (1877, pp. 5–7) noted 3 otocephalic calves, one with sphenocephaly and 2 with triocephaly. Hannover (1882–84, p. 160) found 6 cases in the literature of otocephaly, which he called agnathia with synotia. Taruffi cited 4 or 5 cases of aprosopus (1881–94, vol. 6, pp. 424–29, 433) and others with agnathia (*ibid.*, vol. 8, pp. 403–5), including those of Barrier and Gurlt, many of which were probably otocephalic. Two of the agnathics also had cyclopic features. He also noted (*ibid.*, vol. 2, pp. 310–15) 3 aprosopic duplication monsters.

Marx (1911, p. 618) discussed a calf with aprosopia, i.e., triocephaly; a photograph of the specimen showed a headless animal with ears at the apex of the stump of the body. A 6-month otocephalic calf fetus, with ears fused below its face, had brain defects (Tridon 1909) commonly seen in this condition, including virtual absence of the cerebral hemispheres and other forebrain structures, while the hindbrain as usual was normal. A severe case of possible otocephaly had a very small cranial cavity, which contained a brain reduced to a mere protruberance and a cerebellum (Lesbre and Pécherot 1913*b*).

Riccardi (1924) noted a calf with a grade of otocephaly known as opocephaly, in which there is a single or double median eye, in addition to abnormalities of the lower jaw and ears (Blanc 1895). In this specimen the pinnae met around what was interpreted as being a rudimentary oral opening, above which was the single large eye. The middle ears were also approximated, but the inner ones were well formed. The pons, cerebellum, and mesencephalon were normal, as is usual; the cerebral hemispheres were united, vesicular, and devoid of convolutions. The entire olfactory apparatus comprising the rhinencephalon was missing. Lima (1918*b*) cited Brites' study of a calf with otocephaly of the spherocephalic or triocephalic grade.

Schmincke (1921) observed a calf that may have been otocephalic. The ears were approximated and surrounded a transverse, supposedly oral, opening. Upper and lower jaws were absent. The brain was not mentioned. Wright and Wagner (1934) and Lima (1936) each reported a calf with a high grade of otocephaly. A photograph of an otocephalic, multiply deformed calf's head was presented by Belting (1963). A recently discovered (Irvin 1966) acephalic calf, whose neck ended in 2 large ear flaps, between which was a small, nonpatent buccopharyngeal opening, undoubtedly had a severe grade of otocephaly. A somewhat less extreme form was also reported (Rees 1966).

Duplication Monstrosities

A large number of duplication monstrosities have been observed in cattle. Early examples were summarized by Otto (1816, pp. 9–11) and Saint-Hilaire (1832–37, vol. 3, pp. 121, 123, 130, 144–45, 196–97, 202, 204, 357); some later ones were collected or noted by other writers (B. 1862; Gurlt 1877, pp. 18–19, 36–37, 39, 41–43; Taruffi 1881–94, vol. 2, pp. 310–15; Pouchet and Beauregard 1882; Brand 1883; Sperino 1890; Petit 1893; Mégnin 1896; Voltz 1897; Alexander 1899; Nevermann 1901; Lesbre and Forgeot 1903; Schwalbe 1907, pp. 294–95; Woolridge 1906; Penhale 1907; Hieronymi 1908; Messner 1908–9; Bussano 1909; Lesbre and Pécherot 1912, 1913*c*; Riemer 1913–14; Reese 1914; Reisinger 1915; Levens 1917; Crocker 1919*a*; Zimmerman 1919; Goldsmith 1921; Schlegel 1920*a*, 1921; Smallwood 1921; Krölling 1922; Taylor 1922; Niedoba 1924; Lubosch 1925; Raschke 1927; Meyer 1928; Vau and Richter 1934; Örs and Karátson 1936; Keller and Niedoba 1937; Ehlers 1939; Vor 1940; Frauchiger and Hofmann 1941, p. 174; Davis 1942; Hughes 1946; Weber 1946*a*; Astle 1948; Dutton 1950; Frauchiger and Fankhauser 1957, p. 38; Witt 1963; Mammerickx and Leunen 1964; Bowen 1966; Dozsa 1966; Irvin 1966).

Brain abnormalities were sometimes reported in individuals with cleft face or partial doubling of the head. Gurlt (1877, pp. 7–8, 18–19, 36–37) found several calves with various degrees of facial cleft and brain defects, including those with hydrocephalus, exencephaly, and absent cerebrum and cerebellum. Radasch (1912) described a full-term calf with duplication of the nasal area and mandible that had a fault in the cranium through which the brain was visible. Partial duplication of the forebrain existed in a calf with doubled facial parts (Lesbre and Pécherot 1913c). Lesbre (1912, 1928b) observed calves with cleft face and large encephalocele. A newborn calf with partially duplicated head (diprosopus triophthalmus) was briefly noted by Schlegel (1920a). A bony fault was present in the cranium and the cerebrum and cerebellum were absent. Williams (1931) reported a calf with median cleft face in which the cerebrum was absent except for vestiges; he stated that the condition was suggestive of hydrocephalus after the lateral ventricles have ruptured and the fluid escaped. Andres' (1931) case, a cephalothoracopagic calf with duplication of head structures, had 2 side-by-side, closely compressed brains. Stuhlenmiller's (1933) case had cleft face, which was accompanied by absence of the cerebrum and atrophy of much of the rest of the brain. Spina bifida was found in 2 dicephalic specimens (Krölling 1922; Tagand and Barone 1942). Instances of anencephaly and spina bifida occulta in duplicated cattle (Keller and Niedoba 1937) were already mentioned above. Weber (1946b) noted 2 cases of cleft face, with aplasia of the cerebrum and cerebellum. Recent examples of brain defects in diprosopic individuals were reported by Fehér and Gyürü (1964), Wissdorf (1964), and Dozsa (1966).

Other Defects

Total or partial absence of the corpus callosum, isolated or in association with other abnormalities, has been found several times in cattle. Already mentioned were the cases of Lesbre and Forgeot (1905a); Schellenberg (1909); Houck (1930); Tajima, Yamagiwa, and Iwamori (1951); Saunders et al. (1952); and Baker, Payne, and Baker (1961). In addition, Frauchiger and Fankhauser (1957, p. 48) reported 3 cases of total absence of the corpus callosum.

A fetal calf head was examined by Bradley (1898). The face was absent except for the lower jaw and an imperfect eyelid. The brain appeared to be entirely missing except for the medulla oblongata, which was well developed, and the rudimentary pons. There was no cerebellum, the 4th ventricle being roofed only by cranial meninges. A calf with a similar aprosopia was noted by Schlegel (1914). The cerebral hemispheres consisted of a liquid-filled membranous sac; the olfactory bulbs and nerves and the optic chiasma were absent; and the colliculi and cerebellum were small.

Gurlt (1877, pp. 5–6) recorded a calf with microcephaly, in which the very small cranial cavity contained a tiny brain. A multiply deformed, stillborn calf, with microcephaly, was seen by Lesbre and Forgeot (1905c). The cerebral hemispheres were small, agyric, and vesicular, and the corpus callosum was absent. Despite marked micrognathia and eye and ear defects, the animal was not otocephalic. A microcephalic calf was presented by

Schellenberg (1909). The cerebral hemispheres did not extend to the midbrain, and consequently the pineal gland and colliculi were visible. The hemispheres appeared as 2 vesicles with slightly thickened walls in some places. Cerebellar morphology was reduced in complexity. There were various other changes: the septum pellucidum was absent; the roof of the midbrain was represented by a thin membrane; and the infundibulum as well as the 3rd ventricle as a whole, and possibly also the foramina of Monro, appeared enlarged.

Micrencephaly was seen in 7 Hereford calves by Fielden (1959). The normal-sized cranial cavity was only partly filled by the brain, all parts of which were greatly reduced in size. The most striking deficiencies, however, were presented by the cerebral hemispheres, which showed marked reduction in number of gyri and absence of corpus callosum and fornix. All animals were stillborn or died soon after birth. Six of the calves were from the same herd.

An acephalic calf was dissected by Gripat (1874). Schmincke (1921) listed a large number of calves with different types of acephalus. An abnormal calf head (Rudd 1907) presented meningeal herniations in the frontal region; apparently associated with the latter was possible absence of the olfactory bulbs. Colucci (1912) saw an adult cow with an almost totally absent right cerebral hemisphere and numerous anomalies on the internal face of the left hemisphere. No trace of any inflammatory process could be found. A 12-day-old calf with aplasia of the cerebral hemispheres was mentioned by Frauchiger and Hofmann (1941, pp. 170–71); in place of the absent parts was an amorphous tissue. The pons, medulla oblongata, and cerebellum were normal. One case each of possible syringomyelia was recorded by Bullard (1935) and Martins and Ferri (1951).

Stormont, Kendrick, and Kennedy (1956) presented a preliminary description of a syndrome of lethal defects in Guernsey cattle. In living fetuses taken by cesarian section the most striking feature revealed by histological examination was complete absence of the adenohypophysis. The pedigree suggested a simple autosomal recessive etiology. A fuller description of the abnormalities in 7 animals was given by Kennedy, Kendrick, and Stormont (1957). The fundamental defect was considered to be adenohypophyseal aplasia, but additional abnormalities of the skull and brain were found. The cranium was characteristically domed; fontanelles were present at the summit and the sutures were not fused. There was modest hydrocephalus of the lateral and 3rd ventricles and of the aqueduct of Sylvius, which apparently resulted from occlusion of the 4th ventricle by the anterior lobe of the cerebellum.

The defective young came from prolonged gestations, which were believed (Kennedy, Kendrick, and Stormont 1957) to be due to absence of the fetal pituitary. Two malformed Jersey calves, one with aplasia of the adenohypophysis and hypoplasia of the neurohypophysis, and the other with apparent absence of the entire pituitary, were also products of extended gestations (Blood *et al.* 1957).

17

Horse

Hydrocephalus

Congenital hydrocephalus has not been seen often in horses. The only reference to it in the early literature that I have found is Gurlt's (1877, p. 31) mention of 13 specimens so affected, and Bournay's (1897) of a term foal with an enormously large head. In the latter case, the cranium was well ossified and thus retained its relative dimensions; further, upon its being punctured only a small amount of fluid escaped. Regnault (1901) noted a horse (age unstated) with a large bombose cranium, and Wilson (1902) a newborn foal with a head of immense size. Mahon (1916) delivered a stillborn foal whose cranium was globular and protruberant, and Petiot (1950) delivered 2 animals with immensely enlarged heads. Weber (1946a) listed a horse, and Holý (1959) and Jiřina (1960) each described a case, with this abnormality. Recently Riedel (1963) reported a hydrocephalic foal that was aborted at 8 months. In none of these specimens was the brain described. The severe dystocia that accompanied quite a number of them may be a clue to the comparative rarity of congenital hydrocephalus in horses.

Congenital internal hydrocephalus has occurred in association with hereditary atresia of the colon. Summaries of cases found in Europe and the U.S.A. (Ackerknecht 1914; Nusshag 1925; Yamane 1927) indicated that of 11 horses with atresia coli, apparently only one also had hydrocephalus. The condition was also found in Japan, where Yamane (1927) collected 25 cases. Of these, 3 (including a 7-month fetus) had typical internal hydrocephalus of the lateral ventricles, and 3 others had gliomatous changes at the base of the cerebral hemispheres. This syndrome appeared to be transmitted as a sublethal recessive, homozygotes all dying within 2 to 4 days of birth (Yamane 1927). The gene was introduced into Japan from Ohio, U.S.A., in 1886, through the Percheron stallion Superb. Yamane's 25 cases occurred among the offspring of 6 stallions, all descendants of Superb, mated to related mares.

Spina Bifida

Überreiter (1952) examined an 11-month-old horse with spina bifida occulta in the sacral region. The parents and sibs were normal. At birth a small hollow was noted from the middle of the rump to the base of the tail. The tail was immobile and defecation problems occurred. The 4th and 5th sacral spinal processes were not palpable, and caudal vertebral fusions were present from the 4th sacral downward. The spinal cord apparently ended in the region of the 4th sacral vertebra, in place of which an expanded, liquid-filled sac was found, whose wall contained undifferentiated neural tissue.

Cyclopia

Cyclopia appears to be fairly common in horses. By searching the literature, Saint-Hilaire (1832–37, vol. 2, pp. 386, 402–3; vol. 3, p. 357) unearthed 4 cases; Taruffi (1881–94, vol. 6, pp. 378–79, 433; vol. 8, pp. 357, 395–99), 12 and one cebocephalic (plus 1 cyclopic ass); and Hannover (1882–84, pp. 123, 160), 10. As usual, there was some overlap among the citations of these writers, but since Hannover did not report his sources, the total number of cases cannot be determined. Taruffi's (1881–94, vol. 8, pp. 395–99) sources covered the years 1665 to 1889. Gurlt (1877, pp. 29–30) found 6 foals with cyclopia; a cyclopic animal (*ibid.*, pp. 39–40) with duplicated upper jaw and partly duplicated head and brain (the latter specimen may have been opodymous, i.e., the median eye may have represented the fused middle pair of eyes of the duplicated heads); and another (*ibid.*) with complete absence of the cerebral hemispheres.

Low-grade cyclopia (cebocephaly) in a horse was described by Dareste (1885*a, b*). The eyes were very close together in the midline but were not fused. The nasal region was almost completely absent. A left cleft lip was present. The cranium was flattened in the frontal region and lacked ossification. When the head was opened in this area, a large amount of serous, blood-tinged fluid escaped, in which there floated debris recognizable as nervous matter. After the liquid was drained, the rest of the brain could be seen. Posteriorly, the cerebellum and colliculi were normal; and anteriorly, the olfactory bulbs were rostrally bifurcated, but no olfactory nerves were seen. Between these areas a large pocket was present from which the fluid had originated; in all probability this pocket represented the single cerebral vesicle commonly found in cyclopia. But Dareste, no doubt impressed by the deficiency of brain tissue, considered this feature a form of anencephaly. A cebocephalic horse was also seen by Weber (1885), but the brain was not described.

Orr (1888) recorded a well-formed, newborn colt with a short upper jaw, absent nasal chambers and posterior nares, and a large eye in the center of the forehead (fig. 20). The brain was not described. A statement of the author's is worth quoting. "As the mare has been kept near the railroad, it is believed by some that this strange freak of nature was caused by sudden fright at the train after night as the eye somewhat resembles the head-light of a locomotive."

Lanzillotti-Buonsanti (1889, 1890) described the skull of a cyclopic horse in great detail; the brain, however, was evidently not made available to him. Block (1902) found a near-term fetal horse with a very short upper jaw, absent nasal apparatus, and a single median eye. The brain was small but was not further described. Thieke (1920) also thoroughly outlined the skeleton of a cyclopic newborn horse but did not investigate the brain.

Lyssenkow and Filatow (1925–26) presented what is probably the most complete description of the brain of a cyclopic horse. Externally there was a single median eye, a short upper jaw, an abnormal nasal region, and a vaulted cranium. Dissection revealed complete absence of the cerebral hemispheres, in place of which there was a spacious, liquid-filled cavity. There were no olfactory bulbs and but a single median optic nerve. The diencephalon was rudimentary. The colliculi, cerebellum, pons, medulla oblongata, aqueduct, and 4th ventricle were fairly normal.

Two cyclopic horses were recorded by Lesbre (1928a). The first was a stillborn term specimen with a large, composite, median eye, very short upper jaw, abnormal nasal region, and high-domed skull. The cerebral hemispheres consisted of a hydropic pocket whose thin wall was continuous with the meninges. As usual, a single median optic nerve was present; and the colliculi and cerebellum were normal. The second case was taken from the archives of l'Ecole Vétérinaire de Lyon where it was entered by a *sieur* Lecamus in 1787. A single eye occupied the center of the forehead. Aside from mentioning the singleness of the optic nerve, Lecamus did not remark upon the state of the brain.

Baier (1928) noted arhinencephaly in a newborn horse. The external defects principally involved the nose and mouth and rudimentary development and approximation of the orbits and eyes. The cranium was fairly normal in shape. The rhinencephalon was defective, olfactory bulbs and tracts being absent; but the brain was otherwise normal.

Other Defects

Several duplication monsters were cited by Saint-Hilaire (1832–37, vol. 3, p. 203). A horse with partly duplicated head and brain and cyclopic features was described by Gurlt (1877, pp. 39–40). Panum (1860, p. 126) recorded 6 horses with facial defects, some of which may have represented otocephaly. Gurlt (1877, p. 16) noted a horse with hydrencephalocele, and several others (*ibid.*, pp. 16–19) with different brain defects. Hydromyelomeningocele occurred (Skoda 1909) in a horse with urogenital and anal atresia. Fankhauser (1955) mentioned a specimen with cerebellar atrophy. Frauchiger and Fankhauser (1957, pp. 232–33) included in a table of cases of cerebellar atrophy personally seen, an instance of a horse with agenesis of the vermis and absent corpus callosum. Two cases of absent corpus callosum were referred to by Frauchiger (1959). A photograph of the brain of a horse lacking the corpus callosum was presented by Innes and Saunders (1962, p. 284). Smith (1907) saw a newborn foal with very short legs and a head resembling that of a bulldog, in being large and wide. It is "worthy of note," he said, that "six weeks after service, the mare was sent to an Agricultural Show at which a large and exceptionally ugly young bulldog was repeatedly noticed in the vicinity of the Show buildings."

18

Sheep

Introduction

It is extraordinary that malformations such as hydrocephalus, exencephaly, and spina bifida, which in nearly all other animals discussed are among the commonest defects, are apparently almost unheard-of in sheep. E.g., in 174 malformed lambs collected (Dennis 1965) over a period of 2 years, none of the most frequent defects was apparently of the central nervous system. The predominant malformation was agnathia, often associated with low-set ears and downwardly migrated eyes, i.e., probably otocephaly of low grades. All lambs with this defect died immediately after birth, owing, it was reported, to occluded air passages, i.e., it seems, atretic oral cavity, another sign of otocephaly. Dennis (1965) did find, though, that while apparently uncommon, defects such as small brain, exencephaly, incomplete spine, and spina bifida did occur. It is of interest to note that in the chapter on hereditary defects of sheep, in a book (Sonnenbrodt 1950) devoted to diseases of sheep, not one instance of central nervous system defects was mentioned.

Cyclopia

Cyclopia and the variety of forms it takes in sheep have been recorded and discussed in numerous publications. Early observations were cited by Saint-Hilaire (1832–37, vol. 2, pp. 385–86, 388, 402–4, 406; vol. 3, p. 357), who referred to 12 cases; by Vrolik (1854, pl. 56, figs. 1–10; pl. 57, figs. 7–9), who illustrated and described 2 cyclopic sheep; by Panum (1860, p. 125), who stated that cyclopia occurred in 25/143 sheep with single malformations described by various authors; by Taruffi (1881–94, vol. 6, pp. 378–79, 433; vol. 8, pp. 387–92), who cited 28 cases (and 9 with cephocephaly) from 1684 to 1889, and 8 double monsters with cyclopia (*ibid.*, vol. 2, pp. 310–15); by Hannover (1882–84, p. 123), who stated he found reports of 51 cyclopic sheep but in another place (*ibid.*, p. 160) mentioned only 48 cases, which included 2 double fetuses; and by Gurlt (1878), who referred to 14 specimens described by Otto, one of which was of the rare variety with a suborbital proboscis (see below), cited by Ballantyne (1904, p. 397).

The central nervous system in these animals, and in later cases as well, was, unfortunately, not described as frequently, or as well, as needed for a firm understanding of its role in the syndrome. Apparently, the commonest type of brain abnormality, occurring in intermediate degrees of cyclopia, consisted of a cerebrum not divided into hemispheres and thus composed of one lobe or vesicle, which contained a single, large, liquid-filled ventricle communicating with the 3rd ventricle through a median foramen of Monro. Accompanying these features were a single, median optic nerve and abnormalities or absence of the olfactory bulbs and nerves. In most instances, the mid- and hindbrain were fairly normal.

Otto (1816, pp. 35–40) described a stillborn but full-grown lamb with a median eye, below which was a fleshy proboscis. The brain, he said, was very remarkable. In place of the usual 2 cerebral hemispheres was a single, large, oval body without trace of indentations or convolutions. So fused were the hemispheres, so thinned were they by the pressure of the contained liquid, that a mere membranous sac was formed. The olfactory nerves were absent; only one optic nerve was present; some other cranial nerves were small or absent. The colliculi were close behind the sac but were uncovered. No Sylvian aqueduct was found. The cerebellum and medulla oblongata were normal. Otto (*ibid.*, pp. 32–35) also recorded the skeleton of a partially duplicated sheep whose head showed cyclopic features.

Jaeger (1830) observed a cyclopic animal that lived 2 days (a specimen with cyclocephaly proper according to Saint-Hilaire 1832–37, vol. 2, pp. 402–4). It had a large proboscis situated above the median eye. The cerebrum consisted of a vesicle containing a single, liquid-filled ventricle. The olfactory apparatus was replaced by thin nervous filaments.

Crisp (1856, 1860) saw 2 cases. The first (Crisp 1856) was born alive at full term. It had a single, median eye and no nostrils. "The greater part of the cerebrum was absent, the cavity being occupied by serous fluid. The thalami, corpora striata and corpus callosum were deficient. No olfactory nerves existed. The right optic nerve only was present, and this entered the eye in the usual situation; the other pairs of nerves were in their normal positions, but those to the muscles of the eye could not be clearly traced." The second case (Crisp 1860) was obtained from a sheep killed at a zoo. It was posteriorly duplicated. The head was small and round, lacked mouth and ears, and had a single median eye. The cranial cavity contained serum and a small amount of material of pulpy consistency. The brain was not further described. Proceeding from the head were 2 spinal columns, closely united as far as the lower part of the neck, where they diverged.

In Lombardini's case (cited by Taruffi 1881–94, vol. 8, pp. 387–92), the

2 hemispheres were apparently completely fused into a single mass, forming a large, fluid-filled sac, which may have incorporated the 3rd ventricle as well as the lateral ones. Absent were the olfactory bulbs, corpus callosum, hippocampus, and various other parts of the anterior brain. In Thomson's specimen also (Taruffi, *ibid.*), the hemispheres were fused and the lateral and 3rd ventricles formed one large space; again there was no corpus callosum.

Brotherston (1876–78) was sent a lamb's head with a single median eye. It was said to have been an offspring of a ram that sired 29 others similarly affected. Gurlt (1877, pp. 29–30) observed 17 cyclopic sheep, and 5 duplication monsters with cyclopia (*ibid.*, pp. 54–55); Symington and Woodhead (1886) and Gay (1878) recorded one case each. Lavocat (1885) noted a stillborn premature lamb with a small cyclopic head. Dissection revealed a small cranial cavity, especially anteriorly; and absence of the olfactory bulbs, cerebral hemispheres, and cerebellum. The first 6 cerebral nerves were partly or completely missing, but the last 6 were normal. Mettam (1897) described a cyclopic term lamb with a normal-sized head. A large, single, median eye composed of 2 united irises and pupils was present. The lower jaw was normal. The cerebrum was not divided into hemispheres and contained a single, large, fluid-filled ventricle roofed by thin, cortical material. Only one optic nerve was present. The olfactory bulbs were absent, and the olfactory portion of the cerebrum was not developed. Much the same set of defects was reported by Banchi (1905).

Cyclopia in a duplication monstrosity in sheep was thoroughly described by Lesbre and Pécherot (1913*d*). The abnormal head contained a defective median eye. The hindbrain was doubled but otherwise fairly normal. The forebrain, however, was single and had typical cyclopic abnormalities, such as absent olfactory bulbs, an unconvoluted and liquid-filled, single cerebral vesicle, and a single foramen of Monro. The thalamic area was partly doubled.

Gladstone and Wakeley's (1920) specimen had a trunklike proboscis with blindending nasal cavities situated above its median eye. Sections of the brain showed almost complete obliteration of the 3rd ventricle caused by fusion of the optic thalami. In addition, the corpus callosum was entirely absent, and there was only a single optic nerve.

A detailed description of a cyclopic sheep was given by Thieke (1920). The head was vaulted and shortened. An imperforate proboscis was present in the center of the forehead, beneath which was a large, median, composite orbit and eye. Mainly affected in the central nervous system were the fore- and midbrain, with the latter showing only slight changes. The cerebral hemispheres were undivided and thus formed a vesicle containing a single hydropic ventricle. Other defects were absence of the fornix, corpus callosum, septum pellucidum, corpus striatum, and hippocampus.

Hughes (1936) noted a stillborn cyclopic lamb, from a Welsh Mountain ewe crossed to a Kerry Hill ram. The greater part of its face was occupied by a large, median, composite eye. The cranial cavity was unusually large or may have appeared so because the brain occupied only half of it, the rest being filled with fluid. The cerebral hemispheres formed a single, small, irregular, unconvoluted mass, whose diminutiveness left the colliculi and optic thalamus uncovered and hence visible. A single, median, optic nerve was present. The olfactory bulbs were underdeveloped. The internal anatomy of the brain was not studied. Reese (1937) found a cyclopic lamb of the Hampshire breed. Its brain could not be examined since it was almost completely decomposed. Cyclopia was seen, but apparently only infrequently, among 174 abnormal lambs (Dennis 1965).

Cebocephaly, a milder form of cyclopia, was recorded on a number of occasions. Gurlt (1877, p. 7) described 3 lambs with short upper jaw and one with absent eyes, which Taruffi (1881–94, vol. 6, p. 364) considered ceboce-phalic. Taruffi (*ibid.*, p. 433; vol. 8, pp. 370–72) also cited several other cases. In a sheep fetus with this defect, Phisalix (1889) found the cerebral hemispheres well formed.

Otocephaly

Otocephaly is also fairly common in sheep, and was reported very often, especially in the last century, when, it appears, there was more interest in certain veterinary monsters than in our own time. The great relative frequency of defects of the mandible in sheep struck Ballantyne (1904, p. 428) as so extraordinary that he was drawn to comment on their disproportionate occurrence in this species, in referring to cases seen by Barkow, Otto, Lowne, and numerous others. Saint-Hilaire, *père* (1822, cited by Ballantyne 1904, p. 423) noted a sheep with micrognathia, synotia, and other facial defects. Because of the curious deformity of the sphenoid, he named the condition sphenocephaly.

Saint-Hilaire (1832–37, vol. 2, pp. 423–24, 429, 432) cited a number of authors, who reported a total of about 9 sheep with various degrees of the condition. Vrolik (1854, pl. 58, figs. 11–13; pl. 59, figs. 1–3) illustrated and described 3 cases, one a strophocephalus, in which the mandible was defective and the ears were united beneath the face. Panum (1860, p. 126) found that of 143 sheep with single malformations described by various authors, 50 had micrognathia or agnathia, and 20 others aprosopus, microprosopus, or campylorhini. Arloing (1867) presented a term sheep with agnathia and astomia whose ears were fused beneath the face. In Lavocat's (1885) case the mouth was narrowed, but the eyes and nose were normal. The ears were small and coalesced beneath the head, and the 2 tympanic cavities were fused together.

Taruffi (1881–94) knew of many examples of such abnormalities in sheep: at least 13 cases of agnathia (*ibid.*, vol. 8, pp. 403–5); 27 of aprosopus in single sheep (*ibid.*, vol. 6, pp. 424–29, 433) and 18 in duplication monsters (*ibid.*, vol. 2, pp. 310–15); and 15 with eye and mandibular defects (*ibid.*, vol. 6, p. 433). Gurlt (1877, pp. 4–7) noted many different degrees of otocephaly in 54 or 55 sheep, and remarked (Gurlt 1878) that Otto had collected about 29 possible or certain cases of otocephaly in this species. Hannover's (1882–84, p. 160) prolific search of the literature, which seems to have included just about everything then extant, uncovered 104 cases (including 2 double fetuses) with mandibular defects and fused ears and 44 others with eye defects as well.

A mildly otocephalic lamb (sphenocephaly) was described by Duval and Hervé (1883). It had no mandible and a short upper jaw. The mouth and pharynx did not communicate, being separated by a membrane situated rostral to the Eustachian tubes. The ears and nervous system were not mentioned, but the brain was probably normal. Nicolas and Prenant (1888) described a near-term, mildly otocephalic sheep with an atretic oral cavity and absent lower jaw. The brain was apparently not examined, but Blanc (1895) considered this specimen to be ageniocephalic, and thus the brain was probably normal. A sheep with a similar array of defects was briefly described by Fischer (1955).

Phisalix (1888, 1889) saw a full-term lamb with a single, median eye and no proboscis. The mandible was very short, the mouth small, and the ears low-set. The ossification of the cranium was incomplete, and the fontanelles were wide. When the skull was opened, an abundant, clear liquid escaped. Resting on the base of the skull was a very small brain, occupying about one-quarter of the cranial cavity. All parts of the brain appeared to be represented, with the exception of the cerebral hemispheres, which were totally absent. It seems likely, though, from the author's description, that a thin-layered, fluid-filled cerebral vesicle might have existed, which was torn upon dissection. Dehors (1894) found an otocephalic sheep in which the eyes, though distinct, were approximated. The ears were united under the head, and the lower jaw and mouth were absent.

Blanc (1895) observed 11 sheep with various degrees of otocephaly. He divided these cases and others he collected from the literature into a number of subcategories, according to severity of defectiveness. Following Saint-Hilaire, he considered the essential feature of the condition to be approximation of the external ears toward, or their fusion on, the ventral midline of the neck. But while Saint-Hilaire's (1832–37, vol. 2, pp. 423–24) classification was based entirely on type and degree of abnormalities of eyes, nose, and lower jaw, Blanc refined this system and used the condition of the brain as a further criterion (see p. 242). Five of Blanc's defective sheep were of varieties in which the brain was normal (2 sphenocephaly, 2 agnathocephaly, 1 strophocephaly), and the other 6 were of types with brain defects (4 opocephaly, 1 spherocephaly, 1 triocephaly). Five of the latter had a vesicular forebrain, containing a large, single ventricle and thick walls. The remaining animal, the triocephalic, was aprosopic, and its brain was reduced to a bulbous projection of the spinal cord, topped by a hillock representing an impaired acoustic nerve.

Triocephaly in sheep was also seen by Neveu-Lemaire (1899), Lesbre (1911), and Mercer and Steven (1966). Neveu-Lemaire (1899) described a near-term animal whose head consisted merely of a rudiment topped by 2 large united ears and whose brain was entirely absent except for possible remnants at the end of the spinal cord. Lesbre (1911) presented 2 such sheep with apparent absence of the head and united ears at the anterior end of the neck. As in Neveu-Lemaire's animal, the united ears surrounded an opening that led to the digestive tract. In both animals little more of the brain was present than a spinal elongation capped by parts of the cerebellum. A recent case of triocephaly in a stillborn lamb was noted by Mercer and Steven (1966). The animal was a severely deformed twin to a normal, viable lamb. The head was apparently absent, and the neck ended in 2 membranous ear flaps between which was a small circular orifice. Radiological examination showed that the skull consisted solely of the base of the cranium, the tympanic bulla, and the stylohyoid bone. Dissection revealed that the cerebral hemispheres and midbrain were absent, but the cerebellum was apparently normally developed. The circular orifice mentioned above opened into a muscular buccopharyngeal canal.

Gladstone's (1910) case was that of a lamb with a single, median eye with a proboscis below it. Beneath the latter were external ears connected to each other by an oral depression; when dissected the latter was discovered to be the fused cartilaginous portions of the external auditory canals, closed at each side externally, but continuous with each other in the midline. The cerebral hemispheres were fused together in the midline and, although not examined internally, no doubt contained but a single ventricle. Josephy (1913, pp. 253, 258, 263) presented 3 otocephalic sheep; in a mild case (*ibid.*, p. 258), the only brain defect was arhinencephaly.

Gladstone and Wakeley (1923) described 5 sheep that they believed represented a graded series of otocephalic defects. The least deformed animal merely had brachygnathia; the next, unilateral agnathia (hemignathia); the third, agnathia with approximation of the eyes and orbits and fusion of some facial bones; the fourth, similar to the last, but with fused orbital cavities; and the fifth, a still more extreme variety of the fourth. Obviously, it is contentious whether some of these animals were otocephalic at all.

Another sheep with composite defects was presented by Tillon (1926). The animal was a late fetus with a spherical head and a large, single, median eye; in addition, the lower jaw was atrophied, and beneath the head were located fused ears between which lay an orifice leading to an atretic cavity. The hindbrain was normal, but the cerebral hemispheres were defective.

An otocephalic term sheep was described by Vitu and Houdinière (1934). The head was spherical, had a single, median eye, and no nasal apparatus, mouth or lower jaw. The ears, each possessing an auditory meatus, were united beneath the head. Unfortunately, as was so often the case, the brain was apparently not dissected. In the course of 10 years, Wright (Wright and Wagner 1934) saw 3 cases of otocephaly of various grades in the sheep herds maintained by the U.S. Bureau of Animal Industry at Beltsville, Maryland. Lambs described as "faceless" and "headless" were probably severe otocephalics (Fasten 1932; Winters and Kernkamp 1936).

Lima (1936) presented an otocephalic sheep between whose fused ears there was a double orifice, which communicated with a pharyngeal sac, as did the abnormal, small mouth. The sac in this case was continuous with the esophagus, the limit between them being marked only by a narrow circular ring. The cranium was relatively large, but nevertheless the brain was quite small, with complete agenesis of the prosencephalon and thus apparent absence of the cerebral hemispheres and all interhemispheric connections.

Théret (1948) described a mildly otocephalic (ageniocephalic) lamb, with very reduced mandible and lack of connection between mouth and pharynx. The author was told that 12 other lambs with similar defects were born in 2 years in the same herd from which his specimen came. He concluded that the condition must therefore be inherited and that its mode of transmission was as a recessive lethal.

Millen and Davies (1952) described an otocephalic sheep fetus of 7 weeks gestation age. Externally, the head was rounded and lacked the projection of the snout region. There was no indication of nose, mouth, or eyes, and the pinnae were approximated in the midline of the head, under the "face." The pharynx ended rostrally at the level of attachment of the hyoid cartilage to the auditory cartilages. It was continuous cranially with a very narrow diverticulum, considered as representing the fused tubotympanic cavities, which opened onto the anterior surface of the head, a little above the pinnae. The cartilaginous auditory capsules were closer together than normal. The anterior part of the skull and the ethmoid were missing. Meckel's cartilages were small and fused medially. The upper part of the cranial cavity was empty, with no indication of fore- and midbrain. The cerebellum thus formed the anterior part of the brain, and the 4th ventricle ended blindly, anteriorly. The hindbrain, including cerebellum, pons, medulla, and 4th ventricle, was normal. No pituitary could be recognized. No trace was found of the olfactory, optic, oculomotor, and trochlear nerves.

A 1-day-old lamb with extreme micrognathia was seen by McFarland and Deniz (1964). Signs of otocephaly were absence of the tongue and oral cavity, ventral displacement of ears and eyes, and median union of the external auditory canals where a slitlike opening communicated with a pharyngeal diverticulum. The brain was not described. The lamb was probably the product of a brother–sister mating.

Duplication Monstrosities

Such defects have occurred fairly often in sheep. Otto (1816, pp. 29–30, 32–35) noted 2 such animals. Saint-Hilaire (1832–37, vol. 3, pp. 123, 129, 144, 196–97, 203, 357) recorded about 27 cases; Crisp (1860) noted one; Gurlt (1877, pp. 36–37, 41–43, 54–56) listed 31, including one with absent cranial bones (hemicephaly), 5 with cyclopic defects (i.e., single cerebral ventricle and absent olfactory apparatus), and one with aprosopus; Taruffi (1881–94, vol. 2, pp. 310–15) cited 40, of which 8 had cyclopic features, and 18 aprosopus; and Hannover (1882–84, p. 160) included 2 double fetuses with agnathia and synotia, and 2 with cyclopia. Other duplication monstrosities were observed in sheep by Rayer (1852), Pilcher (1880), Dujon (1897), Alexander (1899), Lesbre (1901), Holding (1904), Schwalbe (1907, p. 230), Wilder (1908), Hübner (1911a), Lesbre and Pécherot (1913d), Schlegel (1916), Reese (1917), Krölling (1922), Lesbre and Tagand (1927), Scaglia (1927), Engel (1931), Pfeffer (1932), Weber (1946a), Marques (1961), and Sachs (1963).

Other Defects

A total of 7 sheep with hydrencephalocele were gathered from the literature by Taruffi (1881–94, vol. 6, pp. 243–47). Sheep with various central nervous system defects were observed by Gurlt (1877): 4 with hydrencephalocele (*ibid.*, p. 16), one with microcephaly, i.e., a very small brain in a very small cranial cavity (*ibid.*, pp. 5–6); one with hydrocephalus of the lateral ventricles and with unconvoluted hemispheres (*ibid.*, p. 38); and one with spina bifida lateralis in the thoracic region (*ibid.*, p. 23).

A multiply deformed fetal sheep was described by Guinard (1891). Various facial and cranial structures were aberrant. The cranium was largely open and consisted of a flat surface comprising an amorphous mass of vascular and nervous tissue containing only vestiges of the brain. A large extent of the spinal canal was open and formed a gutter in which no cord was present.

Complete absence of the cerebellar vermis and possible reduction in size of the cerebellar hemispheres were seen in a 7-day-old lamb with disturbances of equilibrium by Sholl, Sales, and Langham (1939). The cerebellar hemispheres were separated, owing to absence of the vermis, by a fluid-filled space, which was not further described.

In duplication monstrosities, Pfeffer (1932) noted a lamb with lumbosacral spina bifida aperta of the unduplicated part of the spine, one with occipital cranioschisis of the partly doubled head, and an incompletely dicephalic and bispinal sheep with craniorachischisis.

Koens (1945) described a spina bifidous lamb found on the West Frisian island of Texel. The animal had a clinically normal twin. Extending from L4 to S4 was a swelling the size of a chicken egg, which was only partially covered by skin. The part not covered by skin was a dirty red color; this was undoubtedly the area medullovasculosa of the lesion, which was probably originally a rachischisis. Four other such defective lambs occurred in 1944, while none was found in 1945. The author discussed the likelihood of the condition's being hereditary, especially in light of the fact that the animal population of the island was a closed one. He incidentally mentioned that numerous other malformations had also been seen in the sheep of the island, such as microcephaly, anencephaly, and so on. Spina bifida occulta was noted (Grini and Iversen 1948) in 4 sheep sired by a certain ram.

An unusual type of encephalocele was noted in a newborn lamb by Mosimann (1951). Much of the left side of the face, including the eye, maxilla, mandible, and ear, was apparently missing. In its place was a large, skin-covered, liquid-filled cyst, which communicated through a small round opening at the base of the brain with the 3rd ventricle. The only other defects seen were an abnormal pituitary, an enlarged left foramen of Monro, and deficient development of various cranial nerves.

The Arnold–Chiari malformation was observed in 10 sheep by Akker (1962). All had lumbosacral defects ranging from spina bifida occulta to myeloschisis, but these malformations were not described. The rhombencephalon was displaced, but only slightly; the elongation varied in extent from cases in which the cerebellum, which was sometimes very small, reached the foramen magnum, to those in which it extended to the arch of the atlas. The 4th ventricle was also elongated. Hydrocephalus occurred in some animals, but the number so affected was not stated, nor was the condition described. The cerebral hemispheres were large and apparently overgrown, and the convolutions were flattened. An intact skull and spinal column were available for study in only 4 cases. In these specimens the spinal roots immediately cephalic to the spina bifida ran cranially, but the course of the posterior thoracic spinal nerves was normal; hence the effect of traction upon the cord was no longer present in the latter area and could not have been the cause of displacement of the rhombencephalon.

Innes and Saunders (1962, p. 284) mentioned a sheep with absent corpus callosum, and illustrated (*ibid.*, p. 281) another with congenital hydrocephalus. The latter had marked symmetrical dilation of the lateral ventricles from pole to pole; the 3rd ventricle was not involved.

19

Goat

Cyclopia

Early writings contain few records of cyclopia in goats. Jaeger's and Galvagni's cases were cited, respectively, by Saint-Hilaire (1832–37, vol. 2, pp. 402–3) and Taruffi (1881–94, vol. 8, pp. 387–92). Hannover (1882–84, pp. 123, 160) listed 9 cases, which may have included the 5 seen by Gurlt (1877, pp. 29–30). The single-eyed goat with a normal mandible examined by Pigné (1841) had a large cranial cavity, but its brain was unexaminable. Richter (1887) presented a goat with a partly composite eye. The cranial cavity was apparently occupied entirely by an undivided, thin-walled, liquid-filled cerebral vesicle. The rhinencephalon seemed to be missing.

Keil (1911) noted a goat with a composite median eye. The cerebrum was undivided and consisted of a single, large, liquid-filled sac with poorly developed convolutions. Numerous parts of the brain were missing, such as the hippocampus, corpus striatum, corpus callosum, optic tracts, and optic chiasm. The olfactory nerves were maldeveloped and had a deviant origin. The cerebral peduncles were relatively small.

Schwalbe and Josephy (1913, pp. 207, 213–15) illustrated and described 2 cyclopic goats. The first had a small, undivided cerebral sac, almost devoid of convolutions, no olfactory bulbs, and a single optic nerve. The pineal and pituitary glands were absent. The hindbrain was normal. The second animal had a small proboscis near the median eye. The cerebrum was hydrocephalically enlarged, and a large, blister-like encephalocele was associated with the midbrain. The authors (*ibid.*, p. 231) also referred to an ethmocephalic goat with a markedly hydropic brain seen by Otto. Schlegel (1920*b*) noted a macrostomic, arhinencephalic, cyclopic newborn kid with a composite median eye. The skull was balloon-shaped and contained a univentricular, liquid-filled cerebral sac.

Lima (1920) described a stillborn kid with a single, median eye, below which was a deep depression in place of the absent nasal apparatus. An extremely prognathic, upturned mandible was present. Anterior portions of the brain were reduced to a shapeless mass of nervous tissue, but the cerebellum was normal. The greater part of the cranial cavity, between the dura and the upper face of the brain, was filled with fluid. The animal described by Badalà (1927) may have been a severe cyclopic. It had completely absent eyes and nose, abnormal mouth, large lower jaw, and rudimentary external auditory canals. The pinnae were apparently not ectopic. The cranial cavity was very small and was occupied by an anomalous brain mass with no fore- and mid-brain. Essentially, the brain was reduced to a short prolongation of the spinal cord topped rostrally by the cerebellum. A vestige of the 4th ventricle ended blindly, anteriorly.

Stupka's (1931) case had a median eye and no external nasal structures. The ears were normal. The forebrain was very small, which left the cranial cavity mostly empty, except for the liquid it contained. The small, unpaired, poorly convoluted cerebrum lay directly behind the eye. The single anterior ventricle communicated by a pair of foramina of Monro with a somewhat enlarged 3rd ventricle. Found defective, but present, were the olfactory bulbs, septum pellucidum, choroid plexuses of the anterior ventricle, corpus callosum, and hippocampus. The brain was essentially normal from the anterior colliculi back. An extensive description was given of many histological features of the brain.

Monod (1933) noted a near-term cyclopic kid, twin to a normal animal. A single, median eye was situated above a proboscis with rudimentary nostrils. The mouth and oral cavity were very small, but the lower jaw was protruberant. The ears were normal and normally located. The cranium was represented only by the occipital region, and its cavity appeared to contain neither cerebrum nor differentiated cerebellum. The nervous system was not further described.

Cyclopia in duplication monsters was mentioned by Taruffi (1881–94, vol. 2, pp. 310–15).

Otocephaly

Aprosopus was noted in a goat by Brandeberger (1832, cited by Taruffi 1881–94, vol. 6, pp. 424–29), and in duplication monstrosities by Gurlt (1877, pp. 55–56) and Taruffi (1881–94, vol. 2, pp. 310–15). Marx (1911, p. 615) illustrated a goat with close approximation of the eyes (an edocephalic or opocephalic), a proboscis in the forehead area, and low-set fused ears. Josephy (1913, pp. 257–60, 263–65) described 2 otocephalic goats, one a sphenocephalic and the other a triocephalic.

Duplication Monsters

These phenomena have been seen in appreciable numbers in goats (Saint-Hilaire 1832–37, vol. 3, pp. 129, 144, 148–49, 203, 357; Steenkiste 1845;

Gurlt 1877, pp. 41–43, 55–56; Panum 1878; Taruffi 1881–94, vol. 2, pp. 310–15; Bien 1905; Arndt 1925; Corsy and Robert 1925; Weber 1946*a*).

Other Malformations

Malformations common in many other species have been reported only rarely in goats. Gurlt (1877, p. 31) saw 2 kids with congenital hydrocephalus, and reported hydrocephalus and absent cerebral convolutions in an aprosopic duplication monster (*ibid.*, pp. 55–56). Lesbre (1928*b*) described a stillborn term kid with probable hydranencephaly. The head was enormous and had a large frontoparietal fontanelle, which was palpable through the skin. The dura mater could not be recognized, and there was no trace of the arachnoid. The brain consisted of a liquid-filled sac representing the ventricular system, i.e., there was almost total destruction of the brain, and neither cerebrum nor cerebellum could be distinguished as such. This animal and another with similar defects were sired by the same male.

Exencephaly occurred in 2 specimens, one of which also had facial malformations (Gurlt 1877, pp. 16–18). Cohrs (1952, p. 436) presented a photograph of a 3-week-old goat with a frontoparietal encephalocele. Gurlt (1877, pp. 5–6) noted a microcephalic goat with a very small cranial cavity and a very small brain. Curson (1931) briefly described a $5\frac{1}{2}$-week-old kid with eye defects, absent optic nerves, and a grossly hypoplastic, left cerebral hemisphere. Panum (1878) saw a goat with diprosopus and posterior duplication, one part of which presented spina bifida aperta.

Verhaart (1942) recorded a 1-month-old goat with complete motor incapacity, which died 12 days later; its parents and siblings were normal. The whole vermis and the caudal half of the hemispheres of the cerebellum were lacking, and the area of the medulla at the level of the caudal part of the 4th ventricle was abnormally narrow. The 4th ventricle itself was reduced in size, and the lateral parts of its floor were coalesced and enclosed an abnormal central canal. On the other hand, the caudal end of the Sylvian aqueduct was very wide. The cerebrum was apparently normal, but closer examination showed the corpus callosum to be entirely absent.

Weber (1960) examined 6 full-term, probably stillborn, chondrodystrophic dwarf goats of the Saanen breed. The only defect of the central nervous system mentioned was very small olfactory bulbs in all cases. Five of the animals were sired by 2 full-grown but small rams, which, in addition to their chondrodystrophic offspring, also had some (number unstated) young that were small like themselves. Two of the latter were bred together and produced one normal, but nonviable, kid.

Acephalus of various types appears to be relatively common in goats. Numerous authors have recorded, described, and, above all, classified it. The subject was summarized by Koch, Fischer, and Schumann (1957, pp. 246–47).

20

Nonhuman Primates

Because of the potential value of subhuman primates as teratology test animals, interest is growing in the spontaneous congenital malformations they may have. The few estimates that have been made in recent years of the frequency of congenital malformations in such animals seem to indicate that it is not large, but these data are still far too sparse to be trustworthy. For example, Wilson and Gavan (1967) discovered, by means of a questionnaire survey, that only 13 defective animals were seen among 2950 offspring of various primate species bred under conditions permitting detection of external malformations. Five of the defects involved the brain, including 3 anencephaly and 1 hydrocephalus. Wilson and Gavan (1967) thus remarked, "If the information presently available permits any conclusion it is that nonhuman primates are no more prone to spontaneous malformations than man, and it may warrant a statement that they appear to be less likely to show major developmental variations than man."

Koford, Farber, and Windle (1966) reported on 1003 births in rhesus monkeys occurring in Puerto Rico during 1956–63. Of this number, 495 were born, usually spontaneously, in free-ranging colonies, and 508 were born, usually by cesarian section, in laboratory colonies. Stillborn and aborted fetuses were seldom recovered in the former group. Only 3 animals had major congenital malformations, and none of these defects and the several minor ones occurring in a few other newborn monkeys involved the central nervous system.

While it is probable that more systematic and intensive examination of large numbers of newborn monkeys and apes will reveal a higher incidence of malformations than so far discovered, it cannot be predicted what the relative proportions of the different types of defects will be. Past observations are, again, little to be relied on to supply clues to this question. Schultz's (1956) review of teratological conditions in apes and monkeys, e.g., was almost wholly devoted to malformations of the skeleton and dentition. But this is not surprising since the observations reported were mostly based on osteological studies. As far as such studies may relate to the nervous system, it is pertinent to record Schultz's (1938) finding that, of an unstated total examined, 7 gibbons had spina bifida of the atlas and another had fusion of atlas and occiput.

In Ruch's (1959) 600-page book *Diseases of Laboratory Primates*, while the subject of anomalies and agenesis of the nervous system occupies less than 3 pages (pp. 402, 430–31), the intriguing statement was made, without substantiation however, that congenital hydrocephalus was frequently found in zoo-born monkeys.

Lapin and Yakovleva (1963, p. 229) noted that the great majority of the congenital malformations occurring among the liveborn and stillborn primates at the Sukhumi breeding farm in the years 1953–58 were of the central nervous system. But the incidence of defects was not mentioned; and except for one case (*ibid.*, pp. 233–34), the abnormalities of the central nervous system were not listed or described.

Prior to these few population studies, a small number of cases of congenital malformations of the central nervous system were noted and described in primates. A very detailed account was presented by Tumbelaka (1915) of absence of the corpus callosum in a young female cebus monkey (*Cebus hypoleucus*), which, after a year's stay in the Amsterdam zoo, had had frequent convulsive attacks for a week preceding its autopsy.

A firstborn male sacred baboon (*Papio hamadryas*) was found dead the day after its birth in the zoological gardens of Dehiwala, Ceylon (Hill 1939). A small sacrococcygeal spina bifida, without hernial swelling, was found just above the base of the tail. The lesion, measuring 12 mm long by 15 mm transversely, was covered only by a thick vascular membrane, the area medullovasculosa of what was revealed to be a myelomeningocele, i.e., the end product of an unclosed neural plate.

Microscopic study disclosed the following details. Immediately above the deformity and in its anterior region, the central canal was greatly enlarged and filled with extravasated blood. Caudal to this site the central canal was traced to an opening at the base of the central region of the bifidous disc. Ventral to the center of the lesion the ganglia formed a midline mass—a feature reminiscent of the situation in trypan blue-induced spina bifida in rats (see p. 62).

Fourteen years later, further examination (Cameron and Hill 1955) of preserved parts of the baboon showed that in addition to the spina bifida, an Arnold–Chiari malformation was also present. The skull was normal and not obviously enlarged. The cerebral hemispheres were normal, but the hindbrain was small. A large tongue of cerebellar tissue passed caudally on the dorsal surface of the medulla, was indented posteriorly by the bony margin of the foramen magnum, and extended over the entire dorsal surface of the cervical cord. The medulla oblongata and the 4th ventricle were also greatly elongated. The other ventricles were normal except for slight dilatation of the occipital horns of the lateral ventricles.

A captive-bred, male grivet monkey (*Cercopithecus aethiops*), whose growth and behavior were previously apparently normal, died suddenly at 10 months of age, probably because of self-inflicted injury; and was diagnosed as having had internal hydrocephalus (Fox 1941). The skull was not thin or disproportionately large, but the lateral ventricles were widely distended, while the 3rd ventricle and aqueduct were probably within normal limits. The cerebellum and pituitary were normal. The right lateral ventricle had ruptured and formed an irregular opening on the posterior curvature of the right occipital lobe, producing a hemorrhage in the calvaria. The left ventricle had not ruptured, but the cortex of the left occipital lobe was thin and showed localized meningeal thickening.

Urbain, Riese, and Nouvel (1941) examined a female gelada baboon (*Theropithecus gelada*; considered *Papio gelada* by Buettner-Janusch 1966) of more than a year of age that was found dead in her cage in a zoo. No significant clinical signs were noted in the days preceding death. Macroscopic examination of the brain revealed cerebellar and other abnormalities. While the left cerebellar vermis and hemisphere seemed entirely intact, the right hemisphere was almost completely atrophied. Though this very reduced part still had the characteristic lamellar structure of the cerebellar cortex, it was in reality merely a sac filled with a serous fluid, whose wall therefore was all that remained of the cortex. These unilateral cerebellar defects were associated with pathological changes in the overlying bone. Brain defects were also seen in the left cerebral hemisphere, where the basal portion and the pole of the temporal lobe were slightly reduced, compared to the size of the same regions of the right hemisphere. All these facts indicated an early provenance, probably prenatal.

The case described by Lapin and Yakovleva (1963, pp. 233–34), mentioned above, was a nonviable, multiply malformed rhesus monkey, one of a pair of prematurely born twins, whose cotwin was normal. In place of a head there was a cutaneous sac with a funnel-shaped retraction on the ventral surface corresponding to a mouth. On the lateral surfaces were 2 cutaneous folds resembling external ears. The cephalic sac extended into a shapeless torso, the upper limbs of which were handless. Removal of the skin in the region of the sac revealed a cranium about one-third normal size. Moreover, the brain occupied the lesser part of the cranial cavity, most of which contained fluid. The very small cerebrum was composed almost entirely of parietal lobes, which were sharply delimited from the rudiments of the frontal lobes. The cerebellum was also very small. The authors believed that the monster was associated with the fact that the mother had had an almost incessantly recurring dysentery during pregnancy, for which she was repeatedly given massive doses of various antibiotics.

In an electron microscope study of the spinal cord of fetal and neonatal monkeys (*Macaca irus*), Bodian (1966) noticed scattered neuronal degeneration in several otherwise apparently normal animals of a wide spread of prenatal ages. It did not seem that the phenomenon was normal; yet it was inexplicable. All young in the colony were sired by the same male. The youngest fetus (44–47 days, 28 mm) had a severe subependymal defect in the cervical cord, suggesting an early stage of hydromyelia. A case of frank hydromyelia was noted in the cervical cord of an adult rhesus monkey seemingly normal in other physical respects.

Duplication has been found rarely. Partial duplication of the skull of a longtailed monkey (*Cercopithecus sabaeus*), with normal brain and meninges, was recorded by Landois (1879). Bolk (1927) described a symmetrical dicephalic cynomolgus monkey a radiograph of which showed 2 vertebral columns. Hartman (1943) briefly noted a rhesus monkey with 2 partly united heads and doubling of the spinal column from the midthorax region upwards. Apparently in neither of the last 2 cases was the nervous system dissected.

In a recently published book on paleopathology it was stated (Wells 1964, p. 44) that "anencephaly, a monstrosity in which the child is born with total absence of the upper brain and the top of its head, has not yet been reported from antiquity apart from one case of an Egyptian mummified monkey." Although the author did not say where he learned this information, there can be little doubt that he was referring—however garbled his version may be—to the incident originally recorded by Saint-Hilaire (1832–37, vol. 2, pp. 363–65). In my infelicitous translation, the relevant passage is as follows. "A mummy, newly brought from Egypt by M. Passalacque, and belonging to the beautiful archeological collection of that learned traveler, was in 1826 subjected to examination by my father. It came from the catacombs of Hermopolis, the tomb ordinarily of sacred monkeys and ibises. A clay amulet, crude but a faithful representation of a monkey, the cynocephalus of old, had been found near it; and the pose of this figurine was exactly that of the mummy itself. It was concluded from all these signs that the bandages hid a monkey. But as it appeared to differ by its size and form from the other monkeys buried with it, an interesting scientific discovery was expected and a close examination of it was requested of my father. To the great surprise and astonishment of all, the examination revealed the features of a human fetal monstrosity." There follows a description of it, which clearly labels it an anencephalic. He continued.

"We see in effect a human anencephalic excluded from human burial. Though born of a woman, it resembled an animal, but a sacred animal, and of which the religion commanded a pious preservation of the remains. [Thus it was embalmed and buried in the cemetery for animals.] Why all these honors of embalmment accorded to a being that was denied human entombment? Without doubt because this monster, monkey born of a woman, to the eyes of the Egyptians, was one of those prodigies, cited so often by ancient authors, whose apparition presaged celestial vengeance and threw entire populations into terror."

21

Other Species

Malformations and monstrosities in less common and more exotic mammalian species have been noted on quite a few occasions. Deer seem to have been favored by observers. Thoracopagus deer embryos were noted by Morand (1752). Jaeger (1826) described a deer fetus from a Bengal deer cow (which he called *Cervus axis*; Walker 1964, p. 1388, called it *Axis axis*). It was agnathic, had a very small tongue and blind pharyngeal sac, and thus was possibly otocephalic. The brain was normal. Saint-Hilaire (1832–37) recorded an acephalic deer seen by Rudolphi and a dicephalic one by Winslow (*ibid.*, vol. 2, pp. 484–85, and vol. 3, pp. 196–97, respectively). Hannover (1882–84, pp. 123, 160) listed one deer with cyclopia. One of a pair of fetuses carried by a shot deer had a partly duplicated head (Fay 1960), the only case of dicephalism in over 2,300 deer fetuses examined in 8 years. Duplication in other artiodactyla, i.e., dicephalic buffalo calves, was reported by Reddy and Balasubramanyam (1949) and Sapre (1953).

In studies of the effects of abrupt deceleration, one of 8 bears used—a 2-year-old male black bear (*Euarctos americanus*)—died and was found to have congenital internal communicating hydrocephalus (Halstead and Kiel 1962). Its only unusual feature previously noted was bluntness of the anterior face.

At necropsy the skull was enlarged with a sharply rising anterior cranium. A peculiarity noted was that the internal occipital eminence was more than usually prominent, projecting 2 cm inward to encroach on the superior surface of the cerebellum. The brain surface was flattened, and the sulci were narrow. The posterior part of the cerebellum had a 1 cm-wide shelf where tissue had been compressed by the posterior skull. The lateral and 3rd ventricles were greatly expanded and covered by a thin rim of tissue. The volume of each lateral ventricle was about 22 ml, versus a normal capacity of 3 ml. The rostral entrance to the aqueduct was hidden by a fold on the floor of the 3rd ventricle. But a probe was easily passed to the 4th ventricle. The foramina of

Magendie and Luschka of the 4th ventricle were found without difficulty and were patent, it was claimed. The 4th ventricle was only moderately dilated. The hydrocephalus was advanced and had probably been present since birth. The authors believed that the condition was caused by blockage of the foramina of the 4th ventricle by pressure of the overly developed internal occipital eminence. The flap of tissue over the aqueduct was not further mentioned, nor apparently considered as a factor in the development of the hydrocephalus.

A 6-week-old lion cub (*Felis leo*) that had been a weakling from birth died "in fits" and was discovered to have pronounced internal hydrocephalus (Hamerton 1932). Scherer (1944, p. 313) mentioned a tiger with porencephaly and hemiatrophy, due, he said, to birth trauma.

A 10-year autopsy study of foxes turned up 10 cases of hydrocephalus (Chaddock 1948). Defects of the brain in an adult fox from the Basel zoo were noted by Fankhauser (1965). The only clinical symptoms exhibited were circling when excited. Various malformations were found at autopsy, including marked internal hydrocephalus, especially of the left side; a porencephalic opening at the anterior end of the left lateral gyrus; nearly complete absence of the corpus callosum, and of the centrum ovale and internal capsule on the left side; and hypoplasia of several cerebellar tracts.

Duplication in moles (*Talpa europaea*) has been recorded a number of times. Vallisneri (cited by Saint-Hilaire 1832–37, vol. 3, p. 145) noted posterior duplication; Taruffi (1881–94, vol. 2, pp. 310–15), a syncephalus monoprosopus; and Broek (1906, cited by Hübner 1911*b*), a partly duplicated 7-mm embryo, in which the brain was doubled posterior to the lamina terminalis.

The genus Mustela has made several contributions. Good (1915), in passing, mentioned but did not describe an 8-mm ferret embryo with cervical spina bifida. Internal hydrocephalus was observed in several mink (Gorham 1947). The cranium was greatly expanded, soft, and fluctuated on palpation. The lateral ventricles were expanded to such a degree that the hemispheres were flattened against the cranial bones, pressing them outward, and effacing the cerebral convolutions. The cerebral walls were very thin. The 3rd and 4th ventricles were apparently not enlarged. The subarachnoid spaces were distended and hemorrhagic, which may have resulted from stretching and rupture of the pia-arachnoid vessels. Shackelford (1950, p. 74) found the condition to be inherited as a recessive.

Hemmingsen and Venge (1964, cited by Johansson 1965), in Denmark, found that 89 (3.8%) of 2349 mink that were stillborn or died within 24 hours of birth had observable external malformations, included among which were 9 with cerebral hernia, and one with cyclopia.

And, finally, Valenciennes (1848) reported a dolphin (not further identified) with a partly duplicated head, caught in the Antilles (i.e., Caribbean) whose size indicated that it had lived for some time, since these animals are quite small at birth.

References

Ackerknecht, E. 1914. Atresia (s. dysgenesia) coli beim Pferde. Beiträge zur Kenntnis des Missbildungen bei Säugetieren. *Deut. Tierärztl. Wschr.* 22: 65–69, 83–85.

Adametz, L. 1925. Neues über den disproportionierten Zwergwuchs (Achondroplasie) als Rassen bildende Domestikationsmutation. *Z. Tierz. Züchtungsbiol.* 3: 125–40.

Adams, C. E.; Hay, M. F.; and Lutwak-Mann, C. 1961. The action of various agents upon the rabbit embryo. *J. Embryol. Exp. Morph.* 9: 468–91.

Adams, J. M.; Heath, H. D.; Imagawa, D. T.; Jones, M. H.; and Shear, H. H. 1956. Viral infections in the embryo. *Am. J. Dis. Child.* 92: 109–14.

Adelmann, H. B. 1920. An extreme case of spina bifida with dorsal hernia in a calf. *Anat. Rec.* 19: 29–34.

Agarwal, I. P.; Monga, J. N.; Monga, S.; and Dravid, V. 1960. Neutralization of teratogenic activity of trypan blue by cortisone acetate. An experimental study in rats. *Ind. J. Med. Res.* 48: 331–36.

Akker, S. van den. 1962. Arnold–Chiari malformations in animals. *Acta Neuropath. Suppl.* 1: 39–44.

Albrecht. 1911. Eine Missgeburt. *München. Tierärztl. Wschr.* 54: 4–5.

Aldred, J. P.; Stob, M.; and Andrews, F. N. 1961. Effect of high temperature, chlorpromazine and progesterone upon embryonic survival in the mouse. *J. Anim. Sci.* 20: 964. (Abst.)

Alexander, G. 1899. Zur Anatomie der janusartigen Doppelmissbildungen mit besonder Berücksichtigung der Synotie. *Roux Arch. Entwickl.* 8: 642–88.

Alexander, J. E. 1962. Anomaly of craniopharyngeal duct and hypophysis. *Can. Vet. J.* 3: 83.

Alexandrov, V. A. 1964. Pathological effect of myelosan on embryogenesis. [In Russian; English summary in *Exc. Med.* Sect. XXI. 5: 914, 1965.] *Dokl. Akad. Nauk. SSSR.* 159: 918–20.

———. 1965. Teratogenous effect of antileukemic drug—myelosan (mileran) on rat embryo. [In Russian with English summary.] *Arkh. Anat.* 44: 87–94.

———. 1966. Analysis of the lethal effect of "myleran" on rat embryos. *Nature* 209: 1215–16.

Alexandrovskaya, M. M. 1959. Certain morphological changes in the central nervous system of white rats irradiated in the prenatal period. [In Russian; English translation by U.S. Joint Publ. Res. Serv., L-1195-N excerpt.] *Med. Radiol. (U.S.S.R.)* 4: 13–21.

Allen, E., and MacDowell, E. C. 1940. Variation in mouse embryos of 8 days gestation. *Anat. Rec.* 77: 165–73.

Altmann, F. 1955. Congenital atresia of the ear in man and animals. *Ann. Otol. Rhin. Laryng.* 64: 824–58.

Amano, S.; Shimizu, S.; Takaya, M.; Sakagami, T.; and Akiyama, N. 1963. Congenital malformation in rats due to hypervitaminosis A in combination with trypan blue and cortisone acetate. [In Japanese with English summary.] *J. Osaka City Med. Cent.* 12: 303–9.

Ancel, P. 1950. *La chimiotératogenèse. Réalisation des monstruosités par des substances chimiques chez les vertébrés.* Paris: Doin.

350 References

Andersen, D. H. 1941. Incidence of congenital diaphragmatic hernia in the young of rats bred on a diet deficient in vitamin A. *Am. J. Dis. Child.* 62: 888–89. (Abst.)

———. 1949. Effect of diet during pregnancy upon the incidence of congenital diaphragmatic hernia in the rat. *Am. J. Path.* 25: 163–85.

Anderson, I., and Morse, L. M. 1966. The influence of solvent on the teratogenic effect of a folic acid antagonist in the rat. *Exp. Mol. Path.* 5: 134–45.

Anderson, P. K. 1964. Lethal alleles in *Mus musculus*. Local distribution and evidence for isolation of demes. *Science* 145: 177–78.

Anderson, W. A., and Davis, C. L. 1950. Congenital cerebellar hypoplasia in a Holstein–Friesian calf. *J. Am. Vet. Med. Ass.* 117: 460–61.

Andres, J. 1931. Eine seltene Doppelmissbildung beim Kalbe. *Arch. Wiss. Prakt. Tierheilk.* 62: 617–31.

Angervall, L. 1959. Alloxan diabetes and pregnancy in the rat. Effects on offspring. *Acta Endocr. Suppl.* 44: 1–86.

———. 1962. Adrenalectomy in pregnant rats. Effects on offspring. *Acta Endocr.* 41: 546–60.

Angervall, L., and Lundin, P. M. 1962. STH and ACTH administration to hypophysectomized pregnant rats. Effect on growth of offspring. *Path. Microbiol.* 25: 852–58.

Annett, H. E. 1939. A note on a new recessive in cattle. *J. Genet.* 37: 301–2.

Anthony, A. 1955. Harmful effects of sound in mice. *Anat. Rec.* 122: 431. (Abst.)

Antoine, G. 1906. Description d'un veau anencéphalien brachyprosope. *Ann Méd. Vét.* 55: 441–45.

Araki, E. 1958. Morphogenesis of cranial malformation due to excessive vitamin A. [In Japanese with English summary.] *J. Osaka City Med. Cent.* 7: 445–52.

Arbab-Zadeh, A. 1966. Toxische und teratogene Wirkungen des Thalidomid. *Deut. Z. Ges. Gerichtl. Med.* 57: 285–90.

Arloing, S. 1867. Monstre strophocéphale (Geoffroy St.-Hilaire); perocephalus agnathus astomus (Gurlt). *J. Méd. Vét.* 22: 355–60.

Arndt, H. J. 1925. Zur Kenntnis der tierischen Doppelmissbildungen (Cephalo-thorakopagus monosymmetros monoprosopus von der Ziege). *Virchow Arch. Path. Anat.* 255: 1–16.

Arnikar, H. J.; Singh, L. M.; and Udupa, K. N. 1963. Radiation induced congenital defects in albino rats. *Current Sci.* 32: 209.

Arvay, A.; Nagy, T.; and Bazsó, J. 1961. L'importance des excitations cumula-tives neurotrope dans la genèse des malformations congénitales. *Biol. Neonat.* 3: 1–23.

Asling, C. W.; Hurley, L. S.; and Wooten, E. 1960. Abnormal development of the otic labyrinth in young rats following maternal manganese deficiency. *Anat. Rec.* 136: 157. (Abst.)

Asling, C. W.; Nelson, M. M.; Dougherty, H. L.; Wright, H. V.; and Evans, H. M. 1960. The development of cleft palate resulting from maternal pteroylglutamic (folic) acid deficiency during the latter half of gestation in rats. *Surg. Gynec. Obstet.* 111: 19–28.

Astle, N. L. 1948. A living two-headed calf. *Vet. Med.* 43: 34–35.

Atkinson, J. C. 1833. Feline monstrosity. *London Med. Gaz.* 12: 294–95.

Auerbach, R. 1954. Analysis of the developmental effects of a lethal mutation in the house mouse. *J. Exp. Zool.* 127: 305–29.

———. 1955. The development of X-ray induced "spina-bifida" in the mouse. *Anat. Rec.* 121: 258. (Abst.)

———. 1956. Effects of single and fractionated doses of X-rays on mouse embryos. *Nature* 177: 574.

Averill, R. L. W., and Purves, H. D. 1963. Differential effects of permanent hypothalamic lesions on reproduction and lactation in rats. *J. Endocr.* 26: 463–77.

B. 1862. Monstrosity in a calf. *Boston Med. Surg. J.* 66: 26.

Baba, T., and Araki, E. 1959. Morphogenesis of malformation due to excessive vitamin A. I. Morphogenesis of exencephaly. *Osaka City Med. J.* 5: 9–15.

Baba, T., and Goda, S. 1961. The effect of embryonic environment of formation of individual. XV. Embryological study of rachischisis in rat induced by trypan blue injections. *Acta Path. Jap.* 11: 257–58. (Abst.)

Baba, T., and Tsuruhara, T. 1959. Morphogenesis of malformation due to excessive vitamin A. IV. Morphogenesis of congenital hydronephrosis and hydroureter. *Osaka City Med. J.* 5: 219–37.

Babbott, F. L., Jr.; Binns, W.; and Ingalls, T. H. 1962. Field studies of cyclopian malformations in sheep. *Arch. Env. Hlth.* 5: 109–13.

Bacq, Z. M., and Alexander, P. 1961. *Fundamentals of radiobiology.* 2d ed. New York: Pergamon.

Badalà, G. 1927. Prosopo-aplasia con microcefalia in un capretto (Capra hircus) neonato. *Monit. Zool. Ital.* 38: 225–33.

Badtke, G.; Degenhardt, K. H.; and Lund, O. E. 1959. Tierexperimenteller Beitrag zur Ätiologie und Phänogenese kraniofacialer Dysplasien. *Z. Anat. Entwickl.* 121: 71–102.

Bagg, H. J. 1922. Disturbances in mammalian development produced by radium emanation. *Am. J. Anat.* 30: 133–61.

Baier, W. 1928. Arhinencephalie beim Fohlen. *Arch. Wiss. Prakt. Tierheilk.* 57: 586–94.

Bailey, J. H., and Nelson, L. F. 1965. Reproductive performance of sows on a ration devoid of carotene and vitamin A. *J. Am. Vet. Med. Ass.* 147: 1387–92.

Baird, B.; Adey, W. R.; Baird, C. D. C.; Casady, R. B.; and Hagen, K. W. 1964. Congenital malformations of unknown etiology in domestic rabbits. *Anat. Rec.* 148: 257. (Abst.)

Baird, B., and Cook, S. F. 1960. Hypoxia and fetal cardiovascular anomalies. *Circulation* 22: 720. (Abst.)

———. 1962. Hypoxia and reproduction of Swiss mice. *Am. J. Physiol.* 202: 611–15.

———. 1966. Neurologic, musculoskeletal and vascular responses to mountain hypoxia. *Fed. Proc.* 28: 190. (Abst.)

Baird, C. D. C.; Nelson, M. M.; Monie, I. W.; Wright, H. V.; and Evans, H. M. 1955. Congenital cardiovascular anomalies produced with the riboflavin antimetabolite, galactoflavin, in the rat. *Fed. Proc.* 14: 428. (Abst.)

Baker, J. B. E. 1960. The effects of drugs on the foetus. *Pharmacol. Rev.* 12: 37–90.

Baker, M. L.; Blunn, C. T.; and Plum, M. 1951. "Dwarfism," in Aberdeen-Angus cattle. *J. Hered.* 42: 141–43.

Baker, M. L.; Payne, L. C.; and Baker, G. N. 1961. The inheritance of hydro-cephalus in cattle. *J. Hered.* 52: 134–38.

Baker, R. C., and Graves, G. O. 1936. Partial cerebellar agenesis in a dog. *Arch. Neur. Psychiat.* 36: 593–600.

Ball, V., and Auger, L. 1926. Encéphalopathies atrophiques du jeune âge. Porencéphalie vraie unilatérale et idiotie chez un chat. *J. Méd. Vét.* 72: 397–412.

Ballantyne, J. W. 1904. *Manual of antenatal pathology and hygiene. The embryo.* Edinburgh: William Green & Sons.

Banchi, A. 1905. Del cranio e del cervello di due ciclopi. *Sperimentale* 59: 201–20.

Banks, W. C., and Monlux, W. S. 1952. Canine hydrocephalus. *J. Am. Vet. Med. Ass.* 121: 453–54.

Baranov, V. S. 1965. The peculiar features of the injuring effect of aminopterin at different stages of rat embryogenesis. [In Russian.] *Dokl. Akad. Nauk. SSSR.* 163: 1032–35.

————. 1966. The specificity of the teratogenic effect of aminopterin as compared to other teratogenic agents. [In Russian with English summary.] *Bull. Eksp. Biol. Med.* 61: 77–82.

Barashnev, Y. I. 1964. Malformations of fetal brain resulting from alloxan diabetes in mother. [In Russian; English translation in *Fed. Proc. Transl. Suppl.* 24: T382–T386, 1965.] *Arkh. Pat.* 26: 63–71.

Barber, A. N. 1957. The effects of maternal hypoxia on inheritance of recessive blindness in mice. *Am. J. Ophth.* 44: 94–101.

Barber, A. N., and Geer, J. C. 1964. Studies on the teratogenic properties of trypan blue and its components in mice. *J. Embryol. Exp. Morph.* 12: 1–14.

Barber, A. N.; Willis, J.; and Afeman, C. 1961. Changes in the lens induced by maternal hypersensitivity in mice. *Am. J. Ophth.* 51: 949–55.

Barber, C. W. 1936. Unilateral hydrocephalus: A case report. *Cornell Vet.* 26: 350–52.

Barboriak, J. J.; Krehl, W. A.; Cowgill, G. R.; and Whedon, A. D. 1957. Effect of partial pantothenic acid deficiency on reproductive performance of the rat. *J. Nutr.* 63: 591–99.

Barilyak, I. R. 1965. Comparison of the effects produced by oranyl and cyclamide on the embryogenesis in albino rats. [In Russian with English summary.] *Farmakol. Toksik.* 28: 616–20.

Barlow, R. M. 1958. Recent advances in swayback. *Proc. Roy. Soc. Med.* 51: 748–52.

Barlow, R. M., and Donald, L. G. 1963. Hydrocephalus in calves associated with unusual lesions in the mesencephalon. *J. Comp. Path. Ther.* 73: 410–15.

Barnett, S. A., and Manly, B. M. 1954. Breeding of mice at −3°C. *Nature* 173: 355.

Barnicot, N. A. 1947. The supravital staining of osteoclasts with neutral red: their distribution on the parietal bone of normal growing mice, and a comparison with the mutants grey-lethal and hydrocephalus-3. *Proc. Roy. Soc. B.* 134: 467–85.

Barr, M. L. 1948. Observations on the foramen of Magendie in a series of human brains. *Brain* 71: 281–89.

Barrier. 1876. Tératologie vétérinaire—monstre de la famille des otocéphaliens (crotaphocéphale). *C. R. Soc. Biol.*, ser. 6 3: 271–79.

———. 1885. Sur les veaux cynocéphales. *C. R. Soc. Biol.*, ser. 8 2: 213–15.

Barry, A.; Patten, B. M.; and Stewart, B. H. 1957. Possible factors in the development of the Arnold–Chiari malformation. *J. Neurosurg.* 14: 285–301.

Bartelheimer, H., and Kloos, K. 1952. Die Auswirkung des experimentellen Diabetes auf Gravidität und Nachkommenschaft. *Z. Ges. Exp. Med.* 119: 246–65.

Baumgartner, W. J. 1928. A double monster pig—cephalothoracopagus monosymmetros. *Anat. Rec.* 37: 303–16.

Baxter, J. S., and Boyd, J. D. 1938. Abnormal development of the brain in an 8 mm pig embryo. *J. Anat.* 72: 422–29.

Beaudoin, A. R. 1962. Interference of Niagara Blue 2B with the teratogenic action of trypan blue. *Proc. Soc. Exp. Biol. Med.* 109: 709–11.

———. 1963. Serum proteins during normal rat pregnancy and rat pregnancies insulted with a teratogen. *Anat. Rec.* 145: 205. (Abst.)

———. 1964. The teratogenicity of Congo red in rats. *Proc. Soc. Exp. Biol. Med.* 117: 176–79.

———. 1966. The effect of trypan blue on the postnatal development of serum proteins. *Life Sci.* 5: 673–77.

Beaudoin, A. R., and Ferm, V. H. 1961. The effect of disazo dyes on protein metabolism in the pregnant rabbit. *J. Exp. Zool.* 147: 219–26.

Beaudoin, A. R., and Kahkonen, D. 1963. The effect of trypan blue on the serum proteins of the fetal rat. *Anat. Rec.* 147: 387–96.

Beaudoin, A. R., and Pickering, M. J. 1960. Teratogenic action of several synthetic compounds structurally related to trypan blue. *Anat. Rec.* 137: 297–305.

Beaudoin, A. R., and Roberts, J. M. 1965. Serum proteins and teratogenesis. *Life Sci.* 4: 1353–58.

———. 1966. Teratogenic action of the thyroid stimulating hormone and its interaction with trypan blue. *J. Embryol. Exp. Morph.* 15: 281–90.

Beck, F. 1961. Comparison of the different teratogenic effects of three commercial samples of trypan blue. *J. Embryol. Exp. Morph.* 9: 673–77.

Beck, F., and Lloyd, J. B. 1963a. The preparation and teratogenic properties of pure trypan blue and its common contaminants. *J. Embryol. Exp. Morph.* 11: 175–84.

———. 1963b. An investigation of the relationship betewen foetal death and foetal malformation. *J. Anat.* 97: 555–64.

———. 1964. Dosage-response curves for the teratogenic activity of trypan blue. *Nature* 201: 1136–37.

———. 1966. The teratogenic effects of azo dyes. *Adv. Terat.* 1: 131–93.

Beck, F.; Spencer, B.; and Baxter, J. S. 1960. Effect of trypan blue on rat embryos. *Nature* 187: 605–7.

Beck, S. L. 1963. Frequencies of teratologies among homozygous normal mice compared with those heterozygous for anophthalmia. *Nature* 200: 810–11.

———. 1964a. Sub-line differences among C57 Black mice in response to trypan blue and outcross. *Nature* 204: 403–4.

————. 1964*b*. Effect of strain of dam on response to trypan blue. *Am. Zool.* 4: 427. (Abst.)

Begg, H. 1903. Dexter monstrosities. *Vet. Rec.* 15: 414–15.

Belkina, A. P. 1958. The effect of quinine administered to pregnant rabbits on the development of the fetal brain. [In Russian with English summary.] *Arkh. Pat.* 20: 64–69.

Belling, T. H., and Holland, L. A. 1962. Variations of internal hydrocephalus. *Vet. Med.* 57: 405–8.

Belting, H. 1963. Synotie, Peroprosopie, Microcephalie und Cyclopie beim Kalb. *Deut. Tierärztl. Wschr.* 70: 213.

Benda, C. E. 1954. The Dandy–Walker syndrome or the so-called atresia of the foramen Magendie. *J. Neuropath. Exp. Neur.* 13: 14–29.

Bendixen, H. C. 1944. Littery occurrence of anophthalmia or microphthalmia together with other malformations in swine—presumably due to vitamin A deficiency of the maternal diet in the first period of pregnancy and the preceding period. *Acta Path. Microbiol. Scand. Suppl.* 54: 161–79.

————. 1950. Einige Beobachtungen über Schäden, die durch A-vitamin-armes Futter bei Schweinen hervorgerufen werden. *Deut. Tierärztl. Wschr.* 57: 150–55.

Bennett, D. 1956. Developmental analysis of a mutation with pleiotropic effects in the mouse. *J. Morph.* 98: 199–233.

————. 1959. Brain hernia, a new recessive mutation in the house mouse. *J. Hered.* 50: 265–68.

————. 1964*a*. Selection toward normality in genetically tailless mice, and some correlated effects. *Am. Nat.* 98: 5–11.

————. 1964*b*. Abnormalities associated with a chromosome region in the mouse. II. Embryological effects of lethal alleles in the *t*-region. *Science* 144: 263–67.

————. 1966. *Mouse News Letter* 35: 20.

Bennett, D.; Badenhausen, S.; and Dunn, L. C. 1959. The embryological effects of four late-lethal *t*-alleles in the mouse, which affect the neural tube and skeleton. *J. Morph.* 105: 105–43.

Bennett, D., and Dunn, L. C. 1958. Effects on embryonic development of a group of genetically similar lethal alleles derived from different populations of wild house mice. *J. Morph.* 103: 135–57.

————. 1960. A lethal mutant (t^{w18}) in the house mouse showing partial duplications. *J. Exp. Zool.* 143: 203–19.

————. 1964. Repeated occurrences in the mouse of lethal alleles of the same complementation group. *Genetics* 49: 949–58.

Bennett, D.; Dunn, L. C.; and Badenhausen, S. 1959. A second group of similar lethals in populations of wild house mice. *Genetics* 44: 795–802.

Berger, J., and Innes, J. R. M. 1948. "Bull-dog" calves (chondrodystrophy, achondroplasia) in a Friesian herd. *Vet. Rec.* 60: 57–58.

Berry, M.; Clendinnen, B. G.; and Eayrs, J. T. 1963. Electrocortical activity in the rat X-irradiated during early development. *Electroenceph. Clin. Neurophysiol.* 15: 91–104.

Berry, M., and Eayrs, J. T. 1966. The effects of X-irradiation on the development of the cerebral cortex. *J. Anat.* 100: 707–22.

Berry, R. J. 1961. The inheritance and pathogenesis of hydrocephalus-3 in the mouse. *J. Path. Bact.* 81: 157–67.

Bertazzoli, C.; Chieli, T.; and Grandi, M. 1965. Absence of tooth malformation in offspring of rats treated with a long-acting sulphonamide. *Experientia* 21: 151–52.

Bertone, L. L., and Monie, I. W. 1965. Teratogenic effect of methyl salicylate and hypoxia in combination. *Anat. Rec.* 151: 443. (Abst.)

Bertrand, I.; Medynski, C.; and Salles, P. 1936. Etude d'un cas d'agénésie du vermis cérébelleux chez le chien. *Rev. Neur.* 66: 716–33.

Bertrand, M.; Schwam, E.; Frandon, A.; Vagne, A.; and Alary, J. 1966. Sur un effet tératogène systématique et spécifique de la caféine chez les rongeurs. *C. R. Soc. Biol.* 159: 2199–2202.

Bevelander, G., and Cohlan, S. Q. 1962. The effect on the rat fetus of transplacentally acquired tetracycline. *Biol. Neonat.* 4: 365–70.

Bien, G. 1905. Zur Anatomie des Zentralnervensystems einer Doppelmissbildung bei der Ziege. *Arb. Neur. Inst. Wien* 12: 282–96.

Bierwolf, D. 1956. Kleinhirnmissbildungen durch hereditaren Hydrocephalus bei der Hausmaus. *Wiss. Z. Univ. Halle* 5: 1237–82.

———. 1958. Die Embryogenese des Hydrocephalus und der Kleinhirnmissbildungen beim Dreherstamm der Hausmaus. *Morph. Jahrb.* 99: 542–612.

Bignami, G.; Bovet, D.; Bovet-Nitti, F.; and Rosnati, V. 1962. Thalidomide. *Lancet* 2: 1333.

Bignami, G.; Bovet-Nitti, F.; and Rosnati, V. 1963. Effects of thalidomide and related compounds on rat pregnancy. Third International Meeting in Forensic Immunology, Medicine, Pathology and Toxicology, London, April 16–24.

Binns, W. 1965. Discussion. In *Embryopathic activity of drugs*, ed. J. M. Robson, F. M. Sullivan, and R. L. Smith, pp. 114–15. Boston: Little, Brown & Co.

Binns, W.; Anderson, W. A.; and Sullivan, D. J. 1960. Further observations on a congenital cyclopian-type malformation in lambs. *J. Am. Vet. Med. Ass.* 137: 515–21.

Binns, W.; James, L. F.; and Shupe, J. L. 1964. Toxicosis of *Veratrum californicum* in ewes and its relationship to a congenital deformity in lambs. *Ann. N. Y. Acad. Sci.* 111: 571–76.

Binns, W.; James, L. F.; Shupe, J. L.; and Everett, G. 1963. A congenital cyclopian-type malformation in lambs induced by maternal ingestion of a range plant, *Veratrum californicum. Am. J. Vet. Res.* 24: 1164–75.

Binns, W.; James, L. F.; Shupe, J. L.; and Thacker, E. J. 1962. Cyclopian-type malformation in lambs. *Arch. Env. Hlth.* 5: 106–8.

Binns, W.; Shupe, J. L.; Keeler, R. F.; and James, L. F. 1965. Chronologic evaluation of teratogenicity in sheep fed *Veratrum californicum. J. Am. Vet. Med. Ass.* 147: 839–42.

Binns, W.; Thacker, E. J.; James, L. F.; and Huffman, W. T. 1959. A congenital cyclopian-type malformation in lambs. *J. Am. Vet. Med. Ass.* 134: 180–83.

Birkner, R. 1958. Symptomatik und systematik der Strahlenschädigungen. *Strahlentherapie* 106: 335–53.

Bishop, M. 1921. The nervous system of a two-headed pig embryo. *J. Comp. Neur.* 32: 379–428.

Bishop, M. W. H., and Cembrowicz, H. J. 1964. A case of *amputate*, a rare recessive lethal condition of Friesian cattle. *Vet. Rec.* 76: 1049–53.

Blackwell, R. L.; Knox, J. H.; and Cobb, E. H. 1959. A hydrocephalic lethal in Hereford cattle. *J. Hered.* 50: 143–48.

Blahser, S., and Labie, C. 1964. Le diagnostic nécropsique chez le chat. *Econ. Méd. Anim.* 5: 67–77.

Blake, J. A. 1900. The roof and lateral recesses of the fourth ventricle considered morphologically and embryologically. *J. Comp. Neur.* 10: 79–108.

Blanc, L. 1895. Sur l'otocéphalie et la cyclotie. *J. Anat. Physiol. (Paris)* 31: 187–218, 288–309.

Blandau, R. J., and Young, W. C. 1939. The effects of delayed fertilization on the development of the guinea pig ovum. *Am. J. Anat.* 64: 303–20.

Blandau, R. J., and Jordan, E. S. 1941. The effect of delayed fertilization on the development of the rat ovum. *Am. J. Anat.* 68: 275–87.

Block. 1902. Eine Missgeburt—Cyclops arhynchus—beim Pferde. *Z. Veterinärk.* 14: 206–10.

Blood, D. C. 1946. Cerebellar hypoplasia and degeneration in the kitten. *Aust. Vet. J.* 22: 120–21.

———. 1956. Arthrogryposis and hydranencephaly in newborn calves. *Aust. Vet. J.* 32: 125–31.

Blood, D. C.; Hutchins, D. R.; Jubb, K. V.; and Whittem, J. H. 1957. Prolonged gestation of Jersey cows. *Aust. Vet. J.* 33: 329.

Bloom, J. L., and Falconer, D. S. 1966. "Grizzled," a mutant in linkage group X of the mouse. *Genet. Res.* 7: 159–67.

Blunn, C. T., and Hughes, E. H. 1938. Hydrocephalus in swine. A new lethal effect. *J. Hered.* 29: 203–8.

Bodansky, M., and Duff, V. B. 1936. Influence of pregnancy on resistance to thyroxine, with data on creatine content of maternal and fetal myocardium. *Endocrinology* 20: 537–40.

Bodian, D. 1966. Spontaneous degeneration in the spinal cord of monkey fetuses. *Bull. Johns Hopkins Hosp.* 119: 212–34.

Bodmer, W. F. 1961. Effects of maternal age on the incidence of congenital abnormalities in mouse and man. *Nature* 190: 1134–35.

Boisselot, J. 1948. Malformations congénitales provoquées chez le rat par une insuffisance en acide pantothénique du régime maternel. *C. R. Soc. Biol.* 142: 928–29.

———. 1949. Malformations foetales par insuffisance en acide pantothénique. *Arch. Fr. Pédiat.* 6: 225–30.

Boizy and Blanc, L. 1893. Un cas remarquable de monstruosité du cerveau. *J. Méd. Vét.,* ser. 3 18: 656–60.

Bolk, L. 1927. Die Doppelbildung eines Affen. *Beitr. Path. Anat.* 76: 238–53.

Bone, J. F. 1953. Hydrocephalus in calves. *N. Am. Vet.* 34: 25–28.

Bonner, R. B.; Mylrea, P. J.; and Doyle, B. J. 1961. Arthrogryposis and hydranencephaly in calves. *Aust. Vet. J.* 37: 160.

Bonnevie, K. 1934. Embryological analysis of gene manifestation in Little and Bagg's abnormal mouse tribe. *J. Exp. Zool.* 67: 443–520.

———. 1935. Vererbbare Missbildungen und Bewegungsstörungen auf embryonale Gehirnanomalien zurückführbar. *Erbarzt* 2: 145–50.

———. 1936*a*. Vererbbare Gehirnanomalie bei kurzschwänzigen Tanzmäusen. *Acta Path. Microbiol. Scand. Suppl.* 26: 20–26.

———. 1936*b*. Abortive differentiation of the ear vesicles following a hereditary brain-anomaly in the "short-tailed waltzing mice." *Genetica* 18: 105–25.

———. 1936*c*. Pseudencephaly als spontane recessive (?) Mutation bei der Hausmaus. *Skr. Norske Vidensk.-Akad. Oslo,* I. Mat.-nat., Kl., 1936, no. 9, 39 pp.

———. 1943. Hereditary hydrocephalus in the house mouse. I. Manifestation of the *hy*-mutation after birth and in embryos 12 days old or more. *Skr. Norske Vidensk.-Akad. Oslo,* I. Mat.-nat., Kl., 1943, no. 4, 32 pp.

———. 1945. Hereditary hydrocephalus in the house mouse. III. Manifestation of the *hy*-mutation in embryos 9–11 days old, and younger. *Skr. Norske Vidensk.-Akad. Oslo,* I. Mat.-nat., Kl., 1944, no. 10, 60 pp.

Bonnevie, K., and Brodal, A. 1946. Hereditary hydrocephalus in the house mouse. IV. The development of the cerebellar anomalies during foetal life with notes on the normal development of the mouse cerebellum. *Skr. Norske Vidensk.-Akad. Oslo,* I. Mat.-nat., Kl., 1946, no. 4, 60 pp.

Borden, J. van der. 1967. Experimental synotia dorsalis in mouse embryos. *Ann. Otol. Rhin. Laryng.* 76: 129–48.

Born, E. 1962. Über ein Blasenhirn bei einen vietnamesischen Hängebauchschwein. Zugleich ein Beitrag zur vergleichenden Neuropathologie. *Acta Neuropath.* 2: 86–90.

Boucher, D., and Carteret, P. 1965. Action du chlorhydrate de tétracycline, injecté à la mère au cours de la gestation, sur la croissance somatique des descendants. *J. Physiol. (Paris)* 57: 567–68.

Boucher, D., and Delost, P. 1964*a*. Développement post-natal des descendants issus de mères traitées par la streptomycine au cours de la gestation chez la souris. *C. R. Soc. Biol.* 158: 2065–69.

———. 1964*b*. Développement post-natal des descendants issus de mères traitées par la penicilline au cours de la gestion chez la souris. *C. R. Soc. Biol.* 158: 528–32.

Bough, R. G.; Gurd, M. R.; Hall, J. E.; and Lessel, B. 1963. Effect of methaqualone hydrochloride in pregnant rabbits and rats. *Nature* 200: 656–57.

Boulard. 1852*a*. Note sur un foetus monstre de chien, avec encéphalocèle et spina bifida. *Gaz. Méd. Paris* 23: 321.

———. 1852*b*. Note sur un foetus monstre de chien, avec encéphalocèle et spina bifida. *C. R. Soc. Biol.,* ser. 1 4: 60–61.

Bouricius, J. K. 1948. Embryological and cytological studies in rats heterozygous for a probable reciprocal translocation. *Genetics* 33: 577–87.

Bournay, J. 1897. Un cas d'hydrocéphalie avec ossification complète de la paroi cranienne chez un poulain. Dystocie. Accouchement dystocique. *Rev. Vét.* 22: 597–600.

Bovard, K. P., and Priode, B. M. 1965. Snorter dwarfism in an Angus inbred line. *J. Hered.* 56: 243–46.

Bovet-Nitti, F.; Bignami, G.; and Bovet, D. 1963. Antihistamine drugs on rat pregnancy: Effects of pyrilamine and meclizine. *Life Sci.* 2: 303–10.

Bovet-Nitti, F., and Bovet, D. 1959. Action of some sympatholytic agents on pregnancy in the rat. *Proc. Soc. Exp. Biol. Med.* 100: 555–57.

Bowen, D. I. 1966. A double monster. *Vet. Rec.* 78: 669

Braden, A. W. H. 1957. The relationship between the diurnal light cycle and the time of ovulation in mice. *J. Exp. Biol.* 34: 177–88.

Braden, A. W. H., and Austin, C. R. 1954. Fertilization of the mouse egg and the effect of delayed coitus and of hot-shock treatment. *Aust. J. Biol. Sci.* 7: 552–65.

Bradley, O. C. 1898. Defective development of the face and cranium in a calf. *Vet. J.* 46: 393–96.

————. 1899. Two monsters. Congenital cerebral hernia in the pig. *Vet. J.* 47: 177–81.

Brady, G. T. 1904. Specimen of cyclocephalus in a full-term calf. *Pacific Med. J.* 47: 56.

Bragonier, J. R.; Roesky, N.; and Carver, M. J. 1964. Teratogenesis: Effects of substituted purines and the influence of 4-hydroxypyrazolopyrimidine in the rat. *Proc. Soc. Exp. Biol. Med.* 116: 685–88.

Brambell, F. W. R., and Hemmings, W. A. 1949. The passage into the embryonic yolk-sac cavity of maternal plasma proteins in rabbits. *J. Physiol.* 108: 177–85.

Brand. 1883. Dicephalus bispinalis von einer Kuh. *München. Tierärztl. Wschr.* 27: 329–30.

Brandt, G. W. 1941. Achondroplasia in calves. *J. Hered.* 32: 183–86.

Brauer. 1898. Perocephalus aprosopus synotus. *Berlin. Tierärztl. Wschr.* 13: 289–90.

Breglia, A. 1894–95. Su di un canale anomalo in un encefalo di feto di coniglio. *Gior. Ass. Napol. Med. Nat.* 5: 65–77.

Brent, R. L. 1960. The indirect effect of irradiation on embryonic development. II. Irradiation of the placenta. *Am. J. Dis. Child.* 100: 103–8.

————. 1963. Discussion. In *Conference proceedings. Prenatal irradiation effects on CNS development,* ed. J. Werboff, p. 54. Washington, D.C., October 4–6.

————. 1964a. Drug testing in animals for teratogenic effects: Thalidomide in the pregnant rat. *J. Pediat.* 64: 762–70.

————. 1964b. The production of congenital malformations using tissue antisera. II. The spectrum and incidence of malformations following the administration of kidney antiserum to pregnant rats. *Am. J. Anat.* 115: 525–41.

————. 1965. Effect on proteins, antibodies, and autoimmune phenomena upon conception and embryogenesis. In *Teratology: Principles and techniques,* ed. J. G. Wilson, and J. Warkany, pp. 215–33. Chicago: Univ. of Chicago Press.

————. 1966a. The production of congenital malformations using tissue antisera. IV. Evaluation of the mechanism of teratogenesis by varying the route and time of administration of anti-rat-kidney antiserum. *Am. J. Anat.* 119: 555–62.

————. 1966b. Immunologic aspects of developmental biology. *Adv. Terat.* 1: 81–129.

Brent, R. L.; Averich, E.; and Drapiewski, V. A. 1961. Production of congenital malformations using tissue antibodies. I. Kidney antisera. *Proc. Soc. Exp. Biol. Med.* 106: 523–26.

Brent, R. L.; Bolden, B. T.; Weiss, A.; Franklin, J. B.; and George, E. F. 1962. The evaluation of teratogenic agents by means of the uterine vascular clamping technique. *Abst. Terat. Soc.* 2: 17. (Abst.)

Brent, R. L., and Franklin, J. B. 1960. Uterine vascular clamping: New procedure for the study of congenital malformations. *Science* 132: 89–91.

Brent, R. L.; Franklin, J. B.; and Bolden, B. T. 1963. Modification of irradiation effects on rat embryos by uterine vascular clamping. *Radiat. Res.* 18: 58–64.

Brent, R. L., and McLaughlin, M. M. 1960. The indirect effect of irradiation on embryonic development. I. Irradiation of the mother while shielding the embryonic site. *Am. J. Dis. Child.* 100: 94–102.

Brinsmade, A. B. 1957. Entwicklungsstörungen am Kaninchenembryo nach Glukosemangel beim trächtigen Muttertier. *Beitr. Path. Anat.* 117: 140–53.

Brinsmade, A.; Büchner, F.; and Rübsaamen, H. 1956. Missbildungen am Kaninchenembryo durch Insulininjektion beim Muttertier. *Naturwissenschaften* 43: 259.

Brinsmade, A. B., and Rübsaamen, H. 1957. Zur teratogenetischen Wirkung von unspezifischem Fieber auf den sich entwickelnden Kaninchenembryo. *Beitr. Path. Anat.* 117: 154–64.

Brizee, K. R. 1964. Effects of single and fractionated doses of total body X-irradiation *in utero* on growth of the brain and its parts. *Nature* 202: 262–64.

Brizee, K. R.; Jacobs, L. A.; and Kharetchko, X. 1961. Effects of total-body X-irradiation *in utero* on early postnatal changes in neuron volumetric relationships and packing density in cerebral cortex. *Radiat. Res.* 14: 96–103.

Brock, N., and Kreybig, T. von. 1964. Experimenteller Beitrag zur Prüfung teratogener Wirkungen von Arzneimitteln an der Laboratoriumsratte. *Naunyn Schmiedeberg Arch. Exp. Path.* 249: 117–45.

Brodal, A. 1946. Correlated changes in nervous tissues in malformations of the central nervous system. *J. Anat.* 80: 88–93.

Brodal, A.; Bonnevie, K.; and Harkmark, W. 1944. Hereditary hydrocephalus in the house mouse. II. The anomalies of the cerebellum: Partial defective development of the vermis. *Skr. Norske Vidensk.-Akad. Oslo,* I. Mat.-nat. Kl., 1944, no. 8, 42 pp.

Brodal, A., and Hauglie-Hanssen, E. 1959. Congenital hydrocephalus with defective development of the cerebellar vermis (Dandy–Walker syndrome). Clinical and anatomical findings in two cases with particular reference to the so-called atresia of the foramina of Magendie and Luschka. *J. Neur. Neurosurg. Psychiat.* 22: 99–108.

Brotherston, A. 1876–78. Zoological notes. *Trans. Berwickshire Nat. Club* 8: 520–26.

Brouwer, B. 1934. Familial olivo-ponto-cerebellar hypoplasia in cats. *Psychiat. Neur. Blad.* 38: 352–67.

Brown, R. A., and West, G. B. 1964. Effect of acetylsalicylic acid on foetal rats. *J. Pharm. Pharmacol.* 16: 563–65.

Brown, R. V. 1963. *Mouse News Letter* 29: 67.

Brown, S. O.; Krise, G. M.; and Pace, H. B. 1963. Continuous low-dose radiation effects on successive litters of the albino rat. *Radiat. Res.* 19: 270–76.

360   *References*

Brown, W. H., and Pearce, L. 1945. Hereditary achondroplasia in the rabbit. I. Physical appearance and general features. *J. Exp. Med.* 82: 241–60.

Bruch, R. M. 1966. *Mouse News Letter* 35: 20–21.

————. 1967. Congenital head and brain malformations in mice homozygous for a recessive mutation. *Anat. Rec.* 157: 220–21. (Abst.)

Brüggemann, H. 1951. Wasserkopf beim Kalb. *Züchtungskunde* 22: 280–84.

Buck, P.; Clavert, J.; and Rumpler, Y. 1962. Action tératogénique des cortico des chez la lapine. *Ann. Chir. Infant.* 3: 73–87.

Buettner-Janusch, J. 1966. A problem in evolutionary systematics: Nomenclature and classification of baboons, genus *Papio. Folia Primat.* 4: 288–308.

Bujard, E. 1919. A propos d'un cas d'opocéphalie chez le cobaye: Les synotocyclopes et les strophocéphales. *C. R. Soc. Phys. Genève* 36: 43–50.

Bullard, J. F. 1935. Syringomyelia in a Jersey calf. *J. Am. Vet. Med. Ass.* 87: 575–77.

Burns, K. F. 1950. Congenital Japanese B encephalitis infection of swine. *Proc. Soc. Exp. Biol. Med.* 75: 621–25.

Burns, M., and Fraser, M. N. 1966. *Genetics of the dog. The basis of successful breeding.* Philadelphia: Lippincott.

Burris, M. J., and Priode, B. M. 1956. Crossbred dwarfs in beef cattle. *J. Hered.* 47: 245–48.

Bussano, G. 1909. Di un caso di "dicefalia" osservato in un vitello. *Clin. Vet.* (*Milan*) 32: 305–8, 321–27.

Butler, J., and Lyon, M. F. 1967. *Mouse News Letter* 36: 36.

Butz, H., and Böttger, T. 1939. Enzephalozele der Stirngegend bei zwei neugeborenen Ferkeln. *Deut. Tierärztl. Wschr.* 47: 427–28.

Cahen, R. L. 1964. Evaluation of the teratogenicity of drugs. *Clin. Pharmacol. Ther.* 5: 480–514.

Cahen, R. L.; Sautai, M.; Montagne, J.; and Pessonnier, J. 1964. Recherche de l'effet tératogène de la 2-diéthylaminopropiophénone. *Méd. Exp.* 10: 201–24.

Callas, G., and Walker, B. E. 1963. Palate morphogenesis in mouse embryos after X-irradiation. *Anat. Rec.* 145: 61–72.

Cameron, A. H. 1956. The spinal cord lesion in spina bifida cystica. *Lancet* 2: 171–74.

————. 1957. The Arnold-Chiari and other neuro-anatomical malformations associated with spina bifida. *J. Path. Bact.* 73: 195–211.

Cameron, A. H., and Hill, W. C. O. 1955. The Arnold–Chiari malformation in a sacred baboon (*Papio hamadryas*). *J. Path. Bact.* 70: 552–54.

Carey, B. W. 1962. Drugs and deformities. *J. Am. Med. Ass.* 181: 805–6.

Carey, E. 1917. The anatomy of the double pig, syncephalus thoracopagus, with especial consideration of the genetic significance of the circulatory apparatus. *Anat. Rec.* 12: 177–91.

Carmichael, J. 1933. "Bull-dog" calf in African cattle. *Nature* 131: 878.

Carpent, G. 1958. Action tératogène du bleu de trypan chez la rate gestante et régulation hormonale du mécanisme gravidique. *Ann. Endocr.* 19: 904–12.

————. 1962. Le déséquilibre hormonal gravidique et ses répercussions sur la morphologie du foetus chez le rat. *Arch. Anat. Micr. Morph. Exp.* 51: 459–540.

Carpenter, M. B., and Harter, D. H. 1956. A study of congenital feline cerebellar malformations. An anatomic and physiologic evaluation of agenetic defects. *J. Comp. Neur.* 105: 51–93.

Carpenter, M. B., and Penny, S. 1952. Feline truncal ataxia associated with degeneration of the cerebellar cortex and roof nuclei. *J. Neuropath. Exp. Neur.* 11: 421–28.

Carter, T. C. 1956. Genetics of the Little and Bagg X-rayed mouse stock. *J. Genet.* 54: 311–26.

———. 1959. Embryology of the Little and Bagg X-rayed mouse stock. *J. Genet.* 56: 401–35.

Carton, C. A.; Pascal, R. R.; and Tennyson, V. 1961. Hydrocephalus and vitamin-A-deficiency in the rabbit: General considerations. In *Disorders of the developing nervous system,* ed. W. S. Fields, and M. M. Desmond, pp. 214–66. Springfield, Ill.: Thomas.

Carton, C. A.; Perry, J. H.; Winter, A.; and Tennyson, V. 1956. Studies of hydrocephalus in C_{57} black mice. *Trans. Am. Neur. Ass.* 81: 147–49.

Caspari, E., and David, P. R. 1940. The inheritance of a tail abnormality in the house mouse. *J. Hered.* 31: 427–31.

Cattanach, B. 1965. Snaker: A dominant abnormality caused by chromosomal imbalance. *Z. Vererbungsl.* 96: 275–84.

Caujolle, F.; Caujolle, D.; Cros, S.; and Calvet, M. 1967. Limits of toxic and teratogenic tolerance of dimethyl sulfoxide. *Ann. N. Y. Acad. Sci.* 141: 110–25.

Caujolle, F.; Caujolle, D.; Cros, S.; Calvet, M.; and Tollon, Y. 1965. Pouvoir tératogène du diméthylsulfoxyde et du diéthylsulfoxyde. *C. R. Acad. Sci.* 260: 327–30.

Center, E. M. 1960. "Dorsal excrescences" in the mouse—genetic or non-genetic? *J. Hered.* 51: 21–26.

Chaddock, T. T. 1948. Ten-year autopsy study of foxes. *Vet. Med.* 43: 13.

Chai, C. K., and Degenhardt, K. H. 1962. Developmental anomalies in inbred rabbits. *J. Hered.* 53: 174–82.

Chaillous, M. J; Robin, V.; and Mollaret, P. 1931. Cataracte bilatérale et troubles cérébelleux congénitaux chez un jeune chat. *Bull. Soc. Opht. Paris* 43: 53–56.

Chamberlain, J. G. 1964. Prenatal development of hydrocephaly in the rat. *Anat. Rec.* 148: 270. (Abst.)

Chamberlain, J. G., and Nelson, M. M. 1963a. Multiple congenital abnormalities in the rat resulting from acute maternal niacin deficiency during pregnancy. *Proc. Soc. Exp. Biol. Med.* 112: 836–40.

———. 1963b. Congenital abnormalities in the rat resulting from single injections of 6-aminonicotinamide during pregnancy. *J. Exp. Zool.* 153: 285–300.

Chambers, D.; Whatley, J. A., Jr.; and Stephens, D. F. 1954. The inheritance of dwarfism in a Comprest Hereford herd. *J. Anim. Sci.* 13: 956–57. (Abst.)

Chambon, Y. 1955. Action de la chlorpromazine sur l'évolution et l'avenir de la gestation chez la rate. *Ann. Endocr.* 16: 912–22.

Chambon, Y.; Depagne, A.; and Le Veve, Y. 1966. Malformations et déformations foetales par insuffisance hormonale gestative chez le lapin et chez le rat. *Bull. Ass. Anat.* 131: 270–79.

Chang, M. C. 1944. Artificial production of monstrosities in the rabbit. *Nature* 154: 150.

———. 1952. Effects of delayed fertilization on segmenting ova, blastocysts and fetuses in rabbit. *Fed. Proc.* 11: 24. (Abst.)

———. 1957. Effect of pyrogen on embryonic degeneration in the rabbit. *Fed. Proc.* 16: 21. (Abst.)

Chang, M. C., and Fernandez-Cano, L. 1959. Effects of short changes of environmental temperature and low atmospheric pressure on the ovulation of rats. *Am. J. Physiol.* 196: 653–55.

Chang, M. C., and Hunt, D. M. 1960. Effects of in vitro radiocobalt irradiation of rabbit ova on subsequent development in vivo with special reference to the irradiation of maternal organism. *Anat. Rec.* 137: 511–19.

Chang, M. C.; Hunt, D. M.; and Harvey, E. B. 1963. Effects of radiocobalt irradiation of pregnant rabbits on the development of fetuses. *Anat. Rec.* 145: 455–66.

Chang, M. C.; Hunt, D. M.; and Romanoff, E. B. 1958. Effects of radiocobalt irradiation of unfertilized or fertilized rabbit ova in vitro on subsequent fertilization and development in vivo. *Anat. Rec.* 132: 161–79.

Chase, H. B. 1943. A new appearance of pigtail. *Rec. Genet. Soc. Am.* 12: 45. (Abst.)

Chaube, S., and Murphy, M. L. 1963. Teratogenic effect of hadacidin (a new growth inhibitory chemical) on the rat fetus. *J. Exp. Zool.* 152: 67–73.

———. 1964. Teratogenic effects of 5-chlorodeoxyuridine on the rat fetus; protection by physiological pyrimidines. *Canc. Res.* 24: 1986–93.

———. 1966. The effects of hydroxyurea and related compounds on the rat fetus. *Canc. Res.* 26: 1448–57.

Cheng, D. W. 1956. A study of the occurrence of teratogeny in vitamin E-deficient rats and associated abnormalities in blood and tissues. *Iowa St. Coll. J. Sci.* 30: 340–41. (Abst.)

———. 1959. Effect of progesterone and esterone on the incidence of congenital malformations due to maternal vitamin E deficiency. *Endocrinology* 64: 270–75.

Cheng, D. W.; Bairnson, T. A.; Rao, A. N.; and Subbammal, S. 1960. Effect of variations of rations on the incidence of teratogeny in vitamin E-deficient rats. *J. Nutr.* 71: 54–60.

Cheng, D. W.; Chang, L. F.; and Bairnson, T. A. 1957. Gross observations on developing abnormal embryos induced by maternal vitamin E deficiency. *Anat. Rec.* 129: 167–85.

Cheng, D. W., and Thomas, B. H. 1953. Relationship of time of therapy to teratogeny in maternal avitaminosis E. *Proc. Iowa Acad. Sci.* 60: 290–99.

———. 1955. Histological changes in the abnormal rat fetuses induced by maternal vitamin E deficiency. *Anat. Rec.* 121: 274. (Abst.)

Chesley, P. 1932. Lethal action in the short-tailed mutation in the house mouse. *Proc. Soc. Exp. Biol. Med.* 29: 437–38.

———. 1935. Development of the short-tailed mutant in the house mouse. *J. Exp. Zool.* 70: 429–59.

Chesley, P., and Dunn, L. C. 1936. The inheritance of taillessness (anury) in the house mouse. *Genetics* 21: 525–36.

Chiari, H. 1891. Ueber Veränderungen des Kleinhirns infolge von Hydrocephalie des Grosshirns. *Deut. Med. Wschr.* 17: 1172–75

Chidester, F. E. 1914. Cyclopia in mammals. *Anat. Rec.* 8: 355–66.

————. 1924. The anatomy of an otocephalic dog. *Anat. Rec.* 28: 15–30.

Chin, E.; Nelson, M. M.; and Monie, I. W. 1963. Combinations of teratogenic procedures in rat teratogenesis. *Anat. Rec.* 145: 216–17. (Abst.)

Chomette, G. 1955. Entwicklungsstörungen nach Insulinschock beim trächtiger Kaninchen. *Beitr. Path. Anat.* 115: 439–51.

Christie, G. A. 1961. An embryological analysis of certain cardiac abnormalities produced in rats by the injection of trypan blue. *Scot. Med. J.* 6: 465–76.

————. 1964. The teratogenic activity of trypan blue, and its effect on the thyro-hypophyseal axis in the rat. *J. Anat.* 98: 377–84.

————. 1965. Teratogenic effects of synthetic compounds related to trypan blue: The effect of 1,7-diamino-8-naphthol-3,6-disulphonic acid on pregnancy in the rat. *Nature* 208: 1219–20.

————. 1966. Influence of thyroid function on the teratogenic activity of trypan blue in the rat. *J. Anat.* 100: 361–68.

Clark, F. H. 1932. Hydrocephalus, a hereditary character in the house mouse. *Proc. Nat. Acad. Sci. USA.* 18: 654–56.

————. 1934. Anatomical basis of hereditary hydrocephalus in the house mouse. *Anat. Rec.* 58: 225–33.

————. 1935. Two hereditary types of hydrocephalus in the house mouse (*Mus musculus*). *Proc. Nat. Acad. Sci. USA.* 21: 150–52.

Clavert, J.; Buck, P.; and Rumpler, Y. 1961. Actions tératogènes du soludéca-dron chez la lapine. *C. R. Soc. Biol.* 160: 1569–71.

Clavert, J.; Buck, P.; Rumpler, Y.; and Ruch, J. V. 1965. Malformations cardio-vasculaires déterminées chez les embryons par injections de "cortisoniques" à la lapine gestante. *Thérapie* 20: 1579–84.

Clavert, J.; Rumpler, Y.; and Ruch, J. V. 1965. Effets tératogènes du phosphate de dexaméthasone en fonction du stade du développement. *Bull. Ass. Anat.* 125: 465–72.

Clemmer, T. P., and Telford, I. R. 1966. Abnormal development of the rat heart during prenatal hypoxic stress. *Proc. Soc. Exp. Biol. Med.* 121: 800–803.

Cobb, S. 1928. A case of cerebellar aplasia in a cat. *Arch. Neur. Psychiat.* 19: 931–32.

Coben, L. A. 1967. Absence of a foramen of Magendie in the dog, cat, rabbit, and goat. *Arch. Neur.* 16: 524–28.

Cock, A. G. 1950. A case of incomplete twinning in the rabbit. *J. Genet.* 50: 59–66.

Coggi, G. 1965. Embriopatie nel topo da pantoiltaurina, antivitamina dell'acido pantotenico. *Folia Hered. Path.* 14: 147–54.

Cohlan, S. Q. 1953a. Excessive intake of vitamin A during pregnancy as a cause of congenital anomalies in the rat. *Am. J. Dis. Child.* 86: 348–49. (Abst.)

————. 1953b. Excessive intake of vitamin A as a cause of congenital anomalies in the rat. *Science* 117: 535–36.

————. 1954. Congenital anomalies in the rat produced by the excessive intake of vitamin A during pregnancy. *Pediatrics* 13: 556–67.

Cohlan, S. Q., and Kitay, D. 1965. The teratogenic effect of vincaleukoblastine in the pregnant rat. *J. Pediat.* 66: 541–44.

Cohlan, S. Q., and Stone, S. M. 1955. Congenital malformations of the brain produced by exposure of the pregnant rat to rubella virus. *Am. J. Dis. Child.* 90: 616–17. (Abst.)

————. 1961. Observations on the effect of experimental endocrine procedures on the teratogenic action of hypervitaminosis A in the rat. *Biol. Neonat.* 3: 330–42.

Cohrs, P. 1936. Ein weiterer Beitrag zum Vorkommen von eineiiger Zwillingen beim Hausschwein. *Z. Zücht. B.* 36: 295–305.

————. 1952. Das Nervensystem. In *Lehrbuch der speziellen pathologischen Anatomie der Haustiere,* ed. K. Nieberle, and P. Cohrs, pp. 425–72. 3d ed. Jena: Fischer.

Cohrs, P.; Comberg, G.; Meyer, H.; and Trautwein, G. 1963. Erbliche Meningocele cerebralis beim Schwein. *Deut. Tierärztl. Wschr.* 70: 437–40.

Cohrs, P., and Schulz, L. C. 1952. Entwicklungsmechanisch bedingte partielle Aplasien der Rinde und von Windungsteilen des Kleinhirns beim Schwein. *Deut. Z. Nervenheilk.* 168: 135–41.

Cole, C. L., and Moore, L. A. 1942. Hydrocephalus, a lethal in cattle. *J. Agr. Res.* 65: 483–91.

Collet, G.; Ajuriaguerra, J. de.; Fankhauser, R.; and Bogaert, L. van. 1954. L'hypogénésie cérébelleuse chez le chat. *Rev. Neur.* 91: 175–99.

Colton, H. S. 1929. "High brow" albino rats. *J. Hered.* 20: 225–27.

Colucci. 1912. Agenesia di un emisfero cerebrale di un bovino. *Atti Cong. Soc. Ital. Neur.* 3: 178–80.

Conaway, C. H. 1955. Embryo resorption and placental scar formation in the rat. *J. Mammal.* 36: 516–32.

Conn, J. H., and Hardy, J. D. 1959. Experimental production of cardiovascular anomalies in dogs using trypan blue. *Surg. Forum* 9: 294–97.

Conneally, P. M.; Stone, W. H.; Tyler, W. J.; Casida, L. E.; and Morton, N. E. 1963. Genetic load expressed as fetal death in cattle. *J. Dairy Sci.* 46: 232–36.

Conrow, S. B. 1917. A six-legged rat. *Anat. Rec.* 12: 365–70.

Cooper, W. A. 1962. Congenital heart abnormalities in biotin-deficient and pantothenic acid-deficient rats. *Texas J. Sci.* 14: 278–79.

Coppenger, C. J. 1964. Effects of prenatal chronic gamma irradiation on the prenatal and postnatal development of the albino rat. *Diss. Abst.* 25: 705. (Abst.)

Coppenger, C. J., and Brown, S. O. 1965. Postnatal manifestations in albino rats continuously irradiated during prenatal development. *Texas Rep. Biol. Med.* 23: 45–55.

Cordy, D. R., and Shultz, G. 1961. Congenital subcortical encephalopathies in lambs. *J. Neuropath. Exp. Neur.* 20: 554–62.

Cordy, D. R., and Snelbaker, H. A. 1952. Cerebellar hypoplasia and degeneration in a family of Airedale dogs. *J. Neuropath. Exp. Neur.* 11: 324–28.

Cornwall, L. H. 1927. Cerebro-cerebellar agenesis in its relation to cerebellar function. *Brain* 50: 562–72.

————. 1929. Cerebro-cerebellar agenesis in relation to cerebellar function. *Res. Publ. Ass. Nerv. Ment. Dis.* 6: 463–80.

Corsy, F., and Robert, J. 1925. Sur un cas d'iniodyme triote. *Marseille Méd.* 62: 966–70.

Coupin, F. 1920. Sur l'absence de trous de Magendie et de Luschka chez quelques mammifères. *C. R. Soc. Biol.* 83: 954–56.

Courrier, R., and Jost, A. 1939. Sur l'analyse quantitative de l'endocrinologie de la gestation chez la lapine. *C. R. Soc. Biol.* 130: 726–29.

Courrier, R., and Marois, M. 1953. Action de l'hypothermie expérimentale sur le gestation chez le rat. *C. R. Soc. Biol.* 147: 1922–24.

——. 1954. Retard de la nidation et du développement foetal chez la rate en hypothermie. *Ann. Endocr.* 15: 738–45.

Courtney, K. D., and Valerio, D. A. 1967. Experimental teratology in *Macaca mulatta*. *Abst. Terat. Soc.* 7: 21. (Abst.)

Cowen, D., and Geller, L. M. 1960. Long-term pathological effects of prenatal X-irradiation on the central nervous system of the rat. *J. Neuropath. Exp. Neur.* 19: 488–527.

Cozens, D., and Mawdesley-Thomas, L. E. 1966. Reduplication of the pituitary in a dog. *Vet. Rec.* 78: 474–75.

Cozens, D. D. 1965. Abnormalities of the external form and of the skeleton in the New Zealand White rabbit. *Food Cosmet. Toxic.* 3: 695–700.

Crampton, E. W. 1926. Partial twinning in pigs. *J. Hered.* 17: 411–12.

Crary, D. D.; Fox, R. R.; and Sawin, P. B. 1966. Spina bifida in the rabbit. *J. Hered.* 57: 236–43.

Crary, D. D., and Sawin, P. B. 1952. A second achondroplasia in the domestic rabbit. *J. Hered.* 43: 254–59.

Crew, F. A. E. The significance of an achondroplasia-like condition met with in cattle. *Proc. Roy. Soc. B.* 95: 228–55.

——. 1924. The bull-dog calf, a contribution to the study of achondroplasia. *Proc. Roy. Soc. Med.* 17: 39–58.

Crew, F. A. E., and Auerbach, C. 1941. "Pigtail," a hereditary tail abnormality in the house mouse, *Mus musculus*. *J. Genet.* 41: 267–74.

Crisp. 1856. [A monoculus lamb.] *Proc. Zool. Soc. London* 24: 149–50.

——. 1860. A monoculus lamb which had recently been dissected. *Trans. Path. Soc. London* 11: 305–6.

Crocker, W. J. 1919*a*. Monstrosities. *J. Am. Vet. Med. Ass.* 54: 387–88.

——. 1919*b*. Hydrencephalocele, anopia, campylognathia, acheilia superior and sarcodontia (calf). *Cornell Vet.* 9: 55–56.

Croft, P. G. 1962. The EEG as an aid to diagnosis of nervous diseases in the dog and cat. *J. Small Anim. Pract.* 3: 205–13.

Currarino, G., and Silverman, F. N. 1960. Orbital hypotelorism, arhinencephaly, and trigonocephaly. *Radiology* 74: 206–17.

Curry, G. A. 1959. Genetical and developmental studies on droopy-eared mice. *J. Embryol. Exp. Morph.* 7: 39–65.

Curson, H. H. 1931. Anatomical studies, no. 25: Ankyloblepharon, monophthalmia, aplasia N. optici, and hypoplasia cerebri in a kid. *Rep. Dir. Vet. Serv. Anim. Ind.* (Un. S. Afr.) 17: 865–67.

Curtis, R. L.; English, D.; and Kim, Y. J. 1964. Spina bifida in a "stub" dog stock, selectively bred for short tails. *Anat. Rec.* 148: 365. (Abst.)

Dagg, C. P. 1960. Sensitive stages for the production of developmental abnormalities in mice with 5-fluorouracil. *Am. J. Anat.* 106: 89–96.

————. 1963. The interaction of environmental stimuli and inherited susceptibility to congenital deformity. *Am. Zool.* 3: 223–33.

————. 1963–64. Spina bifida production by X-irradiation. *Ann. Rep. Jackson Lab.* 35: 65.

————. 1964. Some effects of X-irradiation on the development of inbred and hybrid mouse embryos. In *Effects of ionizing radiation on the reproductive system,* ed. W. D. Carlson, and F. X. Gassner, pp. 91–102. New York: Macmillan.

————. 1965. Experimental modification of gene penetrance. *Abst. Terat. Soc.* 5: 8. (Abst.)

————. 1966. Teratogenesis. In *Biology of the laboratory mouse,* ed. E. L. Green, pp. 309–28. 2d ed. New York: McGraw-Hill.

Dagg, C. P., and Kallio, E. 1962. Teratogenic interaction of fluorodeoxyuridine and thymidine. *Anat. Rec.* 142: 301–2. (Abst.)

Dagg, C. P.; Schlager, G.; and Doerr, A. 1966. Polygenic control of the teratogenicity of 5-fluorouracil in mice. *Genetics* 53: 1101–17.

D'Agostino, A. N., and Brizzee, K. R. 1966. Radiation necrosis and repair in rat fetal cerebral hemisphere. *Arch. Neur.* 15: 615–28.

D'Agostino, A. N.; Kernohan, J. W.; and Brown, J. R. 1963. The Dandy–Walker syndrome. *J. Neuropath. Exp. Neur.* 22: 450–70.

D'Amato, C. J., and Hicks, S. P. 1965. Effects of low levels of ionizing radiation on the developing cerebral cortex of the rat. *Neurology* 15: 1104–16.

Dandy, W. E. 1921. The diagnosis and treatment of hydrocephalus due to occlusions of the foramina of Magendie and Luschka. *Surg. Gynec. Obstet.* 32: 112–24.

Dandy, W. E., and Blackfan, K. D. 1914. Internal hydrocephalus. An experimental, clinical and pathological study. *Am. J. Dis. Child.* 8: 406–82.

Danforth, C. H. 1925. Hereditary doubling, suggesting anomalous chromatin distribution in the mouse. *Proc. Soc. Exp. Biol. Med.* 23: 145–47.

————. 1930. Developmental anomalies in a special strain of mice. *Am. J. Anat.* 45: 275–88.

Danforth, C. H., and Center, E. 1954. Nitrogen mustard as a teratogenic agent in the mouse. *Proc. Soc. Exp. Biol. Med.* 86: 705–7.

————. 1967. Genetical and embryological basis of the *duplicitas posterior* manifestation in the mouse. *Genetics* 56: 554. (Abst.)

Daniel, P. M., and Stritch, S. J. 1958. Some observations on the congenital deformity of the central nervous system known as the Arnold–Chiari malformation. *J. Neuropath. Exp. Neur.* 17: 255–66.

Dareste, C. 1852. Mémoire sur un chat iléadelphe a tête monstrueuse. *Ann. Sci. Nat., Zool.,* ser. 3 18: 81–94.

————. 1885a. Sur un cas de cébocéphalie avec complication d'anencéphalie partielle, observé chez un poulain. *C. R.' Acad. Sci.* 101: 184–86.

————. 1885b. Mémoire sur un cas de cébocéphalie observé chez un poulain. *J. Anat. Physiol. (Paris)* 21: 346–55.

————. 1887. Les veaux à tête de bouledogue. *Bull. Soc. Anthrop. Paris,* ser. 3 10: 375–83.

Davaine. 1862. Sur une difformité analogue au pied-bot coincidant avec un spina-bifida chez le veau. *C. R. Soc. Biol.,* ser. 3 4: 186–89.

Davey, R. J., and Stevenson, J. W. 1963. Pantothenic acid requirement of swine for reproduction. *J. Anim. Sci.* 22: 9–13.

David, G.; Mercier-Parot, L.; Rain, B.; and Tuchmann-Duplessis, H. 1966. Anomalies dentaires dans l'otocéphalie provoquée par des corps anti-tissulaires. *C. R. Soc. Biol.* 160: 1182–86.

David, G.; Mercier-Parot, L.; and Tuchmann-Duplessis, H. 1963. Action tératogène d'hétéro-anticorps tissulaires. I. Production de malformations chez le rat par action d'un sérum anti-rein. *C. R. Soc. Biol.* 157: 939–42.

Davis, M. E., and Plotz, E. J. 1954. The effects of cortisone acetate on intact and adrenalectomized rats during pregnancy. *Endocrinology* 54: 384–95.

Davis, S. L. 1942. A bovine monster. *Vet. Med.* 37: 95.

Dawson, J. E. 1964. Effect of sodium tolbutamide on pregnant albino rats and their young. *Diabetes* 13: 527–31.

Deganello, U., and Spangaro, S. 1899. Aplasie congénitale du cervelet chez un chien. Résultat de l'examen microscopique des centres nerveux. *Arch. Ital. Biol.* 32: 165–73.

Degenhardt, K. H. 1954. Durch O_2-Mangel induzierte Fehlbildungen der Axialgradienten bei Kaninchen. *Z. Naturforsch.* 9B: 530–36.

———. 1960*b*. Cranio-facial dysplasia induced by oxygen-deficiency in rabbits. *Biol. Neonat.* 2: 93–104.

———. 1960*b*. Die genetische und morphologische Analyse spezieller Entwicklungsstörungen in einem Stamm ingezüchteter Hermelin-Kaninchen. *Akad. Wiss. Lit. Math.-Naturwiss. Kl.*, pp. 917–88.

———. 1963. Experimentelle Missbildungen der Kopfregion in ihrer Bedeutung für die ontogenetische Frühentwicklung. *Berlin. Deut. Ophth. Ges.* 65: 160–68.

Degenhardt, K. H.; Badtke, G.; and Lund, O. E. 1961. Aetiology and pathogenesis of maxillo-facial and mandibulo-facial dysplasias. In *Second International Conference of Human Genetics*, p. E183. Amsterdam: Excerpta Medica Found.

Degenhardt, K. H., and Grüter, H. J. 1959. Durch Röntgenstrahlen induzierte Entwicklungsstörungen bei Kaninchenembryonen. *Z. Naturforsch.* 14B: 753–56.

Degenhardt, K. H., and Kladetzky, J. 1955. Wirbelsäulenmissbildung und Chordaanlage. Experimentelle teratogenetische und embryohistologische Untersuchungen bei Kaninchen. *Z. Menschl. Vererb. Konst.* 33: 151–92.

Degoix. 1879. Un monstre de l'espèce porcine. *Rec. Méd. Vét.* 56: 1237.

Dehors, G. 1894. Quelques cas tératologiques observés à l'abattoir de Santiago. *Act. Soc. Sci. Chili* 4: 313–21.

Dekker, A., and Mehrizi, A. 1964. The use of thalidomide as a teratogenic agent in rabbits. *Bull. Johns Hopkins Hosp.* 115: 223–30.

Delahunt, C. S. 1966. Rubella-induced cataracts in monkeys. *Lancet* 1: 825.

Delahunt, C. S., and Lassen, L. J. 1964. Thalidomide syndrome in monkeys. *Science* 146: 1300–1305.

deLahunta, A., and Cummings, J. F. 1965. The clinical and electroencephalographic features of hydrocephalus in three dogs. *J. Am. Vet. Med. Ass.* 146: 954–64.

Delatour, P.; Dams, R.; and Favre-Tissot, M. 1965. Thalidomide: Embryopathies chez le chien. *Thérapie* 20: 573–89.

DeMyer, W. 1964. Vinblastine-induced malformations of face and nervous system in two rat strains. *Neurology* 14: 806–8.

368 References

————. 1965*a*. Production of major cerebral malformations by drugs with special reference to the holoprosencephalies (cyclopia-arhinencephaly). *Proc. Int. Cong. Neuropath.* 5: 717–21.

————. 1965*b*. Cleft lip and jaw induced in fetal rats by vincristine. *Arch. Anat.* 48: 181–86.

DeMyer, W., and Zeman, W. 1963. Alobar holoprosencephaly (arhinencephaly) with median cleft lip and palate: Clinical, electroencephalographic and nosologic considerations. *Conf. Neur.* 23: 1–36.

Dennis, S. M. 1965. Congenital abnormalities in sheep. *J. Dep. Agr. West Aust.* ser. 4 6: 235–40.

Deol, M. S. 1961. Genetical studies on the skeleton of the mouse. XXVIII. Tail-short. *Proc. Roy. Soc. B.* 155: 78–95.

————. 1964*a*. The origin of the abnormalities of the inner ear in dreher mice. *J. Embryol. Exp. Morph.* 12: 727–33.

————. 1964*b*. The abnormalities of the inner ear in *kreisler* mice. *J. Embryol. Exp. Morph.* 12: 475–90.

————. 1966*a*. Influence of the neural tube on the differentiation of the inner ear in the mammalian embryo. *Nature* 209: 219–20.

————. 1966*b*. The probable mode of gene action in the circling mutants of the mouse. *Genet. Res.* 7: 363–71.

Deol, M. S., and Truslove, G. M. 1963. A new gene causing cerebral degeneration in the mouse. *Proc. XI Int. Cong. Genet.* 1: 183–84. (Abst.)

Dexler, H. 1923. Über die konstitutionelle Hydrozephalie beim Hunde. *Tierärztl. Arch.* 3A: 103–268.

Dickie, M. M. 1964. New Splotch alleles in the mouse. *J. Hered.* 55: 97–101.

Dickie, M. M., and Belden, S. A. 1964–65. Belly spot mutations. *Ann. Rep. Jackson Lab.* 36: 104–5.

Didcock, K. A.; Jackson, D.; and Robson, J. M. 1956. The action of some nucleotoxic substances on pregnancy. *Brit. J. Pharmacol.* 11: 437–41.

Dieckmann, E. M. 1953. Missbildungen beim Schwein. *Mschr. Veterinärmed.* 8: 347–48.

Dijkstra, J., and Gillman, J. 1961. Chromatographic separation of biologically active components from commercial trypan blue. *Nature* 191: 803–4.

DiPaolo, J. A. 1963. Congenital malformation in strain A mice: Its experimental production by thalidomide. *J. Am. Med. Ass.* 183: 139–41.

————. 1964. Polydactylism in the offspring of mice injected with 5-bromodeoxyuridine. *Science* 145: 501–3.

DiPaolo, J. A.; Gatzek, H.; and Pickren, J. 1964. Malformations induced in the mouse by thalidomide. *Anat. Rec.* 149: 149–56.

Dobler, R. 1903. Aus der Praxis. Über congenitale Missbildungen. III. Rachischisis partialis dorso-lumbalis. *Mitt. Ver. Badisch. Tierärzte* 3: 65–66.

Dobrovolskaïa-Zavadskaïa, N. 1927. Sur la mortification spontanée de la queue chez la souris nouveau-née et sur l'existence d'un caractère (facteur) héréditaire "non-viable." *C. R. Soc. Biol.* 97: 114–16.

Dobrovolskaïa-Zavadskaïa, N., and Kobozieff, N. 1927. Sur la reproduction des souris anoures. *C. R. Soc. Biol.* 97: 116–18.

————. 1932. Les souris anoures et à queue filiforme qui se reproduisent entre elle sans disjonction. *C. R. Soc. Biol.* 110: 782–84.

Dobrovolskaïa-Zavadskaïa, N.; Kobozieff, N.; and Veretennikoff, S. 1934. Etude morphologique et génétique de la brachyourie chez les descendants de souris à testicules irradiés. *Arch. Zool.* 76: 249–358.

Dollahon, J. C., and Koger, M. 1960. Inheritance of the guinea trait in the descendants of Florida native cattle. *J. Hered.* 51: 32–34.

Done, J. T. 1957. The pathological differentiation of diseases of the central nervous system of the pig. *Vet. Rec.* 69: 1341–49.

Dow, R. S. 1940. Partial agenesis of the cerebellum in dogs. *J. Comp. Neur.* 72: 569–86.

Downs, W. G., Jr. 1928. An American "Dexter monster." *Anat. Rec.* 37: 365–72.

Dozsa, L. 1966. A case of rare monstrosity in a calf. *Path. Vet.* 3: 226–33.

Drobeck, H. P.; Coulston, F.; and Cornelius, D. 1965. Effects of thalidomide on fetal development in rabbits and on establishment of pregnancy in monkeys. *Toxic. Appl. Pharmacol.* 7: 165–78.

Druckrey, H.; Ivanković, S.; and Preussmann, R. 1966. Teratogenic and carcinogenic effects in the offspring after single injection of ethylnitrosourea to pregnant rats. *Nature* 210: 1378–79.

Dubois and Lapoulot. 1899. A propos de la tête d'un veau atteint de méningocèle et dermoïde cornéen. *J. Méd. Vét.*, ser. 5 3: 205–8.

Duckworth, W. L. H. 1908. Description of a microcephalous new-born pig in which the face and fore-parts of the brain were undeveloped, and the buccopharyngeal membrane remained imperforate. *Proc. Cambridge Phil. Soc.* 14: 447–56 and 2 plates.

Dugès, A. 1827. De monopsie et d'aprosopie. *Rev. Méd. Fr. Etr.* 4: 407–42.

Dujon. 1897. Monstre par fusion de deux foetus de mouton. *Ann. Gynéc. Obstét.* 48: 127–29.

Duke-Elder, S. 1963. *System of ophthalmology.* Vol. 3, *Normal and abnormal development.* Pt. 2, Congenital deformities, pp. 315–1190. St. Louis: Mosby.

Dumas, M. 1964. Effect of maternal hypervitaminosis A on fetal rat development. *Diss. Abst.* 25: 3784–85. (Abst.)

Dunn, L. C. 1934. A new gene affecting behavior and skeleton in the house mouse. *Proc. Nat. Acad. Sci. USA.* 20: 230–32.

————. 1956. Analysis of a complex gene in the house mouse. *Cold Spring Harbor Symp. Quant. Biol.* 21: 187–95.

————. 1957. Studies of the genetic variability of wild house mice. II. Analysis of eight additional alleles at locus *T. Genetics* 42: 299–311.

Dunn, L. C., and Bennett, D. 1960. A comparison of the effects, in compounds, of seven genetically similar *T* alleles from populations of wild house mice. *Genetics* 45: 1531–38.

Dunn, L. C.; Bennett, D.; and Beasley, A. B. 1962. Mutation and recombination in the vicinity of a complex gene. *Genetics* 47: 285–303.

Dunn, L. C., and Caspari, E. 1945. A case of neighboring loci with similar effects. *Genetics* 30: 543–68.

Dunn, L. C., and Gluecksohn-Schoenheimer, S. 1938. A dominant short-tail mutation in the house-mouse with recessive lethal effect. *Genetics* 23: 146–47. (Abst.)

————. 1943. Tests for recombination amongst three lethal mutations in the house mouse. *Genetics* 28: 29–40.

————. 1944. A specific abnormality associated with a variety of genotypes. *Proc. Nat. Acad. Sci. USA.* 30: 173–76.

————. 1947. A new complex of hereditary abnormalities in the house mouse. *J. Exp. Zool.* 104: 25–51.

Dunn, L. C.; Glueksohn-Schoenheimer, S.; and Bryson, V. 1940. A new mutation in the house mouse affecting spinal column and urogenital system. *J. Hered.* 31: 343–48.

Dunn, L. C., and Glueksohn-Waelsch, S. 1951. On the origin and genetic behavior of a new mutation (t^3) at a mutable locus in the mouse. *Genetics* 36: 4–12.

————. 1954. A genetical study of the mutation "Fused" in the house mouse, with evidence concerning its allelism with a similar mutation "Kink." *J. Genet.* 52: 383–91.

Dunn, L. C., and Morgan, W. C., Jr. 1953. Segregation ratios of mutant alleles from wild populations of *Mus musculus*. *Am. Nat.* 87: 327–29.

Dunn, L. C., and Suckling, J. 1956. Studies of genetic variation in wild populations of house mice. I. Analysis of seven alleles at locus *T*. *Genetics* 41: 344–52.

Duplan, J. F., and Monnot, P. 1965. Comparaisons des mortalités prénatales et néonatales provoquées chez la souris par l'irradiation X des seuls foetus ou de la mère seule. *C. R. Soc. Biol.* 159: 17–21.

Dutt, R. H. 1960. Temperature and light as factors in reproduction among farm animals. *J. Dairy Sci.* 43: 123–44.

————. 1963. Critical period for early embryo mortality in ewes exposed to high ambient temperature. *J. Anim. Sci.* 22: 713–19.

Dutton, C. E. 1950. Bovine monstrosity. *Vet. Med.* 45: 507.

Duval, M., and Hervé, G. 1883. Sur un monstre otocéphalien. *C. R. Soc. Biol.*, ser. 7 5: 76–78.

Duzgunes, O., and Tuncay, A. 1962. The amputated condition in Brown Swiss cattle. *J. Hered.* 53: 226.

Dwornik, J. J., and Moore, K. L. 1965. Skeletal malformations in the Holtzman rat embryo following the administration of thalidomide. *J. Embryol. Exp. Morph.* 13: 181–93.

Dyban, A. P.; Akimova, I. M.; and Svetlova, V. A. 1965. Embryonal development of rats acted upon with 2,4-diamino-5-p-chlorophenyl-6-ethylpyrimidine. [In Russian.] *Dokl. Akad. Nauk. SSSR.* 163: 1514–17.

Dyer, I. A.; Cassatt, W. A., Jr.; and Rao, R. R. 1964. Manganese deficiency in the etiology of deformed calves. *Bioscience* 14: 31–32.

Dyer, I. A., and Rojas, M. A. 1965. Manganese requirements and functions in cattle. *J. Am. Vet. Med. Ass.* 147: 1393–96.

Dyrendahl, S., and Hallgren, W. 1956. Nya fall av acroteriasis congenita inom låglandsrasen. *Nord. Vet. Med.* 8: 959–65.

Eaton, O. N. 1952. Abnormalities in the mouse. *J. Hered.* 43: 159–66.

Edwards, M. J. 1967. Congenital defects in guinea pigs following induced hyperthermia during gestation. *Arch. Path.* 84: 42–48.

Ehlers, D. P. 1939. Unusual bovine monster. *Vet. Med.* 34: 96.

Ellinger, T. U. H.; Wotton, R. M.; and Hall, I. J. 1950. A report on the occurrence of a median eye in a partially dicephalic cat. *Anat. Rec.* 107: 67–71.

Ely, F.; Hull, F. E.; and Morrison, H. B. 1939. Agnathia, a new bovine lethal. *J. Hered.* 30: 104–8.

Emerson, J. L., and Delez, A. L. 1965. Cerebellar hypoplasia, hypomyelinogenesis, and congenital tremors of pigs, associated with prenatal hog cholera vaccination of sows. *J. Am. Vet. Med. Ass.* 147: 47–54.

Endo, A. 1966. Teratogenesis in diabetic mice treated with alloxan prior to conception. *Arch. Env. Hlth.* 12: 492–500.

Engel, E. 1931. Einige Cephalothoracopagi bei Säugetieren. *Virchow Arch. Path. Anat.* 280: 706–22.

Ephrussi, B. 1935. The behavior in vitro of tissues from lethal embryos. *J. Exp. Zool.* 70: 197–204.

Epstein, H. 1955. Phlogenetic significance of *spina bifida* in zebu cattle. *Ind. J. Vet. Sci.* 25: 313–16.

Erfurth, F. 1965. Röntgenologische Veränderungen bei der Thalidomidembryopathie des Kaninchens. *Z. Kinderheilk.* 92: 90–97.

Erickson, B. A., and O'Dell, B. L. 1961. Major dietary constituents and vitamin B_{12} requirement. *J. Nutr.* 75: 414–18.

Erickson, B. H., and Murphree, R. L. 1964. Limb development in prenatally irradiated cattle, sheep and swine. *J. Anim. Sci.* 23: 1066–71.

Ericson-Strandvik, B., and Gyllensten, L. 1963. The central nervous system of foetal mice after administration of streptomycin. *Acta Path. Microbiol. Scand.* 59: 292–300.

Ernst, P. 1909. Missbildungen des Nervensystems. In *Die Morphologie der Missbildungen des Menschen und der Tiere*, ed. E. Schwalbe, vol. 3, pt. 2, chap. 2, pp. 67–252. Jena: Fischer, 1906–37.

Ershoff, B. H., and Bajwa, G. S. 1963. Protective effects of a radioprotective agent on testes injury of prenatally X-irradiated rats. *Exp. Med. Surg.* 21: 101–7.

Ershoff, B. H., and Kruger, L. 1962. A neurological defect in the offspring of rats fed a pantothenic acid-deficient diet during pregnancy. *Exp. Med. Surg.* 20: 180–84.

Ershoff, B. H.; Steers, C. W., Jr.; and Kruger, L. 1962. Effects of radioprotective agents on foot deformities and gait defects in the prenatally X-irradiated rat. *Proc. Soc. Exp. Biol. Med.* 111: 391–94.

Escobar, A., and Dow, R. S. 1966. Brain stem nuclei in cerebellar hypoplasia. An anatomical study in kitten and human. *Anat. Rec.* 154: 344. (Abst.)

Evans, H. E.; Ingalls, T. H.; and Binns, W. 1966. Teratogenesis of craniofacial malformations in animals. III. Natural and experimental cephalic deformities in sheep. *Arch. Env. Hlth.* 13: 706–14.

Evans, H. M.; Burr, G. O.; and Althausen, T. L. 1927. The antisterility vitamine—fat soluble E. *Mem. Univ. Calif.* 8: 1–176.

Evans, H. M.; Nelson, M. M.; and Asling, C. W. 1951. Multiple congenital abnormalities resulting from acute folic acid deficiency during gestation. *Science* 114: 479. (Abst.)

Everett, J. W. 1935. Morphological and physiological studies on the placenta in the albino rat. *J. Exp. Zool.* 70: 243–85.

Everson, G. J., and Wang, T. I. 1967. Copper deficiency in the guinea pig and related brain abnormalities. *Fed. Proc.* 26: 633. (Abst.)

Faassen, F. van. 1957. Hypothyreoidie en Aangeboren Misvormingen. Doctoral thesis, Univ. of Utrecht.

Fabro, S.; Schumacher, H.; Smith, R. L.; and Williams, R. T. 1964*a*. Teratogenic activity of thalidomide and related compounds. *Life Sci.* 3: 987–92.

———. 1964*b*. Identification of thalidomide in rabbit blastocysts. *Nature* 201: 1125–26.

Fabro, S.; Schumacher, H.; Smith, R. L.; Stagg, R. B. L.; and Williams, R. T. 1965. The metabolism of thalidomide: Some biological effects of thalidomide and its metabolites. *Brit. J. Pharmacol.* 25: 352–62.

Fabro, S., and Smith, R. L. 1966. The teratogenic activity of thalidomide in the rabbit. *J. Path. Bact.* 91: 511–19.

Fabro, S.; Smith, R. L.; and Williams, R. T. 1965. Persistence of maternally administered [¹⁴C] thalidomide in the rabbit embryo. *Biochem. J.* 97: 14P.

Faigle, J. W.; Keberle, H.; Riess, W.; and Schmid, K. 1962. The metabolic fate of thalidomide. *Experientia* 18: 389–97.

Fainstat, T. 1954. Cortisone-induced cleft palate in rabbits. *Endocrinology* 55: 502–8.

Faix, R. 1950. Hydrocephalia congenita bei einem Kalb. *Tierärztl. Umsch.* 5: 407–8.

Falconer, D. S., and Sierts-Roth, U. 1951. Dreher, ein neues Gen der Tanzmausgruppe bei der Hausmaus. *Z. Ind. Abst. Vererbungsl.* 84: 71–73.

Fankhauser, R. 1955. Cerebellar atrophy in animals. *Schweiz. Arch. Neur. Psychiat.* 75: 378–81.

———. 1957. Bildungsstörungen des Kleinhirns. *Deut. Tierärztl. Wschr.* 64: 225–30.

———. 1959. Hydrocephalus-Studien. *Schweiz. Arch. Tierheilk.* 101: 407–16.

———. 1965. Drei Verbildungen des Gehirns. *Schweiz. Arch. Tierheilk.* 107: 1–10.

Fankhauser, R., and Wyler, R. 1953. Die Nervenkrankheiten des Schweines. *Schweiz. Arch. Tierheilk.* 95: 585–619.

Fasten, N. 1932. A headless lamb. *J. Hered.* 23: 420–21.

Fave, A. 1964. Les embryopathies provoquées chez les mammifères. *Thérapie* 19: 43–164.

Favre-Tissot, M., and Delatour, P. 1965. Psychopharmacologie et tératogénèse à propos du disulfirame: Essai experimental. *Ann. Médicopsych.* 123: 735–40.

Fay, L. D. 1960. A two-headed white-tailed deer fetus. *J. Mammal.* 41: 411–12.

Fehér, G., and Gyürü, F. 1964. Kalb mit doppeltem Gesicht (Diprosopus, Tetraophthalmus, Diotus, Trignatus, Tetracornus). *Acta Vet. Acad. Sci. Hung.* 14: 419–36.

Feigin, I. H. 1956. Arnold–Chiari malformation with associated malformations of the mid-brain. *Neurology* 6: 22–31.

Feild, L. E.; Kreshover, S. J.; and Lieberman, J. E. 1960. Temporary uterine circulatory arrest as a cause of abnormal fetal development. *J. Dent. Res.* 39: 1240–47.

Felisati, D. 1962. Thalidomide and congenital abnormalities. *Lancet* 2: 724–25.

Felisati, D., and Nodari, R. 1963. Effets toxiques et tératogéniques de la thalidomide sur les foetus de lapin. *Schweiz. Med. Wschr.* 93: 1559–62.

Ferm, V. H. 1956. Permeability of the rabbit blastocyst to trypan blue. *Anat.
Rec.* 125: 745–59.

———. 1958. Teratogenic effects of trypan blue on hamster embryos. *J. Embryol.
Exp. Morph.* 6: 284–87.

———. 1959. Relative effect of teratogenic and nonteratogenic azo dyes on
adrenal weight. *Anat. Rec.* 133: 379–80. (Abst.)

———. 1963a. Colchicine teratogenesis in hamster embryos. *Proc. Soc. Exp.
Biol. Med.* 112: 775–78.

———. 1963b. Congenital malformations in hamster embryos after treatment
with vinblastine and vincristine. *Science* 141: 426.

———. 1964. Teratogenic effects of hyperbaric oxygen. *Proc. Soc. Exp. Biol.
Med.* 116: 975–76.

———. 1965a. The rapid detection of teratogenic activity. *Lab. Inv.* 14:
1500–1505.

———. 1965b. Teratogenic activity of hydroxy urea. *Lancet.* 1: 1338–39.

———. 1966a. Severe developmental malformations: Malformations induced
by urethane and hydroxyurea in the hamster. *Arch. Path.* 81: 174–77.

———. 1966b. Teratogenic effect of dimethyl sulphoxide. *Lancet* 1: 208–9.

———. 1966c. Congenital malformations induced by dimethyl sulphoxide in
the golden hamster. *J. Embryol. Exp. Morph.* 16: 49–54.

———. 1967. Potentiation of the teratogenic effect of vitamin A with exposure
to low environmental temperature. *Life Sci.* 6: 493–97.

Ferm, V. H., and Kilham, L. 1963a. Rat virus (RV) infection in fetal and pregnant hamsters. *Proc. Soc. Exp. Biol. Med.* 112: 623–26.

———. 1963b. Mumps virus infection of the pregnant hamster. *J. Embryol.
Exp. Morph.* 11: 659–66.

———. 1964. Congenital anomalies induced in hamster embryos with H-1
virus. *Science* 145: 510–11.

———. 1965. Histopathological basis of the teratogenic effects of H-1 virus on
hamster embryos. *J. Embryol. Exp. Morph.* 13: 151–58.

Ferm, V. H., and Low, R. J. 1965. Herpes simplex virus infection in the pregnant
hamster. *J. Path. Bact.* 89: 295–300.

Fernandez-Cano, L. 1959. The effects of increase or decrease of body temperature or of hypoxia on ovulation and pregnancy in the rat. In *Recent progress in the
endocrinology of reproduction*, ed. C. W. Lloyd, pp. 97–106. New York: Academic
Press.

Ferrario, I. 1957. Il trypanblau e le sue recenti applicazioni in patologia sperimentale con particolare riguardo alla patologia antenatale. *Folia Hered. Path.* 6:
15–49.

Ferrill, H. W. 1943. Effect of chronic insulin injection on reproduction in white
rats. *Endocrinology* 32: 449–50.

Few, A. B. 1966. The diagnosis and surgical treatment of canine hydrocephalus.
J. Am. Vet. Med. Ass. 149: 286–93.

Fielden, E. D. 1959. Micrencephaly in Hereford calves. *New Zealand Vet. J.*
7: 80–82.

Filimonoff, I. N. 1929. Ein Fall von Hydrozephalie beim Hunde. *J. Psych. Neur.* (*Leipzig*) 37: 673–78.

Filippi, B., and Mela, V. 1957*a*. Malformazioni congenite facciali e degli arti da tetracyclina. *Minerva Chir.* 12: 1106–10.

———. 1957*b*. Malformazioni congenite degli arti ottenute sperimentalmente in embrioni di ratto in seguito a trattamento con penicillina et streptomicina. *Minerva Chir.* 12: 1047–52.

Finley, K. H. 1935. An anatomical study in familial olivo-ponto-cerebellar hypoplasia in cats. *Verh. Kon. Akad. Wetensch.* 38: 922–31.

Finn, C. A. 1962. Embryonic death in aged mice. *Nature* 194: 499–500.

Finnie, E. P., and Leaver, D. D. 1965. Cerebellar hypoplasia in calves. *Aust. Vet. J.* 41: 287–88.

Finzi, G. 1919. Atassia cerebellare nel cane per aplasia del lobo vermiano. *Clin. Vet.* (*Milan*) 42: 571–84.

Fischer, E. 1929. Zur Frage der Zwillingsbilding beim Nagetier. (Ein Fall von Duplicitas posterior.) *Roux Arch. Entwickl.* 118: 352–59.

Fischer, H. 1955. Agnathia, a rare lethal malformation in sheep. *Hemera Zoa* 62: 260–62.

———. 1959. Acroteriasis congenita in a Holstein-Friesian calf—fetus. *Hemera Zoa* 66: 91–92.

Fischer, H. 1956. Morphologische und mikroskopisch-anatomische Untersuchungen am Innenohr eines Stammes spontanmutantierter Hausmäuse (Dreher). *Z. Mikr. Anat. Forsch.* 62: 348–406.

———. 1958. Die Embryogenese der Innenohrmissbildungen bei dem spontanmutierten Dreherstamm der Hausmaus. *Z. Mikr. Anat. Forsch.* 64: 476–97.

———. 1959*a*. Morphologische und mikroskopisch-anatomische Untersuchungen an Gehirn einer neuen Mutante der Hausmaus mit autosomal vererbbarer Leukencephalose. *Z. Menschl. Vererb. Konst.* 35: 46–70.

———. 1959*b*. Mikroskopische Untersuchungen am Gehirn einer neuen Hausmausmutante mit Leukodystropie. *Verh. Deut. Zool. Ges.* 64: 519–24.

Forgeot and Nicolas, A. 1906. Hydrocéphalie chez un chien enragé. *Bull. Soc. Sci. Vét. Lyon* 7: 115–16.

Forsheim, A. 1908. Beschreibung der Brust- und Baucheingeweide einiger Doppelmissbildungen (von Mensch, Schwein, Katze und Ente) nebst Bemerkungen über die modernen Ansichten betreffs der Entstehung von Doppelmissbilding im allgemeinen. *Anat. Hefte* 37: 117–42.

Forsthoefel, P. F. 1962. Genetics and manifold effects of Strong's luxoid gene in the mouse, including its interactions with Green's luxoid and Carter's luxate genes. *J. Morph.* 110: 391–420.

———. 1963. The embryological development of the effects of Strong's luxoid gene in the mouse. *J. Morph.* 113: 427–51.

Fox, H. 1941. Matters of medical and laboratory interest. *Rep. Penrose Res. Lab.*, pp. 14–25.

Fox, M. H., and Goss, C. M. 1956. Experimental production of a syndrome of congenital cardiovascular defects in rats. *Anat. Rec.* 124: 189–207.

———. 1957. Experimentally produced malformations of the heart and great vessels in rat fetuses. Atrial and caval abnormalities. *Anat. Rec.* 129: 309–31.

————. 1958. Experimentally produced malformations of the heart and great vessels in rat fetuses. Transposition complexes and aortic arch abnormalities. *Am. J. Anat.* 102: 65–92.

Fox, M. H.; Goss, C. M.; and Bordeaux, L. F. 1958. The effect of trypan blue injections at different stages of pregnancy upon the fetus. *Anat. Rec.* 130: 302–3. (Abst.)

Fox, M. W. 1963a. Low-grade otocephaly in a dog. *J. Am. Vet. Med. Ass.* 143: 289–90.

————. 1963b. Developmental abnormalities of the canine skull. *Can. J. Comp. Med.* 27: 219–22.

————. 1964a. Anatomy of the canine skull in low-grade otocephaly. *Can. J. Comp. Med.* 28: 105–7.

————. 1964b. The otocephalic syndrome in the dog. *Cornell Vet.* 54: 250–59.

————. 1965. Diseases of possible hereditary origin in the dog. A bibliographic review. *J. Hered.* 56: 169–76.

Franklin, J. B., and Brent, R. L. 1960. Interruption of uterine blood flow: A new technique for the production of congenital malformations. Comparison of the eighth, ninth, and tenth days of gestation. *Surg. Forum* 11: 415–16.

————. 1964. The effect of uterine vascular clamping on the development of rat embryos three to fourteen days old. *J. Morph.* 115: 273–90.

Franklin, J. B.; Goldfarb, A. R.; Matsumoto, R.; and Brent, R. L. 1963. Modification by progestational compounds of the teratogenic effect of uterine vascular clamping. *Fertil. Steril.* 14: 365–69.

Fraser, F. C. 1961. Genetics and congenital malformations. *Prog. Med. Genet.* 1: 38–80.

————. 1962. Pregnancy and adrenocortical hormones. *Brit. Med. J.* 2: 479.

————. 1964. Experimental teratogenesis in relation to congenital malformations in man. In *Second International Conference on Congenital Malformations*, pp. 227–87. New York: International Medical Congress.

Fraser, F. C., and Fainstat, T. D. 1951. Production of congenital defects in the offspring of pregnant mice treated with cortisone. *Pediatrics* 8: 527–33.

Fratta, I., and Sigg, E. B. 1965. Teratological studies with thalidomide analogues in rabbits. *Pharmacologist* 7: 162. (Abst.)

Fratta, I. D.; Sigg, E. B.; and Maiorana, K. 1965. Teratogenic effects of thalidomide in rabbits, rats, hamsters, and mice. *Toxic. Appl. Pharmacol.* 7: 268–86.

Frauchiger, E. 1940. Kleinhirnaplasie bei einem Kalb. *Schweiz. Arch. Tierheilk.* 82: 425–27.

————. 1959. Neuropathologie comparée des malformations cérébrales. In *Malformations congénitales du cerveau*, ed. G. Heuyer, M. Feld, and J. Gruner, pp. 41–55. Paris: Masson.

Frauchiger, E., and Fankhauser, R. 1949. *Die Nervenkrankheiten unserer Hunde.* Bern: Huber.

————. 1952. Arnold–Chiari-Hirnmissbildung mit Spina bifida und Hydrozephalus beim Kalb. *Schweiz. Arch. Tierheilk.* 94: 145–48.

————. 1957. *Vergleichende Neuropathologie des Menschen und der Tiere.* Berlin: Springer.

Frauchiger, E., and Hofmann, W. 1941. *Die Nervenkrankheiten des Rindes.* Bern: Huber.

Freye, H., and Freye, H. A. 1959. Experimentelle Untersuchungen über den Einfluss einmaliger kurzfristiger O₂-Mangel-Exposition auf frühe Embryonalstadien von Hausmäusen. *Biol. Zbl.* 78: 789–98.

Frick, E., and Lampl, F. 1953. Über die Entwicklung des Gehirns von Ratten bei Kupfermangel. *Klin. Wschr.* 31: 912–13.

Friedman, M. H. 1957. The effect of o-diazo-acetyl-l-serine (azaserine) on the pregnancy of the dog. *J. Am. Vet. Med. Ass.* 130: 159–62.

Fritz, H. 1966. Failure of thalidomide metabolites to produce malformations in the rabbit embryo. *J. Reprod. Fertil.* 11: 157–59.

Frye, F. L., and McFarland, L. Z. 1965. Spina bifida with rachischisis in a kitten. *J. Am. Vet. Med. Ass.* 146: 481–82.

Fujimori, H.; Yamada, F.; Shibukawa, N.; and Itani, I. 1965. The effect of tuberculostatics on the fetus: An experimental production of congenital anomaly in rats by ethionamide. *Proc. Congen. Anom. Res. Ass. Jap.* 5: 34–35. (Abst.)

Fujita, S.; Horii, M.; Tanimura, T.; and Nishimura, H. 1964. H³-thymidine autoradiographic studies on cytokinetic responses to X-ray irradiation and to thio-TEPA in the neural tube of mouse embryos. *Anat. Rec.* 149: 37–48.

Fuller, J. L. 1956. The inheritance of structural defects in dogs. *Mich. St. Univ. Vet.* 16: 103–8, 125.

Funk and Wagnalls Standard College Dictionary. 1963. New York: Funk & Wagnalls Co.

Gabriélidès, A. 1896. Examen microscopique d'un oeil cyclope observé sur un embryon de suidé. *Arch. Opht. (Paris)* 16: 627–30.

Gaines, T. B., and Kimbrough, R. D. 1966. The sterilizing, carcinogenic and teratogenic effects of metepa in rats. *Bull. Wld. Hlth. Org.* 34: 317–20.

Gall, C. 1959. Impairment in gestation, parturition, and lactation after hypothalmic lesions. *Fed. Proc.* 18: 50. (Abst.)

Gallier. 1898. Monstre cyclocéphalien. *Bull. Soc. Cent. Méd. Vét.* 52: 380–81.

Garber, E. D. 1952. A dominant, sex-linked mutation in the house mouse. *Science* 116: 89.

Gardner, D. L. 1959. Familial canine chondrodystrophia foetalis (achondroplasia). *J. Path. Bact.* 77: 243–47.

Gardner, W. 1923. Hydrocephalus. *Vet. J.* 79: 176–78.

Gardner, W. J. 1959. Anatomic features common to the Arnold–Chiari and the Dandy–Walker malformations suggest a common origin. *Cleveland Clin. Quart.* 26: 206–22.

Garro, F., and Pentschew, A. 1964. Neonatal hydrocephalus in the offspring of rats fed during pregnancy non-toxic amounts of tellurium. *Arch. Psychiat. Nervenkr.* 206: 272–80.

Gates, A. H. 1965a. Rate of ovular development as a factor in embryonic survival. In *Ciba Foundation symposium on preimplantation stages of pregnancy*, ed. G. E. W. Wolstenholme, and M. O'Connor, pp. 270–88. Boston: Little, Brown & Co.

———. 1965b. *Mouse News Letter* 32: 82.

Gatz, A. J., and Allen, L. 1961. A study of amelus guinea pigs. *Anat. Rec.* 139: 302. (Abst.)

Gavrilescu, C. 1924. Hydrocéphalie chez le veau. *Arh. Vet.* (*Bucharest*) 18: 5–6.

Gay, M. 1878. Sopra un mostro ovino (ciclope perostomo arinco). *Gior. Med. Vet.* 27: 193–95.

Gebauer, H. 1954. Zur A-Hypervitaminose und Schwangerschaft. *Pharmazie* 9: 684–85.

Geber, W. F. 1966. Developmental effects of chronic maternal audiovisual stress on the rat fetus. *J. Embryol. Exp. Morph.* 16: 1–16.

Geib, L. W., and Bistner, S. I. 1967. Spinal cord dysraphism in a dog. *J. Am. Vet. Med. Ass.* 150: 618–20.

Gellatly, J. B. M. 1957. Discussion. *Vet. Rec.* 69: 1350–52.

Gentry, J. T. 1962. Developmental disturbances. In *Genetics and dental health*, ed. C. J. Witkop, Jr., pp. 121–28. New York: McGraw-Hill.

George, E. F.; Franklin, J. B.; and Brent, R. L. 1967. Altered embryonic effects of uterine vascular clamping in the pregnant rat by uterine temperature control. *Proc. Soc. Exp. Biol. Med.* 124: 257–60.

George, W. C. 1942. A case of double notochord in a pig embryo. *Anat. Rec.* 82: 465. (Abst.)

Georgi, W. 1936. Über Defektbildungen an Schädeln von kleinen Haushundrassen. *Anat. Anz.* 82: 400–406.

Gepts, W.; Carpent, G.; and Toussaint, D. 1957. Etude de l'effet tératogène du bleu de trypan chez le rat. *C. R. Soc. Biol.* 151: 1776–79.

Gerlinger, P. 1964. Action du cyclophosphamide injecté à la mère sur la réalisation de la forme du corps des embryons de lapin. *C. R. Soc. Biol.* 158: 2154–57.

Gerlinger, P., and Clavert, J. 1965. Anomalies observées chez des lapins issus de mères traitées au cyclophosphamide. *C. R. Soc. Biol.* 159: 1462–66.

Giannotti, D. 1952. Casi di idrocefalo congenito in vitelli. *Mem. Soc. Tosc. Sci. Nat. B.* 59: 34–66.

Gilbert, C., and Gillman, J. 1954. The morphogenesis of trypan blue induced defects of the eye. *S. Afr. J. Med. Sci.* 19: 147–54.

Gillilan, L. A., and Lockard, I. 1954. Correlation of certain neurological dysfunctions with congenital anatomical abnormalities of the central nervous system in five cats. *Anat. Rec.* 118: 302. (Abst.)

Gillman, J.; Gilbert, C.; Gillman, T.; and Spence, I. 1948. A preliminary report on hydrocephalus, spina bifida, and other congenital anomalies in the rat produced by trypan blue. *S. Afr. J. Med. Sci.* 13: 47–90.

Gillman, J.; Gilbert, C.; Spence, I.; and Gillman, T. 1951. A further report on congenital anomalies in the rat produced by trypan blue. *S. Afr. J. Med. Sci.* 16: 125–35.

Gilman, J. P. W. 1956. Congenital hydrocephalus in domestic animals. *Cornell Vet.* 45: 487–99.

Gilmore, L. O. 1949. The inheritance of functional causes of reproductive inefficiency: A review. *J. Dairy Sci.* 32: 71–91.

Giroud, A. 1960. Discussion. In *Ciba Foundation symposium on congenital malformations*, ed. G. E. W. Wolstenholme, and C. M. O'Connor, p. 173. Boston: Little, Brown & Co.

Giroud, A.; Delmas, A.; and Martinet, M. 1959. Etude morphogénétique sur des embryons anencéphales. *Arch. Anat.* 42: 203–30.

———. 1963. Cyclocéphalie: Morphogénèse et mécanisme de sa production. *Arch. Anat.* 47: 295–311.

Giroud, A.; Delmas, A.; Prost, H.; and Lefebvres, J. 1957. Malformations encéphaliques par carence en acide pantothénique et leur interprétation. *Acta Anat.* 29: 209–27.

Giroud, A.; Gounelle, H.; and Martinet, M. 1957. Données quantitatives sur le taux de la vitamine A chez la rat lors d'expériences de tératogénèse par hypervitaminose A. *Bull. Soc. Chim. Biol.* 39: 331–36.

Giroud, A.; Heitz, F.; Martinet, M.; and Deluchat, C. 1965. Au sujet des anomalies du rhinencéphale. *C. R. Soc. Biol.* 159: 606–8.

Giroud, A., and Lefebvres, J. 1951. Anomalies provoquées chez le foetus en l'absence d'acide folique. *Arch. Fr. Pédiat.* 8: 648–56.

Giroud, A.; Lefebvres, J.; and Dupuis, R. 1952. Répercussions sur l'embryon de la carence en acide folique. *Int. Z. Vitaminforsch.* 24: 420–29.

Giroud, A.; Lefebvres-Boisselot, J.; and Dupuis, R. 1957. Un régime polyvitaminé est-il moins tératogène qu'un régime dépourvu d'une seule vitamine B? *C. R. Soc. Biol.* 151: 2085–87.

———. 1961. Carence tératogène en acide pantothénique. Légèreté de la carence. *Bull. Soc. Chim. Biol.* 43: 859–64.

Giroud, A.; Lévy, G.; Lefebvres, J.; and Dupuis, R. 1952. Chute du taux de la riboflavine au stade où se déterminant les malformations embryonnaires. *Int. Z. Vitaminforsch.* 23: 490–94.

Giroud, A., and Martinet, M. 1954. Fentes du palais chez l'embryon de rat par hypervitaminose A. *C. R. Soc. Biol.* 148: 1742–43.

———. 1955*a*. Malformations diverses du foetus de rat suivant les stades d'administration de vitamine A en excès. *C. R. Soc. Biol.* 149: 1088–90.

———. 1955*b*. Hydramnios et anencéphalie. *Gynéc. Obstét.* 54: 391–99.

———. 1956. Tératogénèse par hautes doses de vitamine A en fonction des stades du développement. *Arch. Anat. Micr. Morph. Exp.* 45: 77–99.

———. 1957. Morphogénèse de l'anencéphalie. *Arch. Anat. Micr. Morph. Exp.* 46: 247–64.

———. 1958. Répercussions de l' hypervitaminose A chez l'embryon de lapin. *C. R. Soc. Biol.* 152: 931–32.

———. 1959*a*. Extension à plusieurs espèces de mammifères des malformations embryonnaires par hypervitaminose A. *C. R. Soc. Biol.* 183: 201–2.

———. 1959*b*. Tératogénèse par hypervitaminose A chez le rat, la souris, le cobaye, et le lapin. *Arch. Fr. Pédiat.* 16: 971–75.

———. 1959*c*. Anencéphalie chez la souris par hypervitaminose A. *C. R. Ass. Anat.* 46: 288–91.

———. 1960*a*. Action tératogène de l'hypervitaminose A chez la souris en fonction du stade embryonnaire. *C. R. Soc. Biol.* 154: 1353–55.

———. 1960*b*. Anencéphalie expérimentale chez la souris et comparaisons avec l'anencéphalie chez l'homme. *Acta Anat.* 43: 358–70.

———. 1962. Légèreté de la dose tératogène de la vitamine A. *C. R. Soc. Biol.* 156: 449–50.

Giroud, A.; Martinet, M.; and Deluchat, C. 1965. Mécanisme de développement du bulbe olfactif. *Arch. Anat.* 48: 205–17.

Giroud, A.; Martinet, M.; Deluchat, C.; and Heitz, F. 1966. Au sujet de l'apparition de malformations appartenant au groupe de la cyclocéphalie. *C. R. Soc. Biol.* 160: 1180–82.

Giroud, A.; Martinet, M.; and Lefebvres-Boisselot, J. 1960. Relations entre les anomalies de fermeture du tube nerveux et les déficiences de la voûte osseuse du névraxe et l'indifférenciation de l'épiderme sus-jacent. *Arch. Anat.* 43: 203–16.

Giroud, A.; Martinet, M.; and Solère, M. 1958. Anencéphalie, encéphalocèles, méningocèles par hypervitaminose A. *Arch. Fr. Pédiat.* 15: 835–42.

Giroud, A., and Rothschild, B. de. 1951. Cataracte congénitale après thyroxine. *Bull. Soc. Opht. France*, pp. 543–49.

Giroud, A.; Tuchmann-Duplessis, H.; and Mercier-Parot, L. 1962a. Observations sur les répercussions tératogènes de la thalidomide chez la souris et le lapin. *C. R. Soc. Biol.* 156: 765–68.

———. 1962b. Thalidomide and congenital abnormalities. *Lancet* 2: 298–99.

———. 1962c. Production de malformations congénitales chez la souris après administration de faibles doses de thalidomide. *C. R. Acad. Sci.* 255: 1646–48.

Githens, J. H.; Rosenkrantz, J. G.; and Tunnock, S. M. 1965. Teratogenic effects of azathioprine (Imuran). *J. Pediat.* 66: 962–63.

Gitter, M., and Bowen, P. D. G. 1962. Unusual cerebellar conditions in pigs. Pt. 2. Cerebellar hypoplasia in pigs. *Vet. Rec.* 74: 1152–54.

Giurgea, M., and Puigdevall, J. 1966. Experimental teratology with meclozine. *Med. Pharmacol. Exp.* 15: 375–88.

Gladstone, R. J. 1910. A cyclops and agnathous lamb. *Brit. Med. J.* 2: 1159–60.

Gladstone, R. J., and Wakeley, C. P. G. 1920. A cyclops lamb (C. Rhinocephalus). *J. Anat.* 54: 196–207.

———. 1923. Defective development of the mandibular arch. The etiology of arrested development and an inquiry into the question of the inheritance of congenital defects. *J. Anat.* 57: 149–67.

Glaser, H., 1928. Über die Cephalothoracopagen und einen Prosopothoracopagus disymmetros vom Schwein. *Roux Arch. Entwickl.* 113: 601–39.

Glass, L. E., and Lin, T. P. 1963. Development of X-irradiated and non-irradiated mouse oocytes transplanted to X-irradiated and non-irradiated recipient females. *J. Cell. Comp. Physiol.* 61: 53–60.

Glass, L. E., and McClure, T. R. 1964. Equivalence of X-irradiation *in vivo* or *in vitro* on mouse oocyte survival. *J. Cell. Comp. Physiol.* 64: 347–53.

Gluecksohn-Schoenheimer, S. 1938a. The development of two tailless mutants in the house mouse. Genetics 23: 573–84.

———. 1938b. Time of death of lethal homozygotes in the *T* (Brachyury) series in the mouse. *Proc. Soc. Exp. Biol. Med.* 39: 267–68.

———. 1940. The effect of an early lethal (t^0) in the house mouse. *Genetics* 25: 391–400.

———. 1943. The morphological manifestations of a dominant mutation in mice affecting tail and urogenital system. *Genetics* 28: 341–48.

380   References

―――. 1944. The development of normal and homozygous brachy (*T/T*) mouse embryos in the extra-embryonic coelom of the chick. *Proc. Nat. Acad. Sci. USA.* 30: 134–40.

―――. 1945. The embryonic development of mutants of the *Sd*-strain in mice. *Genetics* 30: 29–38.

―――. 1949. The effects of a lethal mutation responsible for duplications and twinning in mouse embryos. *J. Exp. Zool.* 110: 47–76.

Gluecksohn-Waelsch, S. 1954. Some genetic aspects of development. *Cold Spring Harbor Symp. Quant. Biol.* 19: 41–49.

―――. 1957. The effect of maternal immunization against organ tissues on embryonic differentiation in the mouse. *J. Embryol. Exp. Morph.* 5: 83–92.

―――. 1963. Lethal genes and analysis of differentiation. *Science* 142: 1269–76.

Gluge and Deroubaix. 1840. Observation d'un chien cyclope. *Arch. Méd. Belg.* 3: 115–17.

Godglück, G. 1952. Partielle kongenital Hydrozephalie bei einem Kalbe (Encephalocystomeningocele der Bulbi olfactorii), *Mschr. Veterinärmed.* 7: 250–52.

Goldman, A. S., and Yakovac, W. C. 1963. The enhancement of salicylate teratogenicity by maternal immobilization in the rat. *J. Pharmacol. Exp. Ther.* 142: 351–57.

―――. 1964a. Salicylate intoxication and congenital anomalies. *Arch. Env. Hlth.* 8: 648–56.

―――. 1964b. Prevention of salicylate teratogenicity in immobilized rats by certain central nervous system depressants. *Proc. Soc. Exp. Biol. Med.* 115: 693–96.

―――. 1965. Teratogenic action in rats of reserpine alone and in combination with salicylate and immobilization. *Proc. Soc. Exp. Biol. Med.* 118: 857–62.

Goldschmidt, R. B. 1935. Gen und Ausseneigenschaft. I. *Z. Ind. Abst. Vererdungsl.* 69: 38–69.

Goldsmith, W. M. 1921. A living double-headed calf. *J. Hered.* 12: 237–39.

Goldstein, A., and Hazel, M. M. 1955. Failure of an antihistamine drug to prevent pregnancy in the mouse. *Endocrinology* 56: 215–16.

Goldstein, D. J. 1957. Trypan blue induced anomalies in the genitourinary system of rats. *S. Afr. J. Med. Sci.* 22: 13–22.

Goldstein, F., and Kepes, J. J. 1966. The role of traction in the development of the Arnold–Chiari malformation: An experimental study. *J. Neuropath. Exp. Neur.* 25: 654–66.

Goldstein, M.; Pinsky, M. F.; and Fraser, F. C. 1963. Genetically determined organ specific responses to the teratogenic action of 6-aminonicotinamide in the mouse. *Genet. Res.* 4: 258–65.

Gonţea, I.; Suţescu, P.; Cocora, D.; and Staicu, P. 1964. Malformaţii congenitale prin exces de axeroftol. *Viata Med.* 11: 1315–22.

Good, J. P. 1915. An enquiry into the causation of spina bifida. In *Studies in anatomy*, ed. P. Thompson, pp. 129–80. Anat. Dept., Univ. of Birmingham. Birmingham: Cornish Bros.

Goodwin, R. F. W., and Jennings, A. R. 1958. Mortality of new-born pigs associated with a maternal deficiency of vitamin A. *J. Comp. Path. Ther.* 68: 82–95.

Gordon, H. W.; Peer, L. A.; and Bernhard, W. G. 1961. The relation of the teratogenic action of cortisone to liver transaminase activity. *Biol. Neonat.* 3: 36–48.

Gordon, H. W.; Tkaczyk, W.; Peer, L. A.; and Bernhard, W. G. 1962. The effects of adenosine triphosphate on the teratogenic action of cortisone in mice. *Biol. Neonat.* 4: 340–50.

———. 1963. The effect of adenosine triphosphate and its decomposition products on cortisone induced teratology. *J. Embryol. Exp. Morph.* 11: 475–82.

Gordon, L. 1964. Further report on the morphology of spinal cord defects produced in rats by trypan blue. *Abst. Terat. Soc.* 4: 4–5. (Abst.)

Gorham, J. R. 1947. Hydrocephalus in mink. *Am. Fur Breeder* June, 1947, p. 20.

Gortner, R. A., and Ekwurtzel, J. B. 1965. Incidence of teratogeny induced by vitamin E deficiency in the rat. *Proc. Soc. Exp. Biol. Med.* 119: 1069–71.

Goss, L. J., and Hull, F. E. 1933. Spina bifida (calf). *Cornell Vet.* 29: 239–40.

Gotink, W. M.; Groot, T. De; and Stegenga, T. 1955. Erfelijke gebreken in de rundveefokkerij. *Landbouwk. Tijdschr.* 67: 629–72.

Gottlieb, J. S.; Frohman, C. E.; and Havlena, J. 1958. The effect of antimetabolites on embryonic development. *J. Mich. Med. Soc.* 57: 364–66.

Götze, R. 1923. Die geburtshilfliche Entwicklung eines Hydrocephalus beim Rinde. *Berlin. Tierärztl. Wschr.* 39: 333–34.

Grainger, R. B.; O'Dell, B. L.; and Hogan, A. G. 1954. Congenital malformations as related to deficiencies of riboflavin and vitamin B_{12}, source of protein, calcium to phosphorus ratio and skeletal phosphorus metabolism. *J. Nutr.* 54: 33–48.

Grassnickel, W. 1961. Splanchnocraniopagus beim Schwein. *Berlin. München. Tierärztl. Wschr.* 74: 278.

Gratia, and Antoine, G. 1913. Un cas de spina bifida chez le veau. *Ann. Méd. Vét.* 62: 529–39.

Green, C. R., and Christie, G. S. 1961. Malformations in fetal rats induced by the pyrrolizidine alkaloid, heliotrine. *Brit. J. Exp. Path.* 42: 369–78.

Green, E. L. 1957. Mutant stocks of cats and dogs offered for research. *J. Hered.* 48: 56–57.

———. 1964–65. Mutations in irradiated populations. *Ann. Rep. Jackson Lab.* 36: 67–68.

Green, E. L., ed. 1966. *Biology of the laboratory mouse.* 2d ed. New York: McGraw-Hill.

Greene, H. S. N. 1933. Oxycephaly and allied conditions in man and in the rabbit. *J. Exp. Med.* 57: 967–76.

———. 1940. A dwarf mutation in the rabbit. The constitutional influence on homozygous and heterozygous individuals. *J. Exp. Med.* 71: 839–55.

Greene, H. S. N.; Hu, C. K.; and Brown, W. H. 1934. A lethal dwarf mutation in the rabbit with stigmata of endocrine abnormality. *Science* 79: 487–88.

Gregory, D. 1905. A porcine monstrosity. *Vet. J.* 12: 341–42.

Gregory, P. W., and Carroll, F. D. 1956. Evidence for the same dwarf gene in Herefords, Aberdeen-Angus, and other breeds of cattle. *J. Hered.* 47: 107–11.

Gregory, P. W.; Julian, L. M.; and Tyler, W. S. 1964. Bovine achondroplasia: The progeny test. *Growth.* 28: 191–212.

Gregory, P. W.; Mead, S. W.; and Regan, W. M. 1942. A new type of recessive achondroplasia in cattle. *J. Hered.* 33: 317–22.

Gregory, P. W.; Rollins, W. C.; Pattengale, P. S.; and Carroll, F. D. 1951. Phenotypic expression of homozygous dwarfism in beef cattle. *J. Anim. Sci.* 10: 922–33.

Gregory, P. W.; Tyler, W. S.; and Julian, L. M. 1960. Evidence that the Dexter mutant is genetically related to recessive achondroplasia. *Anat. Rec.* 138: 353–54. (Abst.)

———. 1966. Bovine achondroplasia: The reconstitution of the Dexter components from non-Dexter stocks. *Growth* 30: 393–418.

Griffen, A. B. 1966. Nuclear cytology. In *Biology of the laboratory mouse,* ed. E. L. Green, pp. 51–85. 2d ed. New York: McGraw-Hill.

Griner, L. A.; McCrory, B. R.; Foster, N. M.; and Meyer, H. 1964. Bluetongue associated with abnormalities in newborn lambs. *J. Am. Vet. Med. Ass.* 145: 1013–19.

Grini, O., and Iversen, L. 1948. Spina bifida (rachischisis) hos lam. *Norsk Vet. Tskr.* 60: 253–60.

Gripat, H. 1874. Veau acéphale. Dissection. *Bull. Soc. Anat. Paris* 47: 601–6.

Grote, W. 1965. Störung der Embryonalentwicklung bei erhöhtem CO_2- und O_2-Partialdruck und bei Unterdruck. *Z. Morph. Anthrop.* 56: 165–94.

Gruenwald, P. 1954. Discussion. *J. Cell. Comp. Physiol.* 43 (Suppl.): 28.

Grüneberg, H. 1943*a*. Two new mutant genes in the house mouse. *J. Genet.* 45: 22–28.

———. 1943*b*. Congenital hydrocephalus in the mouse, a case of spurious pleiotropism. *J. Genet.* 45: 1–21.

———. 1947. *Animal genetics and medicine.* New York: Hoeber.

———. 1952*a*. Genetical studies on the skeleton of the mouse. IV. Quasi-continuous variation. *J. Genet.* 51: 95–114.

———. 1952*b*. *The genetics of the mouse.* 2d ed. The Hague: Nijhoff.

———. 1953. Genetical studies on the skeleton of the mouse. VII. Congenital hydrocephalus. *J. Genet.* 51: 327–58.

———. 1954. Genetical studies on the skeleton of the mouse. VIII. Curly-tail. *J. Genet.* 52: 52–67.

———. 1955*a*. Genetical studies on the skeleton of the mouse. XVII. Bent-tail. *J. Genet.* 53: 551–62.

———. 1955*b*. Genetical studies on the skeleton of the mouse. XVI. Tail-kinks. *J. Genet.* 53: 536–50.

———. 1956*a*. An annotated catalogue of the mutant genes of the house mouse. Medical Research Council Memorandum No. 33. London: H.M.S.O.

———. 1956*b*. A ventral ectodermal ridge of the tail in mouse embryos. *Nature* 177: 787–88.

———. 1957*a*. Genetical studies on the skeleton of the mouse. XIX. Vestigial-tail. *J. Genet.* 55: 181–94.

———. 1957*b*. The developmental mechanisms of genes affecting the axial skeleton of the mouse. *Am. Nat.* 91: 95–102.

———. 1958*a*. Genetical studies on the skeleton of the mouse. XXIII. The development of Brachyury and Anury. *J. Embryol. Exp. Morph.* 6: 424–43.

———. 1958*b*. Genetical studies on the skeleton of the mouse. XXII. The development of Danforth's short-tail. *J. Embryol. Exp. Morph.* 6: 124–48.

———. 1963. *The pathology of development. A study of inherited skeletal disorders in animals.* New York: Wiley.

Grüneberg, H., and Lea, A. J. 1940. An inherited jaw anomaly in long-haired dachshunds. *J. Genet.* 39: 285–96.

Grüneberg, H., and Truslove, G. M. 1960. Two closely linked genes in the mouse. *Genet. Res.* 1: 69–90.

Guérin, M. G. 1911. Chien mélomèle. *Rec. Méd. Vét.* 88: 177–80.

Guerrini, G. 1909a. Note di casistica teratologica. [*Syncephalus thoracopagus monoprosopus tribrachius* (Taruffi) *in un gatto.*] *Clin. Vet.* (*Milan*) 32: 593–600.

———. 1909b. Di un caso di *cyclops rhynchaenus* (Gurlt) osservato in un cane. *Clin. Vet.* (*Milan*) 32: 529–35.

Guinard, L. 1891. Monstruosités multiples chez un même animal. *J. Méd. Vét.* ser. 3 16: 8–16.

Gulienetti, R.; Kalter, H.; and Davis, N. C. 1962. Amniotic fluid volume and experimentally-induced congenital malformations. *Biol. Neonat.* 4: 300–309.

Gunberg, D. L. 1954. Spina bifida and herniation of hindbrain in the offspring of trypan blue injected rats. *Anat. Rec.* 118: 387. (Abst.)

———. 1955. Effect of suboptimal protein diets on teratogenic properties of trypan blue administered to pregnant rats. *Anat. Rec.* 121: 398–99. (Abst.)

———. 1956. Spina bifida and the Arnold–Chiari malformation in the progeny of trypan blue injected rats. *Anat. Rec.* 126: 343–67.

———. 1957. Some effects of exogenous hydrocortisone on pregnancy in the rat. *Anat. Rec.* 129: 133–53.

———. 1958. Variations in the teratogenic effects of trypan blue administered to pregnant rats of different strain and substrain origin. *Anat. Rec.* 130: 310. (Abst.)

Gunberg, D. L.; Hawkins, R. G.; Honl, T. C.; and Wirtschafter, D. D. 1962. Variation in trypan blue induced malformations observed in the progeny of two "strains" of rats. *Abst. Terat. Soc.* 2: 15–16. (Abst.)

Gunn, R. M. C. 1924. Chronic internal hydrocephalus. *Vet. Rec.* 4: 511–16.

Gurlt, E. F. 1877. *Ueber thierische Missgeburten. Ein Beitrag zur pathologischen Anatomie und Entwickelungsgeschichte.* Berlin: Hirschwald.

———. 1878. Die neuere Literatur über menschliche und thierische Missgeburten. *Virchow Arch. Path. Anat.* 74: 504–27.

Hackenberger, I., and Kreybig, T. von. 1965. Vergleichende teratologische Untersuchungen bei der Maus und der Ratte. *Arzneimittelforschung* 15: 1456–60.

Hadlow, W. J. 1962. Diseases of skeletal muscle. In *Comparative neuropathology*, J. R. M. Innes and L. Z. Saunders, pp. 147–243. New York: Academic Press.

Hafez, E, S. E. 1960. "Hydrodorsal" and other fetal malformations in swine. *J. Hered.* 51: 77–80.

———. 1964. Effects of over-crowding *in utero* on implantation and fetal development in the rabbit. *J. Exp. Zool.* 156: 269–87.

Hafez, E. S. E.; O'Mary, C. C.; and Ensminger, M. E. 1958. Albino-dwarfism in Hereford cattle, a sublethal character. *J. Hered.* 49: 111–16.

Hain, A. M. 1937. Microphthalmia and other eye-defects throughout fourteen generations of albino rats. *Proc. Roy. Soc. Edinburgh* 57: 64–77.

Hale, F. 1933. Pigs born without eyeballs. *J. Hered.* 24: 105–6.

———. 1935. Relation of vitamin A to anophthalmos in pigs. *Am. J. Ophth.* 18: 1087–93.

———. 1937. Relation of maternal vitamin A deficiency to microphthalmia in pigs. *Texas J. Med.* 33: 228–32.

384   References

Hall, E. K. 1953. Developmental anomalies in the eye of the rat after various experimental procedures. *Anat. Rec.* 116: 383–94.

Halstead, J. R., and Kiel, F. W. 1962. Hydrocephalus in a bear. *J. Am. Vet. Med. Ass.* 141: 367–68.

Hamburgh, M. 1952. Malformations in mouse embryos induced by trypan blue. *Nature* 169: 27.

———. 1954. The embryology of trypan blue induced abnormalities in mice. *Anat. Rec.* 119: 409–27.

———. 1963. Analysis of the postnatal developmental effects of "reeler," a neurological mutation in mice: A study in developmental genetics. *Dev. Biol.* 8: 165–85.

Hamburgh, M., Lynn, E., and Weiss, E. P. 1964. Analysis of the influence of thyroid hormone on prenatal and postnatal maturation of the rat. *Anat. Rec.* 150: 147–62.

Hamburgh, M., and Sobel, E. H. 1960. Observations related to the mechanism of the teratogenic action of trypan blue. Abstracts of Papers Presented at the Teratology Conference, New York, April 9–10, pp. 4–5.

Hamerton, A. E. 1932. Report on the deaths occurring in the society's gardens during 1931. *Proc. Zool. Soc. London* 100: 613–38.

Hannover, A. 1882–84. *Anencephalia, Cyclopia, Synotia.* Copenhagen: Lunos.

Hanson, F. B. 1923. The effects of X-rays on the albino rat. *Anat. Rec.* 24: 415. (Abst.)

Harbitz, F. 1942. Spredte bemerkninger om svulster hos dyr. *Norsk. Vet. Tskr.* 54: 193–224, 277–308.

Harding, J. D. J., and Done, J. T. 1956. Microphthalmia in piglets. *Vet. Rec.* 68: 865–66.

Harding, J. D. J.; Done, J. T.; and Darbyshire, J. H. 1966. Congenital tremors in piglets and their relation to swine fever. *Vet. Rec.* 79: 388–90.

Haring, O. M. 1960. Cardiac malformations in rats induced by exposure of the mother to carbon dioxide during pregnancy. *Circ. Res.* 8: 1218–27.

———. 1965. Effects of prenatal hypoxia on the cardiovascular system in the rat. *Arch. Path.* 80: 351–56.

———. 1966. Cardiac malformations in the rat induced by maternal hypercapnia with hypoxia. *Circ. Res.* 19: 544–51.

Haring, O. M., and Polli, J. F. 1957. Experimental production of cardiac malformations. *Arch. Path.* 64: 290–96.

Harm, H. 1954. Der Einfluss von Trypanblau auf die Nachkommenschaft trächtiger Kaninchen. *Z. Naturforsch.* 9B: 536–40.

Harper, K. H.; Palmer, A. K.; and Davies, R. E. 1965. Effect of imipramine upon the pregnancy of laboratory animals. *Arzneimittelforschung* 15: 1218–21.

Härtel, A., and Härtel, G. 1960. Experimental study of teratogenic effect of emotional stress in rats. *Science.* 132: 1483–84.

Hartman, C. G. 1943. Birth of a two-headed monster in the rhesus monkey. *Science* 98: 449.

Harvey, E. B. 1963. Discussion. In *Conference proceedings. Prenatal irradiation effects on CNS development,* ed. J. Werboff, p. 54. Washington, D.C., October 4–6.

Harvey, E. B., and Chang, M. C. 1962. Effect of radiocobalt irradiation of pregnant hamsters on the development of embryos. *J. Cell. Comp. Physiol.* 59: 293–305.

———. 1964*a*. Effects of single and fractionated X-irradiation of ovarian ova on embryonic development of the hamster. *J. Cell. Comp. Physiol.* 63: 183–88.

———. 1964*b*. Effects of single and fractionated irradiation on the embryonic development of hamsters. *J. Cell. Comp. Physiol.* 64: 445–53.

Hashima, H. 1956. Studies on the prenatal growth of the mouse with special reference to the site of implantation of the embryo. *Tohoku J. Agr. Res.* 6: 307–12.

Haskin, D. 1948. Some effects of nitrogen mustard on the development of external body form in the fetal rat. *Anat. Rec.* 102: 493–511.

Hatziolos, B. C. 1960. A case report—lymphoblastic lymphoma in a bovine fetus. *J. Am. Vet. Med. Ass.* 136: 369–75.

Haumont. 1958. Effets de la cortisone administrée pendant la gestation. *Ann. Endocr.* 19: 442–45.

Hay, M. F. 1964. Effects of thalidomide on pregnancy in the rabbit. *J. Reprod. Fertil.* 8: 59–76.

Hayashi, I.; Yama, T.; and Fujii, H. 1957. Experimental studies on the relationship between embryonic environment and developmental anomalies. Report VII. *Acta Path. Jap.* 7: 444–45. (Abst.)

Healy, M. J. R.; McLaren, A.; and Michie, D. 1960. Foetal growth in the mouse. *Proc. Roy. Soc. B.* 153: 367–79.

Heine, W. 1966. Thalidomidembryopathie im Tierversuch. III. Teratologische Testung von Thalidomidabbauprodukten. *Z. Kinderheilk.* 96: 141–46.

Heine, W., and Kirchmair, H. 1962. Tierexperimentelle Untersuchungen zur Frage der teratogenetischen Wirkung des Contergans. *Deut. Gesundheitsw.* 17: 1429–31.

Heine, W.; Kirchmair, H.; Fiedler, M.; and Stüwe, W. 1965. Thalidomid-Embryopathie bei Kaninchen nach passagerer Leberschädigung der Muttertiere durch Tetrachlorkohlenstoff. *Klin. Wschr.* 42: 592.

Heine, W., and Stüwe, W. 1966. Thalidomidembryopathie im Tierversuch. II. Thalidomidblutspiegelwerte bei lebergesunden und lebergeschädigten Versuchstieren. *Z. Kinderheilk.* 96: 14–18.

Heitz. F., and Martinet, M. 1961. Dualité des stades sensibles dans le développement du palais chez la souris mise en évidence par les rayons X. *C. R. Soc. Biol.* 155: 707–9.

Hemsworth, B. N. and Jackson, H. 1963*a*. Effect of busulphan on the developing gonad of the male rat. *J. Reprod. Fertil.* 5: 187–94.

———. 1963*b*. Effect of busulphan on the developing ovary in the rat. *J. Reprod. Fertil.* 6: 229–33.

Hendrickx, A. G.; Axelrod, L. R.; and Clayborn, L. D. 1966. "Thalidomide" syndrome in baboons. *Nature* 210: 958–59.

Herringham, W. P., and Andrewes, F. W. 1888. Two cases of cerebellar disease in cats, with staggering. *St. Bart. Hosp. Rep.* 24: 241–48.

Herschler, M. S.; Fechheimer, N. S.; and Gilmore, L. O. 1962. Congenital abnormalities in cattle: Their association with hereditary and environmental factors. *J. Dairy Sci.* 45: 1493–99.

Hertwig, P. 1940. Vererbbare Semisterilität bei Mäusen nach Röntgenbestrahlung, verursacht durch reziproke Chromosomentranslokationen. *Z. Ind. Abst. Vererbungsl.* 79: 1–27.

——. 1944. Die Genese der Hirn- und Gehörorganmissbildungen bei röntgenmutierten Kreisler-Mäusen. *Z. Menschl. Vererb. Konst.* 28: 327–54.

——. 1951. Entwicklungsgeschichtliche Untersuchungen über Bewegungsstörungen bei Mäusen. *Verh. Anat. Ges.* 49: 97–107.

——. 1955. Der *Hydrops*-Stamm. Vielfache Auswirkungen einer durch Röntgenbestrahlung von Spermatogonien entstandenen Erbänderung bei der Hausmaus *Züchter* 25: 194–98.

Herzog, A. 1963. Kongenitale, tumoröse Leukose einer Rinderfetus mit besonderer Lokalisation in der Haut. *Mh. Tierheilk.* 12: 201–10.

Heston, W. E. 1951. The "vestigial tail" mouse, a new recessive mutation. *J. Hered.* 42: 71–74.

Hicks, S. P. 1950. Acute necrosis and malformation of developing mammalian brain caused by X-ray. *Proc. Soc. Exp. Biol. Med.* 75: 485–98.

——. 1952. Some effects of ionizing radiation and metabolic inhibition on developing mammalian nervous system. *J. Pediat.* 40: 489–513.

——. 1953. Developmental malformations produced by radiation. *Am. J. Roentgen.* 69: 272–93.

——. 1954*a*. Mechanisms of radiation anencephaly, anophthalmia and pituitary anomalies. Repair in the mammalian embryo. *Arch. Path.* 57: 363–78.

——. 1954*b*. The effects of ionizing radiation, certain hormones, and radiomimetic drugs on the developing nervous system. *J. Cell. Comp. Physiol.* 43 (Suppl.): 151–78.

——. 1958. Radiation as an experimental tool in mammalian developmental neurology. *Physiol. Rev.* 38: 337–57.

Hicks, S. P.; Brown, B. L.; and D'Amato, C. J. 1957. Regeneration and malformation in the nervous system, eye, and mesenchyme of the mammalian embryo after radiation injury. *Am. J. Path.* 33: 459–81.

Hicks, S. P., and D'Amato, C. J. 1961. How to design and build abnormal brains using radiation during development. In *Disorders of the developing nervous system,* ed. W. S. Fields, and M. A. Desmond, pp. 60–93. Springfield, Ill.: Thomas.

——. 1963*a*. Low dose radiation of the developing brain. *Science* 141: 903–5.

——. 1963*b*. Malformation and regeneration of the mammalian retina following experimental radiation. In *Les phakomatoses cérébrales. Deuxième colloque international malformations congénitales de l'encéphale,* ed. L. Michaux, and M. Feld, pp. 45–51. Paris: S.P.E.I.

——. 1966. Effects of ionizing radiations on mammalian development. *Adv. Terat.* 1: 195–250.

Hicks, S. P.; D'Amato, C. J.; and Lowe, M. J. 1959. The development of the mammalian nervous system. I. Malformations of the brain, especially the cerebral cortex, induced in rats by radiation. II. Some mechanism of the malformations of the cortex. *J. Comp. Neur.* 113: 435–69.

Hieronymi, E. 1908. Ein seltener Fall einer Doppelmissbildung eines Kalbes. *Berlin. Tierärztl. Wschr.* 24: 692–93.

Hill, W. C. O. 1939. Spina bifida in a sacred baboon (*Papio hamadryas*). *Ceylon J. Sci. D.* 5: 9–15.

Hippel, E. von. 1907. Über experimentelle Erzeugung von angeborenen Star bei Kaninchen nebst Bemerkungen über gleichzeitig beobachteten Mikrophthalmus und Lidcolobom. *Graefe Arch. Ophth.* 65: 326–60.

Hippel, E. von, and Pagenstecher, H. 1907. Ueber den Einfluss des Cholins und der Röntgenstrahlen auf den Ablauf der Gravidität. *München. Med. Wschr.* 54: 452–56.

Hiraoka, S. 1961. The transplacental effects of the radio-strontium-90 upon the mouse embryos. [In Japanese with English summary]. *Acta Anat. Nippon.* 36: 161–71.

Hjarde, W.; Neimann-Sprensen, A.; Palludan, B.; and Sprensen, P. H. 1961. Investigations concerning vitamin A requirement, utilization and deficiency symptoms in pigs. *Acta. Agr. Scand.* 11: 13–53.

Hjärre, A. 1926. Diastematomyeli och spina bifida occulta hos kalv. *Skand. Vet. Tskr.* 16: 179–204.

Hoar, R. M. 1962. Similarity of congenital malformations produced by hydrocortisone to those produced by adrenalectomy in guinea pigs. *Anat. Rec.* 144: 155–64.

Hoar, R. M., and Salem, A. J. 1961. Time of teratogenic action of trypan blue in guinea pigs. *Anat. Rec.* 141: 173–81.

————. 1962. The production of congenital malformations in guinea pigs by adrenalectomy. *Anat. Rec.* 143: 157–68.

Hodgson, R. E. 1935. An eight generation experiment in inbreeding swine. *J. Hered.* 26: 209–17.

Hoeve, J. van der. 1938. Cyclopie. *Ned. Tijdschr. Geneesk.* 82: 138.

Hofmann, D., and Dietzel, F. 1966. Aborte und Missbildungen nach Kurzwellendurchflutung in der Schwangerschaft. *Geburts. Frauenheilk.* 26: 378–90.

Hogan, A. G.; O'Dell, B. L.; and Whitley, J. R. 1950. Maternal nutrition and hydrocephalus in newborn rats. *Proc. Soc. Exp. Biol. Med.* 74: 293–96.

Höglund, N. J. 1952. Effects of ethyl urethane on reproduction in mice. *Acta Pharmacol.* 8: 82–84.

Holding, R. E. 1904. [Double head of a lamb.] *Proc. Zool. Soc. London* 72: 373–74.

Hollander, W. F. 1966. Hydrocephalic-polydactyl, a recessive pleiotropic mutant in the mouse. *Am. Zool.* 6: 588–89. (Abst.)

Holmdahl, D. E. 1926. Die erste Entwicklung des Körpers bei den Vögeln und Säugetieren, inkl. dem Menschen, besonders mit Rücksicht auf die Bildung des Rückenmarks, des Zöloms und der entodermalen Kloake nebst einem Exkurs über die Entstehung der Spina bifida in der Lumbosakralregion. II–V. *Morph. Jahrb.* 54: 112–208.

Holy, L. 1959. Příspěvek k výskytu a ošetření dystokie u klisen, vyvolané zrůdným utvářením hlavičky. [Treatment of dystokia caused by malformation of the fetal head.] *Veterinářství* 9: 181–83.

Holz, K. 1954. Angeborene Missbildung und akute Entzündung des Zentralnervensystems beim Schwein. *Deut. Tierärztl. Wschr.* 61: 263–66.

————. 1956. Über angeborene Missbildungen des Zentralnervensystems und ihre Bedeutung für die Infektionskrankheiten des Schweines. *Deut. Tierärztl. Wschr.* 63: 260–63.

Holz, K., and Fortuin, V. 1956. Multiple Missbildungen bei einem Schwein. *Deut. Tierärztl. Wschr.* 63: 339–42.

Homburger, F.; Chaube, S.; Eppenberger, M.; Bogdonoff, P. D.; and Nixon, C. W. 1965. Susceptibility of certain inbred strains of hamsters to teratogenic effects of thalidomide. *Toxic. Appl. Pharmacol.* 7: 686–93.

Hommes, O. R. 1959. Trypan blue in the rabbit. *Acta Morph. Neerl. Scand.* 2: 28–37.

Honey, D. P.; Poulson, E.; Robson, J. M.; and Sullivan, F. M. 1964. Reversal by antagonists of the placental and teratogenic effects of 5-hydroxytryptamine. *J. Endocr.* 30: viii–ix.

Hopkins, B. J., and Casarett, B. W. 1964. Gross developmental anomalies induced by strontium-90 in the rat embryo. Univ. Rochester Atomic Energy Report UR-643.

Horii, K. 1964. Prevention of congenital defects in the offspring of alloxan-diabetic mice by insulin treatment. [In Japanese; English summary in *Birth Defects: Abstracts Selected Articles, Nat. Found.* 1(3), abst. 117, 1964.] *Folia Endocr. Jap.* 39: 988–95.

Horii, K.; Watanabe, G.; and Ingalls, H. 1966. Experimental diabetes in pregnant mice. Prevention of congenital malformations in offspring by insulin. *Diabetes* 15: 194–204.

Horsley, J. S., Jr. 1920. A description of a six-legged dog. *Anat. Rec.* 19: 1–27.

Houck, J. W. 1930. Hydrocephalus in lower animals. Congenital occurrence in a calf and an albino rat. *Anat. Rec.* 45: 83–106.

Howell, J. M., and Ritchie, H. E. 1966. Cerebellar malformations in two Ayrshire calves. *Path. Vet.* 3: 159–68.

Howell, J. M., and Siegel, P. B. 1963. Phenotypic variability of taillessness in Manx cats. *J. Hered.* 54: 167–69.

Hsu, C. Y. 1948. Influence of temperature on development of rat embryos. *Anat. Rec.* 100: 79–90.

Hsu, C. Y., and Van Dyke, J. H. 1948. An analysis of growth rates in neural epithelium of normal and spina bifidous (myeloschisis) mouse embryos. *Anat. Rec.* 100: 745. (Abst.)

Hübner, H. 1911a. Zur Kasuistik der tierischen Doppelmissbildungen. (Dicephalus und Cephalothoracopagus Monosymmetros von Lamm.) *Frankfurt. Z. Path.* 8: 135–50.

———. 1911b. Die Doppelbildungen des Menschen und der Tiere. *Erg. Allg. Path.* 15: 650–796.

Hughes, E. H., and Hart, H. 1934. Defective skulls inherited in swine. *J. Hered.* 25: 111–15.

Hughes, H. V. 1936. Cyclopia in the lamb. *J. Comp. Path.* 49: 218–25.

———. 1946. A case of duplicitas in a calf. *Vet. J.* 102: 227–35.

———. 1952. A case of congenital hydrocephalus with hydromyelia in a calf. *Vet. Rec.* 64: 753–55.

Hummel, K. P. 1958. The inheritance and expression of Disorganization, an unusual mutation in the mouse. *J. Exp. Zool.* 137: 389–423.

Hummel, K. P., and Chapman, D. B. 1959. Visceral inversion and associated anomalies in the mouse. *J. Hered.* 50: 9–13.

Hunt, W. L. 1964. Ova transfers in sheep and rabbits: Studies on maternal influences and irradiation damage. *Diss. Abst.* 25: 766. (Abst.)

Hunter, G. W., and Higgins, G. M. 1923. The anatomy of an abnormal double monster (Duroc) pig. *Anat. Rec.* 24: 389. (Abst.)

Hurley, L. S., and Everson, G. J. 1963. Influence of timing of short-term supplementation during gestation on congenital abnormalities of manganese-deficient rats. *J. Nutr.* 79: 23–27.

Hurley, L. S ; Everson, G. J.; and Geiger, J. F. 1958. Manganese deficiency of rats: Congenital nature of ataxia. *J. Nutr.* 66: 309–20.

Hurley, L. S., and Swenerton, H. 1965. Congenital malformations resulting from zinc deficiency in rats. *Fed. Proc.* 24: 568. (Abst.)

———. 1966. Congenital malformations resulting from zinc deficiency in rats. *Proc. Soc. Exp. Biol. Med.* 123: 692–96.

Hurley, L. S., and Tuchmann-Duplessis, H. 1963. Influence de la tétracycline sur le développement pré- et post-natal du rat. *C. R. Acad. Sci.* 257: 302–4.

Hurley, L. S.; Wooten, E.; Everson, G. J.; and Asling, C. W. 1960. Anomalous development of ossification in the inner ear of manganese-deficient rats. *J. Nutr.* 71: 15–19.

Huston, K.; Eldridge, F. E.; and Oberst, F. H. 1961. Congenital hydrocephalus in Ayrshires. *J. Anim. Sci.* 20: 908. (Abst.)

Huston, K., and Gier, H. T. 1958. An anatomical description of a hydrocephalic calf from prolonged gestation and the possible relationships of these conditions. *Cornell Vet.* 48: 45–53.

Hutyra, F., and Marek, J. 1926. *Special pathology and therapeutics of the diseases of domestic animals.* 3d ed. Vol. 3. Chicago: Eger.

Hyde, R. R. 1940. An epidemic of hydrocephalus in a group of experimental rabbits. *Am. J. Hyg. B.* 31: 1–7.

Ibsen, H. L. 1928. Prenatal growth in guinea pigs with special reference to environmental factors affecting weight at birth. *J. Exp. Zool.* 51: 51–91.

Ikeda, Y.; Horiuchi, S.; Yoshimoto, H.; Suzuki, Y.; Furuya, I.; Kawamata, K.; and Kaneko, T. 1965. Effects of thalidomide and aspirin on fetal development of rabbits. *Proc. Congen. Anom. Res. Ass. Jap.* 5: 8. (Abst.)

Ilančić, D. 1940. Ein neuer Letalfaktor beim Rinde. *Züchtungskunde* 15: 129–33.

Inaba, T. 1958. Experimentally reproduced congenital malformations of rats by excessive vitamin-A diet. [In Japanese with English summary.] *J. Osaka City Med. Cent.* 7: 558–66.

Inbred Strains of Mice. 1967. No. 5. (A biennial listing of inbred strains of mice, obtainable from Librarian, Jackson Laboratory, Bar Harbor, Maine).

Ingalls, T. H.; Avis, F. R.; Curley, F. J.; and Temin, H. M. 1953. Genetic determinants of hypoxia-induced congenital anomalies. *J. Hered.* 44: 185–94.

Ingalls, T. H., and Curley, F. J. 1957a. The relation of hydrocortisone injections to cleft palate in mice. *New Eng. J. Med.* 256: 1035–39.

———. 1957b. Principles governing the genesis of congenital malformations induced in mice by hypoxia. *New Eng. J. Med.* 259: 1121–27.

Ingalls, T. H.; Curley, F. J.; and Prindle, R. A. 1950. Anoxia as a cause of fetal death and congenital defect in the mouse. *Am. J. Dis. Child.* 80: 34–45.

————. 1952. Experimental production of congenital abnormalities. Timing and degree of anoxia as factors causing fetal deaths and congenital abnormalities in the mouse. *New Eng. J. Med.* 247: 758–68.

Ingalls, T. H.; Ingenito, E. F.; and Curley, F. J. 1963. Acquired chromosomal anomalies induced in mice by injection of a teratogen in pregnancy. *Science* 141: 810–12.

Inman, O. R., and Markivee, C. R. 1963. Gross effects on rabbit embryos and membranes of X-irradiation in the blastocyst stage. *Anat. Rec.* 147: 139–48.

Innes, J. R. M.; Russell, D. S.; and Wilsdon, A. J. 1940. Familial cerebellar hypoplasia and degeneration in Hereford calves. *J. Path. Bact.* 50: 455–61.

Innes, J. R. M., and Saunders, L. Z. 1962. *Comparative neuropathology.* New York: Academic Press.

Inoue, A.; Ikeda, T.; Imahashi, T.; and Yokota, S. 1964. Analysis of other anomalies accompanied with cardiovascular anomalies induced in rats by maternal trypan blue. [In Japanese with English summary.] *Proc. Res. Inst. Nucl. Med. Biol.* 5: 101–7.

Irvin, A. D. 1966. Monster calves. *Vet. Rec.* 78: 254–55.

Ishii, H.; Kamei, T.; and Omae, S. 1962. Effects of concurrent administrations of chondroitin sulfate with cortisone, vitamin A or noise stimulation on fetal development of the mouse. *Gunma J. Med. Sci.* 11: 259–64.

Ishii, H., and Yokobori, K. 1960. Experimental studies on teratogenic activity of noise stimulation. *Gunma J. Med. Sci.* 9: 153–67.

Jackschath, E. 1899. Fall einer Myelomengocystocele anterior s. inferior bei einem Kalbe. *Berlin. Tierärztl. Wschr.* 15: 455–56.

Jackson, B., and Kinsey, E. 1946. The relation between maternal vitamin A intake, blood levels and ocular abnormalities in the offspring of the rat. *Am. J. Ophth.* 29: 1234–42.

Jackson, C. E.; Johnson, M. L.; Lamar, J. K.; and Goldenthal, E. I. 1967. Effects of hydroxyurea on the axial skeleton of the rat. *Fed. Proc.* 26: 539. (Abst.)

Jackson, D.; Robson, J. M.; and Wander, A. C. E. 1959. The effect of 6-diazo-5-oxo-l-norleucine (DON) on pregnancy. *J. Endocr.* 18: 204–7.

Jacobs, L. A., and Brizee, K. R. 1966. Effects of total-body X-irradiation in single and fractionated doses on developing cerebral cortex in rat foetus. *Nature* 210: 31–33.

Jacobsen, L. 1965. Low-dose embryonic X-irradiation in mice and some seasonal effects in the perinatal period. *Radiat. Res.* 25: 611–25.

Jacoby, M. 1897. Ueber sehr frühzeitige Störungen in der Entwickelung des Centralnervensystem. *Virchow Arch. Path. Anat.* 147: 149–79.

Jaeger, G. 1826. Mangel des Unterkiefers und mangelhafte Entwicklung desselben an dem Fötus eines Hirsches und an zwei Lämmern. *Arch. Anat. Physiol. (Leipzig)* 1: 64–79.

————. 1830. Missbildung des Kopfes eines Kalbes und eines Lammes mit rüsselartigem Fortsatze an der Stirn—und Annäherung dazu bei einem neugeborenen Kinde, als Nachtrag zu den (Jahrg. 1829. III Heft. pag. 202. des Archivs) beschriebenen missgebildeten Schädeln eines Lammes und einer Ziege. *Arch. Anat. Physiol. (Leipzig)* 4: 105–19.

Jakob, H. 1916. Hydrocephalus internus bij den hond. *Tijdschr. Diergeneesk.* 43: 508–9.

James, L. F.; Lazar, V. A.; and Binns, W. 1966, Effects of sublethal doses of certain minerals on pregnant ewes and fetal development. *Am. J. Vet. Res.* 27: 132–35.

Jaworska, M. 1965. Cleft palate produced experimentally in C57/BL strain of mice in two age groups. *Acta. Chir. Plast.* 7: 70–82.

Jefimoff, P. 1898. One-eyed calf. [In Russian.] *Arkh. Vet. Nauk.*, no. 6, pp. 219–20 and plate.

Jelen, P.; Kithierová, E.; Palounková, E.; and Rokos, J. 1964. The morphogenesis of developmental malformations of the central nervous system. I. The influence of trypan blue on the development of the fetus. *Česk. Morf.* 4: 430–41.

Jelgersma, G. 1917. Drei Fälle von Cerebellar-Atrophie bei der Katze; nebst Bemerkungen über das cerebro-cerebellare Verbindungssystem. *J. Psych. Neur. (Leipzig)* 23: 105–36.

Jennings, A. R., and Sumner, G. R. 1951. Cortical cerebellar disease in an Ayrshire calf. *Vet. Rec.* 63: 60–61.

Jensh, R. P., and Magalhaes, H. 1962. The effect of whole body X-irradiation on the central nervous system of golden hamster embryos. *Proc. Penn. Acad. Sci.* 36: 194–99.

Jiřina, K. 1960. Hydrocephalus congenitus internus beim Pferd. *Berlin. München. Tierärztl. Wschr.* 73: 413.

Job, T. T.; Leibold, G. J., Jr.; and Fitzmaurice, H. A. 1935. Biological effects of roentgen rays; determination of critical periods in mammalian development with X-rays. *Am. J. Anat.* 56: 97–117.

Johansson, I. 1953. A new type of achondroplasia in cattle. *Hereditas* 39: 75–87.

———. 1965. Medfödda missbildningar hos mink. *Vara Palsdjur* 36: 93–94, 101.

Johnson, D. R. 1967. *Mouse News Letter* 36: 44.

Johnson, E. M. 1964. Effects of maternal folic acid deficiency on cytologic phenomena in the rat embryo. *Anat. Rec.* 149: 49–55.

Johnson, E. M., and Chepenik, K. P. 1966. Effects of trypan blue on the uptake of tritiated uridine by embryonic rats and their associated membranes. *Abst. Terat. Soc.* 6: 14. (Abst.)

Johnson, E. M.; Nelson, M. M.; and Monie, I. W. 1963. Effects of transitory pterolyglutamic acid (PGA) deficiency on embryonic and placental development in the rat. *Anat. Rec.* 146: 215–24.

Johnson, K. R.; Fourt, D. L.; Ross, R. H.; and Bailey, J. W. 1958. Hereditary congenital ataxia in Holstein–Friesian calves. *J. Dairy Sci.* 41: 1371–75.

Johnson, L. E.; Harshfield, G. S.; and McCone, W. 1950. Dwarfism, an hereditary defect in beef cattle. *J. Hered.* 41: 177–81.

Johnson, P. L. 1926. An anatomical study of abnormal jaws in the progeny of X-rayed mice. *Am. J. Anat.* 38: 281–317.

Johnson, R. H.; Margolis, G.; and Kilham, L. 1967. Identity of feline ataxia virus with feline panleucopenia virus. *Nature* 214: 175–77.

Joly, N. 1857. Sur un nouveau cas de monstruosité offert par un chat monosomien, pour lequel l'auteur propose le nom de *Rhinodyme. C. R. Acad. Sci.* 45: 630-32.

Joly, N., and Lavocat, A. 1855. Sur un anencéphale anoure appartenent à l'espèce bovine. *C. R. Acad. Sci.* 40: 892–94. (Abst.)

Jordan, H. E.; Davis, J. S., Jr.; and Blackford, S. D. 1923. The operation of a factor of spatial relationship in mammalian development, as illustrated by a case of quadruplex larynx and triplicate mandible in a duplicate pig monster. *Anat. Rec.* 26: 311–18.

Josephy. H. 1911. Über Rüsselbildung bei Zyklopie. *Virchow Arch. Path. Anat.* 206: 407–19.

―――. 1913. Missbildungen des Kopfes. III. Otocephalie und Triocephalie. In *Morphologie der Missbildungen des Menschen und der Tiere*, ed. E. Schwalbe, vol. 3, pt. 1, chap. 6, pp. 247–70. Jena: Fischer, 1906–37.

Jost, A. 1956. The age factor in some prenatal endocrine events. *Ciba Found. Coll. Ageing* 2: 18–27.

Jurand, A. 1959. Action of triethanomelamine (TEM) on early and late stages of mouse embryos. *J. Embryol. Exp. Morph.* 7: 526–39.

―――. 1961. Further investigations on the cytotoxic and morphogenetic effects of some nitrogen mustard derivatives. *J. Embryol. Exp. Morph.* 9: 492–506.

Kageyama, M. 1961. Multiple developmental anomalies in offspring of albino mice injected with triethylene melamine (TEM) during pregnancy. [In Japanese with English summary.] *Acta Anat. Nippon.* 36: 10–23.

Kageyama, M., and Nishimura, H. 1961. Developmental anomalies in mouse embryos induced by triethylene melamine (TEM). *Acta Schol. Med. Univ. Kioto Jap.* 37: 318–27.

Kahkonen, D., and Beaudoin, A. R. 1963. Serum proteins in rat fetuses of normal mothers and mothers treated with trypan blue. *Anat. Rec.* 145: 329. (Abst.)

Kajii, T. 1965. Thalidomide experience in Japan. *Ann. Paediat.* 205: 341–54.

Kalinina, N. A. 1957. Some data concerning the mechanism of damage to embryos on irradiation of gravid animals with X-rays. [In Russian; English translation AEC-tr-3361.] In *Experimental medical radiology.* Bk. 1, *Works of the all-union conference on medical radiology, Moscow*, pp. 150–55.

―――. 1961. Some data on the protection of the organism from the action of ionizing radiation during the period of prenatal development. [In Russian; English translation AEC-tr-5427.] *Radiobiologiya* 1: 224–31.

―――. 1964. Mechanism of action of some radioprotective substances on rats during embryogenesis. [In Russian; English summary in *Exc. Med.* Sect. XXI 5: 776–77, 1965.] *Radiobiologiya* 4: 746–51.

Kalter, H. 1953. The genetics and physiology of susceptibility to the teratogenic effects of cortisone in mice. Unpublished Ph.D. thesis, McGill Univ., Montreal.

―――. 1954a. The inheritance of susceptibility to the teratogenic action of cortisone in mice. *Genetics* 39: 185–96.

―――. 1954b. Preliminary studies on the metabolic factors involved in the production of cleft palate in mice. *Genetics* 39: 975. (Abst.)

―――. 1955. The effect of cortisone on the food consumption of pregnant mice. *Can. J. Biochem. Physiol.* 33: 767–72.

————. 1956. Modification of teratogenic action of cortisone in mice by maternal age, maternal weight and litter size. *Am. J. Physiol.* 185: 65–68.

————. 1957*a*. Factors influencing the frequency of cortisone-induced cleft palate in mice. *J. Exp. Zool.* 134: 449–67.

————. 1957*b*. Further evidence of the association between maternal weight and frequency of cleft palate in the offspring of cortisone-treated pregnant female mice. *Genetics* 42: 380. (Abst.)

————. 1959*a*. Attempts to modify the frequency of cortisone-induced cleft palate in mice by vitamin, carbohydrate and protein supplementation. *Plast. Reconstr. Surg.* 24: 498–504.

————. 1959*b*. Seasonal variation in frequency of cortisone-induced cleft palate in mice. *Genetics* 44: 518–19. (Abst.)

————. 1959*c*. Hypervitaminosis A-induced internal congenital malformations in strains of inbred mice. *Anat. Rec.* 134: 589–90. (Abst.)

————. 1960*a*. Teratogenic action of a hypocaloric diet and small doses of cortisone. *Proc. Soc. Exp. Biol. Med.* 104: 518–20.

————. 1960*b*. Congenital malformations of the rectum and urogenital system induced by maternal hypervitaminosis A in strains of inbred mice. *Anat. Rec.* 136: 219. (Abst.)

————. 1960*c*. The teratogenic effects of hypervitaminosis A upon the face and mouth of inbred mice. *Ann. N. Y. Acad. Sci.* 85: 42–55.

————. 1961. The teratogenic action of prednisolone on a genotype resistant to cortisone. *Am. Zool.* 1: 363. (Abst.)

————. 1962. No cleft palate with prednisolone in the rat. *Anat. Rec.* 142: 311. (Abst.)

————. 1963*a*. The uterus in steroid-induced cleft palate. *Abst. Terat. Soc.* 3: 5–6. (Abst.)

————. 1963*b*. Experimental mammalian teratogenesis, a study of galactoflavin-induced hydrocephalus in mice. *J. Morph.* 112: 303–17.

————. 1963*c*. Congenital malformations of the central nervous system. *Am. J. Clin. Nutr.* 12: 264–74.

————. 1965*a*. Interplay of intrinsic and extrinsic factors. In *Teratology: Principles and techniques*, ed. J. G. Wilson and J. Warkany, pp. 57–80. Chicago: Univ. of Chicago Press.

————. 1965*b*. Genes and teratogens. *Abst. Terat. Soc.* 5: 14. (Abst.)

Kalter, H., and Fraser, F. C. 1952. Production of congenital defects in offspring of pregnant mice treated with compound F. *Nature* 169: 665.

Kalter, H., and Warkany, J. 1957. Congenital malformations in inbred strains of mice induced by riboflavin-deficient, galactoflavin-containing diets. *J. Exp. Zool.* 136: 531–66.

————. 1959*a*. Experimental production of congenital malformations in mammals by metabolic procedures. *Physiol. Rev.* 39: 69–115.

————. 1959*b*. Teratogenic action of hypervitaminosis A in strains of inbred mice. *Anat. Rec.* 133: 396–97. (Abst.)

————. 1961. Experimental production of congenital malformations in strains of inbred mice by maternal treatment with hypervitaminosis A. *Am. J. Path.* 38: 1–21.

Kamenoff, R. J. 1935. Effects of the flexed-tail gene on the development of the house mouse. *J. Morph.* 58: 117–55.

Kameswaran, L.; Pennefather, J. N.; and West, G. B. 1962. Possible role of histamine in rat pregnancy. *J. Physiol.* 164: 138–49.

Kameyama, Y. 1959. Experimental study on developmental anomalies produced by X-radiation. *Acta Path. Jap.* 9: 1–16.

Karnes, J. L. 1941. Bulldog calf. *Vet. Med.* 36: 578.

Karnofsky, D. A. 1965. Drugs as teratogens in animal and man. *Ann. Rev. Pharmacol.* 5: 447–72.

Karnofsky, D. A.; Murphy, M. L.; and Lacon, G. R. 1958. Comparative toxicologic and teratogenic effects of 5-fluorosubstituted pyrimidines in the chick embryo and pregnant rat. *Proc. Am. Ass. Canc. Res.* 2: 312–13. (Abst.)

Kato, T. 1958. Embryonic abnormalities of the central nervous system caused by the fuel-gas inhalation of the mother animal. *Folia Psychiat. Neur. Jap.* 11: 301–24.

Kauffman, S. L. 1964. Early morphologic changes in mouse embryo neural tube following transplacental exposure to urethane. *Fed. Proc.* 23: 128. (Abst.)

Kaven, A. 1938*a*. Röntgenmodifikationen bei Mäusen. *Z. Menschl. Vererb. Konst.* 22: 238–46.

———. 1938*b*. Das Auftreten von Gehirnmissbildungen nach Röntgenbestrahlung von Mäuseembryonen. *Z. Menschl. Vererb. Konst.* 22: 247–57.

Keberle, H.; Faigle, J. W.; Fritz, H.; Knüsel, F.; Loustalot, P.; and Schmid, K. 1965. Theories on the mechanism of action of thalidomide. In *Embryopathic activity of drugs*, ed. J. M. Robson, F. M. Sullivan, and R. L. Smith, pp. 210–26. Boston: Little, Brown & Co.

Keeler, C. E. 1933. Absence of the corpus callosum as a mendelizing character in the house mouse. *Proc. Nat. Acad. Sci. USA.* 19: 609–11.

Keeler, R. F., and Binns, W. 1964. Chemical compounds of *Veratrum californicum* related to congenital ovine cyclopian malformations: Extraction of active material. *Proc. Soc. Exp. Biol. Med.* 116: 123–27.

———. 1966*a*. Teratogenic compounds of *Veratrum californicum* (Durand). I. Preparation and characterization of fractions and alkaloids for biologic testing. *Can. J. Biochem.* 44: 819–28.

———. 1966*b*. Teratogenic compounds of *Veratrum californicum* (Durand). II. Production of ovine fetal cyclopia by fractions and alkaloid preparations. *Can. J. Biochem.* 44: 829–38.

———. 1966*c*. Possible teratogenic effects of veratramine. *Proc. Soc. Exp. Biol. Med.* 123: 921–23.

Kehl, R.; Audibert, A.; Gage, G.; and Amarger, J. 1956. Action de la réserpine à différentes périodes de la gestation chez la lapine. *C. R. Soc. Biol.* 150: 2196–99.

Keil, R. 1911. Cyklopie bei einer Ziege. *Arch. Vergl. Ophth.* 2: 12–22.

———. 1912. Cyklopie bei einer neugeborenen Katze. *Arch. Vergl. Ophth.* 3: 30–38.

Keller, K. 1941. Verschiedenartige Missbildungen in einem Wurf beim Schwein. *Wien. Tierärztl. Mschr.* 28: 177–82.

Keller, K., and Niedoba, T. 1937. Untersuchungen an Doppelmonstren des Rindes im Sinne der Zwillingsforschung. *Z. Zücht. B.* 37: 245–93.

Kelly, J. W.; Feagans, W. M.; Parker, J. C., Jr.; and Porterfield, J. M. 1964. Studies on the mechanism of trypan blue-induced congenital malformations. I. Dye fractions and fetal anomalies. *Exp. Mol. Path.* 3: 262–78.

Kendrick, F. J., and King, C. T. G. 1964. Oral anomalies induced in the rat by meclizine hydrochloride. *Oral Surg.* 18: 690–96.

Kendrick, F. J., and Weaver, S. A. 1963. Alteration in amniotic fluid volume and other findings in meclizine hydrochloride induced anomalies. *Proc. Soc. Exp. Biol. Med.* 114: 747–50.

Kennedy, P. C.; Kendrick, J. W.; and Stormont, C. 1957. Adenohypophyseal aplasia, an inherited defect associated with abnormal gestation in Guernsey cattle. *Cornell Vet.* 47: 160–78.

Kernkamp, H. C. H. 1921. Perocephalus in the pig. *J. Am. Vet. Med. Ass.* 59: 625–27.

Kerr, T. 1947. On the effects of colchicine treatment of mouse embryos. *Proc. Zool. Soc. London* 116: 551–64.

Kerruish, D. W. 1964. The Manx cat and spina bifida. *J. Cat Genet.* 1: 16–17.

Kersten, W. 1954. Rückenmarksmissbildung beim Hund und Menschen. *Deut. Tierärztl. Wschr.* 61: 338–46.

Kerville, H. G. de. 1885. Description de quatre monstres doubles (2 chats et 2 poussins) appartenant aux genres synote, iniodyme, opodyme et ischiomèle. *J. Anat. Physiol. (Paris)* 21: 304–8.

———. 1891. Sur un jeune chien monstrueux du genre triocéphale. *Bull. Soc. Etude Sci. Nat. Albeuf* 11: 76–77.

Ketchel, M. M., and Banik, U. K. 1964. Relative radiosensitivities of the maternal reproductive tract and the fertilized ovum. *Nature* 202: 1021–22.

Kilham, L., and Ferm, V. H. 1964. Rat virus (RV) infections of pregnant, fetal and newborn rats. *Proc. Soc. Exp. Biol. Med.* 117: 874–79.

Kilham, L., and Margolis, G. 1966. Viral etiology of spontaneous ataxia of cats. *Am. J. Path.* 48: 991–1011.

Kim, J. N.; Runge, W.; Wells, L. J.; and Lazarow, A. 1960. Effects of experimental diabetes on the offspring of the rat. Fetal growth, birth weight, gestation period, and fetal mortality. *Diabetes* 9: 396–404.

Kimura, S., and Ariyama, H. 1961. Teratogenic effects of pantothenic acid antagonists on animal embryos. *J. Vitamin.* 7: 231–36.

King, C. T. G. 1963. Teratogenic effects of meclizine hydrochloride on the rat. *Science* 141: 353–55.

King, C. T. G., and Howell, J. 1966. Teratogenic effect of buclizine and hydroxyzine in the rat and chlorcyclizine in the mouse. *Am. J. Obstet. Gynec.* 95: 109–11.

King, C. T. G., and Kendrick, F. J. 1962. Teratogenic effects of thalidomide in the Sprague–Dawley rat. *Lancet* 2: 1116.

King, C. T. G ; Weaver, S. A.; and Narrod, S. A. 1965. Antihistamines and teratogenicity in the rat. *J. Pharmacol. Exp. Ther.* 147: 391–98.

King, D. W. 1964. Effect of d-gamma-tocopherol on the incidence of teratogeny in vitamin-E-deficient rats. *Nature* 204: 785–86.

King, J. A. 1965. Malformed calf syndrome on Kodiak Island, Alaska. *J. Am. Vet. Med. Ass.* 147: 239–40.

King, L. S. 1936. Hereditary defects of the corpus callosum in the mouse, *Mus musculus. J. Comp. Neur.* 64: 337–63.

King, L. S., and Keeler, C. E. 1932. Absence of the corpus callosum, a hereditary brain anomaly of the house mouse. Preliminary report. *Proc. Nat. Acad. Sci. USA.* 18: 525–28.

Kinney, C. S., and Morse, L. M. 1964. Effect of a folic acid antagonist, aminopterin, on fetal development and nucleic acid metabolism in the rat. *J. Nutr.* 84: 288–94.

Kisselewa, Z. N. 1934. Ein Fall von Balkenmangel bei der Katze. *Anat. Anz.* 78: 331–35.

Kitchell, R. L.; Sautter, J. H.; and Young, G. A. 1953. The experimental production of malformations and other abnormalities in fetal pigs by means of attenuated hog cholera virus. *Anat. Rec.* 115: 334. (Abst.)

Kitchell, R. L., and Stevens, C. E. 1953. Cardiac, aortic arch and other anomalies in newborn pigs. *Anat. Rec.* 115: 398. (Abst.)

Klatt, B. 1939. Erbliche Missbildungen der Wirbelsäule beim Hund. *Zool. Anz.* 128: 225–35.

————. 1943. Kreuzungen an extremen Rassetypen des Hundes. III. Teil: Der Bulldoggschädel und die Frage der Chondrodystrophie. *Z. Menschl. Vererb. Konst.* 27: 283–345.

Klosovskii, B. N. 1963. *The development of the brain and its disturbance by harmful factors.* New York: Macmillan.

Knobil, E., and Caton, W. L. 1953. The effect of hypophysectomy on fetal and placental growth in the rat. *Endocrinology* 53: 198–201.

Knoche, C., and König, J. 1964. Zur pränatalen Toxizität von Diphenylpyralin-8-chlor-theophyllinat unter Berücksichtigung von Erfahrungen mit Thalidomid und Coffein. *Arzneimittelforschung* 14: 415–24.

Knudsen, P. A. 1965. Congenital malformations of upper incisors in exencephalic mouse embryos, induced by hypervitaminosis A. I. Types and frequency. *Acta. Odont. Scand.* 23: 71–89.

Kobozieff, N. 1935. Recherches morphologiques et génétiques sur l'anourie chez la souris. *Bull. Biol.* 69: 265–405.

Kobozieff, N., and Gruner, J. 1954. Atrophie cérébelleuse familiale du chat. Etude anatomo-clinique, présentation d'un animal. *Rev. Neur.* 91: 63–66.

Kobozieff, N., and Pomriaskinsky-Kobozieff, N. A. 1947. Sur l'hydrocéphalie, mutation nouvelle chez la souris. *C. R. Acad. Sci.* 224: 963–65.

Kobozieff, N.; Pomriaskinsky-Kobozieff, N. A.; and Migne, P. 1955. De l'hydrocéphalie héréditaire chez la souris. Contribution à l'étude de l'hydrocéphalie chez les animaux domestiques et de laboratoire. *Biol. Bull.* 89: 189–210.

Kobozieff, N.; Tuchmann-Duplessis, H.; Mercier-Parot, L.; and Pomriaskinsky-Kobozieff, N. A. 1959. Influence du bleu trypan sur la fréquence d'apparition et la gravité des malformations chez des souris présentant une polydactylie héréditaire. *Rec. Méd. Vét.* 135: 317–24.

Koch, P.; Fischer, H.; and Schumann, H. 1957. *Erbpathologie der landwirtschaftlichen Haustiere.* Berlin: Parey.

Koch, P.; Fischer, H.; and Stubbe, A. E. 1955. Die kongenitale cerebellare Ataxie bei Felis domestica als Erbleiden. *Berlin. München. Tierärztl. Wschr.* 68: 246–49.

Kochhar, D. M. 1965. Effects of maternal hypervitaminosis A on cleft palate formation in rat embryos. *Diss. Abst.* 25: 5490–91. (Abst.)

Koens, H. 1945. Spina bifida (rachischisis posterior) bij het lam. *Tijdschr. Diergeneesk.* 70: 307–13.

Koford, C. B.; Farber, P. A.; and Windle, W. F. 1966. Twins and teratisms in rhesus monkeys. *Folia Primat.* 4: 221–26.

Kohno, J. 1960. Embryological studies on experimental cleft palate due to hydrocortisone. [In Japanese with English summary.] *J. Osaka City Med. Cent.* 9: 253–63.

Kollath, J., and Trautmann, J. 1965. Wirkungen von 200 R 200-kV-Röntgen-sowie 200 R Co^{60}-Gammaganzkörperbestrahlung auf in utero bestrahlte Mäuse. 1. Mitteilung: Hirn- und Skelettmissbildungen nach Einzeitbestrahlungen am 10. Schwangerschaftstag. *Strahlentherapie* 126: 253–57.

Koller, P. C. 1944. Segmental interchange in mice. *Genetics* 29: 247–63.

Koller, P. C., and Auerbach, C. A. 1941. Chromosome breakage and sterility in the mouse. *Nature* 148: 501–2.

Kosaka, S. 1927. Effects of roentgen rays upon the fetus. I. Investigation of the influence and effect of roentgen rays upon the mouse fetus. *Jap. J. Obstet. Gynec.* 10: 34–39.

———. 1928*a*. Die extrauterine Entwickelung und die Geschlechtsfunktion der röntgenbestrahlten Feten. [In Japanese with German summary.] *Okayama Igakkai Zasshi* 40: 2553–68.

———. 1928*b*. Der Einfluss der Röntgenstrahlen auf die Foeten. Dritte Mitteilung: Untersuchungen an weissen Ratten. [In Japanese with German summary.] *Okayama Igakkai Zasshi* 40: 1893–1919.

———. 1928*c*. Der Einfluss der Röntgenstrahlen auf die Feten. IV. Mitteilung: Untersuchungen an Meerschweinchen. [In Japanese with German summary.] *Okayama Igakkai Zasshi* 40: 2214–34.

———. 1928*d*. Der Einfluss der Röntgenstrahlen auf die Feten. V. Mitteilung: Zusammenfassende Betrachtung der Resultate der Untersuchungen an allen bisher berichteten Versuchstieren [In Japanese with German summary.] *Okayama Igakkai Zasshi* 40: 2259–74.

Koskenoja, M. 1961. Alloxan diabetes in the pregnant mouse. Its effects on offspring and particularly on their eyes. *Acta Ophth. Suppl.* 68: 1–92.

Kosterlitz, H. W. 1960. Discussion. In *Ciba Foundation symposium on congenital malformations*, ed. G. E. W. Wolstenholme, and C. M. O'Connor. Boston: Little, Brown & Co.

Kotani, S.; Araki, E.; Yukioka, K.; Inaba, T.; Nakamura, S.; and Miyoshi, T. 1958. Experimentally produced congenital anomalies through folic acid deficiency. [In Japanese with English summary.] *J. Osaka City Med. Cent.* 7: 353–59.

Kowalczyk, M. 1964. Congenital malformations and chromosomal abnormalities in the golden hamster (*Mesocricetus auratus*) induced by low doses of X-rays. *Folia Biol.* 12: 23–38.

Kraft, C. 1959. Untersuchungen über die Wirkung von Röntgenstrahlen auf Mäuseembryonen. *Berlin. Med.* 10: 125–29.

Krementz, E. T.; Hooper, R. G.; and Kempson, R. L. 1957. The effect on the rabbit fetus of the maternal administration of propylthiouracil. *Surgery* 41: 619–31.

Kreshover, S. J., and Clough, O. W. 1953. Prenatal influences on tooth development. II. Artificially induced fever in rats. *J. Dent. Res.* 32: 565–77.

Kreshover, S. J.; Clough, O. W.; and Bear, D. M. 1953. Prenatal influences on tooth development. I. Alloxan diabetes in rats. *J. Dent. Res.* 32: 246–61.

Kreshover, S. J., and Hancock, J. A., Jr. 1956. The effect of lymphocytic choriomeningitis on pregnancy and dental tissues in mice. *J. Dent. Res.* 35: 467–78.

Kreshover, S. J.; Knighton, H. T.; and Hancock, J. A., Jr. 1957. The influence of systemically administered trypan blue on prenatal development of rats and mice. *J. Dent. Res.* 36: 677–83.

Kreybig, T. von. 1965a. Die teratogene Wirkung von Cyclophosphamid während der embryonalen Entwicklungsphase bei der Ratte. *Naunyn Schmiedeberg Arch. Exp. Path.* 252: 173–95.

―――. 1965b. Zur Wirkung von Teratogenen auf frühe Stadien der vorgeburtlichen Entwicklung der Ratte. *Naunyn Schmiedeberg Arch. Exp. Path.* 252: 196–204.

―――. 1965c. Verschiedene Wirkmechanismen in teratologischen Experiment. *Naunyn Schmiedeberg Arch. Exp. Path.* 251: 197–98.

―――. 1965d. Die Wirkung einer carcinogenen Methylnitroso-Harnstoff-Dosis auf die Embryonalentwicklung der Ratte. *Z. Krebsforsch.* 67: 46–50.

Kriegel, H., and Langendorff, H. 1964. Die Wirkung einer fraktionierten Röntgenbestrahlung auf die Embryonalentwicklung der Maus. *Strahlentherapie* 123: 429–37.

Kriegel, H.; Langendorff, H.; and Kunick, I. 1962. Die Einwirkung von Röntgenstrahlen auf die Embryonalentwicklung der Maus. *Embryologia* 6: 291–318.

Kriegel, H.; Langendorff, H.; and Shibata, K. 1962. Die Beeinflussung der Embryonalentwicklung bei der Maus nach einer Röntgenbestrahlung. *Strahlentherapie* 119: 349–70.

Krohn, W. O. 1892. Atrophy of the cerebellum in a cat. *J. Nerv. Ment. Dis.* 17: 731–41.

Krölling, O. 1922. Beitrag zur abnormalen Entwicklung der Wiederkäuer. *Wien. Tierärztl. Mschr.* 9: 140–43.

Kröning, F. 1939. Ein neuer Fall erblichem Zwergwuchs beim Kaninchen. *Biol. Zbl.* 59: 363–65.

Kubik, J. 1923. Idiotypischer doppelseitiger kompletter Anophthalmus infolge von Aplasie des Vorder- und Mittelhirns bei einem 12 Tage alten Kaninchenembryo. *Graefe Arch. Ophth.* 112: 234–51.

Kuminek, K. 1960, Die Genetik einer neu aufgetretenen spontanen Kurzschwanzmutationen bei der Hausmaus. *Z. Vererbungsl.* 91: 182–200.

―――. 1959. Die Morphologie der unteren Wirbelsäule bei einer spontanen Kurzschwanzmutation der Hausmaus. *Biol. Zbl.* 78: 719–58.

Kundrat, H. 1882. Arhinencephalie als typische Art von Missbildung. *Wien. Med. Blad.* 5: 1395–97.

Labík, K. 1965. Contribution to the study of the heredity of cranioschisis in piglets. *Sborn. Vysok. Škol. Zeměd. Brně Rada B.* 13: 313–26.

Lalonde, L. M. 1940. A new type of bovine agnathia. *J. Hered.* 31: 80–81.

Lamb, H. D. 1936. Cyclopia in a new-born kitten: Anatomic findings. *Arch. Ophth.* 15: 998–1003.

Lamming, G. E.; Salisbury, G. W.; Hays, R. L.; and Kendall, K. A. 1954. Effect of incipient vitamin A deficiency on reproduction in the rabbit. II. Embryonic and fetal development. *J. Nutr.* 52: 227–39.

Lamming, G. E.; Woollam, D. H. M.; and Millen, J. W. 1954. Hydrocephalus in young rabbits associated with maternal vitamin A deficiency. *Brit. J. Nutr.* 8: 363–69.

Landauer, W. 1954. On the chemical production of developmental abnormalities and of phenocopies in chicken embryos. *J. Cell. Comp. Physiol.* 43 (Suppl.): 261–305.

———. 1959. The phenocopy concept: Illusion or reality? *Experientia.* 15: 409–12.

———. 1960. Nicotine-induced malformations of chick embryos and their bearing on the phenocopy problem. *J. Exp. Zool.* 143: 107–22.

Landois, H. 1879. Ueber einen Affenschädel mit doppeltem Schädeldache. *Jahresber. Westf. Prov. Ver. Wiss.* 8: 24–26.

———. 1902. Ein Doppelschweinchen mit Januskopf. *Jahresber. Westf. Prov. Ver. Wiss.* 30: 66–68.

Langelaan, J. W. 1907. On congenital ataxia in a cat. *Verh. Kon. Akad. Wetensch.* 13: 1–22.

Langman, J., and Drunen, H. van. 1959. The effect of trypan blue upon maternal protein metabolism and embryonic development. *Anat. Rec.* 133: 513–25.

Langman, J., and Faassen, F. van. 1955. Congenital defects in the rat embryo after partial thyroidectomy of the mother animal: A preliminary report on the eye defects. *Am. J. Ophth.* 40: 65–76.

Langman, J., and Welch, G. W. 1966. Effect of vitamin A on development of the central nervous system. *J. Comp. Neur.* 128: 1–16.

Lanzillotti-Buonsanti, A. 1889. Studio intorno allo scheletro della testa di un puledro ciclope (*Cyclops megalostomus arrhynchus*, Gurlt; *Cyclocephalus*, J. [sic] Geoffroy Saint-Hilaire). *Clin. Vet.* (*Milan*) 12: 396–405, 447–50.

———. 1890. Studio intorno allo scheletro della testa di un puledro ciclope (*Cyclops megalostomus arrhynchus*, Gurlt; *Cyclocephalus*, I. Geoffroy Saint-Hilaire). *Clin. Vet.* (*Milan*) 13: 11–16.

Lapin, B. A., and Yakovleva, L. A. 1963. *Comparative pathology in monkeys.* Springfield. Ill.: Thomas.

Lapointe, R., and Harvey, E. B. 1964. Salicylamide-induced anomalies in hamster embryos. *J. Exp. Zool.* 156: 197–200.

Larsen, V. 1963. The teratogenic effects of thalidomide, imipramine HCl and imipramine-N-oxide HCl on White Danish rabbits. *Acta Pharmacol.* 20: 186–200.

Larsson, K. S., and Boström, H. 1965. Teratogenic action of salicylates related to the inhibition of mucopolysaccharide synthesis. *Acta. Paediat* 54: 43–48.

Larsson, K. S.; Boström, H.; and Ericson, B. 1963. Salicylate-induced malformations in mouse embryos. *Acta Paediat.* 52: 36–40.

Larsson, K. S., and Eriksson, M. 1966. Salicylate-induced fetal death and malformations in two mouse strains. *Acta Paediat.* 55: 569–76.

Lassartesse. 1894. Un cas de dystocie par hydrocéphalie anencéphalique congénitale. *Rev. Vét.* 19: 79–82.

Laurenson, R. D., and Kropp, B. N. 1959. Use of alizarin red S with trypan blue in teratological studies in the rat. *Anat. Rec.* 133: 402. (Abst.)

Lauvergne, J. J., and Cuq, P. 1963. Ectromélie et otocéphalie héréditaires en race Française Frisonne Pie Noire. *Ann. Zootech.* 12: 181–92.

Lavocat, A. 1885. Agneau cyclocéphalien, ophthalmocéphale. (Nouveau genre.) *Rev. Vét.* 10: 233–44 and plate.

Lazarow, A.; Kim, J. N. K.; and Wells, L. J. 1960. Birth weight and fetal mortality in pregnant subdiabetic rats. *Diabetes* 9: 114–17.

Lazarus, S. H., and Volk, B. W. 1963. Absence of teratogenic effect of tolbutamide in rabbits. *J. Clin. Endocr.* 23: 597–99.

Lecyk, M. 1965. The effect of hypothermia applied in the given stages of pregnancy on the number and form of vertebrae in the offspring of white mice. *Experientia* 21: 452–53.

———. 1966. The effect of hyperthermia applied in the given stages of pregnancy on the number and form of vertebrae in the offspring of white mice. *Experientia* 22: 254–55.

Lefebvres-Boisselot, J. 1951. Role tératogène de la déficience en acide pantothénique chez le rat. *Ann. Méd.* 52: 225–98.

———. 1955. Contribution à l'étude des besoins en acide pantothénique de l'embryon et du foetus. Résultats expérimentaux obtenus chez le rat. *Arch. Sci. Physiol.* 9: 145–55.

Lejour-Jeanty, M. 1966. Becs-de-lièvre provoqués chez le rat par un dérivé de la pénicilline, l'hadacidine. *J. Embryol. Exp. Morph.* 15: 193–211.

Lengerová, A. 1957. Effects of intrauterine irradiation in rats in relation to the stage of embryogenesis at the time of exposure. *Folia Biol.* 3: 321–32.

Lenz, W. 1961. Diskussionsbemerkung. Tagung der Rhein.-Westfäl. Kinderärzteverinigung, Düsseldorf, November 11.

———. 1964. Chemicals and malformations in man. In *Second international conference on congenital malformations*, pp. 263–76. New York: International Medical Congress.

Léonard, A.; Maisin, J. R.; and Malfait, L. 1964. Etude de la descendance de rats irradiés dans le jeune âge. *C. R. Soc. Biol.* 158: 391–95.

Lesbre, F. X. 1894. Etude anatomique d'un porc synote et sphénocéphale. Considérations générales sur les monstres sycéphaliens. *J. Méd. Vét.*, ser. 3 19: 532–46.

———. 1901. Etude d'un agneau déradelphe. *J. Anat. Physiol.* (*Paris*) 37: 409–23.

———. 1911. Etude de deux agneaux jumeaux triocéphales, suivie de considérations générales sur les monstres otocéphaliens. *J. Méd. Vét.*, ser. 5 15: 69–86.

———. 1912. Etude de quelques cas de division complète du nez et de la mâchoire supérieure chez des veaux. Considérations générales sur cette monstruosité, appelée schistocéphalie. *J. Méd. Vét.*, ser. 5 16: 451–61.

———. 1928a. Les monstres cyclocéphaliens. Trois cas nouveaux chez des animaux. Considerations générales sur cette monstruosité. *Rec. Méd. Vét.* 104: 540–43, 597–616.

———. 1928b. Sur les encéphalocèles et, d'une manière générale, l'hydropisie ventriculaire d l'encéphale, chez l'homme et les animaux. *Rec. Méd. Vét.* 104: 269–85.

Lesbre, F. X., and Forgeot. 1903. Etude anatomique d'un foetus bovin sycéphalien d'un genre intermédiaire aux genres janiceps at iniope d'Is. Geoffroy Saint-Hilaire. *J. Anat. Physiol. (Paris)* 39: 11–38.

————. 1904. Etude anatomique de deux veaux achondroplases, suivie de considérations générales sur l'achondroplasie. *J. Méd. Vét.*, ser. 5 8: 1–16, 82–95.

————. 1905*a*. Anomalies multiples chez un veau. *Rev. Gén. Méd. Vét.* 6: 198–207.

————. 1905*b*. Etude d'un veau mort-né affecté d'hydrocéphalie, d'ectrodactylie et de nombreuses autres anomalies. *J. Méd. Vét.*, ser. 5 9: 449–60.

————. 1905*c*. Monstruosité complexe chez un veau (ectromélie, microcéphalie, brachygnathie inférieure, etc.). *Rec. Méd. Vét.* 82: 158–66.

Lesbre, F. X., and Guinard, L. 1891. Etude anatomique et physiologique d'un jeune chat opodyme. *Bull. Soc. Anthrop. Lyon* 10: 191–214.

Lesbre, F. X., and Jarricot, J. 1908. Etude anatomique de deux chats hétéradelphes suivie de considérations générales sur l'hétéradelphie. *Bibl. Anat. (Paris)* 17: 128–57.

Lesbre, F. X., and Pécherot, R. 1912. Etude d'un boeuf rhinodyme avec considérations générales sur les monstres du même genre. *J. Anat. Physiol. (Paris)* 48: 377–403.

————. 1913*a*. Note sur un chien otocéphalien opocéphale. *J. Méd. Vét.*, ser. 5 17: 262–65.

————. 1913*b*. Sur un veau généiocephale; nouveau genre de cyclocéphalien. *C. R. Acad. Sci.* 157: 301–2.

————. 1913*c*. Etudes d'un veau opodyme. *J. Anat. Physiol. (Paris)* 49: 555–64.

————. 1913*d*. Etude anatomique d'un agneau synote et cyclocéphale. *J. Méd. Vét.*, ser. 5 17: 144–57.

Lesbre, F. X., and Tagand, R. 1927. Etude anatomique d'un monstre triple de l'espèce ovine. *Rec. Méd. Vét.* 103: 885–89.

Levens, H. 1917. Mitteilungen aus der Praxis. *Deut. Tierärztl. Wschr.* 25: 165–67.

Lichtenstein, B. W. 1942. Distant neuroanatomic complications of spina bifida (spinal dysraphism): Hydrocephalus, Arnold–Chiari deformity, stenosis of the aqueduct of Sylvius, etc.; pathogenesis and pathology. *Arch. Neur. Psychiat.* 47: 195–214.

————. 1959. Atresia and stenosis of the aqueduct of Sylvius with comments on the Arnold–Chiari complex. *J. Neuropath. Exp. Neur.* 18: 3–21.

Lichtenstein, H.; Guest, G. M.; and Warkany, J. 1951. Abnormalities in offspring of white rats given protamine zinc insulin during pregnancy. *Proc. Soc. Exp. Biol. Med.* 78: 398–402.

Liénaux, E. 1897. Un cas de syringomyélie chez le chien. *Ann. Méd. Vét.* 46: 486–95.

Lima, J. A. P. de. 1918*a*. Study of an opodymous kitten. *J. Anat.* 52: 276–81.

————. 1918*b*. Etude d'un monstre otocéphalien. *Bull. Soc. Port. Sci. Nat.* 8: 61–71.

————. 1920. Anatomy of a fetus of a cyclopean goat. *Anat. Rec.* 19: 73–81.

————. 1936. Les monstres otocéphaliens. *C. R. 12me Cong. Int. Zool. (Lisbon)*, pp. 721–33 and 3 plates.

Lin, T. P., and Glass, L. E. 1963. Cause of pre-implantation death of mouse oocytes X-irradiated *in vitro. Anat. Rec.* 142: 253. (Abst.)

Lindsay, J. 1900. Dissection of a cyclopean monster. *Veterinarian* 73: 243–47.

Lipton, J. M. 1966. Locomotor behavior and neuromorphologic anomalies in prenatally and postnatally irradiated rats. *Radiat. Res.* 28: 822–29.

List, C. F. 1941. Neurologic syndromes accompanying developmental anomalies of occipital bone, atlas and axis. *Arch. Neur. Psychiat.* 45: 577–616.

Little, C. C. 1948. Genetics in cocker spaniels. Observations on heredity and on physiology of reproduction in American cocker spaniels. *J. Hered.* 39: 181–85.

Little, C. C., and Bagg, H. J. 1923. The occurrence of two heritable types of abnormality among the descendants of X-rayed mice. *Am. J. Roentgen.* 10: 975–89.

———. 1924. The occurrence of four inheritable morphological variations in mice and their possible relation to treatment with X-rays. *J. Exp. Zool.* 41: 45–91.

Lloyd, J. B., and Beck, F. 1963. An evaluation of acid disazo dyes by chloride determination and paper chromatography *Stain Tech.* 38: 165–71.

———. 1964a. Teratogenic activity of Niagara blue 2B and Afridol blue. *Biochem. J.* 91: 14P–15P.

———. 1964b. The relationship between serum levels and teratogenic potency of two acid disazo dyes in the rat. *Abst. Terat. Soc.* 4: 11. (Abst.)

———. 1966. The relationship of chemical structure to teratogenic activity among bisazo dyes: A re-evaluation. *J. Embryol. Exp. Morph.* 16: 29–39.

Lloyd, J. B., Beck, F., and Griffiths, A. 1965. Structure-activity studies for teratogenic effects of disazo dyes. *J. Pharm. Pharmacol.* 17 (Suppl.): 126A–128A.

Loawhakasetr, P. 1965. Influence of certain chemicals on the sensitivity of rat embryos to X-irradiation. *Diss. Abst.* 25: 7352. (Abst.)

Lockard, I., and Gillilan, L. A. 1956. Neurologic dysfunctions and their relation to congenital abnormalities of the central nervous system in cats. *J. Comp. Neur.* 104: 403–71.

Lohmeyer, H. 1961. Cortison, Schwangerschaft und Missbildungen des Neugeborenen. *Geburts. Frauenheilk.* 21: 560–65.

Loosli, R. 1964. Erzeugung fötaler Missbildungen am Kaninchen mit Thalidomid. *Path. Microbiol.* 27: 1003–11.

Loosli, R., and Theiss, E. 1964. Methodik und Problematik der medikamentösexperimentellen Teratogenese. *Bull. Schweiz. Akad. Med. Wiss.* 20: 398–416.

Lorke, D. 1965. Embryotoxische Wirkungen an der Ratte. *Naunyn Schmiedeberg Arch. Exp. Path.* 250: 360–82.

Loustalot, P. 1964. Tierexperimentelle Abklärung teratogener Nebenwirkungen von Pharmaka. In *Medikamentöse Pathogenese fetaler Missbildungen,* ed. T. Koller, and H. Erb., pp. 29–39. Basel: Karger.

Love, E. J.; Kinch, R. A. H.; and Stevenson, J. A. F. 1964. The effect of protamine zinc insulin on the outcome of pregnancy in the normal rat. *Diabetes* 13: 44–48.

Lubosch, W. 1925. Präparationsbefund an einer Duplicitas anterior vom Kalbe. *Verh. Phys. Med. Ges. (Würzburg),* n.s. 50: 223–29.

Lucey, J. F., and Behrman, R. E. 1963. Thalidomide: Effect upon pregnancy in the rhesus monkey. *Science* 139: 1295–96.

Lund, O. E. 1966. Combinations of ocular and cerebral malformations with cranio-facial dysplasia. *Ophthalmologica* 152: 13–36.

Lutwak-Mann, C. 1964. Observations of progeny of thalidomide-treated male rabbits. *Brit. Med. J.* 1: 1090–91.

Lutwak-Mann, C.; Schmid, K.; and Keberle, H. 1967. Thalidomide in rabbit semen. *Nature* 214: 1018–19.

Lyngdoh, O. 1950. Production of congenital abnormalities in offspring of trypan blue injected rats. *Anat. Rec.* 106: 281. (Abst.)

Lyon, M. F. 1959. A new dominant T-allele in the house mouse. *J. Hered.* 50: 140–42.

Lyon, M. F.; Phillips, R. J. S.; and Searle, A. G. 1964. The overall rates of dominant and recessive lethal and visible mutation induced by spermatogonial x-irradiation of mice. *Genet. Res.* 5: 448–67.

Lyssenkow, N. K., and Filatow, W. P. 1925–26. Ein Fall von Zyklopie beim Pferde. *Arch. Augenheilk.* 97: 314–40.

Macalister, A. 1867. Notes on an instance of cranial deformity in a domestic cat, with remarks on its probable origin. *Med. Pr. Circ. (Dublin)*, n.s. 4: 290–92.

MacFarlane, W. V.; Pennycuik, P. R.; and Thrift, E. 1957. Resorption and loss of foetuses in rats living at 35°C. *J. Physiol.* 135: 451–59.

Mackensen, J. A., and Stevens, L. C. 1960. Rib fusions, a new mutation in the mouse. *J. Hered.* 51: 264–68.

Magendie, F. 1821. Anatomie d'un chien cyclope et astome. *Rev. Méd. Hist. Phil. (Paris)* 6: 323–28.

Magnusson, H. 1917. Überzahlige Extremitäten und spina bifida mit Inklusion von Lungengewebe bei einem Kalbe. *Berlin. Tierärztl. Wschr.* 33: 533–34.

————. 1918. Övertaliga extremiteter och spina bifida hos en kalv. *Sven. Veterinärt.* 23: 58–61.

Mahon, F. C. 1916. A hydrocephalous monster (foal) with a few remarks on parturition in the mare. *Vet. J.* 72: 152–59.

Mainland, D. 1929. Posterior duplicity in a dog, with reference to mammalian teratology in general. *J. Anat.* 63: 473–95.

Maisin, H.; Dunjic, A.; Maldague, P.; and Maisin, J. 1955. Au sujet de la protection des embryons irradiés *in utero* par la mercaptoéthylamine. *C. R. Soc. Biol.* 149: 1687–90.

Majima, A. 1961. Eye-abnormalities in mouse embryos caused by X-radiation of mothers. On changes in the initial stage of development by irradiation on the 8th day of pregnancy. *Nagoya J. Med. Sci.* 24: 85–96.

————. 1962. Eye-abnormalities in mouse embryos and fetuses caused by X-radiation of mothers. Processes of production in case of exposure with 200 r on the 8th day of pregnancy. *Nagoya J. Med. Sci.* 24: 171–82.

Malet, J. 1885. Un cas de proencéphalie chez le veau. *Rev. Vét.* 10: 599–603.

Mammerickx, M., and Leunen, J. 1964. Anomalies foetales dans l'espèce bovine. Rapport concernant l'observation de 1008 foetus prélevés aux abattoirs de Cureghem-Bruxelles. *Rev. Agr. (Brussels)* 17: 1077–94.

Mandel, G. H. 1967. Antibiotics. In *The encyclopedia of biochemistry*, ed. R. J. Williams, Jr., and E. M. Lansford, pp. 75–80. New York: Reinhold.

404   References

Marin-Padilla, M. 1966. Mesodermal alterations induced by hypervitaminosis A. *J. Embryol. Exp. Morph.* 15: 261–69.

Marin-Padilla, M., and Benirschke, K. 1963. Thalidomide induced alterations in the blastocyst and placenta of the armadillo, *Dasypus novemcinctus mexicanus,* including a choriocarcinoma. *Am. J. Path.* 43: 999–1016.

Marin-Padilla, M., and Ferm, V. H. 1965. Somite necrosis and developmental malformations induced by vitamin A in the golden hamster. *J. Embryol. Exp. Morph.* 13: 1–8.

Marques, P. 1961. Um caso de lambdoidia (deradelfia) em carneiro. *An. Esc. Sup. Med. Vet.* 3: 63–70.

Martins, E. O., and Ferri, A. G. 1951. Siringomielia em bovina. *Rev. Fac. Med. Vet. Univ. São Paulo* 4: 399–405.

Marx, H. 1911. Die Missbildungen des Ohres. In *Die Morphologie der Missbildungen des Menschen und der Tiere,* ed. E. Schwalbe, vol. 3, pt. 2, chap. 6, pp. 565–632. Jena: Fischer, 1906–37.

Mason, K. E. 1935. Foetal death, prolonged gestation, and difficult parturition in the rat as a result of vitamin A-deficiency. *Am. J. Anat.* 57: 303–49.

Mather, G. W. 1956. Achondroplasia in a litter of pups. *J. Am. Vet. Med. Ass.* 128: 327–28.

Mauer, I. 1963. *Mouse News Letter* 29: 92.

———. 1964a. Vitamin A-induced congenital defects in hairless mice. *Biol. Neonat.* 6: 26–37.

———. 1964b. *Mouse News Letter* 31: 59.

Mauss, H. J., and Stumpe, K. 1963. Tierexperimentelle Untersuchungen zur Frage der Thalidomid-Embryopathie. *Klin. Wschr.* 41: 21–25.

McBride, W. G. 1961. Thalidomide and congenital abnormalities. *Lancet* 2: 1358.

McCafferty, R. E.; Wood, M. L.; and Knisely, W. H. 1965. Morphological and physiological effects of thalidomide and trypan blue on uteri and concepti of gravid mice. *Am. J. Obstet. Gynec.* 91: 260–69.

McClellan, R. O.; Kerr, M. E.; and Bustad, L. K. 1963. Reproductive performance of female miniature swine ingesting strontium-90 daily. *Nature* 197: 670–71.

McColl, J. D. 1966. Teratogenicity studies. *Appl. Ther.* 8: 48–52.

McColl, J. D.; Globus, M.; and Robinson, S. 1965. Effect of some therapeutic agents on the developing rat fetus. *Toxic. Appl. Pharmacol.* 7: 409–17.

McColl, J. D.; Robinson, S.; and Globus, M. 1967. Effect of some therapeutic agents on the rabbit fetus. *Toxic. Appl. Pharmacol.* 10: 244–52.

McFarland, L. Z. 1959. Spina bifida with myelomeningocele in a calf. *J. Am. Vet. Med. Ass.* 134: 32–34.

McFarland, L. Z., and Deniz, E. 1964. Extreme agnathia in a ewe lamb. *Cornell Vet.* 54: 541–44.

McFee, A. F.; Murphree, R. L.; and Reynolds, R. L. 1965. Skeletal defects in prenatally irradiated sheep, cattle and swine. *J. Anim. Sci.* 24: 1131–35.

McGrath, J. T. 1956. *Neurological examination of the dog with clinicopathological observations.* Philadelphia: Lea & Febiger.

———. 1965. Spinal dysraphism in the dog. With comments on syringomyelia. *Path. Vet.* 2 (Suppl.): 1–36.

McIntosh, W. C. 1868. Notes on the structure of a monstrous kitten. *J. Anat. Physiol.* 2: 366–73.

McLaren, A. 1965. Genetic and environmental effects on foetal and placental growth in mice. *J. Reprod. Fertil.* 9: 79–98.

McLaren, A., and Michie, D. 1959. The spacing of implantations in the mouse uterus. *Mem. Soc. Endocr.* 6: 65–75.

McLaren, F. D. 1903. Dexter monstrosities. *Vet. Rec.* 15: 414.

McLaurin, R. L. 1964. Partial cephaloceles. *Neurology* 14: 764–72.

McNutt, W. 1957. Influence of genetic background on the incidence of spina bifida in two strains of mice. *Anat. Rec.* 127: 434–35. (Abst.)

Mead, S. W.; Gregory, P. W.; and Regan, W. M. 1942. Proportionate dwarfism in Jersey cows. *J. Hered.* 33: 411–16.

———. 1946a. Deleterious recessive genes in dairy bulls selected at random. *Genetics* 31: 574–88.

———. 1946b. A recurrent mutation of dominant achondroplasia in cattle. *J. Hered.* 37: 183–88.

Meckel, J. F. 1826. Ueber die Verschmelzungsbildungen. *Arch. Anat. Physiol. (Leipzig)* 1: 238–310.

Mégnin. P. 1878. Sur un exemple d'otocéphalie, chez une chienne. *Bull. Acad. Vét. France* 35: 151.

———. 1879. Monstre cyclocéphalien rhinocéphale (cochon). *Rec. Méd. Vét.* 56: 328–30.

———. 1896. Sur un veau a deux têtes vivant. *C. R. Soc. Biol.*, ser. 10 3: 448–49.

Meier, H., and Hoag, W. G. 1962. The neuropathology of "reeler," a neuromuscular mutation in mice. *J. Neuropath. Exp. Neur.* 21: 649–54.

Mellin, G. W., and Katzenstein, M. 1962. The saga of thalidomide: Neuropathy to embryopathy, with case reports of congenital anomalies. *New Eng. J. Med.* 267: 1184–93, 1238–44.

Menschow, G. B. 1934. Fattori letali nel coniglio cincilla. *Rev. Coniglicolt.* 6: 8–9.

Mercer, R., and Steven, D. H. 1966. Synotia in a stillborn lamb. *Vet. Rec.* 78: 94–96.

Mercier-Parot, L. 1957. Influence de la cortisone et de l'hormone corticotrope sur la gestation et le développement post-natal du rat. *Biol. Méd.* 46: 1–95.

Mercier-Parot, L., David, G., and Tuchmann-Duplessis, H. 1963. Action tératogène d'hétéro-anticorps tissulaires. II. Etude de l'action tératogène chez la souris de sérums anti-rein. *C. R. Soc. Biol.* 157: 974–77.

Messner, E. 1908–9. Das Zentralnervensystem eines Dicephalus monauchenos vom Kalbe. *J. Psych. Neur. (Leipzig)* 12: 124–34.

Mettam, A. E. 1897. Cyclopia. *Veterinarian* 70: 194–203.

Meyer, B. 1928. Interessante Zwillingsgeburt beim Kalbe. *Berlin. Tierärztl. Wschr.* 44: 386.

Meyer, H., and Trautwein, G. 1966. Experimentelle Untersuchungen über erbliche Meningocele cerebralis beim Schwein. I. Zuchtversuche und genetische Analyse. *Path. Vet.* 3: 529–42.

Meyer, R. de. 1961. *Etude expérimentale de la glycorégulation gravidique et de l'action teratogène des perturbations du métabolisme glucidique.* Paris: Masson.

406   References

Meyer, R. de, and Isaac-Mathy, M. 1958. A propos de l'action tératogène d'un sulfamide hypoglycémiant (N-sulfanilil-N' butyluree-BZ[55]). *Ann. Endocr.* 19: 167–72.

Micucci, T. 1926. Di alcune monstruositá anatomiche. *Clin. Vet.* (*Milan*) 49: 107–10.

Miessner. 1899. Defectbildung am Gehirn, verbunden mit Hydrocephalus internus chronicus congenitus beim Hunde. *Berlin. Tierärztl. Wschr.* 15: 239–40.

Miklashevskiy, V. E., and Gol'dberg, M. B. 1961. Conditioned-reflex activity of white rats exposed to the effect of X-rays in the pre-implantation stage of embryonic development. In *Effects of ionizing radiation on the functions of the higher nervous system of progeny*, ed. I. A. Piontkovskiy, pp. 21–39. Moscow: Medgiz. Translation Series AEC-tr-5553, USAEC.

Milks, H. J. 1918. Hydrocephalus. *Cornell Vet.* 8: 298.

Millar, R., and Tucker, R. 1952. Nervous symptoms developed in the chondrodystrophic dog. *Brit. Vet. J.* 108: 293–98.

Millen, J. W., and Davies, J. 1952. Neuro-mesodermal relationships as illustrated by a specimen of synotia in the sheep. *Acta Anat.* 16: 148–59.

Millen, J. W., and Dickson, A. D. 1957. The effect of vitamin A upon the cerebrospinal-fluid pressures of young rabbits suffering from hydrocephalus due to maternal hypovitaminosis A. *Brit. J. Nutr.* 11: 440–46.

Millen, J. W., and Woollam, D. H. M. 1956. The effect of the duration of vitamin A deficiency in female rabbits upon the incidence of hydrocephalus in their young. *J. Neur. Neurosurg. Psychiat.* 19: 17–20.

———. 1957. Influence of cortisone on teratogenic effects of hypervitaminosis A. *Brit. Med. J.* 2: 196–97.

———. 1958a. Vitamins and cerebrospinal fluid. In *Ciba Foundation symposium on the cerebrospinal fluid*, ed. G. E. W. Wolstenholme, and C. M. O'Connor, pp. 168–85. Boston: Little, Brown & Co.

———. 1958b. Insulin-cortisone relationship in experimental teratogenesis. *Nature* 181: 418.

———. 1958c. Effect of vitamin B complex on the teratogenic activity of hypervitaminosis A. *Nature* 182: 940.

———. 1959. Observations on the experimental production of malformations of the central nervous system. *J. Ment. Defic. Res.* 3: 23–32.

———. 1960. Potency of parental vitamin A. *Nature* 185: 249–50.

———. 1962. *The anatomy of the cerebrospinal fluid*. London: Oxford Univ. Press.

Millen, J. W.; Woollam, D. H. M.; and Lamming, G. E. 1953. Hydrocephalus associated with deficiency of vitamin A. *Lancet* 2: 1234–36.

———. 1954. Congenital hydrocephalus due to experimental hypovitaminosis A. *Lancet* 2: 679–83.

Miller, J. R. 1958. Some embryological consequences of maternal fasting and their relation to the phenocopy concept. *Proc. X Int. Cong. Genet.* 2: 190. (Abst.)

———. 1962a. A strain difference in response to the teratogenic effect of maternal fasting in the house mouse. *Can. J. Genet. Cytol.* 4: 69–78.

———. 1962b. Effect of cortisone on the developing mouse foetus. *Nature* 194: 891–92.

Milne, A. H. 1942. A congenital deformity affecting the skull and brain of a piglet. *Vet. Rec.* 54: 367–68.

Mintz, B. 1964. Gene expression in the morula stage of mouse lethals, as observed during development of t^{12}/t^{12} lethal mutants *in vitro*. *J. Exp. Zool.* 157: 267–72.

Mohr, O. L. 1926. Über Letalfaktoren, mit Berücksichtigung ihres Verhaltens bei Haustieren und beim Menschen. *Z. Ind. Abst. Verebungsl.* 41: 59–109.

Mohr, U.; Althoff, J.; and Wrba, H. 1964. Morphologische Veränderungen der Rattenplazenta beim Alloxandiabetes. *Naturwissenschaften* 51: 440.

Molinier, M. 1879. Monstre cyclocéphale. Preuves tératologiques de la construction vertébrale de la tête. *Rev. Vét.* 4: 405–9.

Monell, G. C. 1846. Case of a deformed calf. *N. Y. J. Med.* 7: 43–45.

Monie, I. W. 1961. Chlorambucil-induced abnormalities of the urogenital system of rat fetuses. *Anat. Rec.* 139: 145–53.

———. 1965. Comparative development of rat, chick and human embryos. In *Supplement to teratology workshop manual. A collection of lectures and demonstrations from the second workshop in teratology*, pp. 146–62. Chicago: Pharmaceutical Manufacturers Association.

Monie I. W.; Armstrong, R. M.; and Nelson, M. M. 1961. Hydrocephalus and other abnormalities in rat young resulting from maternal pteroylglutamic acid deficiency from the 8th to 10th days of pregnancy. *Abst. Terat. Soc.* 1: 8. (Abst.)

Monie, I. W., and Khemmani, M. 1967. Facial and other malformations in rat fetuses resulting from maternal administration of retinoic (vitamin A) acid during pregnancy. *Abst. Terat. Soc.* 7: 35–36. (Abst.)

Monie, I. W.; Takacs, E.; and Warkany, J. 1966. Transposition of the great vessels and other cardiovascular abnormalities in rat fetuses induced by trypan blue. *Anat. Rec.* 156: 175–90.

Monod, R. 1933. Chevreau cyclocéphalien, monophtalme, rhinocéphale. *Rec. Méd. Vét.* 109: 21–22.

Montanari, G. 1961. Malformazioni congenite da carenza: Avitaminosi B_{12}. *Riv. Anat. Pat. Oncol.* 20: 390–400.

Monti, F., and Guarda, F. 1961. Atassia cerebellare congenita in un vitello da ipoplasia del cervelletto. *Clin. Vet.* (*Milan*) 84: 65–75.

Moore, K. L.; Dwornik, J. J.; and Dalton, R. D. 1964. Congenital defects produced in the rat by thalidomide. *Anat. Rec.* 148: 313–14. (Abst.)

Morand. 1752. Description d'un petit faon de biche, monstrueux, envoyé par le Roi à l'Académie. *Hist. Acad. Roy. Sci.* (*Paris*), pp. 23–24.

Morgan, W. C., Jr. 1950. A new tail-short mutation in the house mouse whose lethal effects are conditioned by the residual genotype. *J. Hered.* 41: 208–15.

———. 1952. *Mouse News Letter* 6: 33.

———. 1953. A new crooked tail mutation involving distinctive pleiotropism. *J. Genet.* 52: 354–73.

———. 1954. Eventration and exencephaly in mouse embryos. *Genetics* 39: 984. (Abst.)

Morot, C. 1889. Note sur un foetus porcin opocéphale. *J. Méd. Vét.*, ser. 3 14: 593–95.

Morrill, C. V. 1932. Internal hydrocephalus in pure-bred and hybrid dogs. *Anat. Rec.* 52 (Suppl.): 27. (Abst.)

Morris, J. M.; van Wagenen, G.; Hurteau, G. D.; Johnston, D. W.; and Carlsen, R. A. 1967a. Compounds interfering with ovum implantation and development. I. Alkaloids and antimetabolites. *Fertil. Steril.* 18: 7–17.

Morris, J. M.; van Wagenen, G.; McCann, T.; and Jacob, D. 1967b. Compounds interfering with ovum implantation and development. II. Synthetic estrogens and antiestrogens. *Fertil. Steril.* 18: 18–34.

Morsier, G. de. 1962. La dysplasie olfacto-génitale. Trois cas observés chez le veau. Essai de tératogénèse. *Acta Neuropath.* 1: 433–49.

Morton, N. E.; Crow, J. F.; and Muller, H. J. 1956. An estimate of the mutational damage in man from data on consanguineous marriages. *Proc. Nat. Acad. Sci. USA.* 42: 855–63.

Moscarella, A. A.; Stark, R. B.; and de Forest, M. 1962. Anemia, cortisone, and maternal stress as teratogenic factors in mice. *Surg. Forum.* 13: 469–71.

Mosher, H. P. 1938. Does animal experimentation show similar changes in the ear of mother and fetus after the ingestion of quinine by the mother? *Laryngoscope* 48: 361–95.

Mosimann, W. 1951. Ein eigenartiger Fall von Encephalocele beim Schaf. *Schweiz. Arch. Tierheilk.* 93: 389–97.

Moussu. 1899. Porcelet cyclocéphale. *Rec. Méd. Vét.* 76: 47–48.

Müller, M. 1966. Does nitrogen mustard affect the foetus directly or secondarily by its effects on the mother? *Experientia* 22: 247.

Müller, M. and Škreb N. 1964. Does nitrogen mustard mimic the X-ray effects in any case? *Experientia* 20: 70–71.

Murakami, U. 1953. Artificial induction of pseudencephaly, short-tail, taillessness, myelencephalic blebs and some fissure formations (phenocopies) of mice. *Proc. Jap. Acad.* 29: 138–42.

Murakami, U., and Kameyama, Y. 1954. Malformations resulted from insults in the early stage of pregnancy of the mouse. *Proc. Jap. Acad.* 30: 409–13.

———. 1958. Effects of low-dose X-radiation in the mouse. *Am. J. Dis. Child.* 96: 272–77.

———. 1965. Malformations of the mouse fetus caused by hypervitaminosis-A of the mother during pregnancy. *Arch. Env. Hlth.* 10: 732–41.

Murakami, U.; Kameyama, Y.; and Kato, T. 1954. Basic processes seen in disturbance of early development of the central nervous system. *Nagoya J. Med. Sci.* 17: 74–84.

———. 1956a. Effects of a vaginally applied contraceptive with phenylmercuric acetate upon developing embryos and their mother animals. *Ann. Rep. Res. Inst. Env. Med. Nagoya Univ.* 4: 88–99.

———. 1956b. Effects of maternal anoxia upon the development of embryos. *Ann. Rep. Res. Inst. Env. Med. Nagoya Univ.* 4: 76–87.

Murakami, U.; Kameyama, Y.; and Majima, A. 1960. A dynamic observation on the formation of developmental abnormalities of the fetus caused by X-radiation. *Ann. Rep. Res. Inst. Env. Med. Nagoya Univ.* 8: 101–15.

Murakami, U.; Kameyama, Y.; Majima, A.; and Sakurai, T. 1961. Patterns of radiation malformations of the mouse fetus and subjected stage of development. *Ann. Rep. Res. Inst. Env. Med. Nagoya Univ.* 9: 71–81.

———. 1962. Radiation malformations belonging to the cyclopia-arrhinencephalia-otocephalia group in the mouse foetus. *J. Embryol. Exp. Morph.* 10: 64–72.

Murakami, U.; Kameyama, Y.; and Nogami, H. 1962. Skeletal malformation in the mouse fetus caused by maternal hypoxia during early stages of pregnancy. *Ann. Rep. Res. Inst. Env. Med. Nagoya Univ.* 10: 45–55.

———. 1963. Malformation of the extremity in the mouse foetus caused by X-radiation of the mother during pregnancy. *J. Embryol Exp. Morph.* 11: 549–69.

Murkibhavi, G. R.; Hattangady, S. R.; Jamkhedkar, P. P.; and Kulkarni, P. E. 1964. Some congenital abnormalities. Congenital external hydrocephalus in a litter of Doberman pinscher. *Ind. Vet. J.* 41: 732–34.

Murphree, O. D.; Monroe, B. L.; and Seager, L. D. 1962. Survival of offspring of rats administered phenothiazines during pregnancy. *J. Neuropsychiat.* 3: 295–97.

Murphree, R. L., and Pace, H. B. 1960. The effects of prenatal radiation on postnatal development in rats. *Radiat. Res.* 12: 495–504.

Murphy, M. L. 1960. Teratogenic effects of tumour-inhibiting chemicals in the foetal rat. In *Ciba Foundation symposium on congenital malformations*, ed. G. E. W. Wolstenholme, and C. M. O'Connor, pp. 78–107. Boston: Little, Brown & Co.

———. 1962. Teratogenic effects in rats of growth inhibiting chemicals, including studies on thalidomide. *Clin. Proc. Child. Hosp. (Washington, D.C.)* 18: 307–22.

———. 1965. Dose-response relationships in growth-inhibiting drugs in the rat: Time of treatment as a teratological determinant. In *Teratology: Principles and techniques*, ed. J. G. Wilson, and J. Warkany, pp. 161–84. Chicago: Univ. of Chicago Press.

Murphy, M. L., and Chaube, S. 1964. Preliminary survey of hydroxyurea (NSC-32065) as a teratogen. *Canc. Chemother. Rep.* 40: 1–7.

Murphy, M. L.; Dagg, C. P.; and Karnofsky, D. A. 1957. Comparison of teratogenic chemicals in the rat and chick embryos. *Pediatrics* 19: 701–14.

Murphy, M. L.; Dagg, C. P.; and Runner, C. C. 1961. Teratogenic effects of 5-fluorodeoxyuridine and fluorodeoxycytidine in inbred strains of mice. *Abst. Terat. Soc.* 1: 7. (Abst.)

Murphy, M. L., and Karnofsky, D. A. 1956. Effect of azaserine and other growth-inhibiting agents on fetal development of the rat. *Cancer* 9: 955–62.

Murphy, M. L.; Moro, A. D.; and Lacon, C. 1958. Comparative effects of five polyfunctional alkylating agents on the rat fetus, with additional notes on the chick embryo. *Ann. N. Y. Acad. Sci.* 68: 762–81.

Myers, L. 1955. Experimentally induced anomalies of the internal ears of albino rat embryos. *S. Afr. J. Sci.* 51: 214–16.

Nachtsheim, H. 1931. Über eine erbliche Nervenkrankheit (Syringomyelie) beim Kaninchen. *Z. Pelztier Rauchwarenk.* 3: 254–59.

———. 1937a. Erbpathologische Untersuchungen am Kaninchen. *Z. Ind. Abst. Vererbungsl.* 73: 463–66.

———. 1937b. Erbpathologie des Kaninchens. *Erbarzt* 4: 25–30.

———. 1939. Erbleiden des Nervensystems bei Säugetieren. In *Handbuch der Erbbiologie des Menschen*, ed. G. Just, vol. 5, pp. 1–58. Berlin: Springer.

410   References

――――. 1958. Erbpathologie der Nagetiere. In *Pathologie der Labora-toriumstiere*, ed. P. Cohrs, R. Jaffe, and H, Meesen, pp. 310–452. Berlin: Springer.

Nagahama, M.; Akiyama, N.; and Miki, T. 1965. Experimental production of malformations with salicylates (acetyl salicylate and phenyl salicylate) in rats. *Proc. Congen. Anom. Res. Ass. Jap.* 5: 35. (Abst.)

Nanjo, H. 1964. Maldevelopment of the fetuses caused by maternal administration of thio-TEPA in relation to maternal age. [In Japanese with English summary.] *Acta Anat. Nippon.* 39: 258–62.

Narrod, S. A.; Wilk, A. L.; and King, C. T. G. 1965. Metabolism of meclizine in the rat. *J. Pharmacol. Exp. Ther.* 147: 380–84.

Nebel, L., and Hamburgh, M. 1966. Observations on the penetration and uptake of trypan blue in embryonic membranes of the mouse. *Z. Zellforsch.* 75: 129–37.

Neel, J. V. 1961. Some genetic aspects of congenital defect. In *First international conference on congenital malformations*, pp. 63–69. Philadelphia: Lippincott.

Nelson, M. M. 1955. Mammalian fetal development and antimetabolites. In *Antimetabolites and cancer*, ed. C. P. Rhoads, pp. 107–28. Washington, D.C.: American Association for the Advancement of Science.

――――. 1957. Production of congenital anomalies in mammals by maternal dietary deficiencies. *Pediatrics* 19: 764–76.

Nelson, M. M.; Asling, C. W.; and Evans, H. M. 1952. Production of multiple congenital abnormalities in young by maternal pteroylglutamic acid deficiency during gestation. *J. Nutr.* 48: 61–80.

Nelson, M. M.; Baird, C. D. C.; Wright, H. V.; and Evans, H. M. 1956*a*. Multiple congenital abnormalities in the rat resulting from riboflavin deficiency induced by the antimetabolite galactoflavin. *J. Nutr.* 58: 125–34.

Nelson, M. M., and Evans, H. M. 1948. Effect of desoxypyridoxine on reproduction in the rat. *Proc. Soc. Exp. Biol. Med.* 68: 274–76.

――――. 1951. Effect of pyridoxine deficiency on reproduction in the rat. *J. Nutr.* 43: 281–94.

――――. 1955. Relation of thiamine to reproduction in the rat. *J. Nutr.* 55: 151–63.

Nelson, M. M.; Wright, H. V.; Asling, C. W.; and Evans, H. M. 1955. Multiple congenital abnormalities resulting from transitory deficiency of pteroylglutamic acid during gestation in the rat. *J. Nutr.* 56: 349–70.

Nelson, M. M.; Wright, H. V.; Baird, C. D. C.; and Evans, H. M. 1956*b*. Effect of a 36-hour period of pteroylglutamic acid deficiency on fetal development in rats. *Proc. Soc. Exp. Biol. Med.* 92: 554–56.

――――. 1957. Teratogenic effects of pantothenic acid deficiency in the rat. *J. Nutr.* 62: 395–405.

Nes, N. 1959. Spina bifida ledsaget av muskelkontraktur og andre defekter hos kalv. *Nord. Vet. Med.* 11: 33–54.

Neuweiler, W., and Richter, R. H. H. 1964. Beitrage zur Frage der Entstehung kongenitaler Anomalien. Bisherige Ergebnisse unserer Versuche über die Wirkung verschiedener Substanzen auf die embryonale und foetale Entwicklung der Ratte. In *Medikamentöse Pathogenese fetaler Missbildungen*, ed. T. Koller, and H. Erb, pp. 47–79. Basel: Karger.

Nevermann. 1901. Eine Kalbsmissgeburt und deren Entwicklung. *Berlin. Tierärztl. Wschr.* 17: 705–7.

Neveu-Lemaire, M. 1899. Description anatomique d'un mouton triocéphale. *Bull. Soc. Zool. France* 24: 74–87.

———. 1902. Description anatomique d'un jeune chat monstrueux du genre synote. *Bull. Soc. Zool. France* 27: 123–28.

Newberne, P. M. 1962. The subcommissural organ of the vitamin B_{12}-deficient rat. *J. Nutr.* 76: 393–413.

Newberne, P. M., and O'Dell, B. L. 1958. Histopathology of hydrocephalus resulting from a deficiency of vit. B_{12}. *Proc. Soc. Exp. Biol. Med.* 97: 62–65.

———. 1959. Pathology of vitamin B_{12} deficiency in infant rats. *J. Nutr.* 68: 343–57.

Nickerson, W. S. 1917. Achondroplasia in a calf with a thymus in place of a thyroid. *J. Lancet.* 27: 7–10.

Nicolas, A., and Prenant, A. 1888. Observations d'une monstruosité rare. (Absence du maxillaire inférieur. Défaut de communication entre la bouche et les fosses nasales d'une part, le pharynx et pharynx d'autre part.) *J. Anat. Physiol. (Paris)* 24: 113–41.

Niedoba, T. 1924. Über den Haarstrich einiger Doppelmissbildungen des Rindes. *Anat. Anz.* 58: 564–72.

Nishikawa, M. 1963. Influence of maternal fasting for a short period upon the development of mouse embryos. [In Japanese with English summary.] *Acta Anat. Nippon.* 38: 181–84.

———. 1964. Teratogenic effect of combined administration of fasting and thio-TEPA upon mouse embryos. [In Japanese with English summary.] *Acta Anat. Nippon.* 39: 252–57.

Nishimura, H. 1963. Interstrain differences in susceptibility to the teratogenic effects of mitomycin C in mice. *Abst. Terat. Soc.* 3: 16. (Abst.)

Nishimura, H., and Kuginuki, M. 1958. Congenital malformations induced by ethyl-urethan in mouse embryos. *Folia Anat. Jap.* 31: 1–10.

Nishimura, H., and Nakai, K. 1960. Congenital malformations in offspring of mice treated with caffeine. *Proc. Soc. Exp. Biol. Med.* 104: 140–42.

Nishimura, H., and Takagaki, S. 1959*a*. Congenital malformations in mice induced by nitrogen mustard. *Acta Schol. Med. Univ. Kioto Jap.* 36: 20–26.

———. 1959*b*. Developmental anomalies in mice induced by 2,3-dimercapto-propanol (BAL). *Anat. Rec.* 135: 261–68.

Nobele, de, and Lams, H. 1927. Über die Wirkung der Röntgenstrahlen auf die Schwangerschaft und die Entwicklung des Fötus. *Strahlentherapie* 25: 702–7.

Nordby, J. E. 1929. An inherited skull defect in swine. A preliminary report on the inheritance of a fronto-parietal skeletal defect involving the meningocoele and proencephalus types of cranioschisis in swine. *J. Hered.* 20: 228–32.

Nordby, J. E., and Taylor, B. L. 1928. A syncephalus thoracopagus monster in swine. *Am. Nat.* 62: 34–47.

Nuss, J. I. L. 1966. Evidence for unrelated multiple-gene mutations as the cause of a hydrocephalus syndrome in newborn calves. *Diss. Abst.* 26: 6323–24. (Abst.)

Nusshag, W. 1925. Ueber das gehaüfte Auftreten einer Missbildung am Fohlendarm. *Berlin. Tierärztl. Wschr.* 41: 646–48.

Obbink, H. J. K. 1955/57. Bijdrage tot de kennis omtrent de oorzaken van aangeboren misvormingen van niet-erfelijke oorsprong. Een experimenteel onderzoek bij ratten over het verband tussen foliumzuurdeficientie tijdens de zwangerschap en het onstaan van aangeboren hydrocephalus. [In Dutch with English summary.] *Mededel. Lab. Physiol. Chem. Univ. Amsterdam Ned. Inst. Volksvoed* 16: 1–132.

Obbink, H. J. K., and Dalderup, L. M. 1964. Effect of acetylsalicylic acid on foetal mice and rats. *Lancet* 1: 565.

O'Brien, C. A.; Hupp, E. W.; Austin, J. W.; Szabuniewicz, M.; and Sorensen, A. M., Jr. 1963. Multiple anomalies occurring in a new-born Spanish goat following prenatal gamma-radiation. *Nature* 200: 906–7.

O'Brien, C. A.; Hupp, E. W.; Sorensen, A. M., Jr.; and Brown, S. O. 1964. The response of Spanish goats to prenatally administered gamma radiation. *J. Anim. Sci.* 23: 911. (Abst.)

O'Dell, B. L.; Hardwick, B. C.; and Reynolds, G. 1961. Mineral deficiencies of milk and congenital malformations in the rat. *J. Nutr.* 73: 151–57.

O'Dell, B. L.; Whitley, J. R.; and Hogan, A. G. 1948. Relation of folic acid and vitamin A to incidence of hydrocephalus in infant rats. *Proc. Soc. Exp. Biol. Med.* 69: 272–75.

———. 1951. Vitamin B_{12}, a factor in prevention of hydrocephalus in infant rats. *Proc. Soc. Exp. Biol. Med.* 76: 349–53.

Oettel, H., and Frohberg, H. 1964. Teratogene Wirkung einfacher Säureamide im Tierversuch. *Naunyn Schmiedeberg Arch. Exp. Path.* 247: 363.

O'Hara, P. J., and Shortridge, E. H. 1966. Congenital anomalies of the porcine central nervous system. *New Zealand Vet. J.* 14: 13–18.

Ohba, N. 1958. Formation of embryonic abnormalities of the mouse by a viral infection of mother animals. *Acta Path. Jap.* 8: 127–38.

———. 1959a. Formation of embryonic abnormalities of the mouse by a viral infection of mother animals (second report). *Acta Path. Jap.* 9: 149–57.

———. 1959b. Embryonic abnormalities caused by the endotoxin injection of mother animals. *Acta Path. Jap.* 9: 141–48.

Ohzu, E. 1965. Effects of low dose X-irradiation on early mouse embryos. *Radiat. Res.* 26: 107–113.

Ohzu, E., and Makino, S. 1964. Some abnormalities produced by low dose X-irradiations in early mouse embryos. *Proc. Jap. Acad.* 40: 670–73.

Ohzu, E., and Shoji, R. 1965. Preliminary notes on abnormalities induced by velban in developing mouse embryos. *Proc. Jap. Acad.* 41: 321–25.

Okano, K.; Esumi, K.; Ito ,S.; Kashiyama, S.; Fujita, H.; Toba, T.; and Ito, H. 1958. Influences of nitromin on rat embryo. *Acta Path. Jap.* 8: 561. (Abst.)

Okano, K.; Fujita, H.; Ito, T.; Kashiyama, S.; Esumi, K.; Ito, H.; and Toba, T. 1959. Effects of thio-TEPA on fetus of albino rats. *Acta Path. Jap.* 9: 644–45. (Abst.)

Okano, K.; Ito, T.; Kashiyama, S.; Esumi, K.; Fujita, H.; Ito, H.; and Toba, T. 1957. Histochemical studies on experimental anencephaly and absence of kidney caused by irradiation. *Acta Path. Jap.* 7: 445–46. (Abst.)

Okuda, K. 1964. Noise-stimulation effects on pregnant rats and its fetuses. [In Japanese with English summary.] *J. Otorhinolaryng. Soc. Jap.* 67: 843–48.

Olivecrona, H. 1964. Embryo-destroying effect of injected phenobarbital in the mouse. *Acta Anat.* 58: 217–21.

Onions, C. T., ed. 1956. *The shorter Oxford English dictionary on historical principles.* 3d ed. rev. with addenda. London: Oxford Univ. Press.

Ordy, J. M.; Latanick, A.; Johnson, R.; and Massopust, L. 1963. Chlorpromazine effects on pregnancy and offspring in mice. *Proc. Soc. Exp. Biol. Med.* 113: 833–36.

Orr, S. C. 1888. Strange freak of nature. *J. Comp. Med. Surg.* 10: 377–78.

Örs, T., and Karátson, D. 1936. Ritka borjútorz. (Dicephalus tetrabrachius.) [In Hungarian.] *Allatorv. Lapok* 59: 244–48.

Osipovskiy, A. I.; Afanas'ev, Y. I.; Pauper, A. I.; and Sukhanov, Y. S. 1963. Central nervous system developmental anomalies and deformities in successive generations of gamma-ray-irradiated animals. [In Russian; English translation AEC-tr-5434.] *Radiobiologiya* 3: 120–27.

Osipovskiy, A. I., and Kunicheva, G. S. 1959. Developmental anomalies in the offspring of guinea pigs irradiated by gamma-rays and the inheritance of them by a number of generations. [In Russian.] *Med. Radiol. (U.S.S.R.)* 4: 65–76.

Ostertag, B. 1930*a*. Die Syringomyelie als erbbiologisches Problem. *Verh. Deut. Path. Ges.* 25: 166–74.

———. 1930*b*. Weitere Untersuchungen über vererbbare Syringomyelie des Kaninchens. *Deut. Z. Nervenheilk.* 116: 147–54.

———. 1934. Neuere Ergebnisse bei der vererbbaren Syringomyelie des Kaninchens. *Atti X Cong. Mond. Pollicolt.* 3: 526–32.

Otis, E. M. 1953. Prenatal mortality rates of seventeen radiation induced translocations in mice. Univ. of Rochester Atomic Energy Report UR-291.

Otto, A. W. 1816. *Seltene Beobachtungen zur Anatomie, Physiologie und Pathologie gehörig.* Breslau: Holäufer.

———. 1824. *Neue seltene Beobachtungen zur Anatomie, Physiologie und Pathologie gehörig.* Berlin: Rücker.

Oules, M. 1909. Sur un cas d'hydrocéphalie chez un chien. *Toulouse Méd.*, ser. 2 11: 250–56.

Overholser, M. D.; Whitley, J. R.; O'Dell, B. L.; and Hogan, A. G. 1954. The ventricular system in hydrocephalic rat brains produced by a deficiency of vitamin B_{12} or of folic acid in the maternal diet. *Anat. Rec.* 120: 917–34.

Ozawa, G. 1899. Diprosopus triophthalmos in a newborn cat. *Tokyo Med. J.*, pp. 1372–75.

Paget, G. E., and Thorpe, E. 1964. A teratogenic effect of a sulphonamide in experimental animals. *Brit. J. Pharmacol*, 23: 305–12.

Pahnish, O. F.; Stanley, E. B.; and Safley, C. E. 1955. The inheritance of a dwarf anomaly in beef cattle. *J. Anim. Sci.* 14: 200–7.

Pahnish, O. F.; Stanley, E. B.; Safley, C. E.; and Roubicek, C. B. 1955. Dwarfism in beef cattle. *Agr. Exp. Sta. Univ. Arizona Bull.* 268.

Pai, A. C., and Gluecksohn-Waelsch, S. 1961. Interactions of *t* alleles at the *T* locus in the house mouse. *Experientia* 17: 372–74.

414   References

Palludan, B. 1961. The teratogenic effect of vitamin A deficiency in pigs. *Acta Vet. Scand.* 2: 32–59.

————. *A-Avitaminosis in swine: A study on the importance of vitamin A for reproduction.* Copenhagen: Munksgaard.

Pálsson, P. A., and Grímsson, H. 1953. Demyelination in lambs from ewes which feed on seaweeds. *Proc. Soc. Exp. Biol. Med.* 83: 518–20.

Pantelouris, E. M. 1958. Protection of foetuses against radiation injury. *Nature* 181: 563–64.

Panu, A., and Adamşteanu, I. 1937. Hydrocéphalie interne, cyphose et autres anomalies congénitales chez le chien. *Arh. Vet. (Bucharest)* 29: 16–21.

Panu, A.; Mihailesco, M.; and Adamşteanu, I. 1939. Hypoplasie cérébelleuse et pachygyrie chez la chatte. *Arh. Vet. (Bucharest)* 31: 18–27.

Panum, P. L. 1860. *Untersuchungen über die Entstehung der Missbildungen zunächst in den Eiern der Vögel.* Berlin: Reimer.

————. 1878. Beiträge zur Kenntnis der physiologischen Bedeutung der Angebornen Missbildungen. *Virchow Arch. Path. Anat.* 72: 69–91.

Paoletti, C.; Riou, G.; and Truhaut, R. 1962. Electrophoretic pattern of plasma proteins in rats treated with trypan blue and ethionine. *Nature* 193: 784–85.

Papez, J. W., and Rundles, R. W. 1938. Thalamus of a dog without a hemisphere due to unilateral congenital hydrocephalus. *J. Comp. Neur.* 69: 89–102.

Parrott, M. W.; Johnston, M. E.; and Durbin, P. W. 1960. The effect of thyroid and parathyroid deficiency on reproduction in the rat. *Endocrinology* 67: 467–83.

Parsons, P. A. 1963. Congenital abnormalities and competition in man and other mammals at different maternal ages. *Nature* 198: 316–17.

Patt, H. M., and Brues, A. M. 1954. The pathological physiology of radiation injury in the mammal. I. Physical and biological factors in radiation injury. In *Radiation biology,* ed. A. Hollaender, vol. 1, pt. 2, pp. 919–58. New York: McGraw-Hill.

Patten, B. M. 1952. Overgrowth of the neural tube in young human embryos. *Anat. Rec.* 113: 381–93.

————.1953. Embryological stages in the establishing of myeloschisis with spina bifida. *Am. J. Anat.* 93: 365–95.

Pearce, L. 1950. Hereditary osteopetrosis of the rabbit. IV. Pathologic observations; general features. *J. Exp. Med.* 92: 601–24.

Pearce, L., and Brown, W. H. 1945*a*. Hereditary achondroplasia in the rabbit. II. Pathologic aspects. *J. Exp. Med.* 82: 261–80.

————. 1945*b*. Hereditary achondroplasia in the rabbit. III. Genetic aspects; general considerations. *J. Exp. Med.* 82: 281–95.

————. 1948. Hereditary osteopetrosis of the rabbit. I. General features and course of disease; genetic aspects. *J. Exp. Med.* 88: 579–96.

Pearn, J. H., and Vickers, T. H. 1966. The rabbit thalidomide embryopathy. *Brit. J. Exp. Path.* 47: 186–92.

Pellegrin, J. 1901. Présentation d'un foetus de chat monstre synote. *Bull. Soc. Zool. France* 26: 153–55.

Penhale, R. E. L. 1907. Monstrosity. *Vet. Rec.* 19: 772.

Pennycuik, P. R. 1964. The effects on rats of chronic exposure to 34°C. IV. Reproduction. *Aust. J. Biol. Sci.* 17: 245–60.

————. 1965. The effects of acute exposure to high temperatures on prenatal development in the mouse with particular reference to secondary vibrissae. *Aust. J. Biol. Sci.* 18: 97–113.

Perry, J. H. 1961. Alterations in blood-brain barrier in experimental hydrocephalus. In *Disorders of the developing nervous system*, ed. W. S. Fields, and M. M. Desmond, pp. 326–42. Springfield, Ill. Thomas.

Persaud, T. V. N. 1965. Tierexperimentelle Untersuchungen zur Frage der teratogenen Wirkung von Barbituraten. *Acta Biol. Med. Ger.* 14: 89–90.

Petiot, M. P. 1950. Hydrocéphalie du poulain. *Rec. Méd. Vét.* 126: 467–70.

Petit, G. 1893. Description d'un monstre double sysomien du genre dérodyme. *Rec. Méd. Vét.* 70: 292–96.

Pfaltz, H., and Severinghaus, E. L. 1956. Effects of vitamin deficiencies on fertility, course of pregnancy, and embryonic development in rats. *Am. J. Obstet. Gynec.* 72: 265–76.

Pfeffer, W. 1932. Über Zweiköpfigkeit bei Tier und Mensch. *Beitr. Path. Anat.* 89: 575–601.

Phillips, J. M. 1945. "Pig jaw" in cocker spaniels. Retrognathia of the mandible in the cocker spaniel and its relationship to other deformities of the jaw. *J. Hered.* 36: 177–81.

Phisalix, C. 1888. Note sur la cyclopie chez les mammifères. *C. R. Soc. Biol.*, ser. 8 5: 667–69.

————. 1889. Monstres cyclopes. *J. Anat. Physiol.* (*Paris*) 25: 67–105.

Pickard, J. N. 1933. Some heritable defects in rabbits. *Vet. J.* 89: 23–24.

Pigné. 1841. Tête d'un chevreau cyclocéphale. *Bull. Soc. Anat. Paris* 16: 138.

Pike, R. L.; Kirksey, A.; and Callahan, J. 1959. Effects of 6-aminonicotinamide administration during pregnancy upon the maternal rat and her offspring. *Fed. Proc.* 18: 541. (Abst.)

Pilcher, L. S. 1880. Double monsters. *Ann. Anat. Surg. Soc. Brooklyn* 2: 19–33.

Pinsky, L., and DiGeorge, A. M. 1965. Cleft palate in the mouse: A teratogenic index of glucocorticoid potency. *Science* 147: 402–3.

Pinsky, L., and Fraser, F. C. 1959. Production of skeletal malformations in the offspring of pregnant mice treated with 6-aminonicotinamide. *Biol. Neonat.* 1: 106–12.

————. 1960. Congenital malformations after a two-hour inactivation of nicotinamide in pregnant mice. *Brit. Med. J.* 2: 195–97.

Pisani, J. F., and Kerr, W. E. 1961. Lethal equivalents in domestic animals. *Genetics* 46: 773–86.

Plagens, G. M. 1933. An embryological study of a special strain of deformed x-rayed mice, with special reference to the etiology and morphogenesis of the abnormalities. *J. Morph.* 55: 151–83.

Pobedinskiy, N. M. 1961. The influence of ionizing radiation on pregnancy and the development of the fetus. [In Russian; English translation by U.S. Joint Publ. Res. Serv., No. 10884.] *Med. Radiol.* (*U.S.S.R.*) 6: 111–31.

Pobisch, R. 1960. Die Einwirkung der Röntgenstrahlen auf den Kaninchenembryo mit besonderer Berücksichtigung der postnatalen Entwicklung. Untersuchung zur Festellung der wichtigsten kritischen Perioden des Kaninchenembryos von 8. bis 24. graviditätstag. *Radiol. Austriac.* 11: 19–82.

Poenaru, L., and Vechiu, A. 1922. Sur un cas d'ataxie cérébelleuse congénitale chez le chat. *Arh. Vet.* (*Bucharest*) 16: 1–4.

Poswillo, D. 1966. Observations of fetal posture and causal mechanisms of congenital deformity of palate, mandible, and limbs. *J. Dent. Res.* 45: 584–96.

Potter, E. L. 1961. *Pathology of the fetus and infant.* 2d. ed. Chicago: Year Book Medical Publ.

Pouchet, and Beauregard. 1882. Veau monstrueux iniodyme. *C. R. Soc. Biol.*, ser. 7 4: 521–23.

Poulson, E., and Robson, J. M. 1964. Effect of phenelzine and some related compounds on pregnancy and on sexual development. *J. Endocr.* 30: 205–15.

Poulson, E., Robson, J. M., and Sullivan, F. M. 1963. Teratogenic effects of 5-hydroxytryptamine in mice. *Science* 141: 717–18.

Pozhidayev, E. A. 1961. Effects of X-ray irradiation of rats prior to pregnancy upon subsequent embryogenesis. [In Russian, English translation by U.S. Joint Publ. Res. Serv., No. 12387.] *Radiobiologiya* 1: 316–42.

Prior, G. P. U.; Hunter, J. I.; and Latham, O. 1924. Atavism and endocrine pecularities in pigs. *Med. J. Aust.* 2: 89–92.

Pullig, T. 1952. Inheritance of a skull defect in cocker spaniels. *J. Hered.* 43: 97–99.

Punnett, R. C. 1936. The experiments of T. H. Riches concerning the production of monsters in cattle. *J. Genet.* 32: 65–72.

Rabaud, E. 1905. Etudes anatomiques sur les monstres composés. I. Chat monocéphalien déradelphe. *Bull. Soc. Philom. Paris*, ser. 9 7: 323–47.

Radasch, H. E. 1912. A contribution to the teratology of the domestic animals; incomplete duplication. *Anat. Anz.* 42: 481–98.

Ranström, S. 1956. Stress and pregnancy. *Acta Path. Microbiol. Scand. Suppl.* 111: 113–14.

Raschke, O. 1922. Kephalothorakopagus vom Hund. *Deut. Tierärztl. Wschr.* 30: 441–42.

———. 1927. Kleine pathologisch-anatomische Mitteilungen. *Deut. Tierärztl. Wschr.* 35: 468–70.

Rayer, P. 1852. Sur deux cas rares de monstruosité. *C. R. Soc. Biol.*, ser. 1 4: 341–48.

———. 1862. Sur plusieurs monstres de lièvre et de perdreau. *C. R. Soc. Biol.*, ser. 3 4: 111–12.

Rebollo, M. A. 1958. Rôle des pressions liquidiennes dans la morphogenèse de l'encéphale. *C. R. Soc. Biol.* 152: 312–14.

Reddy, D. S., and Balasubramanyam. 1949. A case of bicephalous monstrosity [*sic*] in a buffalo-calf. *Ind. Vet. J.* 26: 421–22.

Reddy, D. V.; Adams, F. H.; and Baird, C. 1963. Teratogenic effects of serotonin. *J. Pediat.* 63: 394–97.

Reed, S. C. 1937. The inheritance and expression of Fused, a new mutation in the house mouse. *Genetics* 22: 1–13.

Rees, H. G. 1966. Aprosopus: A synotia-like condition in a stillborn calf. *Vet. Rec.* 79: 484–85.

Reese, A. M. 1911. The anatomy of a double cat. *Anat. Rec.* 5: 383–90.

———. 1914. The osteology of a double-headed calf. *Am. Nat.* 48: 701–4.

———. 1917. The anatomy of a two-headed lamb. *Anat. Rec.* 13: 179–97.

———. 1937. Another lamb cyclops. *Anat. Anz.* 84: 198–203.

Regan, W. M.; Mead, S. W.; and Gregory, P. W. 1947. The relation of inbreeding to calf mortality. *Growth* 11: 101–31.

Regnault, F. 1901. Forme du crâne dans l'hydrocéphalie chez les animaux. *Bull. Soc. Anat. Paris* 76: 460.

Reisinger, L. 1915. Konfiguration der Rückenmarke einer Doppelmissbildung des Kalbes. *München. Tierärztl. Wschr.* 66: 277–81.

Rhodes, M. B.; Urman, H. K.; Marsh, C. L.; and Grace, O. D. 1962. Serum enzyme studies of a hydrocephalic syndrome of newborn calves. *Proc. Soc. Exp. Biol. Med.* 111: 735–37.

Riccardi, A. 1924. Di un feto bovino ciclope otocefalo (opocefalo). *Clin. Vet.* (*Milan*) 47: 405–14.

Richardson, L. R. 1951. Nutritional hydrocephalus in infant rats. *Proc. Soc. Exp. Biol. Med.* 76: 142–44.

Richardson, L. R., and DeMottier, J. 1947. Inadequate maternal nutrition and hydrocephalus in infant rats. *Science* 106: 644.

Richardson, L. R., and Hogan, A. G. 1946. Diet of mother and hydrocephalus in infant rats. *J. Nutr.* 32: 459–65.

Richman, S. M.; Thomas, W. A.; and Konikov, N. 1957. Survival of rats with induced congenital cardiovascular anomalies. *Arch. Path.* 63: 43–48.

Richter. 1887. Cyclopie, Arhinencephalie und einblasiges Gehirn. *Zbl. Nervenheilk. Psychiat.* 10: 398–99.

Riedel, P. 1963. Der Hydrocephalus congenitus internus als Geburtshindernis beim Pferd. *Mh. Veterinärmed.* 18 (Suppl.): 27–28.

Riemer, G. 1913–14. Vergleich der Gehirne einer Duplicitas anterior von Kalbe. *Stud. Path. Entwickl.* 1: 220–37.

Riggs, H. E.; McGrath, J. J.; and Schwartz, H. P. 1956. Malformation of the adult brain (albino rat) resulting from prenatal irradiation. *J. Neuropath. Exp. Neur.* 15: 432–47.

Ritter, W. 1963. Durch Röntgenstrahlen induzierte Kopfmissbildungen bei Mäuseembryonen. *Deut. Zahnärzt.* 17: 245–49.

Robertson, G. G. 1959. Embryonic development following maternal hypoxia in the rat. *Anat. Rec.* 133: 420–21. (Abst.)

Robertson, J. M.; Samankova, L.; and Ingalls, T. H. 1966. Hydrocephalus and cleft palate in an inbred rabbit colony. *J. Hered.* 57: 142–48.

Robin, M. V. 1911. Atrophie du cervelet chez un veau nouveau-né. *Rev. Vét.* 36: 601–5.

Robinson, R. 1958. Genetic studies of the rabbit. *Bibl. Genet.* 17: 229–558.

———. 1959. Genetics of the domestic cat. *Bibl. Genet.* 18: 273–362.

———. 1965. *Genetics of the Norway rat.* Oxford: Pergamon.

Robson, J. M. 1963. The problem of teratogenicity. *Practitioner* 191: 136–42.

Robson, J. M.; Poulson, E.; and Sullivan, F. M. 1965. Pharmacological principles of teratogenesis. In *Embryopathic activity of drugs,* ed. J. M. Robson, F. M. Sullivan, and R. L. Smith, pp. 21–35. Boston: Little, Brown & Co.

Robson, J. M., and Sullivan, F. M. 1963a. Mechanism of lethal action of 5-hydroxytryptamine on the foetus. *J. Endocr.* 25: 553–54.

————. 1963*b*. The production of foetal abnormalities in rabbits by imipramine. *Lancet* 1: 638–39.

Rogers, L. L.; Lloyd, A. J.; and Fowler, A. C. 1965. Teratogenic effects of drugs combined with a mild nutritional deficiency. *Fed. Proc.* 24: 443. (Abst.)

Roizin, L.; Rugh, R.; and Kaufman, M. A. 1962. Neuropathologic investigations of the x-irradiated embryo rat brain. *J. Neuropath. Exp. Neur.* 21: 219–43.

Rokkones, T. 1955. Experimental hydrocephalus in young rats. *Int. Z. Vitaminforsch.* 26: 1–10.

Rosa, F. M. da. 1946. Hidrocefalia, uma nova mutação no coelho. *Rev. Med. Vet.* (*Lisbon*) 41: 1–55.

Rosahn, P. D., and Greene, H. S. N. 1935. Birth weight criterion of dwarfism in the rabbit. *Proc. Soc. Exp. Biol. Med.* 32: 1580–83.

————. 1936. The influence of intrauterine factors on the fetal weight of rabbits. *J. Exp. Med.* 63: 901–21.

Rosenkrantz, J. G.; Githens, J. H.; Cox, S. M.; and Kellum, D. L. 1967. Azathioprine (imuran) and pregnancy. *Am. J. Obstet. Gynec.* 97: 387–94.

Ross, O. A., and Spector, S. 1952. Production of congenital abnormalities in mice by alloxan. *Am. J. Dis. Child.* 84: 647–48. (Abst.)

Ross, O. B.; Phillips, P. H.; Bohstedt, G.; and Cunha, T. J. 1944. Congenital malformations, syndactylism, talipes, and paralysis agitans of nutritional origin in swine. *J. Anim. Sci.* 3: 406–14.

Rothenbacher, H. 1962. Congenital heart, skeletal and other defects in Michigan calves. *Mich. St. Univ. Vet.* 23: 32–36.

Roux, C. 1959. Action tératogène de la prochlorpémazine. *Arch. Fr. Pédiat.* 16: 968–71.

————. 1962. A propos de la morphogénèse de la tête chez les monstres doubles. *C. R. Soc. Biol.* 156: 1759–61.

————. 1964. Action tératogène du triparanol chez l'animal. *Arch. Fr. Pédiat.* 21: 451–64.

Roux, C., and Aubry, M. 1966. Action tératogène chez le rat, d'un inhibiteur de la synthèse du cholesterol, le AY 9944. *C. R. Soc. Biol.* 160: 1353–57.

Roux, C.; Cahen, R.; and Dupuis, R. 1965. Malformations viscérales provoquées par le thalidomide chez le lapin. *C. R. Soc. Biol.* 159: 1059–63.

Roux, C., and Dupuis, R. 1961. Action tératogène du triparanol. *C. R. Soc. Biol.* 155: 2255–57.

————. 1966. Action tératogène du triparanol chez la souris. *C. R. Soc. Biol.* 160: 923–28.

Roux, C.; Fournier, R.; Dupuis, Y.; and Dupuis, R. 1962. Carence tératogène en vitamine A. *Biol. Neonat.* 4: 371–78.

Ruch, T. C. 1959. *Diseases of laboratory primates*. Philadelphia: Saunders.

Rudd, T. W. 1907. Abnormal head of a calf. *Vet. J.* 63: 354–55.

Ruffolo, P. R., and Ferm, V. H. 1965*a*. The teratogenicity of 5-bromodeoxyuridine in the pregnant Syrian hamster. *Life Sci.* 4: 633–37.

————. 1965*b*. The embryocidal and teratogenic effects of 5-bromodeoxyuridine in the pregnant hamster. *Lab. Inv.* 14: 1547–53.

Rugh, R. 1962. Low levels of X-irradiation and the early mammalian embryo. *Am. J. Roentgen.* 87: 559–66.

————. 1965. Effect of ionizing radiations, including radioisotopes, on the placenta and embryo. *Birth Defects Original Article Series* 1: 64–73.

Rugh, R.; Caveness, W. F.; Duhamel, L.; and Schwartz, G. S. 1963. Structural and functional (electro-encephalographic) changes in the post-natal mammalian brain resulting from X-irradiation of the embryo. *Milit. Med.* 128: 392–408.

Rugh, R., and Clugston, H. 1955. Protection of mouse fetus against X-irradiation death. *Science* 123: 28–29.

Rugh, R.; Duhamel, L.; Chandler, A.; and Varma, A. 1964. Cataract development after embryonic and fetal X-irradiation. *Radiat. Res.* 22: 519–34.

Rugh, R.; Duhamel, L.; Skaredoff, L.; and Somogyi, C. 1966. Gross sequelae of fetal x-irradiation of the monkey (*Macaca mulatta*). I. Effect on body and organ weights at 23 months. *Atompraxis* 12: 468–73.

Rugh, R., and Grupp, E. 1959a. X-irradiation exencephaly. *Am. J. Roentgen.* 81: 1026–52.

————. 1959b. Exencephalia following x-irradiation of the pre-implantation embryo. *J. Neuropath. Exp. Neur.* 18: 468–81.

————. 1959c. Response of the very early mouse embryo to low levels of ionizing radiation. *J. Exp. Zool.* 141: 571–87.

————. 1960a. Fractionated x-irradiation of the mammalian embryo and congenital anomalies. *Am. J. Roentgen.* 84: 125–44.

————. 1960b. Protection of the embryo against the congenital and lethal effects of x-irradiation (pt. I and pt. II). Atompraxis 6: 143–48, 209–17.

————. 1961. Neuropathological effects of low-level X-irradiation of the mammalian embryo. *Milit. Med.* 126: 647–64.

Rugh, R.; Grupp, E.; and Wohlfromm, M. 1961. Evidence of prenatal heterosis relating to X-ray induced congenital anomalies. *Proc. Soc. Exp. Biol. Med.* 106: 219–21.

Rugh, R., and Wohlfromm, M. 1962. Can the mammalian embryo be killed by X-irradiation? *J. Exp. Zool.* 151: 227–44.

————. 1963a. X-irradiation-induced congenital anomalies in hybrid mice. *Biol. Bull.* 124: 303–10.

————. 1963b. Age of the mother and previous breeding history and the incidence of X-ray-induced congenital anomalies. *Radiat. Res.* 19: 261–69.

————. 1966. Previous reproductive history and the susceptibility to X-ray-induced congenital anomalies. *Nature* 210: 969–70.

Rugh, R., and Wolff, J. 1955a. Resilience of the fetal eye following radiation insult. *Proc. Soc. Exp. Biol. Med.* 89: 248–53.

————. 1955b. Reparation of the fetal eye following radiation insult. *Arch. Ophth.* 54: 351–59.

Rumpf, T. 1885. Beiträge zur pathologischen Anatomie des centralen Nervensystems. *Arch. Psychiat. Nervenkr.* 16: 410–41.

Runner, M. N. 1954. Inheritance of susceptibility to congenital deformity— embryonic instability. *J. Nat. Canc. Inst.* 15: 637–49.

————. 1959. Inheritance of susceptibility to congenital deformity. Metabolic clues provided by experiments with teratogenic agents. *Pediatrics* 23: 245–51.

————. 1965. Syndrome response to interaction of teratogenic treatments. *Congen. Anom.* 5: 219–21.

Runner, M. N. and Dagg, C. P. 1960. Metabolic mechanisms of teratogenic agents during morphogenesis. *Nat. Canc. Inst. Monogr.* 2: 41–54.

Runner, M. N., and Miller, J. R. 1956. Congenital deformity in the mouse as a consequence of fasting. *Anat. Rec.* 124: 437–38. (Abst.)

Russell, D. S. 1949. Observations on the pathology of hydrocephalus. Medical Research Council Special Report Series, No. 285, London: H.M.S.O.

Russell, D. S., and Donald, C. 1935. The mechanism of internal hydrocephalus in spina bifida. *Brain* 58: 203–15.

Russell, E. S. 1954. Search for new cases of parental and seasonal influences upon variations within inbred strains. *Ann. N. Y. Acad. Sci.* 57: 597–605.

Russell, J. S. R. 1895a. Defective development of the central nervous system in a cat. *Brain* 18: 37–53.

———. 1895b. Defective development of the cerebellum in a puppy. *Brain* 18: 523–30.

Russell, L. B. 1950. X-ray induced developmental abnormalities in the mouse and their use in the analysis of embryological patterns. I. External and gross visceral changes. *J. Exp. Zool.* 114: 545–601.

———. 1954. The effects of radiation on mammalian prenatal development. In *Radiation biology*, ed. A. Hollaender, vol. 1 pt. 2, pp. 861–918. New York: McGraw-Hill.

———. 1956. X-ray-induced developmental abnormalities in the mouse and their use in the analysis of embryological patterns. II. Abnormalities of the vertebral column and thorax. *J. Exp. Zool.* 131: 329–95.

———. 1965. Death and chromosome damage from irradiation of preimplantation stages. In *Ciba Foundation symposium on preimplantation stages of pregnancy*, ed. G. E. W. Wolstenholme, and C. M. O'Connor, pp. 217–41. Boston: Little, Brown & Co.

Russell, L. B.; Badgett, S. K.; and Saylors, C. L. 1960. Comparison of effects of acute, continuous, and fractionated irradiation during embryonic development. In *Immediate and low level effects of ionizing radiation*, ed. A. A. Buzzati-Traverso, pp. 343–59. London: Taylor & Francis.

Russell, L. B., and Major, M. H. 1957. Radiation-induced presumed somatic mutations in the house mouse. *Genetics* 42: 161–75.

Russell, L. B., and Montgomery, C. S. 1965. Radiation-sensitivity differences within cell-division cycles during mouse cleavage. *Int. J. Radiat. Biol.* 10: 151–64.

Russell, L. B., and Russell, W. L. 1950. The effects of radiation on the preimplantation stages of the mouse embryo. *Anat. Rec.* 108: 521. (Abst.)

———. 1952. Radiation hazards to the embryo and fetus. *Radiology* 58: 369–76.

———. 1954a. An analysis of the changing radiation response of the developing mouse embryo. *J. Cell. Comp. Physiol.* 43 (Suppl.): 103–47.

———. 1954b. Pathways of radiation effects in the mother and the embryo. *Cold Spring Harbor Symp. Quant. Biol.* 14: 50–58.

Russell, L. B.; Russell, W. L.; and Major, M. H. 1951. The effect of hypoxia on the radiation induction of developmental abnormalities in the mouse. *Anat. Rec.* 11: 455. (Abst.)

Russell, W. L. 1947. Splotch, a new mutation in the house mouse, *Mus musculus*. *Genetics* 32: 102. (Abst.)

————. 1954. Genetic effects of radiation in mammals. In *Radiation biology*, ed. A. Hollaender, vol. 1, pt. 2, pp. 825–59. New York: McGraw-Hill.

Russell, W. L., and Gower, J. S. 1950. Offspring from transplanted ovaries of fetal mice homozygous for a lethal gene (*Sp*) that kills before birth. *Genetics* 53: 133–34. (Abst.)

Sachs, R. 1963. Missbildungen, Entwicklungsstörungen und Anomalien beim Karakulschaf. With a summary in English. Sammlung einiger tierärztlich-tierzüchterisch interessanter pathologisch-anatomischer Präparate und Gedanken zur Karakulzucht in Südwestafrika von der Warte des praktischen Tierarztes. *Yearb. S.W. Afr. Karakul Breeders Ass.* 6: 21–27, 29–31, 33–37, 39, 101, 103.

Saint-Hilaire, I. G. 1832–37. *Histoire générale et particulière des anomalies de l'organisation chez l'homme et les animaux, ouvrage comprenant des recherches sur les caractères, la classification, l'influence physiologique et pathologique, les rapports généraux, les lois et les causes des monstruosités, des variétés et vices de conformation, ou traité de tératologie.* 3 vols. and atlas. Paris: Baillière.

————. 1850. Rapport sur un veau phocomèle et hydrocéphale, et sur des figures de ce monstre transmises à l'Académie par M. le Ministre de l'Agriculture et du Commerce. *C. R. Acad. Sci.* 31: 668–70.

Salzgeber, B., and Wolff, E. 1964. Experimental production of malformations of the limbs by means of chemical substances. *Int. Rev. Exp. Path.* 3: 329–63.

Sansone, G., and Zunin, C. 1953. Embriopatie sperimentali da deficienza di acido folico nel ratto, prodotte mediante somministrazione di aminopterina. *Bull. Soc. Ital. Biol. Sper.* 29: 1697–99.

Sansone, G., and Zunin, C. 1954. Embriopatie sperimentali da somministrazione di antifolici. *Acta Vitamin.* 8: 73–79.

Sapre, M. V. 1953. Dicephalous monstrosity in a murrah buffalo. *Ind. Vet. J.* 29: 549.

Sarvella, P. A., and Russell, L. B. 1956. Steel, a new dominant gene in the house mouse with effects on coat pigment and blood. *J. Hered.* 47: 123–28.

Sato, A. 1963. On some effects of ionizing radiations upon developing polyovulated mouse eggs. *Embryologia* 7: 320–30.

Saunders, L. Z.; Sweet, J. D.; Martin, S. M.; Fox, F. H.; and Fincher, M. G. 1952. Hereditary congenital ataxia in Jersey calves. *Cornell Vet.* 42: 559–91.

Sautter, J. H.; Young, G. A.; Luedke, A. J.; and Kitchell, R. L. 1953. The experimental production of malformations and other abnormalities in fetal pigs by means of attenuated hog cholera virus. *Proc. Am. Vet. Med. Ass.* 90: 146–50.

Sawin, P. B. 1955. Recent genetics of the domestic rabbit. *Adv. Genet.* 7: 183–226.

Sawin, P. B., and Crary, D. D. 1955. Hereditary scoliosis in the rabbit. *Anat. Rec.* 121: 449–50. (Abst.)

————. 1957. Morphogenetic studies of the rabbit. XVII. Disproportionate adult size caused by the *Da* gene. *Genetics* 42: 72–91.

————. 1964. Genetics of skeletal deformities in the domestic rabbit (*Oryctolagus cuniculus*). *Clin. Orthopaed.* 33: 71–90.

Sawin, P. B.; Crary, D. D.; Fox, R. R.; Trask, M.; and Wuest, H. M. 1964. A pilot study of thalidomide effects on the rabbit. *Abst. Terat. Soc.* 4: 17–18. (Abst.)

Sawin, P. B.; Crary, D. D.; Fox, R. R.; and Wuest, H. M. 1965. Thalidomide malformations and genetic background in the rabbit. *Experientia* 21: 672–77.

Scaglia, G. 1927. Osservazioni sugli encefali di un agnello dicefalo monoaucheno. Contributo alla conoscenza delle somiglianze fra gemelli uniovulari. *Monit. Zool. Ital.* 38: 110–20.

Scaglione, S. 1962. Osservazioni e ricerche sull'azione dell'insulina sugli embrioni di ratte gravide con microfotografie. *Acta Genet. Med.* (*Rome*) 11: 418–29.

Schaible, R. H. 1961. *Mouse News Letter* 24: 38–39.

Scheidy, S. F. 1953. Familial cerebellar hypoplasia in cats. *N. Am. Vet.* 34: 118–19.

Schellenberg, K. 1909. Über Hochdifferenzierte Missbildungen des Grosshirns bei Haustieren. Ein Beitrag zur vergleichenden pathologischen Anatomie der Entwicklungsstörungen des Zentralnervensystems. *Arb. Hirnanat. Inst. Zürich.* 3: 1–48.

Scherer, H. J. 1944. *Vergleichende Pathologie des Nervensystems der Säugetiere unter besonderer Berücksichtigung der Primaten.* Leipzig: Thieme.

Schindler, H. 1956. "Amputated" calves in local herds. [In Hebrew.] *Refuah Vet.* 13: 78–79.

Schlegel, M. 1909. Bericht über die Tätigkeit des tierhygienischen Instituts der Universität Freiburg i. Br. im Jahre 1908. *Z. Tiermed.* 13: 337–53.

———. 1912. Kephalothorakopagus s. Synkephalus mit asymmetrischem Januskopf bei einem Schweinezwilling. *Z. Tiermed.* 16: 356–57.

———. 1913. Bericht über die Tätigkeit des tierhygienischen Instituts der Universität Freiburg i. Br. im Jahre 1912. *Z. Tiermed.* 17: 369–99.

———. 1914. Bericht über die Tätigkeit des tierhygienischen Instituts der Universität Freiburg i. Br. im Jahre 1913. *Z. Tiermed.* 18: 364–405.

———. 1916. Mitteilungen aus dem tierhygienischen Institut der Universität Freiburg i. Br. im Jahre 1914. *Z. Infektionskr. Haustier.* 17: 246–89.

———. 1920*a*. Akrania et Anencephalia, Diprosopus triophthalmus makrostomus diotus, Palatoschisis und Dignathia inferior beim Kalb. *Z. Infektionskr. Haustier.* 20: 316–18.

———. 1920*b*. Kyklenkephalie, Hydrocephalus congenitus, Arhinenkephalie, Synophthalmia bei einem neugeborenen Zicklein. *Z. Infektionskr. Haustier.* 20: 318–19.

———. 1921. Die Missbildungen der Tiere. *Erg. Allg. Path.* 19: 650–732.

Schlotthauer, C. F. 1934. Internal hydrocephalus in a dog. *J. Am. Vet. Med. Ass.* 85: 788–94.

———. 1936. Internal hydrocephalus in dogs. *J. Am. Vet. Med. Ass.* 89: 141–49.

———. 1959. Diseases affecting the nervous system. In *Canine medicine*, ed. H. P. Hoskins, J. V. Lacroix, and K. Mayer, pp. 573–94. Santa Barbara, Calif.: American Veterinary Publ.

Schmidt, J. 1904. Ein seltener Fall von Cyclopie beim Schwein. *Arch. Wiss. Prakt. Tierheilk.* 30: 466–71.

Schmincke, A. 1921. Vergleichende Untersuchungen über die Anlage des Skelettsystems in tierischen Missbildungen mit einem Beitrag zur makro- und mikroskopischen Anatomie derselben. (Hemiacardius acephalus vom Schwein, Holocardius amorphus vom Rind.) *Virchow Arch. Path. Anat.* 230: 564–607.

Schnecke, C. 1941. Zwergwuchs beim Kaninchen und seine Vererbung. *Z. Menschl. Vereb. Konst.* 25: 425–57.

Schnürer. L. B. 1963. Maternal and foetal responses to chronic stress in pregnancy. *Acta Endocr. Suppl.* 80: 1–96.

Schoop, G. 1955. Die Bedeutung des Vitamin A für die Entwicklung der Ferkel vor und nach der Geburt. *Tierärztl. Umsch.* 10: 194–200.

Schroeder, H. 1924. Mitteilungen aus der Klinik für kleine Haustiere der tierärztlichen Hochschulte zu Berlin. *Berlin. Tierärztl. Wschr.* 40: 471–73.

Schultz, A. H. 1938. To Asia after apes. *Am. J. Anthrop.* 23: 499. (Abst.)

———. 1956. The occurrence and frequency of pathological and teratological conditions and of twinning among non-human primates. In *Primatologia. Handbuch der primatenkunde*, ed. H. Hofer, A. H. Schultz, and D. Starck, vol. 1, pp. 965–1014. Basel: Karger.

Schulz, L. C. 1955. Merencephalie (anencephalia partialis) und Meroacranie bei einem Kalb. *Deut. Tierärztl. Wschr.* 62: 189–90.

Schumacher, H., and Gillette, J. 1966. Embryotoxic effects of thalidomide. *Fed. Proc.* 25: 353. (Abst.)

Schut, J. W. 1946. Olivopontocerebellar atrophy in a cat. *J. Neuropath. Exp. Neur.* 5: 77–81.

Schutte, J. A. 1963. Case report: Bovine cerebellar hypoplasia associated with vicarious hydrocephalus. *J. S. Afr. Vet. Med. Ass.* 34: 441–43.

Schwalbe, E. 1907. *Die Doppelbildungen.* Vol. 2 of *Die Morphologie der Missbildungen des Menschen und der Tiere*, ed. E. Schwalbe. Jena: Fischer, 1906–37.

Schwalbe, E., and Gredig, M. 1906. Ueber Entwicklungsstörungen des Kleinhirns, Hirnsstamms und Halsmarks bei spina bifida (Arnoldsche und Chiarische Missbildung). *Beitr. Path. Anat.* 40: 132–94.

Schwalbe, E., and Josephy, H. 1913. Die Missbildungen des Kopfes. II. Die Cyclopie. In *Die Morphologie der Missbildungen des Menschen und der Tiere*, ed. E. Schwalbe, vol. 3, pt. 1, chap. 5, pp. 205–46. Jena: Fischer, 1906–37.

Scott, J. P. 1937. The embryology of the guinea pig. III. The development of the polydactylous monster. A case of growth accelerated at a particular period by a semi-dominant lethal gene. *J. Exp. Zool.* 77: 123–57.

———. 1938. The embryology of the guinea pig. II. The polydactylous monster. A new teras produced by the genes *PxPx*. *J. Morph.* 62: 299–321.

Searle, A. G. 1965. *Mouse News Letter* 32: 39.

———. 1966. Curtailed, a new dominant *T*-allele in the house mouse. *Genet. Res.* 7: 86–95.

Seefelder, R. 1910. Die angeborenen Anomalien und Missbildungen des Auges. Kritischer Literatur bericht, umfassend den Zeitraum vom Jahre 1898 bis 1. April 1910. *Erg. Allg. Path.* 14: 615–786.

Seligmann, C. G. 1904. Cretinism in calves. *J. Path. Bact.* 9: 311–22.

Seller, M. J. 1962. Thalidomide and congenital abnormalities. *Lancet* 2: 249.

———. 1964. Serotonin as a teratogen. *Brit. Med. J.* 1: 308–9.

Serrano, M. S. 1933. Un caso de hidrocefalia con ceguera consecutiva en el perro. *Rev. Hig. San. Pec.* 23: 28–32.

Setälä, K., and Nyyssönen, O. 1965. Hypnotic sodium pentobarbital as a teratogen for mice. *Naturwissenschaften.* 51: 413.

Setokoesoemo, B. R., and Gunberg, D. L. 1966. The effect of fasting on trypan blue induced congenital malformations in the rat. *Anat. Rec.* 154: 488. (Abst.)

Sever, J. L.; Meier, G. W.; Windle, W. F.; Schiff, G. M.; Monif, G. R.; and Fabiyi, A. 1966. Experimental rubella in pregnant rhesus monkeys. *J. Infect. Dis.* 116: 21–26.

Shackelford, R. M. 1950. *Genetics of the ranch mink.* New York: Pilsbury Publ. Inc.

Shah, M. K. 1956. Reciprocal egg transplantations to study the embryo-uterine relationship in heat-induced failure of pregnancy in rabbits. *Nature* 177: 1134–35.

Shapira, R.; Doherty, D. G.; and Burnett, W. T., Jr. 1957. Chemical protection against ionizing radiation. III. Mercaptoalkylguanidines and related isothiuronium compounds with protective activity. *Radiat. Res.* 7: 22–34.

Shaw, A. O. 1938. A skull defect in cattle. *J. Hered.* 29: 319–20.

Shelesnyak, M. C., and Davies, A. M. 1955. Disturbance of pregnancy in mouse and rat by systemic antihistaminic treatment. *Proc. Soc. Exp. Biol. Med.* 89: 629–32.

Shelton, M. 1964. Relation of environmental temperature during gestation to birth weight and mortality of lambs. *J. Anim. Sci.* 23: 360–65.

Shidara, T. 1963. Experimental studies on the mechanism of teratogenic activity of noise; the role of the maternal adrenals. [In Japanese with English summary.] *Jap. J. Otol.* 66: 532–47.

Shimizu, T.; Kawakami, Y.; Fukuhara, S.; and Matumoto, M. 1954. Experimental stillbirth in pregnant swine infected with Japanese encephalitis virus. *Jap. J. Exp. Med.* 24: 363–75.

Shoji, R., and Makino, S. 1966. Preliminary notes on the teratogenic and embryocidal effects of colchicine on mouse embryos. *Proc. Jap. Acad.* 42: 822–27.

Sholl, L. B. 1931. Hydrocephalus in a calf. *J. Am. Vet. Med. Ass.* 78: 867–68.

Sholl, L. B.; Sales, E. K.; and Langham, R. 1939. Three cases of cerebellar agenesia. *J. Am. Vet. Med. Ass.* 95: 229–30.

Shrode, R. R., and Lush, J. L. 1947. The genetics of cattle. *Adv. Genet.* 1: 209–61.

Shultz, G., and DeLay, P. D. 1955. Losses in newborn lambs associated with bluetongue vaccination of pregnant ewes. *J. Am. Vet. Med. Ass.* 127: 224–26.

Shute, E. 1936. The relation of deficiency of vitamin E to the anti-proteolytic factor found in the serum of aborting women. *J. Obstet. Gynec. Brit. Emp.* 43: 74–86.

Sidman, R. L.; Green, M. C.; and Appel, S. H. 1965. *Catalog of the neurological mutants of the mouse.* Cambridge: Harvard Univ. Press.

Sidman, R. L.; Lane, P. W.; and Dickie, M. M. 1962. Staggerer, a new mutation in the mouse affecting the cerebellum. *Science* 137: 610–12.

Sikov, M. R., and Lofstrom, J. E. 1961. Sensitization and recovery phenomena after embryonic irradiation. *Am. J. Roentgen.* 85: 145–51.

———. 1962. Influence of energy and dose rate on the responses of rat embryos to radiation. *Radiology* 79: 302–9.

Sikov, M. R., and Noonan, T. R. 1958. Anomalous development induced in the embryonic rat by the maternal administration of radiophosphorus. *Am. J. Anat.* 103: 137–61.

Silagi, S. 1962. A genetical and embryological study of partial complementation between lethal alleles at the *T* locus of the house mouse. *Dev. Biol.* 5: 35–67.

————. 1963. Some aspects of the relationship of RNA metabolism to development in normal and mutant mouse embryos cultivated *in vitro. Exp. Cell. Res.* 32: 149–52.

Silvestri, A., and Lughi, G. C. 1959. Consanguineita' e teratologia. *Prog. Vet.* (*Turin*) 14: 725–28.

Silvestrini, B., and Garau, A. 1964. Malformazioni fetali prodotte dalla talidomide nel topo. *Boll. Chim. Farmacol.* 103: 804–14.

Sinclair, J. G. 1950. A specific transplacental effect of urethane in mice. *Texas Rep. Biol. Med.* 8: 623–32.

Sinclair, J. G., and Abreu, B. E. 1965. Transplacental effects of drugs in mice. *Texas Rep. Biol. Med.* 23: 849–53.

Sippel, W. L. 1951. Unusual cases seen at Tifton diagnostic lab. *Georgia Vet. J.* 3: 4–5.

Skalko, R. G. 1965. The effect of Co^{60}-radiation on development and DNA synthesis in the 11-day rat embryo. *J. Exp. Zool.* 160: 171–81.

Skoda, C. 1909. Atresia ani et urogenitalis bei Perocormus acaudatus (Pferd). *Z. Tiermed.* 13: 144–55.

Škreb, N. 1965. Température critique provoquant des malformations pendant le développement embryonnaire du rat et ses effets immédiats. *C. R. Acad. Sci.* 261: 3214–16.

Škreb, N.; Bijělić, N.; and Luković, G. 1963. Weight of rat embryos after X-ray irradiation. *Experientia* 19: 263–64.

Škreb, N., and Frank, Z. 1963. Developmental abnormalities in the rat induced by heat shock. *J. Embryol. Exp. Morph.* 11: 445–57.

Slatis, H. M. 1960. An analysis of inbreeding in the European bison. *Genetics* 45: 275–87.

Slotnick, V., and Brent, R. L. 1966. The production of congenital malformations using tissue antisera. V. Fluorescent localization of teratogenic antisera in the maternal and fetal tissue of the rat. *J. Immun.* 96: 606–10.

Smallwood, W. M. 1914. Another cyclopian pig. *Anat. Anz.* 46: 441–45.

————. 1921. Notes on a two-headed calf. *Anat. Rec.* 22: 27–35.

Smith, A. U. 1957. The effects on foetal development of freezing pregnant hamsters (*Mesocricetus auratus*). *J. Embryol. Exp. Morph.* 5: 311–23.

Smith, L. J. 1956. A morphological and histochemical investigation of a preimplantation lethal (t^{12}) in the house mouse. *J. Exp. Zool.* 132: 51–84.

Smith, L. J., and Stein, K. F. 1961. Retarded shortening of the primitive streak in homozygous Looptail mice. *Anat. Rec.* 139: 321 (Abst.).

————. 1962. Axial elongation in the mouse and its retardation in homozygous Looptail mice. *J. Embryol. Exp. Morph.* 10: 73–87.

Smith, S. 1907. A malformed equine foetus. *Vet. Rec.* 19: 446.

Smith, W. N. A. 1963a. The site of action of trypan blue in cardiac teratogenesis. *Anat. Rec.* 147: 507–23.

————. 1963b. Influence of trypan blue on resorption of rat embryos. *Nature* 200: 699–700.

Smithberg, M. 1961. Teratogenic effects of some hypoglycemic agents in mice. *Univ. Minn. Med. Bull.* 33: 62–72.

Smithberg, M., and Runner, M. N. 1963. Teratogenic effects of hypoglycemic treatments in inbred strains of mice. *Am. J. Anat.* 113: 479–89.

Smithberg, M.; Sanchez, H. W.; and Runner, M. N. 1956. Congenital deformity in the mouse induced by insulin. *Anat. Rec.* 124: 441. (Abst.)

Snell, G. D. 1935. The induction by X-rays of hereditary changes in mice. *Genetics* 20: 545–67.

————. 1946. An analysis of translocations in the mouse. *Genetics* 31: 157–80.

Snell, G. D., and Ames, F. B. 1939. Hereditary changes in the descendants of female mice exposed to roentgen rays. *Am. J. Roentgen.* 41: 248–55.

Snell, G. D.; Bodemann, E.; and Hollander, W. 1934. A translocation in the house mouse and its effect on development. *J. Exp. Zool.* 67: 93–104.

Snell, G. D., and Picken, D. I. 1935. Abnormal development in the mouse caused by chromosome unbalance. *J. Genet.* 31: 213–35.

Sobin, S. 1955. Experimental creation of cardiac defects. *Proc. M. R. Pediat. Res. Conf.* 14: 13–16.

Soiva, K.; Grönroos, M.; and Aho, A. J. 1959. Effect of audiogenic-visual stimuli on pregnant rats. *Ann. Med. Exp. Fenn.* 37: 464–70.

Solomon, F. 1959. Embryomegaly and increased fetal mortality in pregnant rats with mild alloxan diabetes. *Diabetes* 8: 45–50.

Somers, G. F. 1962. Thalidomide and congenital abnormalities. *Lancet* 1: 912–13.

————. 1963. The foetal toxicity of thalidomide. *Proc. Eur. Soc. Study Drug Toxic.* 1: 49–58.

Sonnenbrodt, A. 1950. Erbfehler und Erbkrankheiten bei Schafen. In *Lehrbuch der Krankheiten des Schafes*, ed. T. Opperman, pp. 304–21. 5th ed. Hannover: Schaper.

Spatz, M.; Dougherty, W. J.; and Smith, D. W. E. 1967. Teratogenic effects of methylazoxymethanol. *Proc. Soc. Exp. Biol. Med.* 124: 476–78.

Sperino, G. 1890. Sul midollo spinale di un vitello dicephalus dipus dibrachius. *Int. Mschr. Anat. Physiol.* 7: 386–95.

Spuhler, V. 1944. Über kongenitale, zerebellare Ataxie mit gleichzeitiger Affektion der Grosshirnrinde bei Felis domestica. *Schweiz. Arch. Tierheilk.* 86: 359–78, 422–34, 463–73.

Staats, J. 1964. Standardized nomenclature for inbred strains of mice. Third listing. *Canc. Res.* 24: 147–68.

Steenkiste, C. van. 1845. Description anatomico-tératologique d'un chevreau diplocéphale a corps simple (2ᵐᵉ genre de la diplogénèse). *Ann. Soc. Méd. Chir. Bruges* 6: 85–98.

Stefanelli, S., and Grignolo, A. 1950. Idrocefalia congenita sperimentale in seguito a trattamento con trypanblau. *Ann. Ostet. Ginec.* 72: 806–12.

Stefani, A. 1897. Aplasie congénitale du cervelet chez un chien. *Arch. Ital. Biol.* 30: 235–40.

Stegenga, T. 1964. Aangeboren afwijkingen bij rundvee. *Tijdschr. Diergeneesk.* 89: 286–93.

Stein, K. F.; Lievre, F.; and Smoller, C. G. 1960. Abnormal brain differentiation in the homozygous Loop-tail embryo. *Anat. Rec.* 136: 324–25. (Abst.)

Stein, K. F., and Mackensen, J. A. 1957. Abnormal development of the thoracic skeleton in mice homozygous for the gene for looped-tail. *Am. J. Anat.* 100: 205–24.

Stein, K. F., and Rudin, I. A. 1953. Development of mice homozygous for the gene for looptail. *J. Hered.* 44: 59–69.

Steiner, G.; Bradford, W.; and Craig, J. M. 1965. Tetracycline-induced abortion in the rat. *Lab. Inv.* 14: 1456–63.

Stempak, J. G. Maternal hypothyroidism and its effects on fetal development. *Endocrinology* 70: 443–45.

———. 1964. Etiology of trypan blue induced antenatal hydrocephalus in the albino rat. *Anat. Rec.* 148: 561–71.

———. 1965. Etiology of antenatal hydrocephalus induced by folic acid deficiency in the albino rat. *Anat. Rec.* 151: 287–95.

Šterk, V., and Sofrenović, D. 1958. Meningocele—congenital anomaly of pigs. [In Yugoslav with English summary.] *Acta. Vet.* (*Belgrade*) 8: 109–14.

Stock, R. A. 1902. The Dexter breed "monstrosities." *Vet. Rec.* 15: 402.

Stockard, C. R. 1921. Developmental rate and structural expression: An experimental study of twins, "double monsters" and single deformities, and the interaction among embryonic organs during their origin and development. *Am. J. Anat.* 28: 115–277.

———. 1941. *The genetic and endocrinic basis for differences in form and behavior.* Philadelphia: Wistar.

Storch, C. 1884. Ein Fall von Cyclopie bei einem Kalb. *Oesterr. Vrtljschr. Wiss. Veterinärk.* 62: 112–15.

Stormont, C. 1958. Genetics and disease. *Adv. Vet. Sci.* 4: 137–62.

Stormont, C.; Kendrick, J. W.; and Kennedy, P. C. 1956. A "new" syndrome of inherited lethal defects associated with abnormal gestation in Guernsey cattle. *Genetics* 41: 663. (Abst.)

Strandskov, H. H. 1932. Effects of x-rays in an inbred strain of guinea pigs. *J. Exp. Zool.* 63: 175–202.

Strong, L. C., and Hardy, L. B. 1956. A new "luxoid" mutant in mice. *J. Hered.* 47: 277–84.

Strong, L. C., and Hollander, W. F. 1949. Hereditary loop-tail in the house mouse accompanied by imperforate vagina and with lethal craniorachischisis when homozygous. *J. Hered.* 40: 329–34.

Strong, R. M., and Alban, H. 1932. The development of the lateral apertures of the fourth ventricle in the albino rat brain. *Anat. Rec.* 52: 39. (Abst.)

Stuhlenmiller, M. 1933. Interessante Hemmungsmissbildung am Kopfe eines Kalbes. *Berlin. Tierärztl. Wschr.* 49: 85–86.

Stupka, W. 1931. Über die Bauverhältnisse des Gehirns einer zyklopischen Ziege. *Arb. Neur. Inst. Wien* 33: 315–94.

———. 1933. Zur Histologie und Pathogenese einiger schwererer Fehlbildungen der Nase. *Acta Otolaryng.* 19: 1–5.

Sugawa, Y.; Mochizuki, H.; and Tsubahara, H. 1951. Studies on the hydrocephalus of calves. [In Japanese with English summary.] *Exp. Rep. Gov. Exp. Sta. Anim. Hyg.* (*Tokyo*) 23: 187–98.

Sumi, T. 1960. Experimental studies on the congenital hydrocephalus due to excessive sugar. [In Japanese with English summary.] *J. Osaka City Med. Cent.* 9: 351–59.

428   *References*

Surrarrer, T. C. 1943. Bulldog and hairless calves. *J. Hered.* 34: 175–78.

Suu, S. 1956. Studies on the short-spine dogs. I. Their origin and occurrence. [In Japanese with English summary.] *Res. Bull. Fac. Agr. Gifu Univ.* 7: 127–34.

———. 1962. A gross-anatomical study on the skeleton of the short-spine dog. [In Japanese with English summary.] *Res. Bull. Fac. Agr. Gifu Univ.* 15: 1–72.

Symington, J., and Woodhead, G. S. 1886. Observation on cyclopea in the human subject and in the lower animals. *Proc. Roy. Phys. Soc.* 9: 268–79.

Tabuchi, A.; Kinutani, K.; Nakagawa, S.; Hirata, M,; Fujiwara, T.; Yoshinaga, H.; and Antoku, S. 1962. Fetal disturbances due to radiation (neutron, X-ray, and ^{137}Cs). *Hiroshima J. Med. Sci.* 11: 101–15.

Tabuchi, E.; Narita, R.; Ebi, Y.; and Hosoda, T. 1953. Studies on hydrocephalus of new born calves in Aomori, Akita and Iwate prefectures. *Exp. Rep. Gov. Exp. Sta. Anim. Hyg. (Tokyo)* 26: 21–26.

Tagand, R., and Barone, R. 1942. Trois observations de spina bifida chez les animaux domestiques. *Bull. Soc. Sci. Vét. Lyon* 43: 118–23.

———. 1943. Une nouvelle observation clinique de spina bifida chez le chien. *Bull. Soc. Sci. Vét. Lyon* 44: 47–48.

Taggart, J. K., Jr., and Walker, A. E. 1942. Congenital atresia of the foramens of Luschka and Magendie. *Arch. Neur. Psychiat.* 48: 583–612.

Tajima, M.; Yamagiwa, S.; and Iwamori, H. 1951. Histo-pathological studies on the hydromicrencephalia of calves. [In Japanese with English summary.] *Jap. J. Vet. Sci.* 13: 43–54.

Takakusu, A.; Hidaka, T.; Shinoda, H.; and Ban, Y. 1962. Experimental studies on the malformation induced by stimulation or destruction of the hypothalamus of pregnant rabbits. *Med. J. Osaka Univ.* 12: 321–53.

Takano, K.; Tanimura, T.; and Nishimura, H. 1965. The susceptibility of the offspring of alloxan-diabetic mice to a teratogen. *J. Embryol. Exp. Morph.* 14: 63–73.

Takano, K.; Yamamura, H.; Suzuki, M.; and Nishimura, H. 1966. Teratogenic effect of chlormadinone acetate in mice and rabbits. *Proc. Soc. Exp. Biol. Med.* 121: 455–57.

Takaori, S.; Tanabe, K.; and Shimamoto, K. 1966. Developmental abnormalities of skeletal system induced by ethylurethan in the rat. *Jap. J. Pharmacol.* 16: 63–73.

Takaya, M. 1963. Teratogenic effect of the antitumor antibiotics. *Proc. Congen. Anom. Res. Ass. Jap.* 3: 47–48. (Abst.)

Takekoshi, S. 1961. Teratogenesis due to hypervitaminosis A in combination with other teratogenic factors (cortisone, trypan blue, noise-stimulation, urethan and chondroitinsulfate). [In Japanese with English summary.] *J. Otorhinolaryng. Soc. Jap.* 64: 1489–97.

———. 1964. The mechanism of vitamin A induced teratogenesis. *J. Embryol. Exp. Morph.* 12: 263–71.

———. 1965a. Effects of hydroxymethylpyrimidine on isoniazid- and ethionamide-induced teratosis. *Gunma J. Med. Sci.* 14: 233–44.

———. 1965b. Effects of urethan on the teratogenic action of hypervitaminosis A. *Gunma J. Med. Sci.* 14: 210–12.

Talbert, G. B., and Krohn, P. L. 1966. Effect of maternal age on viability of ova and uterine support of pregnancy in mice. *J. Reprod. Fertil.* 11: 399–406.

Tanimura, T., and Nishimura, H. 1962. Teratogenic effect of thio-TEPA, a potent antineoplastic compound, upon the offspring of pregnant mice. [in Japanese.] *Acta Anat. Nippon.* 37: 66–67.

Taruffi, C. 1881–94. *Storia della teratologia.* 8 vols. Bologna: Regia Tipografia.

Tatum, E. L. 1961. Some molecular aspects of congenital malformations. In *First international conference on congenital malformations*, pp. 281–90. Philadelphia: Lippincott.

Taylor, J. 1922. A bovine monstrosity. *Vet. Rec.* 34: 163.

Tennyson, V. M., and Pappas, G. D. 1961. Electronmicroscope studies of the developing telencephalic choroid plexus in normal and hydrocephalic rabbits. In *Disorders of the developing nervous system*, ed. W. S. Fields, and M. M. Desmond, pp. 267–318. Springfield, Ill: Thomas.

Thalhammer, O., and Heller-Szöllösy, E. 1955. Exogene Bildungsfehler ("Missbildungen") durch Lostinjection bei der graviden Maus. *Z. Kinderheilk.* 76: 351–65.

Theiler, K. 1959. Anatomy and development of the "truncate" (boneless) mutation in the mouse. *Am. J. Anat.* 104: 319–43.

Theiler, K., and Glücksohn-Waelsch, S. 1956. The morphological effects and the development of the Fused mutation in the mouse. *Anat. Rec.* 125: 83–104.

Theiler, K., and Stevens, L. C. 1960. The development of rib fusions, a mutation in the house mouse. *Am. J. Anat.* 106: 171–83.

Théret, M. 1948. Une mutation léthale récessive chez le mouton. (Micrognathie et imperforation bucco-pharyngienne.) *Rec. Méd. Vét.* 124: 445–57.

Thieke, A. 1920. Beitrag zur Kasuistik der Zyklopie. *Arch. Wiss. Prakt. Tierheilk.* 46: 34–61.

Thiernesse. 1850–51. Rapport sur un monstre double monomphalien de l'espèce porcine, compliqué de rhinocéphalie chez l'un des sujets composant. Formation d'un nouveau genre appelé gastropage. *Bull. Acad. Roy. Méd. Belg.* 10: 240–50.

Thiersch, J. B. 1954a. Effect of certain 2,4-diaminopyrimidine antagonists of folic acid on pregnancy and rat fetus. *Proc. Soc. Exp. Biol. Med.* 87: 571–77.

———. 1954b. The effect of 6-mercaptopurine on the rat fetus and on reproduction of the rat. *Ann. N. Y. Acad. Sci.* 60: 220–27.

———. 1957a. Effect of 2,4,6 triamino-"s"-triazene (TR), 2,4,6 "tris" (ethyleneimino)-"s"-triazene (TEM) and N, N′, N″-triethylenephosphoramide (TEPA) on rat litter *in utero. Proc. Soc. Exp. Biol. Med.* 94: 36–40.

———. 1957b. Effect of 2-6 diaminopurine (2-6 DP): 6 chloropurine (ClP) and thioguanine (ThG) on rat litter *in utero. Proc. Soc. Exp. Biol. Med.* 94: 40–43.

———. 1957c. Effect of o-diazo acetyl-l-serine on rat litter. *Proc. Soc. Exp. Biol. Med.* 94: 27–32.

———. 1957d. Effect of 6 diazo 5 oxo l-norleucine (DON) on the rat litter *in utero. Proc. Soc. Exp. Biol. Med.* 94: 33–35.

———. 1958. Effect of N-desacetyl thio colchicine (TC) and N-desacetylmethyl-colchicine (MC) on rat fetus and litter *in utero. Proc. Soc. Exp. Biol. Med.* 98: 479–85.

———. 1960. Discussion. In *Ciba Foundation symposium on congenital malformations*, ed. G. E. W. Wolstenholme, and C. M. O'Connor, p. 111. Boston: Little, Brown & Co.

————. 1962*a*. Effect of 6-(1'-methyl-4'-nitro-5'-imidazolyl)-mercaptopurine and 2-amino-6-(1'-methyl-4'-nitro-5'-imidazolyl)-mercaptopurine on the rat litter *in utero*. *J. Reprod. Fertil.* 4: 297–302.

————. 1962*b*. Effect of substituted mercaptopurines on the rat litter *in utero*. *J. Reprod. Fertil.* 4: 291–95.

————. 1962*c*. Effects of acetamides and formamides on the rat litter *in utero*. *J. Reprod. Fertil.* 4: 219–20.

————. 1964. The effect of substituted 2,4-diamino-pyrimidines on the rat fetus *in utero*. *Proc. Int. Cong. Chemother.* 3: 367–72.

Thiersch, J. B., and Philips, F. S. 1950. Effect of 4-amino-pteroyl-glutamic acid (aminopterin) on early pregnancy. *Proc. Soc. Exp. Biol. Med.* 74: 204–8.

Thomas, B. H., and Cheng, D. W. 1952. Congenital abnormalities associated with vitamin E malnutrition. *Proc. Iowa Acad. Sci.* 59: 218–26.

Thoonen, J., and Hoorens, J. 1960. Zenuwziekten van niet infectieuse of niet parasitaire aard bij het varken. [In Flemish with English summary.] *Vlaams Diergeneesk. Tijdschr.* 29: 67–86.

Thuringer, J. M. 1919. The anatomy of dicephalic pig, monosomus diprosopus. *Anat. Rec.* 15: 359–67.

Tiedemann, F. 1826. Observation de cyclopie, ou réunion des deux yeux en un seul, chez un foetus de cochon, avec organisation anormale du cerveau. *Rec. Méd. Vét.* 3: 377–81.

Tihen, J. A.; Charles, D. R.; and Sipple, T. O. 1948. Inherited visceral inversion in mice. *J. Hered.* 39: 29–31.

Tillon. 1926. Otocéphalie sur un foetus de mouton. *Rec. Méd. Vét.* 102: 669–72.

Tobin, C. E. 1941. Some effects of thyrotropic hormone on the pregnant rat. *Proc. Soc. Exp. Biol. Med.* 48: 592–95.

Todd, N. B. 1961. The inheritance of taillessness in Manx cats. *J. Hered.* 52: 228–32.

————. 1964. The Manx factor in domestic cats. *J. Hered.* 55: 225–30.

Toussaint, M. D. 1958. L'effet tératogène du bleu de trypan sur l'oeil de rat. *Bull. Soc. Belge Opht.* 114: 460–73.

Trasler, D. G. 1958. Genetic and other factors influencing the pathogenesis of cleft palate in mice. Unpublished Ph.D. thesis, McGill Univ., Montreal.

————. 1960. Influence of uterine site on occurrence of spontaneous cleft lip in mice. *Science* 132: 420–21.

————. 1965. Aspirin-induced cleft lip and other malformations in mice. *Lancet* 1: 606–7.

Trasler, D. G., and Fraser, F. C. 1958. Factors underlying strain, reciprocal cross, and maternal weight differences in embryo susceptibility to cortisone-induced cleft palate in mice. *Proc. X Int. Cong. Genet.* 2: 296–97. (Abst.)

Trasler, D. G.; Naylor, A. F.; and Miller, J. R. 1964. Interactions in the effects of dose, strain, maternal weight, and food on the frequency of cortisone-induced cleft palate in the mouse. *Abst. Terat. Soc.* 4: 20–21. (Abst.)

Trasler, D. G.; Walker, B. E.; and Fraser, F. C. 1956. Congenital malformations produced by amniotic-sac puncture. *Science* 124: 439.

Trautwein, G., and Meyer, H. 1966. Experimentelle Untersuchungen über erbliche Meningocele cerebralis beim Schwein. II. Pathomorphologie der Gehirnmissbildungen. *Path. Vet.* 3: 543–55.

Tridon, J. 1909. Otocéphalie et anencéphalie. *Rev. Gén. Méd. Vét.* 13: 64–65.

Troussier, M. 1904. Observation sur deux veaux jumeaux hydrocéphales. *Bull. Soc. Sci. Vét. Lyon.* 7: 7–8.

Truslove, G. M. 1946. The anatomy and development of the fidget mouse. *J. Genet.* 54: 64–86.

Tsiroyannis, E.; Brouwers, J.; Bienfet, V.; and Kaeckenbeeck, A. 1957. Agénésie du cervelet chez un veau ataxique. *Ann. Méd. Vét.* 101: 223–30.

Tsuchikawa, K., and Akabori, A. 1964. Differences of the response to teratogens between inbred strains of mice. (1) Differences of the response to ethylurethane between strain CBA and C3HeB/Fe. *Proc. Congen. Anom. Res. Ass. Jap.* 4: 48. (Abst.)

Tsuchikawa, K., and Akabori, H. 1965. Strain differences of susceptibility to induced congenital anomalies in mice. *Proc. Congen. Anom. Res. Ass. Jap.* 5: 2. (Abst.)

Tuchmann-Duplessis, H. 1960. Discussion. In *Ciba Foundation symposium on congenital malformations*, ed. G. E. W. Wolstenholme, and C. M. O'Connor, p. 18. Boston: Little, Brown & Co.

Tuchmann-Duplessis, H.; Gershon, R.; and Mercier-Parot, L. 1957. Troubles de la gestation chez la ratte, provoqués par la résperpine et essais d'hormonothérapie compensatrice. *J. Physiol. (Paris)* 49: 1007–19.

Tuchmann-Duplessis, H., and Lefebvres-Boisselot, J. 1957a. Malformations produites chez le rat par l'acide x-méthylfolique. *C. R. Ass. Anat.* 44: 738–41.

———. 1957b. Les effets tératogènes de l'acide x-méthylfolique chez la chatte. *C. R. Soc. Biol.* 151: 2005–8.

Tuchmann-Duplessis, H., and Mercier-Parot, L. 1955. Influence du bleu trypan et de l'azobleu sur le développement de l'embryon du rat. *C. R. Ass. Anat.* 42: 1326–30.

———. 1957. Production de malformations chez la souris par administration d'acide x-méthylfolique. *C. R. Soc. Biol.* 151: 1855–57.

———. 1958a. Sur l'action tératogène de quelques substances antimitotiques chez le rat. *C. R. Acad. Sci.* 247: 152–54.

———. 1958b. Influence d'un sulfamide hypoglycémiant, l'aminophénurobutane BZ55, sur la gestation de la ratte. *C. R. Acad. Sci.* 246: 156–58.

———. 1958c. Influence de trois sulfamides hypoglycémiants sur la ratte gestante. *C. R. Acad. Sci.* 247: 1134–37.

———. 1958d. Sur l'activité tératogène chez le rat de l'actinomycine D. *C. R. Acad. Sci.* 247: 2200–3.

———. 1959a. A propos de malformations produites par le bleu trypan. *Biol. Méd.* 48: 238–51.

———. 1959b. Sur l'action abortive et tératogène de la 6-chloropurine. *C. R. Acad. Sci.* 153: 1133–36.

———. 1959c. Sur l'action tératogène d'un sulfamide hypoglycémiant. *J. Physiol. (Paris)* 51: 65–83.

———. 1959d. Action de la chlorpropamide, sulfamide hypoglycémiant, sur la gestation et le développement foetal du rat. *C. R. Acad. Sci.* 249: 1160–62.

432   References

————. 1959*e*. A propos de l'action tératogène de l'actinomycine. *C. R. Soc. Biol.* 153: 1697–1700.

————. 1960*a*. The teratogenic action of the antibiotic actinomycin D. In *Ciba Foundation symposium on congenital malformations*, ed. G. E. W. Wolstenholme, and C. M. O'Connor, pp. 115–28. Boston: Little, Brown & Co.

————. 1960*b*. Influence de l'actinomycine D sur la gestation et le développement foetal du lapin. *C. R. Soc. Biol.* 154: 914–16.

————. 1961*a*. Malformations foetales chez le rat traité par de fortes doses de déserpidine. *C. R. Soc. Biol.* 155: 2291–93.

————. 1961*b*. Répercussions sur la gestation et le développement foetal du rat d'un hypoglycémiant, le chlorhydrate de N, N-diméthylbiguanide. *C. R. Acad. Sci.* 253: 321–23.

————. 1963*a*. Production de malformations chez la souris et le lapin par administration d'un sulfamide hypoglycémiant, la carbutamide. *C. R. Soc. Biol.* 157: 1193–97.

————. 1963*b*. Action du chlorhydrate de cyclizine sur la gestation et le développement embryonnaire du rat, de la souris et du lapin. *C. R. Acad. Sci.* 256: 3359–62.

————. 1964*a*. Répercussions des neuroleptiques et des antitumoraux sur le développement prénatal. *Bull. Schweiz. Akad. Med. Wiss.* 20: 490–526.

————. 1964*b*. Production de malformations des membres chez le lapin par administration d'un antimétabolite: L'azathioprine. *C. R. Acad. Sci.* 259: 3648–51.

————. 1964*c*. Considérations sur les tests tératogènes. Différences de réaction de trois espèces animales à l'égard d'un antitumoral. *C. R. Soc. Biol.* 158: 1984–90.

————. 1964*d*. Influence d'une perturbation du métabolisme des lipides sur la gestation et le développement prénatal de la souris. *C. R. Soc. Biol.* 158: 1025–28.

————. 1964*e*. Avortements et malformations sous l'effet d'un agent provoquant une hyperlipémie et une hypercholestérolémie. *Bull. Acad. Nat. Méd.* 148: 392–98.

————. 1964*f*. A propos des tests tératogénes. Malformations spontanées du lapin. *C. R. Soc. Biol.* 158: 666–70.

————. 1965. Production chez le rat d'anomalies après applications cutanées d'un solvent industriel: La mono-méthyl-formamide. *C. R. Acad. Sci.* 261: 241–43.

————. 1966. Production chez le lapin de malformations des membres par administration d'azathioprine et de 6-mercaptopurine. *C. R. Soc. Biol.* 160: 501–6.

Tucker, R., and Millar, R. 1954. The patterns of nervous symptoms in the chondrodystrophic dog. *Brit. Vet. J.* 110: 359–65.

Tumbelaka, R. 1915. Das Gehirn eines Affen, worin die interhemisphäriale Balkenverbindung fehlt. *Folia Neurobiol.* 9: 1–64.

Turbow, M. M. 1965. Teratogenic effect of trypan blue on rat embryos cultivated *in vitro. Nature* 206: 637.

————. 1966. Trypan blue induced teratogenesis of rat embryos cultivated *in vitro J. Embryol. Exp. Morph.* 15: 387–95.

Tyler, W. J., and Chapman, A. B. 1948. Genetically reduced prolificacy in rats. *Genetics* 33: 565–76.

Überreiter, O. 1952. Spina bifida occulta bei einem Fohlen. *Tierärztl. Umsch.* 7: 351–55.

Ueshima, T. 1961. A pathological study of the vertebral column in the "short-spine dog." *Jap. J. Vet. Res.* 9: 155–78.

Ullrey, D. E.; Becker, D. E.; Terrill, S. W.; and Notzold, R. A. 1955. Dietary levels of pantothenic acid and reproductive performance of female swine. *J. Nutr.* 57: 401–14.

Urbain, A.; Riese, W.; and Nouvel, J. 1941. Atrophie cérébelleuse observée chez un gélada (*Theropithecus gelada* Rüppel). *Rev. Path. Comp.* 41: 176–79.

Urman, H. K., and Grace, O. D. 1964. Hereditary encephalomyopathy. A hydrocephalus syndrome in newborn calves. *Cornell Vet.* 54: 229–49.

Valenciennes, A. 1848. Notice sur un dauphin à deux têtes rapporté des Antilles. *C. R. Acad. Sci.* 27: 249–50.

Val'shtrem, E. A. 1960. The pathogenesis of radiation injuries and repair processes in rat embryos after the irradiation of the females on the 10th day of pregnancy. [In Russian; English translation by U. S. Joint Publ. Res. Serv., No. 5985.] *Arkh. Anat.* 38: 72–79.

———. 1961. An analysis of injuries and reparative processes in rat embryogenesis after X-ray exposure. [In Russian.] *Dokl. Akad. Nauk. SSSR.* 140: 1434–36.

Van Dyke, J. H., and Ritchey, M. G. 1947. Colchicine influence during embryonic development in rats. *Anat. Rec.* 97: 375. (Abst.)

Vankin, G. L., and Grass, H. J. 1966. Colcemid-induced teratogenesis in hybrid mouse embryos. *Am. Zool.* 6: 551. (Abst.)

Vau, E., and Richter, H. 1934. Beschreibung einer Doppelmissbildung von bos (dicephalus bicaudatus sive thoraco-ileo-omphalo-pagus) und Erörterungen neuer Theorien zur Erklärung der Doppelbildungen. (Teilkörper- und Protomerentheorie nach M. Heidenhain, Strukturprinzip: "Dimerie" nach H. Richter.) *München. Tierärztl. Wschr.* 85: 185–89.

Vaupel, M. R.; Nelson, H. A., Jr.; and Roux, K. L., Jr. 1961. Nervous system abnormalities in the progeny of trypan blue injected rats. *Anat. Rec.* 139: 325. (Abst.)

Veerappa, T. R. S., and Bourne, G. H. 1966. Double central canal in spinal cord of rat. *Nature* 209: 729.

Verhaart, W. J. C. 1942. Partial agenesis of the cerebellum and medulla and total agenesis of the corpus callosum in a goat. *J. Comp. Neur.* 77: 49–60.

———. 1948. Cerebellar and cerebral cortical hypoplasia in a cat. *Acta Neerl. Morph.* 6: 169–74.

Verlinde, J. D. 1949. Congenitale cerebellaire ataxie bij katten in samenhang met een vermoedelijke virusinfectie bij de moeder gedurende de graviditeit. *Tijdschr. Diergeneesk.* 74: 659–61.

Verlinde, J. D., and Ojemann, J. G. 1946. Eenige aangeboren misvormingen van het centrale zenuwstelsel. *Tijdschr. Diergeneesk.* 71: 557–64.

Verma, K., and King, D. W. 1966. Disorders of the developing nervous system in avitaminosis E. *Anat. Rec.* 154: 493. (Abst.)

Via, W. F., Jr.; Elwood, W. K.; and Bebin, J. 1959. The effect of maternal hypoxia upon fetal dental enamel. *Henry Ford Hosp. Med. Bull.* 7: 94–101.

Vichi, F.; Masi, P. L.; Pierleoni, P.; and Orlando, S. 1965a. Malformazioni congenite sperimentalmente indotte mediante triparanolo. *Sperimentale* 115: 168–75.

434 References

Vichi, F.; Masi, P. L.; Pierleoni, P.; Orlando, S.; Pagni, L.; and Tollaro, I. 1966. *I fattori metagenetici esogeni nelle malformazioni congenite (oro-maxillo-faciali): Teratogenesi sperimentale e riferimenti clinici.* Saluzzo, Minerva Medica.

Vichi, F.; Pierleoni, P.; Masi, P. L.; and Tollaro, I. 1965*b*. Ipervitaminosi A e malformazioni congenite in feto di ratto. *Riv. Ital. Stomat.* 20: 717–32.

Vichi, G. F., and Bufalini, G. N. 1962. L'idrocefalo congenito da atresia dei forami di Luschka e Magendie. *Radiolog. Med.* 48: 1174–1203.

Vickers, T. H. 1961*a*. Concerning the mechanism of hydrocephalus in the progeny of trypan blue treated rats. *Roux Arch. Entwickl.* 153: 255–61.

————. 1961*b*. Die experimentelle Erzeugung der Arnold–Chiari Missbildung durch Trypan blau. *Beitr. Path. Anat.* 124: 295–310.

————. 1967. The thalidomide embryopathy in hybrid rabbits. *Brit. J. Exp. Path.* 48: 107–17.

Vidovic, V. 1952. Kälte- und Hypoxietoleranz von Rattenembryonen. *Experientia* 8: 304–6.

Vierck, C. J., Jr., and Meier, G. W. 1963. Effects of prenatal hypoxia upon locomotor activity of the mouse. *Exp. Neur.* 7: 418–25.

Ville, de. 1755. Histoire anatomique d'un chat monstrueux. *Collect. Acad. Mém., etc. (Dijon)* 1: 286–87.

Vincent, C. K., and Ulberg, L. C. 1965. Survival of sheep embryos exposed to high temperature. *J. Anim. Sci.* 24: 931–32. (Abst.)

Vitu, P., and Houdinière, A. 1934. Otocéphalie. Variété opocéphalie chez l'agneau. Variété édocéphalie chez le porcelet. *Rec. Méd. Vét.* 110: 398–409.

Voltz. 1897. Ueber eine Missbildung mit überzähliger Bildung. *Wschr. Thierheilk. Viehz.* 41: 455–58.

Vor, D. W. J. de. 1940. Een geval von dicephalus bicollis, waargenomen bij een pasgeboren kalf. *Hemera Zoa* 52: 321.

Voute, E. J., and Dussen, E. E. van der. 1951. Monstrosity in a cat. *J. Am. Vet. Med. Ass.* 118: 150.

Vrolik, W. 1854. *Tabulae ad illustrandam embryogenesin hominis et mammalium tam naturalem quam abnormem.* Leipzig: Weigel.

Vulpian. 1855. Note sur un chat monstrueux (groupe des monstres doubles monosomiens, genre opodyme—Isid. Geoffroy-Saint-Hilaire). *Gaz. Méd. Paris* 26: 18–19.

Wachsmann, F.; Utreras, A.; and Schreiner, E. 1963. Einfluss der Zeit zwischen Bestrahlung und Befruchtung auf die F_1-Generation von Mäusen. *Strahlentherapie* 122: 91–102.

Waddington, C. H., and Carter, T. C. 1952. Malformations in mouse embryos induced by trypan blue. *Nature* 169: 27–28.

————. 1953. A note on abnormalities induced in mouse embryos by trypan blue. *J. Embryol. Exp. Morph.* 1: 167–80.

Waldorf, D. P.; Foote, W. C.; Self, H. L.; Chapman, A. B.; and Casida, L. E. 1957. Factors affecting fetal pig weight late in gestation. *J. Anim. Sci.* 16: 976–85.

Waletzky, E., and Owen, R. 1942. A case of inherited partial sterility and embryonic mortality in the rat. *Genetics* 27: 173. (Abst.)

Walker, B. E. 1959. Effects on palate development of mechanical interference with the fetal environment. *Science* 130: 981.

————. 1965. Cleft palate produced in mice by human-equivalent dosage with triamcinolone. *Science* 149: 862–63.

————. 1966. Production of cleft palate in rabbits by glucocorticoids. *Abst. Terat. Soc.* 6: 27. (Abst.)

Walker, B. E., and Crain, B., Jr. 1960. Effects of hypervitaminosis A on palate development in two strains of mice. *Am. J. Anat.* 107: 49–58.

————. 1961. Abnormal palate morphogenesis in mouse embryos induced by riboflavin deficiency. *Proc. Soc. Exp. Biol. Med.* 107: 404–6.

Walker, B. E., and Fraser, F. C. 1957. The embryology of cortisone-induced cleft palate. *J. Embryol. Exp. Morph.* 5: 201–9.

Walker, E. P. 1964. *Mammals of the world.* Baltimore: Johns Hopkins Press.

Walley. 1875. On a congenital cranial tumour in a calf. *Trans. Edinburgh Obstet. Soc.* 3: 68–70.

Warburton, D.; Trasler, D. G.; Naylor, A.; Miller, J. R.; and Fraser, F. C. 1962. Pitfalls in tests for teratogenicity. *Lancet* 2: 1116–17.

Warkany, J. 1960. Experimental production of congenital malformations of the central nervous system. In *Mental retardation. Proceedings of the 1st international conference on mental retardation,* ed. P. W. Bowman, and H. V. Mautner, pp. 44–64. New York: Grune & Stratton.

Warkany, J., and Kalter, H. 1961. Congenital malformations. *New Eng. J. Med.* 265: 993–1001, 1046–52.

————. 1962. Maternal impressions and congenital malformations. *Plast. Reconstr. Surg.* 30: 628–37.

Warkany, J.; Kalter, H.; and Geiger, J. F. 1957. Experimental teratology with special reference to congenital malformations of the central nervous system. *Pediat. Clin. N. Am.* 4: 983–94.

Warkany, J., and Nelson, R. C. 1940. Appearance of skeletal abnormalities in the offspring of rats reared on a deficient diet. *Science* 92: 383–84.

————. 1941. Skeletal abnormalities in offspring of rats reared on deficient diets. *Anat. Rec.* 79: 83–100.

Warkany, J., and Roth, C. B. 1948. Congenital malformations induced in rats by maternal vitamin A deficiency. II. Effect of varying the preparatory diet upon the yield of abnormal young. *J. Nutr.* 35: 1–12.

Warkany, J., and Schraffenberger, E. 1944. Congenital malformations of the eyes induced in rats by maternal vitamin A deficiency. *Proc. Soc. Exp. Biol. Med.* 57: 49–52.

————. 1947. Congenital malformations induced in rats by roentgen rays. Skeletal changes in the offspring following a single irradiation of the mother. *Am. J. Roentgen.* 57: 455–63.

Warkany, J., and Takacs, E. 1959. Experimental production of congenital malformations in rats by salicylate poisoning. *Am. J. Path.* 35: 315–31.

————. 1965. Congenital malformations in rats from streptonigrin. *Arch. Path.* 79: 65–79.

Warkany, J.; Wilson, J. G.; and Geiger, J. F. 1958. Myeloschisis and myelo-meningocele produced experimentally in the rat. *J. Comp. Neur.* 109: 35–64.

Warwick, E. J.; Chapman, A. B.; and Ross, B. 1943. Some anomalies in pigs. *J. Hered.* 34: 349–52.

436   References

Watanabe, G., and Ingalls, T. H. 1963. Congenital malformations in the offspring of alloxan-diabetic mice. *Diabetes* 12: 66–72.

Webb, R. M. 1944. Congenital communicating hypertensive hydrocephalus in a dog. *Aust. Vet. J.* 20: 231–33.

Weber. 1885. Cébocéphalie. *Rec. Méd. Vét.* 62: 483–84.

Weber, W. 1946a. Über Art, Häufigkeit und Genfrequenz der Missbildungen unserer Haustiere, nebst einem Fall von Agenesie des Geruchsapparates bei einem Kalb. *Schweiz. Arch. Tierheilk.* 88: 497–507.

————. 1946b. Gross- und Kleinhirnaplasie bei einem Kalbe. *Schweiz. Arch. Tierheilk.* 88: 369–71.

————. 1948. Acranie und Anencephalus partialis bei einem Hündchen. *Schweiz. Arch. Tierheilk.* 90: 443–47.

————. 1949. Gehirnmissbildung bei einem Rinderföten. *Acta Anat.* 7: 207–12.

————. 1960. Bulldog-Zicklein bei der Saanenrasse. *Schweiz. Arch. Tierheilk.* 102: 667–70.

Weed, L. H. 1917. The development of the cerebro-spinal spaces in pig and in man. *Carnegie Inst. Contr. Embryol.* 5: 1–116.

Wegener, V. K. 1961. Über die experimentelle Erzeugung von Herzmissbildungen durch Trypanblau. *Arch. Kreislaufforsch.* 34: 99–144.

Wegner, G., and Damminger, K. 1963. Früh- und Spätschäden der Nachkommenschaft von Wistar-Ratten nach Ganzkörperbestrahlung am 9. Graviditätstag. Missbildungen, Beobachtungen der ersten beiden Generationen. *Strahlentherapie* 121: 374–82.

Wegner, G.; Stutz, E.; and Büchner, F. 1961. Tumoren und Missbildungen bei der Wistar-Ratte in der ersten Generation nach Ganzbestrahlung des Muttertieres mit 270 r am 18. Graviditätstag. *Beitr. Path. Anat.* 124: 396–414.

Weidman, W. H.; Young, H. H.; and Zollman, P. E. 1963. The effect of thalidomide on the unborn puppy. *Proc. Mayo Clin.* 38: 518–22.

Weinkopff, P. 1927. Eine Hemmungsbildung bei einem Kalb mit Mikrognathia und Brachymelie. *Berlin. Tierärztl. Wschr.* 43: 62–63.

Wells, C. 1964. *Bones, bodies, and disease. Evidence of disease and abnormality in early man.* New York: Praeger.

Wells, L. J.; Kim, J. N.; and Lazarow, A. 1960. Effects of insulin on the complications of diabetes and pregnancy in the rat. *Diabetes* 9: 490–93.

Werthemann, A., and Reiniger, M. 1950. Über Augenentwicklungsstörungen bei Rattenembryonen durch Sauerstoffmangel in der Frühschwangerschaft. *Acta Anat.* 11: 329–49.

Weyenbergh, H. 1875. Remarques sur un monstre hydrocéphalique extrait mort d'une vache. *Bol. Acad. Nac. Cienc.* (*Cordoba*) 2 (pt. 1): 58–65.

Whittem, J. H. 1957. Congenital abnormalities in calves: Arthrogryposis and hydranencephaly. *J. Path. Bact.* 73: 375–87.

Widmaier, R. 1959. Ein Fall von Hernia Cerebralis [*sic*] beim Schwein. *Deut. Tierärztl. Wschr.* 66: 47.

Wiersig, D. O., and Swenson, M. J. 1967. Teratogenicity of vitamin A in the canine. *Fed. Proc.* 26: 486. (Abst.)

Wiesner, B. P.; Wolfe, M.; and Yudkin, J. 1958. The effects of some antimitotic compounds on pregnancy in the mouse. *Stud. Fertil.* 9: 129–36.

Wilder, B. G. 1883. On the brain of a cat lacking the callosum—preliminary notice. *Am. J. Neur. Psychiat.* 2: 490–99.

Wilder, H. H. 1908. The morphology of cosmobia; speculations concerning the significance of certain types of monsters. *Am. J. Anat.* 8: 355–440.

Williams, R. T.; Schumacher, H.; Fabro, S.; and Smith, R. L. 1965. The chemistry and metabolism of thalidomide. In *Embryopathic activity of drugs*, ed. J. M. Robson, F. M. Sullivan, and R. L. Smith, pp. 167–82. Boston: Little, Brown & Co.

Williams, S. R., and Rauch, R. W. 1917. The anatomy of a double pig (syncephalus thoracopagus). *Anat. Rec.* 13: 273–80.

Williams, W. L. 1909. *Veterinary obstetrics*. Ithaca, New York.

———. 1931. Studies in teratology. *Cornell Vet.* 21: 25–56.

———. 1936. The problem of teratology in clinical veterinary practice. *Cornell Vet.* 26: 1–33.

Williams, W. L., and Frost, J. N. 1938. Subdural hydrocephalus in a calf. *Cornell Vet.* 28: 340–45.

Wilson, J. 1909. The origin of the Dexter-Kerry breed of cattle. *Proc. Roy. Soc. Dublin* 12: 1–17.

Wilson, J. G. 1953. Influence of severe hemorrhagic anemia during pregnancy on development of the offspring in the rat. *Proc. Soc. Exp. Biol. Med.* 84: 66–69.

———. 1954a. Congenital malformations produced by injecting azo blue into pregnant rats. *Proc. Soc. Exp. Biol. Med.* 85: 319–22.

———. 1954b. Withdrawal of claim that azo blue causes congenital malformations. *Proc. Soc. Exp. Biol. Med.* 87: 1.

———. 1954c. Influence on the offspring of altered physiologic status during pregnancy in the rat. *Ann. N. Y. Acad. Sci.* 57: 517–25.

———. 1954d. Differentiation and reaction of rat embryos to radiation. *J. Cell. Comp. Physiol.* 43 (Suppl.): 11–37.

———. 1955. Teratogenic activity of several azo dyes chemically related to trypan blue. *Anat. Rec.* 123: 313–33.

———. 1964. Teratogenic interaction of chemical agents in the rat. *J. Pharmacol. Exp. Ther.* 144: 429–36.

———. 1965. Embryological considerations in teratology. *Ann. N. Y. Acad. Sci.* 123: 219–27.

———. 1966. Effects of acute and chronic treatment with actinomycin D on pregnancy and the fetus in the rat. *Harper Hosp. Bull.* 24: 109–18.

Wilson, J. G.; Beaudoin, A. R.; and Free, H. J. 1959. Studies on the mechanism of teratogenic action of trypan blue. *Anat. Rec.* 133: 115–28.

Wilson, J. G.; Brent, R. L.; and Jordan, H. C. 1953. Differentiation as a determinant of the reaction of rat embryos to X-irradiation. *Proc. Soc. Exp. Biol. Med.* 82: 67–70.

Wilson, J. G., and Gavan, J. A. 1967. Congenital malformations in nonhuman primates: Spontaneous and experimentally induced. *Anat. Rec.* 158: 99–110.

Wilson, J. G.; Jordan, H. C.; and Brent, R. L. 1953. Effects of irradiation on embryonic development. II. X-rays on the ninth day of gestation in the rat. *Am. J. Anat.* 92: 153–88.

438 References

Wilson, J. G., and Karr, J. W. 1951. Effects of irradiation on embryonic development. I. X-rays on the tenth day of gestation in the rat. *Am. J. Anat.* 88: 1–34.

Wilson, J. G.; Roth, C. B.; and Warkany, J. 1953. An analysis of the syndrome of malformations induced by maternal vitamin A deficiency. Effects of restoration of vitamin A at various times during gestation. *Am. J. Anat.* 92: 189–217.

Wilson, J. G.; Shepard, T. H.; and Gennaro, J. F. 1963. Studies on the site of teratogenic action of C^{14}-labeled trypan blue. *Anat. Rec.* 145: 300. (Abst.)

Wilson, J. H. 1902. Maldevelopment in a foal. *Vet. Rec.* 14: 710.

Wimer, R. E. 1965. *Mouse News Letter* 33: 32.

Winfield, J. B. 1966. Actinomycin D teratogenesis in the young mouse embryo. *Am. Zool.* 6: 551. (Abst.)

Winsser, J. 1945. Rachischizis bij een pasgeboren hondje. *Tijdschr. Diergeneesk.* 70: 313.

Winters, L. M. 1948. *Animal breeding.* 4th ed. New York: Wiley & Sons.

Winters, L. M., and Kernkamp, H. C. H. 1935. A faceless lamb. *J. Hered.* 26: 33–34.

Wissdorf, H. 1964. Osteologische Befunde an einem Diprosopus Tetrophthalmus mit Akranie, Merencephalie und beidseitiger Rammsnasenbildung bei einem Kalb. *Zbl. Veterinärmed.* 11: 677–84.

Witt, M. 1963. Doppelgesicht (Diprosopus) beim Kalb. *Deut. Tierärztl. Wschr.* 70: 327.

Wolff, E., and Kirrmann, J. M. 1954. L'influence protectrice de la cysteamine contre l'action tératogène des irradiations localisées. *C. R. Soc. Biol.* 148: 1629–31.

Woodard, J. C., and Newberne, P. M. 1966. Relation of vitamin B_{12} and one-carbon metabolism to hydrocephalus in the rat. *J. Nutr.* 88: 375–81.

Woollam, D. H. M., and Millen, J. W. 1957. Effect of cortisone on the incidence of cleft-palate induced by experimental hypervitaminosis-A. *Brit. Med. J.* 2: 197–98.

———. 1958a. Influence of 4-methyl-2-thiouracil on the teratogenic activity of hypervitaminosis-A. *Nature* 181: 992–93.

———. 1958b. Protection of cysteamine on the teratogenic action of X-irradiation. *Nature* 182: 1801.

———. 1960. The modification of the activity of certain agents exerting a deleterious effect on the development of the mammalian embryo. In *Ciba Foundation symposium on congenital malformations*, ed. G. E. W. Wolstenholme, and C. M. O'Connor, pp. 158–72. Boston: Little, Brown & Co.

———. 1961. Influence of uterine position on the response of the mouse embryo to the teratogenic effects of hypervitaminosis A. *Nature* 190: 184–85.

———. 1962. Influence of uterine position on the response of the mouse embryo to anoxia. *Nature* 194: 990–91.

Woollam, D. H. M.; Millen, J. W.; and Fozzard, J. A. F. 1959. The influence of cortisone on the teratogenic activity of X radiation. *Brit. J. Radiol.* 32: 47–48.

Woollam, D. H. M.; Pratt, C. W. M.; and Fozzard, J. A. F. 1957. Influence of vitamins upon some teratogenic effects of radiation. *Brit. Med. J.* 1: 1219–21.

Woolridge, G. H. 1906. Double-headed calf monstrosity. *Vet. J.* 13: 643–44.

Wriedt, C. 1925. Letale Faktoren. (Todbringende Vererbungsfaktoren.) *Z. Tierz. Züchtungsbiol.* 3: 223–30.

————. 1930. *Heredity in live stock.* London: Macmillan.

Wriedt, C., and Mohr, O. L. 1928. Amputated, a recessive lethal in cattle; with a discussion on the bearing of lethal factors on the principles of live stock breeding. *J. Genet.* 20: 187–215.

Wright, S. 1922. The effects of inbreeding and crossbreeding on guinea pigs. I. Decline in vigor. II. Differentiation among inbred families. U. S. Dep. Agr. Bull. No. 1090.

————. 1934*a*. On the genetics of subnormal development of the head (otocephaly) in the guinea pig. *Genetics* 19: 471–505.

————. 1934*b*. Genetics of abnormal growth in the guinea pig. *Cold Spring Harbor Symp. Quant. Biol.* 2: 137–47.

————. 1934*c*. Polydactylous guinea pigs. Two types respectively heterozygous and homozygous in the same mutant gene. *J. Hered.* 25: 359–62.

————. 1935. A mutation of the guinea pig, tending to restore the pentadactyl foot when heterozygous, producing a monstrosity when homozygous. *Genetics* 20: 84–107.

————. 1960. The genetics of vital characters of the guinea pig. *J. Cell. Comp. Physiol.* 56 (Suppl.): 123–51.

Wright, S., and Eaton, O. N. 1923. Factors which determine otocephaly in guinea pigs. *J. Agr. Res.* 26: 161–81.

Wright, S., and Wagner, K. 1934. Types of subnormal development of the head from inbred strains of guinea pigs and their bearing on the classification and interpretation of vertebrate monsters. *Am. J. Anat.* 54: 383–447.

Wyman, J. 1858. Cyclopism in a pig. *Boston Med. Surg. J.* 59: 121–23.

————. 1861. Double pig. *Boston Med. Surg. J.* 64: 535.

Yakovlev, P. 1959. Pathoarchitectonic studies of cerebral malformations. III. Arhinencephalies (holotelencephalies). *J. Neuropath. Exp. Neur.* 18: 22–55.

Yakovleva, A. I., and Shakhnazarova, N. G. 1965. Teratogenic action of triparanol. [In Russian with English summary.] *Farmakol. Toksik.* 28: 108–11.

Yamada, T. 1959. Abnormal serum protein observed in trypan blue-treated rats. *Proc. Soc. Exp. Biol. Med.* 101: 566–68.

Yamane, J. 1927. Über die "Atresia coli," ein letale, erbliche Darmissbildung beim Pferde, und ihre Kombination mit Gehirngliomen. *Z. Ind. Abst. Vererbungsl.* 46: 188–207.

Yashon, D.; Small, E.; and Jane, J. A. 1965. Congenital hydrocephalus and chronic subdural hematoma in a dog. *J. Am. Vet. Med. Ass.* 147: 832–36.

Yeary, R. A. 1964. Teratogenic agents in man and in animals. *Lancet* 1: 831.

Yeates, N. T. M. 1958. Foetal dwarfism in sheep—an effect of high atmospheric temperature during gestation. *J. Agr. Sci.* 51: 84–89.

Young, G. A.; Kitchell, R. L.; Luedke, A. J.; and Sautter, J. H. 1955. The effect of viral and other infections of the dam on fetal development in swine. I. Modified live hog cholera viruses—immunological, virological, and gross pathological studies. *J. Am. Vet. Med. Ass.* 126: 165–71.

Young, G. B. 1951. Observations on the frequency and sex ratio of Dexter "bulldog" calves. *Vet. Rec.* 63: 635–36.

Young, S., and Cordy, D. R. 1964. An ovine fetal encephalopathy caused by bluetongue vaccine virus. *J. Neuropath. Exp. Neur.* 26: 635–59.

440   References

Younger, R. L. 1965. Probable induction of congenital anomalies in a lamb by apholate. *Am. J. Vet. Res.* 26: 991–95.

Zayed, I. E., and Ghanem, Y. S. 1964. Untersuchungen über einige kongenitale Missbildungen in einer schwartzbunten Rinderherde. *Deut. Tierärztl. Wschr.* 71: 93–95.

Zimmerman. 1919. Zweikopfigkeit als interessante Doppelmissbildung bei einem Braunviehkalbe. *Jahrb. Wiss. Prakt. Tierz.* 13: 128–33.

Zimmermann, K. 1933. Eine neue Mutation der Hausmaus: *"hydrocephalus."* *Z. Ind. Abst. Vererbungsl.* 64: 176–80.

———. 1935. Erbliche Gehirnkrankungen der Hausmaus. *Erbarzt* 2: 119–20.

Zunin, C., and Borrone, C. 1954. Embriopatie da carenza di acido pantotenico. *Acta Vitamin.* 8: 263–68.

———. 1955. L'effetto teratogeno della 6-mercaptopurina. *Minerva Pediat.* 7: 66–71.

Zunin, C.; Borrone, C.; and Cuneo, P. 1960. Prednisone e gravidanza. Richerche sperimentali e osservazioni cliniche sull'effetto teratogeno de prednisone. *Minerva Pediat.* 12: 127–28.

Indexes

Author Index

NOTE: Italicized numerals indicate reference pages.

452   *Author Index*

Subject Index

49132